Unlocking Medical Terminology

Unlocking Medical Terminology

Bruce Wingerd

San Diego State University
San Diego, California

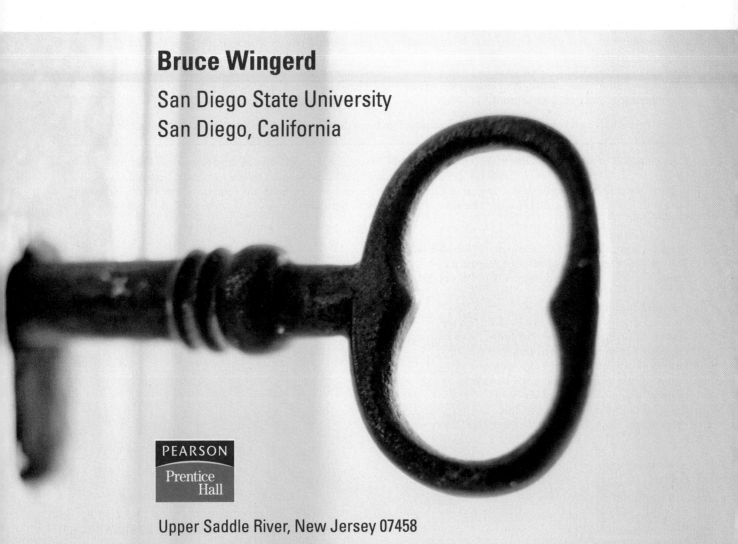

PEARSON
Prentice
Hall

Upper Saddle River, New Jersey 07458

Library of Congress Cataloging-in-Publication Data

Wingerd, Bruce
  Unlocking medical terminology / Bruce Wingerd.
    p. ; cm.
  Includes index.
  ISBN 0-13-048840-2
  1. Medicine—Terminology—Programmed instruction.
  2. Terminology—Computer-assisted instruction I. Title.

  R123.W53 2006
  610'.1'4—dc22
                                        2005005115

Publisher: Julie Levin Alexander
Assistant to Publisher: Regina Bruno
Executive Editor: Mark Cohen
Associate Editor: Melissa Kerian
Editorial Assistant: Jaquay Felix
Media Product Manager: John J. Jordan
Development Editors: Janine Nameny Cannell and Elena Mauceri
Director of Production and Manufacturing: Bruce Johnson
Managing Production Editor: Patrick Walsh
Production Liaison: Christina Zingone
Production Editor: Jessica Balch, Pine Tree Composition
Manufacturing Manager: Ilene Sanford

Manufacturing Buyer: Pat Brown
Design Director: Cheryl Asherman
Design Coordinator: Christopher Weigand
Interior Design: Cheryl Asherman
Cover Design: Solid State Graphics
Director of Marketing: Karen Allman
Channel Marketing Manager: Rachele Strober
Manager of Media Production: Amy Peltier
New Media Project Managers: Stephen Hartner and Tina Rudowski
Composition: Pine Tree Composition, Inc.
Printer/Binder: R.R. Donnelley & Sons
Cover Printer: Phoenix Color Corp.

Netter illustrations used with permission of Icon Learning Systems, a division of MediMedia USA, Inc. All rights reserved.

Pearson Education Ltd., *London*
Pearson Education Australia Pty. Limited, *Sydney*
Pearson Education Singapore, Pte. Ltd.
Pearson Education North Asia Ltd., *Hong Kong*
Pearson Education Canada, Ltd., *Toronto*
Pearson Educación de Mexico, S.A. de C.V.
Pearson Education—Japan, *Tokyo*
Pearson Education Malaysia, Pte. Ltd.
Pearson Education, Upper Saddle River, New Jersey

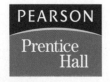

10 9 8 7 6 5 4 3 2 1
ISBN 0-13-048840-2

DEDICATION

For Mala, Josh, and Ryan, all of whom
taught me how to teach with heart.

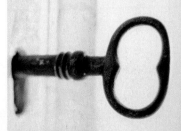

[brief contents]

Chapter 1   Word Parts: The Building Blocks of Medical Terminology   **1**

Chapter 2   The Human Body in Health and Disease   **23**

Chapter 3   Cells, Tissues, and Cancer   **57**

Chapter 4   The Integumentary System   **87**

Chapter 5   The Skeletal and Muscular Systems   **123**

Chapter 6   The Nervous System and Mental Health   **175**

Chapter 7   The Special Senses: The Eyes   **221**

Chapter 8   The Special Senses: The Ears   **253**

Chapter 9   The Endocrine System   **279**

Chapter 10   The Cardiovascular System   **317**

Chapter 11   Blood and the Lymphatic System   **369**

Chapter 12   The Respiratory System   **413**

Chapter 13   The Digestive System   **465**

Chapter 14   The Urinary System   **515**

Chapter 15   The Male Reproductive System   **557**

Chapter 16   The Female Reproductive System   **591**

Chapter 17   Obstetrics and Human Development   **635**

Appendix A   Word Parts   **673**

Appendix B   Abbreviations   **681**

Appendix C   Endings in Medical Terminology   **688**

Appendix D   Pharmacology Terms   **690**

Appendix E   Alternative Medicine: Therapies and Treatments   **694**

Appendix F   Answers to Chapter Review Exercises   **696**

Appendix G   Answers to Self Quiz Exercises   **713**

Index   **739**

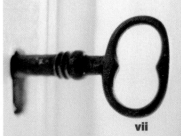

[table of contents]

Preface		**xix**
Acknowledgments		**xxiii**
Reviewers		**xxv**
Chapter 1	**Word Parts: The Building Blocks of Medical Terminology**	**1**
	Learning Objectives	**1**
	The Four Word Parts	**3**
	Defining Medical Terms	**10**
	Constructing Medical Terms	**12**
	Pronunciation of Medical Terms	**14**
	Spelling	**14**
	Singular and Plural Endings	**14**
	Helpful Study Tips	**15**
	Chapter Review	**18**
Chapter 2	**The Human Body in Health and Disease**	**23**
	Learning Objectives	**23**
	Word Parts Focus	**24**
	Anatomy and Physiology Overview	**26**
	Getting to the Root of It—Anatomy and Physiology Terms	**33**
	Medical Terms of the Human Body	**41**
	Let's Construct Terms!	**42**
	Symptoms and Signs	**42**
	Diseases and Disorders	**43**
	Disease Focus—Diagnosis	**44**
	Treatments, Procedures, and Devices	**48**
	Abbreviations	**51**
	Chapter Review	**52**
	Word Parts Checklist	**52**
	Medical Terminology Checklist	**52**
	Show What You Know!	**53**
	Piece It All Together!	**55**
Chapter 3	**Cells, Tissues, and Cancer**	**57**
	Learning Objectives	**57**
	Word Parts Focus	**58**
	Anatomy and Physiology Overview	**61**

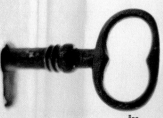

	Getting to the Root of It—Anatomy and Physiology Terms	65
	Medical Terms of Cells, Tissues, and Cancer	69
	Let's Construct Terms!	71
	Symptoms and Signs	71
	Diseases and Disorders	73
	Disease Focus—The Genetics of Cancer	74
	Treatments, Procedures, and Devices	78
	Abbreviations of Cells, Tissues, and Cancer	80
	Chapter Review	81
	Word Parts Checklist	81
	Medical Terminology Checklist	81
	Show What You Know!	82
	Piece It All Together!	84
Chapter 4	**The Integumentary System**	87
	Learning Objectives	87
	Word Parts Focus	89
	Anatomy and Physiology Overview	91
	Getting to the Root of It—Anatomy and Physiology Terms	94
	Medical Terms of the Integumentary System	97
	Let's Construct Terms!	98
	Symptoms and Signs	98
	Diseases and Disorders	104
	Disease Focus—Wound Repair	110
	Treatments, Procedures, and Devices	112
	Abbreviations of the Integumentary System	115
	Chapter Review	116
	Word Parts Checklist	116
	Medical Terminology Checklist	116
	Show What You Know!	117
	Piece It All Together!	120
Chapter 5	**The Skeletal and Muscular Systems**	123
	Learning Objectives	123
	Word Parts Focus	124
	Anatomy and Physiology Overview	127
	Getting to the Root of It—Anatomy and Physiology Terms	136
	Medical Terms of the Skeletal and Muscular Systems	143

	Let's Construct Terms!	144
	Symptoms and Signs	144
	Diseases and Disorders	146
	Disease Focus—Fractures	156
	Treatments, Procedures, and Devices	159
	Abbreviations of the Skeletal and Muscular Systems	165
	Chapter Review	167
	Word Parts Checklist	167
	Medical Terminology Checklist	168
	Show What You Know!	169
	Piece It All Together!	171
Chapter 6	**The Nervous System and Mental Health**	**175**
	Learning Objectives	175
	Word Parts Focus	176
	Anatomy and Physiology Overview	178
	Getting to the Root of It—Anatomy and Physiology Terms	186
	Medical Terms of the Nervous System	190
	Let's Construct Terms!	192
	Symptoms and Signs	192
	Diseases and Disorders	194
	Disease Focus—Accumulation of Fluids in the Brain	202
	Treatments, Procedures, and Devices	205
	Abbreviations of the Nervous System	212
	Chapter Review	213
	Word Parts Checklist	213
	Medical Terminology Checklist	213
	Show What You Know!	214
	Piece It All Together!	217
Chapter 7	**The Special Senses: The Eyes**	**221**
	Learning Objectives	221
	Word Parts Focus	222
	Anatomy and Physiology Overview	224
	Getting to the Root of It—Anatomy and Physiology Terms	226
	Medical Terms of the Eyes	229
	Let's Construct Terms!	229
	Symptoms and Signs	230

	Diseases and Disorders	233
	Disease Focus—Glaucoma and Intraocular Pressure	238
	Treatments, Procedures, and Devices	241
	Abbreviations of the Eyes	246
	Chapter Review	247
	Word Parts Checklist	247
	Medical Terminology Checklist	247
	Show What You Know!	248
	Piece It All Together!	250
Chapter 8	**The Special Senses: The Ears**	**253**
	Learning Objectives	253
	Word Parts Focus	254
	Anatomy and Physiology Overview	255
	Getting to the Root of It—Anatomy and Physiology Terms	258
	Medical Terms of the Ears	261
	Let's Construct Terms!	262
	Symptoms and Signs	262
	Diseases and Disorders	264
	Disease Focus—Otitis Media in Children	266
	Treatments, Procedures, and Devices	269
	Abbreviations of the Ears	273
	Chapter Review	274
	Word Parts Checklist	274
	Medical Terminology Checklist	274
	Show What You Know!	275
	Piece it All Together!	276
Chapter 9	**The Endocrine System**	**279**
	Learning Objectives	279
	Word Parts Focus	280
	Anatomy and Physiology Overview	282
	Getting to the Root of It—Anatomy and Physiology Terms	287
	Medical Terms of the Endocrine System	290
	Let's Construct Terms!	290
	Symptoms and Signs	290
	Diseases and Disorders	293
	Disease Focus—Diabetes Mellitus	302

	Treatments, Procedures, and Devices	305
	Abbreviations of the Endocrine System	310
	Chapter Review	311
	Word Parts Checklist	311
	Medical Terminology Checklist	311
	Show What You Know!	312
	Piece It All Together!	314
Chapter 10	**The Cardiovascular System**	**317**
	Learning Objectives	317
	Word Parts Focus	318
	Anatomy and Physiology Overview	320
	Getting to the Root of It—Anatomy and Physiology Terms	325
	Medical Terms of the Cardiovascular System	332
	Let's Construct Terms!	332
	Symptoms and Signs	333
	Diseases and Disorders	335
	Disease Focus—Heart Disease	340
	Treatments, Procedures, and Devices	346
	Abbreviations of the Cardiovascular System	359
	Chapter Review	361
	Word Parts Checklist	361
	Medical Terminology Checklist	361
	Show What You Know!	362
	Piece It All Together!	365
Chapter 11	**Blood and the Lymphatic System**	**369**
	Learning Objectives	369
	Word Parts Focus	370
	Anatomy and Physiology Overview	372
	Getting to the Root of It—Anatomy and Physiology Terms	378
	Medical Terms of Blood and the Lymphatic System	383
	Let's Construct Terms!	384
	Symptoms and Signs	385
	Diseases and Disorders	387
	Disease Focus—HIV Mode of Infection	394
	Treatments, Procedures, and Devices	398
	Abbreviations of Blood and the Lymphatic System	404

Chapter Review		406
Word Parts Checklist		406
Medical Terminology Checklist		406
Show What You Know!		407
Piece It All Together!		411
Chapter 12	**The Respiratory System**	**413**
	Learning Objectives	413
	Word Parts Focus	414
	Anatomy and Physiology Overview	417
	Getting to the Root of It—Anatomy and Physiology Terms	422
	Medical Terms of the Respiratory System	426
	Let's Construct Terms!	426
	Symptoms and Signs	427
	Diseases and Disorders	431
	Disease Focus—Tuberculosis	438
	Treatments, Procedures, and Devices	442
	Abbreviations of the Respiratory System	455
	Chapter Review	457
	Word Parts Checklist	457
	Medical Terminology Checklist	457
	Show What You Know!	458
	Piece It All Together!	462
Chapter 13	**The Digestive System**	**465**
	Learning Objectives	465
	Word Parts Focus	466
	Anatomy and Physiology Overview	469
	Getting to the Root of It—Anatomy and Physiology Terms	474
	Medical Terms of the Digestive System	478
	Let's Construct Terms!	478
	Symptoms and Signs	479
	Diseases and Disorders	481
	Disease Focus—The Common Cause of GI Ulcers	491
	Treatments, Procedures, and Devices	496
	Abbreviations of the Digestive System	507
	Chapter Review	508
	Word Parts Checklist	508

	Medical Terminology Checklist	**508**
	Show What You Know!	**509**
	Piece It All Together!	**512**
Chapter 14	**The Urinary System**	**515**
	Learning Objectives	**515**
	Word Parts Focus	**516**
	Anatomy and Physiology Overview	**518**
	Getting to the Root of It—Anatomy and Physiology Terms	**521**
	Medical Terms of the Urinary System	**524**
	Let's Construct Terms!	**525**
	Symptoms and Signs	**525**
	Diseases and Disorders	**528**
	Disease Focus—Renal Failure and Dialysis	**533**
	Treatments, Procedures, and Devices	**538**
	Abbreviations of the Urinary System	**549**
	Chapter Review	**550**
	Word Parts Checklist	**550**
	Medical Terminology Checklist	**550**
	Show What You Know!	**551**
	Piece It All Together!	**554**
Chapter 15	**The Male Reproductive System**	**557**
	Learning Objectives	**557**
	Word Parts Focus	**558**
	Anatomy and Physiology Overview	**559**
	Getting to the Root of It—Anatomy and Physiology Terms	**562**
	Medical Terms of the Male Reproductive System	**566**
	Let's Construct Terms!	**567**
	Symptoms and Signs	**567**
	Diseases and Disorders	**569**
	Disease Focus—Enlarged Prostate	**574**
	Treatments, Procedures, and Devices	**577**
	Abbreviations of the Male Reproductive System	**584**
	Chapter Review	**585**
	Word Parts Checklist	**585**
	Medical Terminology Checklist	**585**

	Show What You Know!	**586**
	Piece It All Together!	**589**
Chapter 16	**The Female Reproductive System**	**591**
	Learning Objectives	**591**
	Word Parts Focus	**592**
	Anatomy and Physiology Overview	**594**
	Getting to the Root of It—Anatomy and Physiology Terms	**598**
	Medical Terms of the Female Reproductive System	**603**
	Let's Construct Terms!	**603**
	Symptoms and Signs	**604**
	Diseases and Disorders	**607**
	Disease Focus—Cancers of Female Organs	**613**
	Treatments, Procedures, and Devices	**617**
	Abbreviations of the Female Reproductive System	**627**
	Chapter Review	**629**
	Word Parts Checklist	**629**
	Medical Terminology Checklist	**629**
	Show What You Know!	**630**
	Piece It All Together!	**633**
Chapter 17	**Obstetrics and Human Development**	**635**
	Learning Objectives	**635**
	Word Parts Focus	**636**
	Anatomy and Physiology Overview	**638**
	Getting to the Root of It—Anatomy and Physiology Terms	**643**
	Medical Terms of Obstetrics and Human Development	**647**
	Let's Construct Terms!	**648**
	Symptoms and Signs	**649**
	Diseases and Disorders	**651**
	Disease Focus—Crossing the Placental Blood Barrier	**656**
	Treatments, Procedures, and Devices	**660**
	Abbreviations of Obstetrics and Human Development	**666**
	Chapter Review	**667**
	Word Parts Checklist	**667**
	Medical Terminology Checklist	**667**
	Show What You Know!	**668**
	Piece It All Together!	**670**

Appendix A   **Word Parts**   673

Appendix B   **Abbreviations**   681

Appendix C   **Endings in Medical Terminology**   688

Appendix D   **Pharmacology Terms**   690

Appendix E   **Alternative Medicine: Therapies and Treatments**   694

Appendix F   **Answers to Chapter Review Exercises**   696

Appendix G   **Answers to Self Quiz Exercises**   713

Index   739

[preface]

Welcome to *Unlocking Medical Terminology!*

In the exciting and ever-changing field of health care, there are two constants. One is the human body itself. While scientists discover more about our bodies and develop treatments and procedures to treat the diseases that affect our bodies, the cells, tissues, muscles, and bones that are the basic components of anatomy and physiology remain unchanged. The other constant is the way we construct many of the words related to our bodies. These words establish a medical language used by health care professionals to communicate information accurately.

This book serves as a key to discovering this new language in a fun and eye-catching, yet scientifically precise way. Using word-building techniques, readers will discover that learning medical language is like solving a puzzle. Likewise, readers will understand how the various components of the human body fit together into a series of integrated systems. Along these lines, throughout the activities here, we will present all the pieces (known as word parts), as well as tips for putting them together to construct different combinations of words.

Unlocking Medical Terminology may be used as a text to support lectures or as an independent student workbook. The flexibility of its application is made possible by the book's text-like format, combined with its self-guided, exercise-driven learning program. The text discussions are basic, clear, and concise, and are followed immediately by blocks of review exercises called Self Quizzes. The frequent self quizzes are an effective way of reinforcing content with a minimum of required instructor guidance before readers move to the next section. The answers to all self quiz exercises appear hidden in the red margins and are also listed in full in Appendix G. You can use the decoder included with this book to read the hidden answers in the margins.

Key Features

To help readers navigate this new, exciting journey, we have designed a special *"Keying Interest!"* section that provides a visual walkthrough of the important elements in this novel learning system.

DECODER KEY

You may have noticed that a unique decoder key is packaged in the back of this book. Use this key to reveal the hidden answers that appear within the red column in each Self Quiz section. We designed this feature to provide students with a quick reference to the answers without requiring them to turn to the appendix in the back of the book. Yet at the same time, we did not want to reveal the answers too obviously; thereby forestalling the temptation of looking at the answer before filling in the blank. With this key, learners can enjoy the convenience of on-page answers with less distraction.

Just for fun, try this example:

The suffix meaning "study of" is

NETTER ART

Underscoring our fascination with the precision and beauty of the human body, we have chosen a special collection of artwork to help convey key anatomical concepts. We have richly illustrated the book using the Netter library of images, which is the most comprehensive collection of hand-painted medical illustrations in the world. Healthcare professionals recognize Dr. Frank Netter's work, with its half-century history of classic renderings, as the standard in the field of medical education.

Look for this symbol: *f Netter* to identify those pieces of art that we have selected from the Netter collection.

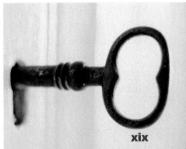

PUZZLE CHALLENGE

Occasionally within the Self Quiz sections of each chapter, you will come across puzzle pieces that look like this: ✦. These symbols serve as clues to the color-coded crossword puzzle called *Piece It All Together,* which appears at the end of the chapter and is designed to reinforce the concepts of fun, active learning and word building. The clues provide encouragement to revisit the chapter information as incentive to complete the puzzle. Once learners have read the chapter and completed the exercises and the puzzle, they can confidently say that they have unlocked the language in that section.

WORD-BUILDING APPROACH

Each chapter presents three tiers of word-building instruction.

- First, we present basic word parts and corresponding exercises in the *Word Parts Focus* section. By starting with the most basic word components, we aim to lay a strong foundation for further study.

- Second, we build upon our foundation by concentrating specifically on the word roots that form many anatomy and physiology terms. In the *Anatomy and Physiology Overview,* we provide an optional "Enrichment Module" that presents key information about each body system. This section is followed by *Getting to the Root of It,* where we analyze and review important word roots related to the corresponding body system.

- Third, we bridge from anatomical structure names to the diseases related to them in the *Let's Construct Terms!* section. Here we assemble prefixes, roots, combining vowels, and suffixes into words pertaining to Symptoms and Signs; Diseases and Disorders; and Treatments, Procedures, and Devices.

DISEASE FOCUS

These short passages profile relevant and interesting pathologies affecting the body system being discussed in the chapter, thus providing deeper context.

FYI AND THINKING CRITICALLY! BOXES

These sidebars appear throughout each chapter to evoke reader interest and investigation. Through these brief sections, we hope to infuse some of our own fascination and curiosity about the human body and medical language.

Organization

We lead off the book with three introductory chapters that establish the fundamentals of medical terminology, anatomy and physiology, and the basic building blocks of human structure, cells and tissues. Then we delve into the human body systems in a sequence that matches most standard anatomy and physiology textbooks. Each chapter begins with *Word Parts Focus,* presenting the word parts that form many of the terms in the chapter. The body system chapters follow with a concise narrative *Anatomy and Physiology Overview* module that concludes with *Getting to the Root of It* word tables and Self Quiz exercises. This section features a demonstration of how anatomy and physiology terms are formed from the word roots listed in the preceding section, providing a bridge between the terms and their word parts and meanings. The next section, *Let's Construct Terms!* is the learning emphasis of each chapter, presenting word part construction, a pronunciation guide, and a definition of each term, followed again by Self Quiz exercises. *Let's Construct Terms!* is subdivided by symptoms, diseases, and treatments. Next *Abbreviations* and a Self Quiz conclude the chapter content before the *Chapter Review* begins. The capstone review section provides several exercises that enable the student to review the information in the chapter. They include short answer questions, fill-ins, case history studies, a crossword puzzle, and a word unscramble.

The appendices provide a ready reference to supplement the chapters:

- Appendix A: prefixes, combining forms, and suffixes for most medical words
- Appendix B: abbreviations
- Appendix C: word endings
- Appendix D: glossary of pharmacology terms
- Appendix E: glossary of terms frequently used in alternative medicine
- Appendix F: answers to the Chapter Review exercises
- Appendix G: answers to the Self Quiz exercises

Comprehensive Teaching and Learning Package

Unlocking Medical Terminology offers a rich array of ancillary materials to benefit instructors and students alike. The full complement of supplemental teaching materials is available to all qualified instructors from your Prentice Hall Health sales representative.

STUDENT CD-ROM

The Student CD-ROM is packaged FREE with every copy of the textbook. It includes:

- A custom flashcard generator
- An audio glossary with pronunciations of the terms presented in the text
- Disease investigation videos, with additional content related to diseases and conditions
- Interactive medical terminology exercises, games, and activities that quiz students on spelling, word-building concepts, anatomy, and more

COMPANION WEBSITE

Students and faculty will both benefit from the FREE Companion Website at www.prenhall.com/wingerd. This website serves as a text-specific interactive online workbook to *Unlocking Medical Terminology*. The Companion Website includes:

- A variety of quizzes in multiple-choice, true/false, labeling, fill-in-the-blank, and essay formats
- Internet links that relate to chapter content
- An audio glossary in which key terms in the book are pronounced.

INSTRUCTOR'S RESOURCE MANUAL (IRM)

This manual contains a wealth of material to help faculty plan and manage the medical terminology course. It includes lecture suggestions and outlines, learning objectives, a 629-question test bank, and more for each chapter. The IRM also guides faculty how to assign and use the text-specific Companion Website, www.prenhall.com/wingerd, and the CD-ROM that accompany the textbook.

INSTRUCTOR'S RESOURCE CD-ROM

Packaged along with the Instructor's Resource Manual, this cross-platform CD-ROM provides many resources in an electronic format. First, the CD-ROM includes the complete 629-question test bank, which allows instructors to generate customized exams and quizzes. Second, it includes a comprehensive, turn-key lecture package in PowerPoint format. The lectures contain discussion points, embedded color images from the textbook, and bonus animations and videos to help infuse an extra spark into the classroom experience. Instructors may use this presentation system as it is provided or they may opt to customize it for their specific needs.

COMPANION WEBSITE SYLLABUS MANAGER™

Faculty adopting this textbook have *free* access to the online **Syllabus Manager** feature of the Companion Website, www.prenhall.com/wingerd. It offers a host of features that facilitate the students' use of the Companion Website and allows faculty to post syllabi and course information online for their students. For more information or a demonstration of **Syllabus Manager,** please contact your Prentice Hall sales representative.

Online Course Management Systems

ONEKEY

Finally, those instructors wishing to facilitate on-line courses will be able to access our premium on-line course management option, which is available in WebCT, Blackboard, or CourseCompass formats. OneKey is an integrated online resource that brings a wide array of supplemental resources together in one convenient place for both students and faculty. OneKey features everything instructors and students need for out-of-class work, conveniently organized to match the syllabus. OneKey's online course management solution features interactive modules, text and image PowerPoint slides, animations, videos, case studies, and more. OneKey also provides course management tools so faculty can customize course content, build online tests, create assignments, enter grades, post announcements, communicate with students, and much more. Testing materials, gradebooks, and other instructor resources are available in a separate section that can be accessed by instructors only. OneKey content is available in three different platforms. A nationally hosted version is available in the reliable, easy-to-use **CourseCompass** platform. The same content is also available for download to locally hosted versions of **BlackBoard** and **WebCT.** Please contact your Prentice Hall sales representative for a demonstration or go online to http://www.prenhall.com/onekey.

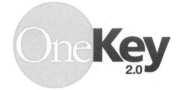

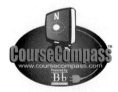

[acknowledgments]

Although I am the only author indicated on the cover of this textbook, this is by no means an independent effort. It was a tremendous team effort involving an amazing group of talented and knowledgeable folks.

My consultants combined many years of teaching medical terminology with their clinical practices to help make this text accurate and current. I appreciate the help of Dr. Harry Plymale, who shared his 40+ years of teaching experience with his medical training and clinical work, and provided a critical eye in every chapter throughout the text's early stages. I also appreciate the efforts of Dan Courson, who applied his recent medical education and clinical experience as a physician's assistant by spending many hours going over every medical term and definition to ensure that the text reflected current and correct clinical usage.

The text also benefited from my students, who pointed out their preferred ways of learning the material, which influenced many of the decisions. In particular, I appreciate the efforts of Marina Procktor, who examined every chapter in the final draft and provided valuable input.

The text would not be in your hands right now if it were not for the vision and leadership of my publisher, Julie Levin Alexander, to whom I am indebted for her faith in my ability to write this book. The executive editor, Mark Cohen, was the book's primary visionary and my early source of encouragement. He was brilliant throughout the project and served as a refreshing source of inspiration and leadership. Mark provided a river of fresh ideas and brought in the creative team of editors lead by Elena Mauceri of Dynamic WordWorks. Elena's contributions to the finished manuscript are substantial, and the text reflects many of her suggestions. I especially appreciate the hard, diligent work of Janine Nameny, who applied a directed problem-solving approach to many of the technical problems associated with the text and contributed her superb creative talents as well. Other contributing members of the editorial team included Sara Wilson and Lynda Hatch, to whom I also owe a debt of gratitude for their special efforts. A special word of thanks goes to Belen Poltorak, who introduced the idea of writing this book with Prentice Hall several years ago, providing the seed that germinated into this incredible project.

There are many other talented people who worked hard to make this book a valuable teaching and learning resource, including Melissa Kerian and Christina Zingone at Prentice Hall, as well as Jessica Balch and the staff of Pine Tree Composition. Special thanks also go to Cheryl Asherman and Mary Siener of Prentice Hall for their work on the design and the decoder feature. I extend to each of them my warmest gratitude.

During the peer review process of the book, many eyes scrutinized every chapter for accuracy, clarity, correctness, and organization. Their helpful suggestions proved to be valuable contributions to the book, and I appreciate their time and efforts.

As a final note, I invite and welcome your reactions, comments, and suggestions to be sent to me directly so that subsequent editions may reflect your educational needs better:

Bruce Wingerd
Biology Department
San Diego State University
San Diego, CA 92182-4614
bwingerd@sciences.sdsu.edu

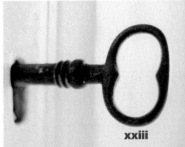

[reviewers]

Linda Andrews, MS, RN
Department Head and Assistant Professor
Health Sciences Department
Rogers State University
Claremore, OK

Nancy Burke, BA, MS, EdD
Adjunct Faculty
Harrisburg Area Community College
Harrisburg, PA

Toni Cade, MBA, RHIA, CCS
Assistant Professor
University of Louisiana at Lafayette
Lafayette, LA

Les Chatelain, MS
Director—Center for Emergency
    Programs
Department of Health Promotion
    and Education
University of Utah
Salt Lake City, UT

Charlotte Creason, RHIA
Program Chair
Health Information Technology
    and Medical Transcription
Tyler Junior College
Tyler, TX

John Doyle, RN, BSN, BS
Professor of Allied Health and Nursing
Victor Valley College
Victorville, CA

Pamela Eugene, BAS, RT
Associate Professor
Delgado Community College—Allied
    Health Division
New Orleans, LA

Kathleen A. Folson, RN, MS, BSN
Whidbey Island Campus
Skagit Valley College
Oak Harbor, WA

Jamie Flower, RN, MSN
Department of Nursing
University of Arkansas—Fort Smith
Fort Smith, AR

Genese M. Gibson, MA
Department Chairperson of Radiologic
    Sciences
Florida Hospital College of Health
    Sciences
Orlando, FL

Lynn Grommet, MNSc, RNC
Allied Health Science—Nursing
East Arkansas Community College
Forrest City, AR

Judith B. Johnson, RN
Nashville State Community College
Nashville, TN

Amy R. Kapanka, MS, MT (ASCP) SC
Program Director of Medical Laboratory
    Technology
Hawkeye Community College
Waterloo, IA

Carol Klinger
Hocking College
School of Health and Nursing
Nelsonville, OH

Jennifer Lamé, MPH, BS, RHIT
Health Information Instructor
Clinical Coordinator
Idaho State University
Pocatello, ID

Sylvia Pickard, MS, RN
Instructor
South Dakota State University
    College of Nursing
Brookings, SD

**Janet Roberts-Andersen, MS, MT
(ASCP)**
Director of Medical Assistant Programs
Hamilton College
Urbandale, IA

Helen Reid, RN, MSN, EdD
Dean of Health Occupations
Trinity Valley Community College
Kaufman, TX

Scott R. Sechrist, EdD, CNMT
Associate Professor and Program Director
Nuclear Medicine Technology
Old Dominion University
Norfolk, VA

Brenda Sewell, RN, MS, HEd
Medical Assistant Program
North Texas Professional Career Institute
Dallas, TX

Joan A. Verderame, RN, MA
Director of Surgical Technology
Bergen Community College
Paramus, NJ

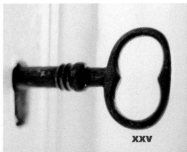

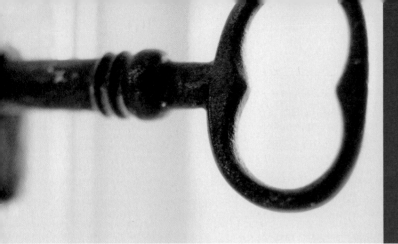

Keying Interest!

We know that learning Medical Terminology can be challenging. Unlocking Medical Terminology provides **two keys** to ensure you have a successful experience:

- Stair-Step Approach to Word Building
- FUN!

Stair-Step Approach to Word Building

The key to medical terminology is learning how to build words. Because no matter how hard you try you'll never be able to memorize all the words you need to know.

The stair-step approach makes this possible! The information is broken down into chunks that build upon each other.

The nervous system is a complex part of the body that has been studied extensively, yet there is still much more to learn. It is composed of the brain, spinal cord, and nerves. Together, these important organs enable you to sense the world around you, integrate this information to form thoughts and memories, and control your body movements and many internal functions.

In this chapter, we will explore the terms of the healthy, normal nervous system before proceeding with the medical terms of neurology. But first we will examine the word parts that are associated with the nervous system.

word parts focus

Let's look at word parts. The following table contains a list of word parts that when combined build many of the terms of the nervous system.

PREFIX	DEFINITION	PREFIX	DEFINITION
a-	without	mono-	single
di-	two	pan-	all, entire
dys-	bad, abnormal	para-	near, alongside
hemi-	one-half	poly-	many
hydro-	water	pre-	before
hyper-	excessive	tetra-	four

WORD ROOT	DEFINITION	WORD ROOT	DEFINITION
alges	pain	lys	break apart, dissolution
astheni	weakness	mening	membrane, meninges
cephal	head	ment	the mind
cerebell	little brain, cerebellum	myel	spinal cord, or bone marrow, or
cerebr	brain, cerebrum		medulla, or myelin sheath
cran, crani	skull, cranium	neur	sinew or cord, nerve
dur	hard	phas	speech
embol	a throwing in	plegi	paralysis
encephal	brain	psych	the mind
esthes	sensation, perception	quad, quadri	four
gangli / ganglion	knot, swelling	radic, radicul	nerve root
gli	glue, neuroglia	somat	the body
gnos	knowledge	thalam	inner chamber, thalamus

1st

Word Part Focus

Familiarize yourself with the word parts covered in chapter text to follow. Then take a quick self-quiz to see what you know. You're the only one who will see your answers.

let's construct terms!

In this section, we will assemble all of the word parts to construct medical terminology related to the nervous system. Abbreviations are used to indicate each word part: **p** = prefix, **r** = root, **cv** = combining vowel, and **s** = suffix. Recall from chapter one that the addition of a combining vowel to the word root creates the combining form for the term. Note that some terms are not constructed from word parts, but they are included here to expand your vocabulary.

The medical terms of the nervous system are listed in the following three sections:

- Symptoms and Signs
- Diseases and Disorders
- Treatments, Procedures, and Devices

Each section is followed by review exercises. Study the lists in these tables and complete the review exercises that follow.

Symptoms and Signs

WORD PARTS (WHEN APPLICABLE)			TERM	DEFINITION
Part	Type	Meaning		
a-	p	without	**aphasia**	inability to speak
phas	r	to speak	(ah FAY zee ah)	
-ia	s	condition of		
cephal	r	head	**cephalalgia**	a headache, or general pain to the head
-algia	s	pain	(seff al AL jee ah)	
dys-	p	difficult, pain	**dysphasia**	difficulty speaking
phas	r	to speak	(dis FAY zee ah)	
-ia	s	condition of		
hyper-	p	excessive	**hyperesthesia**	increased sensitivity to stimulation such as touch or
esthes	r	sensation	(HIGH per ess THEE	pain
-ia	s	condition of	zee ah)	
neur	r	nerve	**neuralgia**	pain in a nerve
-algia	s	pain	(noo RAL jee ah)	
neur	r	nerve	**neurasthenia**	a vague condition of body fatigue often associated
astheni	r	weakness	(noo ras THEE nee ah)	with depression
-a	s	condition of		
par-	p	beside, around	**paresthesia**	abnormal sensation of numbness and tingling
esthes	r	sensation	(par ess THEE zee ah)	without an objective cause
-ia	s	condition of		

getting to the root of it | anatomy and physiology terms

Many of the anatomy and physiology terms are formed from roots that are used to construct the more complex medical terms of the nervous system, including symptoms, diseases, and treatments. In this section, we will review the terms that describe the structure and function of the nervous system *in relation to their word roots*, which are shown in **bold**.

Study the word roots and terms in this list and complete the review exercises that follow.

Word Root (Meaning)	Terms Formed from the Word Root (Pronunciation)	Definition
arachn spider	**arachn**oid (ah RAK noyd)	the middle meninx, it surrounds a space filled with CSF known as the subarachnoid space
	sub**arachn**oid space (sub ah RAK noyd)	the space within the arachnoid, which is filled with CSF
cerebell little brain	**cerebell**um (ser eh BELL um)	the lower posterior part of the brain that is the center of muscle coordination and equilibrium
cerebr brain, cerebrum	**cerebr**ospinal fluid (ser eh broh SPY nal FLOO id)	a colorless fluid produced within the ventricles of the brain that provides liquid shock absorption and a source of nourishment for the brain and spinal cord; abbreviated CSF
	cerebrum (SER eh brum)	the largest part of the brain, it includes the right and left cerebral hemispheres, the corpus callosum, the cerebral cortex, and the lobes
	cerebral hemispheres (seh REE bral HEM iss feerz)	the right and left portions of the cerebrum, separated by the longitudinal fissure
	cerebral cortex (seh REE bral KOR teks)	the outer fringe of the cerebrum, which is composed of gray matter and is the site of nerve pathway termination and origin
	cerebral lobes	functional regions of the cerebral cortex
crani skull, cranium	**crani**um (KRAY nee um)	the dome-shaped part of the skull, which houses the cranial cavity
	cranial nerves (KRAY nee al)	12 pairs of nerves that unite with the brain
encephal brain	di**encephal**on (dye en SEFF ah lon)	the central part of the brain located beneath the cerebrum, which contains the thalamus and the hypothalamus
gangli / ganglion swelling, knot	**gangli**a (GANG lee ah)	clusters of neuron cell bodies that lie outside the CNS
mening membrane	**mening**es (men IN jeez)	the dura mater, arachnoid, and pia mater membranes surrounding the brain and spinal cord; the singular form is *meninx*
myel spinal cord, bone marrow, medulla, myelin sheath	**myel**in sheath (MY eh lin)	a white, fatty membrane that partially wraps the axons of certain neurons
neur sinew or cord, nerve	**neur**oglia (noo ROH glee ah)	supportive cells of nervous tissue
	neuron (NOO ron)	a functional cell of nervous tissue, which generates and transmits nerve impulses; each neuron consists of numerous dendrites, a centralized cell body, and a single axon
	neurotransmitter (noo roh TRANS mit ter)	a chemical that is released into a synapse from one neuron to cause a change in another neuron

3rd

Let's Construct Terms

Finally, you put it all together. In this section you will assemble word parts and roots to form highly useful terms that apply to pathology, treatment procedures, and diagnostic techniques. Once again, a self quiz concludes the section.

2nd

Getting to the Root of It!

Next you learn about word roots. Roots are the basis of most medical terms and they generally refer to anatomy and physiology concepts. Again, a self-assessment quiz follows this learning section to help you confirm your understanding.

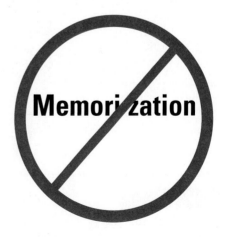

Memorization

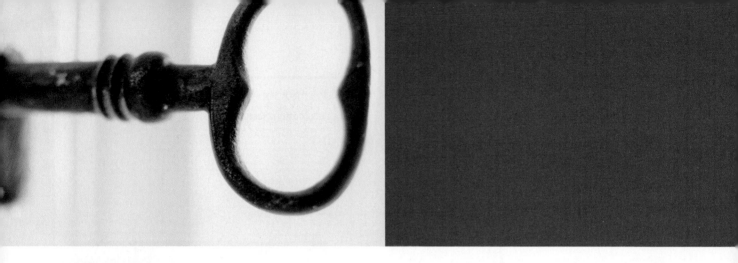

Fun!

You'll remember more if you're enjoying what you are doing. That's why this book is infused with a vivid and engaging approach.

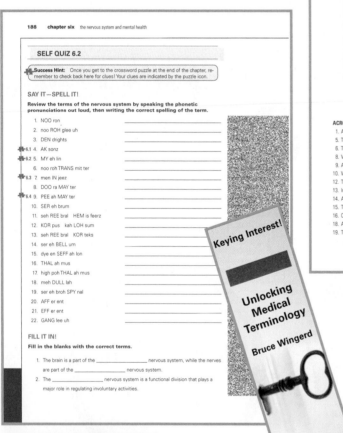
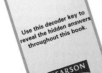

Keying Interest!

Unlocking Medical Terminology

Bruce Wingerd

Use this decoder key to reveal the hidden answers throughout this book.

PEARSON
Prentice Hall

Crossword Puzzle

The color coding in the crossword puzzle gives you hints for the word jumble that follows. You'll need to solve the puzzle in order to solve the jumble, and when you've successfully pieced it all together, you have mastered the chapter.

Puzzle Icons

Puzzle icons throughout the self-quizzes give you hints to the crossword puzzle at the end of each chapter.

Decoder

Use the decoder (found in the back of the book) to reveal the self-quiz answers within each chapter.

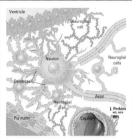

Ventricle

Neuroglial cell

Neuron

Neuroglial cells

Dendrites

Axon

Neuroglial Cell

J. Perkins
MS, MFA

Pia mater

Capillary

Figure 6.2 ::::
Neurons and nervous tissue organization. The neuron is shown in yellow, and three types of neuroglial cells are shown in various colors.
Source: Icon Learning Systems.

Central Nervous System

The central nervous system is the "central station" for incoming and outgoing nerve impulses. As you have just learned, it includes the brain and spinal cord. Both organs are protected by bones, including the cranium and the vertebral column, and by a thick set of membranes called the **meninges.** The meninges are located between the soft nervous tissue of the brain and spinal cord and the hard bones, forming a protective cover that is several layers in thickness (Figure 6.3::::). The layers include an outer tough fibrous **dura mater,** a middle **arachnoid,** and an inner thin **pia mater.** A narrow space exists between the arachnoid and pia mater, called the **subarachnoid space.**

THE BRAIN

The brain receives sensory information, interprets and integrates this information, and controls muscle and glandular responses. Its nerve impulse activity also provides you with your memory, thoughts, dreams, and personality. It receives a large blood supply to fuel its constant activity. The blood flow is critical; if it is restricted for more than a few minutes, neurons begin to expire. The brain is located in the cranial cavity, and weighs about 1.4 kg (3 pounds). Extending from the brain are 12 pairs of nerves, called **cranial nerves.**

In general, the brain is composed of nervous tissue that includes both gray matter and white matter. Gray matter consists mainly of neuron cell bodies and dendrites, whereas white matter consists of axons that are covered with the white insulative myelin sheath. The axons carry nerve impulses to adjacent neurons. Thus, white matter carries nerve impulses, while gray matter serves as integrative centers.

[thinking critically!]

Some drugs cause neurotransmitters to be released more readily, while other drugs inhibit the release of neurotransmitters. Do you think an inhibitory drug would be likely to cause a state of mental depression, or mental attentiveness? Why?

FYI Boxes

FYI boxes provide memory hints, fun facts, points of interest, and alert you to common mistakes to avoid.

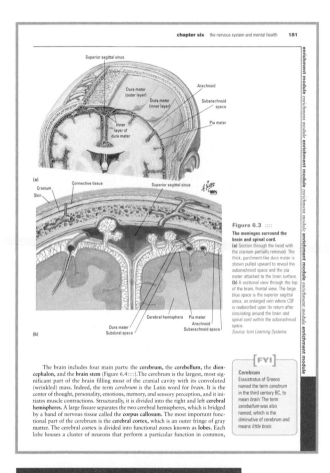

Superior sagittal sinus

Dura mater (outer layer)

Dura mater (inner layer)

Inner layer of dura mater

Arachnoid

Subarachnoid space

Pia mater

(a)

Cranium

Skin

Connective tissue

Superior sagittal sinus

Cerebral hemisphere

Pia mater

Arachnoid

Subarachnoid space

Dura mater

Subdural space

(b)

Figure 6.3 ::::
The meninges surround the brain and spinal cord.
(a) Section through the head with the cranium partially removed. The thick, parchment-like dura mater is shown pulled upward to reveal the subarachnoid space and the pia mater attached to the brain surface. **(b)** A sectional view through the top of the brain, frontal view. The large blue space is the superior sagittal sinus, an enlarged vein where CSF is reabsorbed upon its return after circulating around the brain and spinal cord within the subarachnoid space.
Source: Icon Learning Systems.

The brain includes four main parts: the **cerebrum,** the **cerebellum,** the **diencephalon,** and the **brain stem** (Figure 6.4::::). The cerebrum is the largest, most significant part of the brain filling most of the cranial cavity with its convoluted (wrinkled) mass. Indeed, the term *cerebrum* is the Latin word for *brain.* It is the center of thought, personality, emotions, memory, and sensory perception, and it initiates muscle contractions. Structurally, it is divided into the right and left **cerebral hemispheres.** A large fissure separates the two cerebral hemispheres, which is bridged by a band of nervous tissue called the **corpus callosum.** The most important functional part of the cerebrum is the **cerebral cortex,** which is an outer fringe of gray matter. The cerebral cortex is divided into functional zones known as **lobes.** Each lobe houses a cluster of neurons that perform a particular function in common,

Netter Art

Celebrated as the foremost medical illustrator of the human body and how it works, Dr. Frank H. Netter's incredibly detailed, lifelike renderings bring a rich new dimension to your medical terminology understanding.

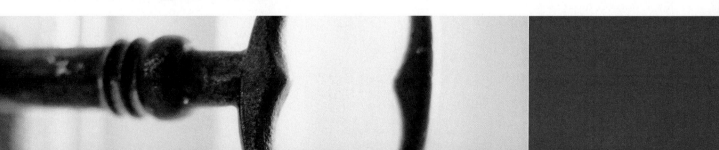

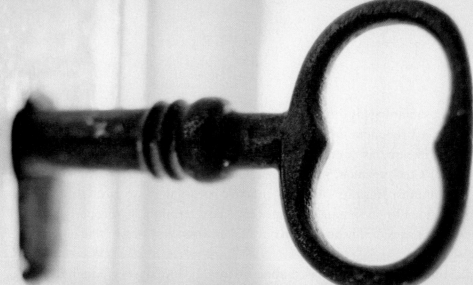

CHAPTER

1

Word Parts: The Building Blocks of Medical Terminology

LEARNING OBJECTIVES

After completing this chapter, you will be able to:

- Discuss the origins and purpose of medical terminology

- Identify the four basic word parts that form many medical terms

- Construct medical terms by assembling word parts

- Define medical terms by breaking them down into word parts

- Use the pronunciation resources available in this text and on the CD and CW

- Use study techniques to practice spelling medical terms correctly

Medical terminology is the language of medicine, spoken in clinics and hospitals throughout the world by people in the health professions. It is a language, like Spanish and German, that includes rules of pronunciation, vocabulary, and grammar. Similar to learning any other language around the world, you must learn its rules and practice speaking its words. Only then can you hope to understand and speak medical terminology properly. By opening the pages of this book, you have taken your first step in this direction.

Medical terminology has a fascinating history. It developed gradually over the years, mainly from older languages. It began nearly 3,000 years ago when Hippocrates, the ancient Greek father of medicine, and Aristotle, the ancient Greek father of philosophy, began describing ailments and parts of the body. They used their language to describe what they saw. For example, Aristotle used the Greek word *diaphragm*, which means *partition* or *barrier*, for the sheet of muscle dividing the thoracic cavity from the abdominal cavity. During the Roman era that followed, the dominant language was Latin. As Romans and their contemporaries expanded their knowledge of the body, they used the Greek words that were already established and added their own Latin words to describe what they saw. In post-Roman Europe, Greek and Latin word parts were still used to build new terms, but occasionally French, Italian, English, and other language word parts were also used as knowledge of the body and medicine gradually expanded.

By the end of the 19th century, the spectacular growth of medical knowledge created the need to add many more terms. To keep the expanding terminology understandable throughout the world, the medical community agreed to continue with the established method of creating new names by using mainly Greek and Latin word parts.

The medical community also began using *eponyms*, which are words based on the personal names of people to describe a disease or body part. For example, Hodgkin's lymphoma is a type of cancer that was first described by William Hodgkin, a British physician. In more recent times, *acronyms*, which are words created from abbreviations or the first letter of a group of words, were also used to form a medical term. An example of an acronym is CAT scan, which is built from the words *c*omputed *a*xial *t*omography scan.

In today's world, medical and scientific knowledge continues advancing at a rapid rate, and new terms are being added to keep pace with the changes. For the most part, new terms are created using the old formulas of Greek and Latin word parts for the sake of consistency. As you are about to learn, the use of these word parts enables people in the health fields to understand the meanings of terms, reducing the need to rely on their skills of memorization.

For the purpose of learning the language of medical terminology, we can divide medical terms into two basic groups: terms that are constructed from

---

[FYI]

Latin and Greek
Some Latin and Greek words are very similar to words used in everyday English, and in fact are the origin of many English words. For example, the Latin word for curve is *curvo*, which means to bend, and the contemporary word plastic comes from the Greek word *plasticos*, which means *capable of being molded*. Some other examples of English words that are derived from other languages are roof from the Old Norse *hrof*, law from the Anglo Saxon word *lagu*, and plate from the Old French word for a flat object, *plat*.

[thinking critically!]

Can you think of another example of an eponym? How about another example of an acronym?

multiple Greek and Latin word parts, and terms that are not. Terms in the first group are called *constructed terms.*

The key to understanding constructed terms is to first learn the meanings of the various word parts. It may be helpful to think of constructed terms as if they were written in code. Once you have the key to a code it is a fairly simple process to decode messages or to use the code to form messages yourself. In the same way, once you know the meanings of the individual word parts, you have the key to the medical terminology code.

You can crack the code by breaking complex terms down into their individual word parts and you can use the code to form medical terms by assembling word parts yourself.

The second group of medical terms consists of words that are composed of only one Greek or Latin word part, and common language terms. They also include words derived from other languages, eponyms, acronyms, and abbreviations. To learn these terms, you must commit them to memory. Word association is often helpful to remember word meanings; so word association clues are provided throughout this text to help you with memorization when necessary. The two divisions of medical terms are illustrated in Figure 1.1▒▒▒.

The Four Word Parts

As you have just learned, many medical terms are constructed from one or more word parts that have Greek or Latin origins. There are four types of word parts:

- Word roots
- Prefixes
- Suffixes
- Combining vowels

For the purpose of clarification, in this text word parts are often separated from one another within a word by a fore-slash so that you may see how the word is constructed. For example, the word *shirttail* has two word parts and may be shown as *shirt/tail*. Also, the medical term *appendicitis* has two word parts and may be shown as *appendic/itis*. The term *antineoplastic* (anti/neo/plast/ic) has four word parts.

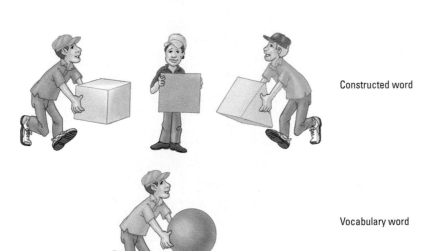

Constructed word

Vocabulary word

Figure 1.1 ▒▒▒

Medical terms are either constructed words, which are composed of more than one word part, or words you must memorize, which include terms that are a single Latin or Greek word part, eponyms, acronyms, abbreviations, etc.

In the following sections, you will learn about the four types of word parts and how they may be assembled to form a constructed term.

WORD ROOTS

A **word root** is the part of a word that contains its primary meaning. The word root is the main body or core of the word. Because it carries the word's primary meaning, a medical term usually contains at least one and sometimes more word roots. For example, the word *abnormal* can be shown as:

ab/norm/al

It means *away from a normal state*. The word root is *norm* since it carries the word's primary meaning.

The medical term *bilateral* can be shown as:

bi/later/al

It literally means *two sides*. The word part *later,* which means *side,* is the root since it contains the word's primary meaning.

The medical term *hypertension* can be shown as:

hyper/tens/ion

The word root is *tens,* because it contains the word's primary meaning, *to stretch.*

Because the Greeks and the Romans used their languages to describe body structures as they learned about them, there is a fundamental relationship between word roots—which carry a term's primary meaning—and the names given to anatomical structures by the Greeks and Romans. Let's look at some structures of the body to illustrate this concept.

The term *cochlea* is a Latin word that means *snail shell*. The cochlea of the ear as shown in Figure 1.2 :::: closely resembles the shape and look of a snail shell. Another example is the term *appendix,* which is a Latin word that means *to hang onto*. The appendix is a small structure that seems to hang onto one end of the large intestine, as Figure 1.3 :::: reveals. Similarly, the term *uvula* is derived from the Latin word that means *grape*. The uvula looks like a grape attached to the roof of the mouth, as shown in Figure 1.4 ::::.

> **[thinking critically!]**
>
> How many word roots can you find in the term *osteoarthritis?* How many word roots are in the term *gastrohepatovenous?*

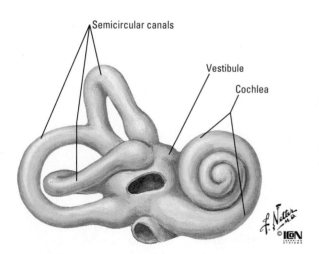

Figure 1.2 :::: **The inner ear.** The coiled structure that resembles the shell of a garden snail is the cochlea. *Source: Icon Learning Systems.*

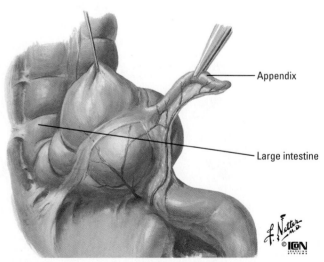

Figure 1.3 :::: The appendix is connected to one end of the large intestine, as shown, and looks like it "hangs onto" the larger structure. *Source: Icon Learning Systems.*

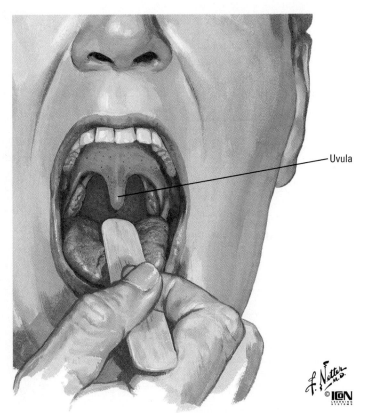

Uvula

Figure 1.4 ⁞⁞⁞⁞

The uvula looks like a grape hanging down from the roof of the mouth.
Source: Icon Learning Systems.

Some word roots that are commonly used to construct medical terms are listed and defined in the following table. This list represents a small sample of the word roots that you will learn in the chapters that follow in this textbook. Study this list and then complete the exercises that follow.

WORD ROOT	DEFINITION	WORD ROOT	DEFINITION
arter, arteri	artery	norm	a common state
arthr	joint	oste	bone
card, cardi	heart	path	disease
gastr	stomach	tens	to stretch
hepat	liver	ven	vein
later	side		

SELF QUIZ 1.1

A. Provide the definition for each of the following word roots.

Success Hint: Once you get to the crossword puzzle at the end of the chapter, remember to check back here for clues! Your clues are indicated by the puzzle icon.

1. later _____

1.1 2. hepat _____

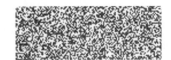

3. norm   _____

4. cardi   _____

5. ven   _____

6. arthr   _____

-1.2 7. arteri   _____

8. gastr   _____

9. oste   _____

-1.3 10. tens   _____

-1.4 11. path   _____

B. Provide the word root for each of the following terms.

1. abnormal   _____

2. bilateral   _____

3. hypertension   _____

4. arthrology   _____

5. hepatitis   _____

6. osteopathy   _____

7. cardiac   _____

8. intravenous   _____

9. gastric   _____

10. arterial   _____

11. pathology   _____

PREFIXES

A **prefix** is the word part that is placed before the root to modify its meaning. The word *prefix* literally means *to fix at the beginning of a word.* The following sentences contain some examples of prefixes.

The familiar word *abnormal,* which can be shown as:

ab/norm/al

includes the prefix ab-, which means *away from.* It is the prefix because it is placed before the root to modify the word meaning.

The medical term *intravenous* can be shown as:

intra/ven/ous

and means *pertaining to within a vein.* The prefix is intra-, which means *within.* It is the prefix because it is placed before the root to modify the word's meaning.

The word *hypertension* can be shown as:

hyper/tens/ion

The prefix is hyper-, which means *excessive or beyond.*

Some of the prefixes that are commonly used to construct medical terms are listed and defined in the following table. Study this list now; then work through the exercises that follow.

PREFIX	DEFINITION	PREFIX	DEFINITION
ab-	away from	intra-	within
bi-	two	pre-	to come before
endo-	within	post-	to follow after
hyper-	above, beyond, excessive	sub-	under
hypo-	below, under, deficient		

SELF QUIZ 1.2

A. Provide the definition of the following prefixes.

1. intra- _____

1.5 2. hyper- _____

3. ab- _____

4. endo- _____

5. pre- _____

6. sub- _____

7. post- _____

8. hypo- _____

9. bi- _____

B. Provide the prefix for each of the following terms.

1. abnormal _____

2. hypertension _____

3. intravenous _____

4. bilateral _____

1.6 5. hypohepatic _____

6. endocardial _____

7. postvenous _____

8. prefix _____

9. subdermal _____

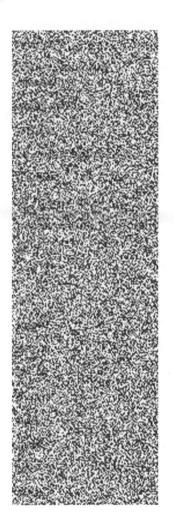

SUFFIXES

A **suffix** is the word part that is attached to the end of the word root. Like the prefix, the suffix modifies the word meaning. The following sentences contain examples of suffixes.

In the familiar word *abnormal*, which can be shown as:

ab/norm/al

the suffix is -al, which means *pertaining to*. It is the suffix because it is placed at the end of the root and modifies the word meaning.

The medical term *endocarditis* can be shown as:

endo/card/itis

It means *inflammation of the inner heart lining*. The suffix is -itis, which means *inflammation*. It is a suffix because it is placed at the end of the root and modifies the word meaning.

The medical term *arthropathy* can be shown as:

arthr/o/pathy

It means *disease of the joint*. The suffix is -pathy, which means *disease*.

The medical term *gastritis* can be shown as:

gastr/itis

It means *inflammation of the stomach*. The suffix is -itis, and the root word *gastr* means stomach.

Some of the suffixes that are commonly used to construct medical terms are listed and defined in the following table. Study this list now; then proceed with your study of word parts. Soon, we will review the information in this table by working through exercises that follow.

SUFFIX	DEFINITION	SUFFIX	DEFINITION
-al	pertaining to	-meter	measure
-ic	pertaining to	-pathy	disease
-ous	pertaining to	-scope	an instrument used for viewing
-itis	inflammation (swelling)	-scopy	use of an instrument for viewing
-logy	study of		

SELF QUIZ 1.3

A. Provide the definition of the following suffixes.

1. -scopy   _____

✚ 1.7 2. -itis   _____

✚ 1.8 3. -pathy   _____

✚ 1.9 4. -ic   _____

5. -logy   _____

6. -ous   _____

7. -meter   _____

8. -scope   _____

9. -al   _____

B. Provide the suffix for each of the following terms.

1. abnormal   _____

2. endocarditis   _____

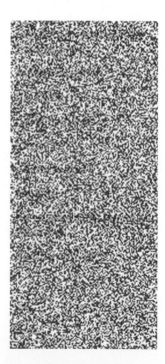

3. osteopathy _____

4. gastric _____

5. pathology _____

6. arteriovenous _____

7. diameter _____

8. endoscope _____

9. angioscopy _____

COMBINING VOWELS AND COMBINING FORMS

A **combining vowel** is a word part that is used to connect other word parts in the formation of a word, but it does not modify the meaning of the word. The combining vowel is usually an *o*, although *i* and *e* are sometimes used. The vowel is used between two word roots or between a word root and a suffix. In most cases, the vowel is used when the suffix or second word root begins with a consonant. It is not used between a prefix and a word root. In each case, a combining vowel is used to ease pronunciation of a word. For example, the medical term *gastrology* can be shown as:

gastr/o/logy

Here *gastr* is the word root, *-logy* is the suffix, and *o* is the combining vowel. It means *study of the stomach*. Notice that using the combining vowel eases the pronunciation of the term. It is much easier to say "gastrology" than "gastrlogy"!

The medical term *arteriovenous* can be shown as:

arteri/o/ven/ous

In this term, the combining vowel connects the two word roots, *arteri* and *ven*.

The medical term *osteopathy* can be shown as:

oste/o/pathy

This term means *disease of bone*. The word root is *oste*, the suffix is *pathy*, and the combining vowel is *o*.

When a word root is shown with the combining vowel attached, it is called a **combining form**. The combining form is written with a slash separating the word root from the combining vowel. Examples of combining forms include:

oste/o

arteri/o

cardi/o

arthr/o

Some combining forms that are commonly used to construct medical terms are listed and defined in the following table. This list represents a small sample of the combining forms that you will see in the chapters that follow in this textbook. Study this list now; then review the information on word parts by working through the exercises that follow.

COMBINING FORM	DEFINITION	COMBINING FORM	DEFINITION
arteri/o	artery	hepat/o	liver
arthr/o	joint	oste/o	bone
cardi/o	heart	path/o	disease
gastr/o	stomach	ven/o	vein

SELF QUIZ 1.4

A. Provide the definition for each of the following combining forms.

1. cardi/o   _____

1.10 2. hepat/o   _____

3. ven/o   _____

1.11 4. arthr/o   _____

5. arteri/o   _____

6. gastr/o   _____

7. oste/o   _____

8. path/o   _____

B. Provide the combining form for each of the following terms.

1. arthrology   _____

2. hepatology   _____

3. osteopathy   _____

4. cardiology   _____

5. venopathy   _____

6. gastrology   _____

7. arteriovenous   _____

8. pathology   _____

Defining Medical Terms

If the word parts to a medical term are known, the term's definition can usually be determined. You can define a medical term by applying the meaning of each part in the term. The simplest method to define a term uses three steps. As an example, we'll break down the medical term *arteriopathy* using word parts listed in the tables presented earlier:

1. Break the medical term down into its individual word parts

     arteri/o/pathy

2. Define each word part

     arteri/o = artery

     pathy = disease

3. Combine and interpret the definitions of the word parts

disease of arteries

Now we'll break down a more complicated term that includes a prefix. The same steps apply:

1. Break the medical term down into its individual word parts

intra/ven/ous

2. Define each word part

ous = pertaining to

intra = within

ven = vein

3. Combine and interpret the definitions of the word parts

pertaining to within vein

In these examples, the meaning of the suffix precedes the meaning of the prefix, which precedes the meaning of the word root. This is the case for most medical terms. The process of defining a medical term by looking at its word parts is illustrated in Figure 1.5⁙.

Practice defining medical terms in this way by working carefully through the next exercise.

Interpreting Medical Terms

When interpreting medical terms, start with the suffix, then the prefix, and then add the word root. Write out the meaning for a term like osteopathy as *disease of bone* or a term like intravenous as *pertaining to within a vein.*

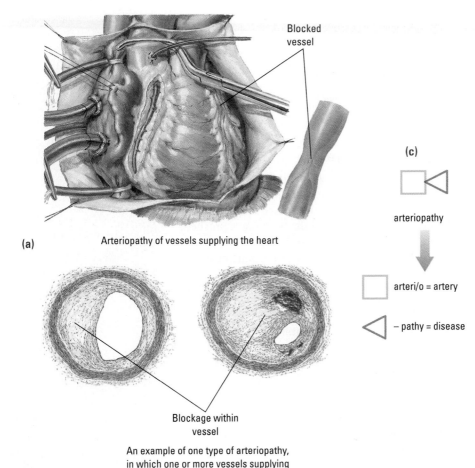

Blocked vessel

(c)

arteriopathy

arteri/o = artery

– pathy = disease

(a)   Arteriopathy of vessels supplying the heart

Blockage within vessel

An example of one type of arteriopathy, in which one or more vessels supplying the heart becomes blocked

(b)

Figure 1.5 ⁙

A medical term can be defined by looking at the meanings of its word parts.
(a) Heart surgery to correct the arteriopathy.
(b) Cross sections of arteries with arteriopathy.
(c) Construction of the term.

SELF QUIZ 1.5

DEFINE IT!

Define these medical terms using the word part definitions listed in the word part tables presented earlier.

1. arteriology   _____

2. hypergastric   _____

3. osteology   _____

4. osteoarthropathy   _____

5. cardiopathic   _____

6. postvenous   _____

MATCH IT!

Match the term on the left with the correct definition on the right.

_____1. hypogastric   a. pertaining to coming before a vein

_____2. cardiopathy   b. study of joints

_____3. gastrology   c. pertaining to a disease of bone

_____4. osteopathic   d. pertaining to below the stomach

_____5. prehepatic   e. inflammation of a joint

_____6. arthrology   f. a disease of the heart

_____7. prevenous   g. study of the stomach

_____8. arthritis   h. pertaining to coming before the liver

Constructing Medical Terms

Most medical terms are formed by assembling various word parts to construct a term. The process is similar to using toy blocks that come in various shapes and sizes to construct a miniature building. Starting with a mental image of the finished building, each block is selected to fit a particular space until the building is finished. When constructing a medical term, start with the definition; determine what you want to communicate. Then select word parts based on their particular meanings until the medical term is constructed.

As an example, let's construct a term for a disease of bone using information from the word part tables presented earlier in the chapter:

1. Start with the definition of what you want to communicate:

2. Find the suffix for *disease:*

3. Find the word root and combining vowel for *bone:*

4. Arrange the word parts properly:

In this example, the combining form (word root with a combining vowel) for bone, *oste/o,* is used because the suffix begins with a consonant.

Now we will construct a more complicated term that contains a prefix and means *pertaining to within a vein.* The same steps apply, plus we add a step for the prefix:

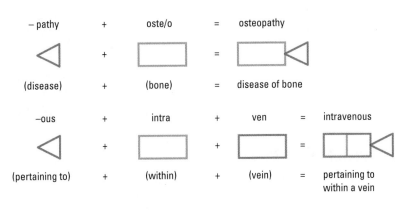

Figure 1.6 ::::

Most medical terms are formed by assembling word parts.

1. Start with the definition of what you want to communicate:

2. Find the suffix that means *pertaining to*:

3. Find the prefix that means *within*:

4. Find the word root for *vein*:

5. Arrange the word parts properly:

In this example, the word root is used without a combining vowel because the suffix starts with a vowel already.

An illustration of the process of assembling word parts to form a term is shown in Figure 1.6::::.

SELF QUIZ 1.6

Practice assembling word parts by working carefully through the exercises that follow.

WORD BUILDING

Using the word parts listed earlier, construct medical terms from the following meanings.

1. disease of a joint _____

1.12 2. inflammation of bone _____

3. study of the heart _____

4. pertaining to the stomach _____

5. pertaining to below the liver _____

6. pertaining to the stomach and liver _____

BREAK IT DOWN!

Analyze and separate each term into its word parts by labeling each word part using p = prefix, r = root, cv = combining vowel, and s = suffix.

1. arthropathy _____

2. osteitis _____

3. cardiology _____

4. gastric   _____

5. hypohepatic   _____

6. gastrohepatic   _____

Pronunciation of Medical Terms

Learning the correct pronunciation of medical terms is important if you are to use them properly. Also, once you learn how to pronounce medical terms, you will find that it will be easier to remember them.

In the following chapters, pronunciations for new medical terms will be provided in parentheses immediately following the term. Remember to use the audio glossary on the CD and CW for additional help with pronunciation of these terms.

In this text, we will use a phonetic (sounds like) pronunciation system, in which the term is spelled out using English letters to create sounds with which you should be familiar. To pronounce a new word, just say it as it is spelled out in parentheses. Note that the syllable with the most spoken emphasis is shown in all capital letters. Here are some examples:

- The term cardiology is pronounced kar dee ALL oh jee. Note that the middle syllable *ALL* carries the most emphasis.

- The term gastrohepatic is pronounced GAS troh heh PAT ik. Note that the long *o* sound in the second syllable is demonstrated when spelled phonetically as *oh*, and the short *e* sound is demonstrated when spelled *eh*.

- The term osteopathic is pronounced oss tee oh PATH ik. Note that the long *e* sound in the second syllable is shown as *tee*.

When in doubt about the correct pronunciation of a term, consult the CD and CW available with this text. Please note that a medical dictionary is another excellent source for correct pronunciations. If you have access to a medical dictionary, it's a great idea to become familiar with it now.

Spelling

Spelling is *very* important! A spelling error that changes just one or two letters in a term can completely change its meaning. For example, *ileum* is part of the small intestine, while *ilium* is part of the hip bone. In this example, the two terms sound the same but are spelled differently by a single letter.

One technique to help you learn how to spell medical terms is to write each term down a number of times until you are able to visualize its correct spelling. Practice this and the other study techniques discussed later in this chapter until you are confident that your spelling is accurate. Remember, medical terminology is a language, and communicating a language clearly and correctly is important—especially in medicine, where the health of a patient may depend on it!

Singular and Plural Endings

Since most medical terms are composed of Latin or Greek word parts, the rules for changing a singular word into a plural form are quite different than they are for the English language. Here are some helpful guidelines:

- If the term ends in *a*, the plural is usually formed by adding an *e*. For example, the plural form of vertebra is vertebrae.

- If the term ends in *is*, the plural form is usually formed by changing the *is* to *es*. For example, the plural form of diagnosis is diagnoses.

- If the term ends in *itis,* the plural form is usually formed by changing the *itis* to *itides.* For example, the plural form of gastritis is gastritides.

- If the term ends in *on* or *um,* the plural is usually formed by changing the *on* or *um* to *a.* For example, the plural form of ganglion is ganglia, and that of myocardium is myocardia.

Additional guidelines of endings that are less frequently encountered are provided in Appendix C. When an unusual ending is encountered in this text, both singular and plural endings will be explained. Again, when in doubt, a medical dictionary is an excellent source for answers—don't hesitate to use one!

Helpful Study Tips

You've just been introduced to the basics of medical terminology. In the coming chapters, the terms will increase in numbers and complexity, making learning a challenge. Included here are some helpful study tips that should make the learning of medical terminology easier and, hopefully, more enjoyable.

ORGANIZE YOUR TIME

The most common obstacle to finding time to study is not a lack of hours in a day, although it may seem like it—rather, it is procrastination (putting tasks off until later). If you are no stranger to the art of procrastination, you, along with many others, must overcome this behavior. Think about your professional and personal goals and the timeline within which you wish to achieve them. If you sincerely want to achieve your goals, you will find the necessary time for study. Try implementing the following techniques to strengthen your study habits:

- Organize your schedule to enable you to find enough time to study in a calm, peaceful manner.

- Identify blocks of time each day that you are willing to set aside for studying; then use them to study.

- Don't wait until the last minute, but spend time throughout the week or weeks preceding your next exam to study the material. Studying a little material each day is much more effective than studying a chapter or more at once.

- Set time aside that you consider a prime time for study: the time that you are most alert and fresh. For some it is in the early morning, for others it is midday, and for others it is in the evening or late night. Find which time of day suits your learning skills the best, and use it.

FLASH CARDS

Flash cards are a terrific way to learn medical terminology, and the CD that comes with this book has a flash card generator feature that you can use to create your own version of this valuable study aid.

Use this feature to print flash cards. You can include a sample word or drawing of your own that will help you to associate the word part with its meaning. Also, you might consider printing the flash cards using different paper colors and building your word part flash card library with color identification. For example, use blue paper for prefixes, red paper for word roots or combining forms, and green paper for suffixes. Print whole terms on yet another color to differentiate them from your flash cards that are word parts.

Once you make your flash cards, don't stuff them in a drawer—use them! Bring them with you wherever you go, using time in between classes, during lunch, waiting for friends, etc. You'll find that studying them for a few minutes here and there will help you learn the terms much more effectively than cramming the night before an exam.

OTHER TIPS

Spelling is often the most difficult part of learning medical terminology. But if you take the time to break down a term into its word parts, you'll find that spelling works itself out. Another tip for learning to spell difficult terms is to write them down. By writing them, sometimes over and over again, the connection between your hand and your mind helps to integrate the spelling of the term into your long-term memory. If you are using flash cards, write the difficult words down on a separate sheet of paper until you are able to visualize the correct spelling in your mind.

Drawing pictures provides an experience for your learning capacity similar to writing down the words repetitively. Draw pictures of not only the term's meaning, but also anything that you believe will help you to find an association with the term. Often the silliest ideas and drawings can help you remember.

Another device that can help is to make up rhymes with melodies of songs with which you are familiar. Take a song that you like and exchange the words with medical terms. Share it with friends, and create rounds. Be creative and have fun!

Using audio is another device that can help, especially with pronunciation. Use the audio glossary on the CD and CW for help with pronunciation of these terms. Hearing the pronunciation of the term will incorporate it into your thoughts for later recall.

A final suggestion is to study with a partner from class. Quiz each other with flash cards, compare notes and study techniques, and review the chapters together. Bouncing new information and ideas back and forth often helps considerably.

SELF QUIZ 1.7

SAY IT—SPELL IT!

Practice pronunciation and spelling of medical terms by speaking the phonetic pronunciations out loud, then writing the correct spelling of the term.

> **Success Hint:**   Use the audio glossary on the CD and CW for additional help with pronunciation of these terms.

1. KAR dee ALL oh jee   _____

2. kar DYE tiss   _____

3. ar TEE ree oh kar DYE tiss   _____

4. my oh KAR dee um   _____

5. oss tee oh PATH ik   _____

FILL IT IN!

Fill in the blanks with the correct terms.

1. In the term cardiology (kar dee ALL oh jee), the _____ syllable is emphasized more than any other.

1.13 2. In the term carditis (kar DYE tiss), the _____ syllable is emphasized.

3. In the term myocardium (MY oh KAR dee um), the *o* is pronounced as a _____ (long or short) vowel.

4. Look up the term endocarditis in the Audio Glossary for this book or in a medical dictionary and write its phonetic translation: _____

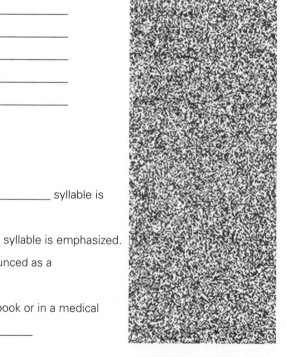

END IT!

Write the correct singular or plural form of each term in the space provided.

Singular Form	Plural Form
1. carditis	_____
2. _____	papillae
3. ovum	_____
4. _____	gastrolyses
5. osteitis	_____
6. _____	axillae

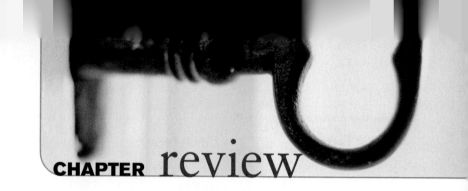

In this section, we will review all the word parts and medical terms from this chapter. As in earlier tables, the word roots are shown in **bold.**

Check each word part and medical term to be sure you understand the meaning. If any are not clear, please go back into the chapter and review that term. Then, complete the review exercises that follow.

[word parts **checklist**]

Prefixes	Word Roots/Combining Vowels	Suffixes
❑ ab-	❑ **arteri**/o	❑ -al
❑ endo-	❑ **arthr**/o	❑ -ic
❑ hyper-	❑ **cardi**/o	❑ -ous
❑ hypo-	❑ **gastr**/o	❑ -itis
❑ intra-	❑ **hepat**/o	❑ -logy
❑ pre-	❑ **later**/o	❑ -meter
❑ post-	❑ **norm**/o	❑ -pathy
❑ sub-	❑ **oste**/o	❑ -scope
	❑ **path**/o	❑ -scopy
	❑ **tens**/o	
	❑ **ven**/o	

[medical terminology **checklist**]

❑ ab**norm**al	❑ **cardi**o**path**ic	❑ hypo**hepat**ic
❑ **appendic**itis	❑ **cardi**opathy	❑ intra**ven**ous
❑ **arteri**al	❑ **card**itis	❑ my**o****cardi**a
❑ **arteri**o**card**itis	❑ **card**itides	❑ my**o****cardi**um
❑ **arteri**ology	❑ endo**cardi**al	❑ **oste**itis
❑ **arteri**opathy	❑ endo**cardi**tis	❑ **oste**itides
❑ **arteri**o**ven**ous	❑ **gastr**ic	❑ **oste**o**arthr**opathy
❑ **arthr**itis	❑ **gastr**itis	❑ **oste**ology
❑ **arthr**ology	❑ **gastr**itides	❑ **oste**opathy
❑ **arthr**opathy	❑ **gastr**o**hepat**ic	❑ **oste**o**path**ic
❑ **axill**a	❑ **gastr**ology	❑ **path**ology
❑ **axill**ae	❑ **hepat**itis	❑ post**ven**ous
❑ bi**later**al	❑ hyper**gastr**ic	❑ pre**hepat**ic
❑ **cardi**ac	❑ hyper**tens**ion	❑ pre**ven**ous
❑ **cardi**ology	❑ hypo**gastr**ic	

[show what **you know!**]

BREAK IT DOWN!

Analyze and separate each term into its word parts by labeling each word part using p = prefix, r = root, cv = combining vowel, and s = suffix.

Example:

1.	venous	r s ven/ous
2.	hypotension	_____
3.	arthritis	_____
4.	gastrology	_____
5.	prehepatitis	_____
6.	hepatogastropathy	_____
7.	osteopathic	_____

WORD BUILDING

Using the word parts listed earlier, construct or recall medical terms from the following meanings.

Example:

1.	disease of a bone	osteopathy
2.	inflammation of a joint	_____
3.	pertaining to the liver	_____
4.	pertaining to before the stomach	_____
5.	pertaining to below the heart	_____
6.	study of joints	_____
7.	pertaining to within a vein	_____
8.	pertaining to a deficiency of the liver	_____
9.	study of disease of bone and joint	_____
10.	inflammation of the stomach	_____

FILL IT IN!

Fill in the blanks.

1. In the medical term osteoarthritis (OSS tee oh ar THRY tis), the emphasis is on the (a) _____ and the

   (b) _____. The first letter *o* in this term is pronounced as a (c) _____ vowel.

2. In the medical term cardioarterial (KAR dee oh ar TEE ree al), the three *e* letters are pronounced as

   (d) _____ vowels.

3. In the medical term hypercapnia (high per KAP nee ah), the *y* is pronounced as a long (e) _____ and

   the primary emphasis is on the (f) _____ syllable.

[piece it all **together!**]

CROSSWORD

From the chapter material, fill in the crossword puzzle with answers to the following clues.

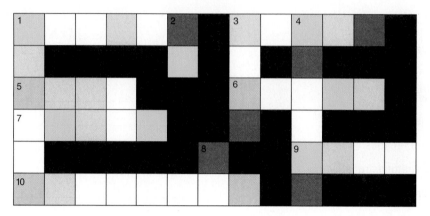

ACROSS

1. What word root means artery? (Find puzzle piece 1.2)
3. What is the prefix in the word hypertension? (Find puzzle piece 1.5)
5. What is the root in the word hypertension? (Find puzzle piece 1.3)
6. What is the suffix in the term osteopathy? (Find puzzle piece 1.8)
7. What word root means liver? (Find puzzle piece 1.1)
9. What suffix means inflammation? (Find puzzle piece 1.7)
10. What is the term for inflammation of bone? (Find puzzle piece 1.12)

DOWN

1. What is the combining form for the term that means joint? (Find puzzle piece 1.11)
2. What is a suffix that means pertaining to? (Find puzzle piece 1.9)
3. What is the prefix in the term hypohepatic? (Find puzzle piece 1.6)
4. What word root and suffix together mean pertaining to disease? (Find puzzle pieces 1.4 and 1.9)
8. What syllable in the term carditis carries the most emphasis? (Find puzzle piece 1.13)
10. What is the most common combining vowel? (Find puzzle piece 1.10)

WORD UNSCRAMBLE

From the completed crossword puzzle, unscramble:

1. All of the letters that appear in **red** squares

   _ ☐ _ _ _ ☐

   Clue: combining form of the term for heart

2. All of the letters that appear in **blue** squares

   ☐ ☐ ☐ _

   Clue: a suffix that means to follow after

3. All of the letters that appear in **yellow** squares

   ☐ ☐ _ _ _ ☐ _ _ _ _

   Clue: greater than normal tension

4. All of the letters that appear in **green** squares

   _ ☐ _ _ ☐ _ _

   Clue: pertaining to the liver

Now write down each of the letters that are boxed and unscramble them to find the hidden medical term:

_ _ _ _ _ _ _ _ _ _ _

MEDmedia wrap-up

www.prenhall.com/wingerd

Before you go on to the next chapter, take advantage of the free CD-ROM and study guide website that accompany this book. Simply load the CD-ROM for additional activities, games, animations, videos, and quizzes linked to this chapter. Then visit www.prenhall.com/wingerd for even more!

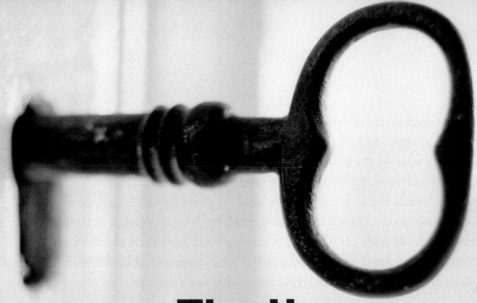

CHAPTER

2

The Human Body in Health and Disease

LEARNING OBJECTIVES

After completing this chapter, you will be able to:

- Define and spell the word parts used to create terms for the human body

- Identify the building blocks, organ systems, and cavities of the body

- Identify the anatomical planes and regions, and directional terms used to describe areas of the body

- Break down and define common medical terms used for symptoms, diseases, disorders, procedures, treatments, and devices associated with the human body

- Build medical terms from the word parts associated with the human body

- Pronounce and spell common medical terms associated with the human body

MEDmedia

www.prenhall.com/wingerd
Enhance your study with the power of multimedia! Each chapter of this book links to activities, games, animations, videos, and quizzes that you'll find on your CD-ROM. Plus, you can click on www.prenhall.com/wingerd, to find a free chapter-specific companion website that's loaded with additional practice and resources.

 CD-ROM

- Audio Glossary
- Exercises & Activities
- Flashcard Generator
- Animations
- Videos

 Companion Website

- Exercises & Activities
- Audio Glossary
- Drug Updates
- Current News Updates

A secure distance learning course is available at www.prenhall.com/onekey.

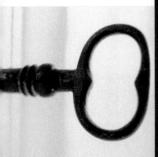

A study of medical terminology includes learning about the human body in a healthy state, as well as in a diseased state. In this chapter, you will learn some basics about the building blocks of the body and body structure and function, which is necessary for understanding many medical terms. You will also learn about the language that is used to describe the location of body parts, known as directional terminology and anatomical planes, as well as information about body cavities and organ systems. To launch you in the right direction, the chapter also introduces the basic concepts of health and disease, including some important terms associated with disease.

word parts focus

Let's look at word parts. The following table contains a list of word parts that when combined build many of the terms of the human body.

PREFIX	DEFINITION	PREFIX	DEFINITION
ana-	up, toward, apart	hypo-	beneath
bi-	two	uni-	one
epi-	upon		

WORD ROOT	DEFINITION	WORD ROOT	DEFINITION
abdomin	abdomen	hom, home	sameness or unchanging
anter	front	iatr	to heal
brach	arm	idi	person, self
card, cardi	heart	ili	flank or groin
caud	tail, downward	infect	to enter, invade
cephal	head	infer	below
cervic	neck	inguin	groin
chondr	gristle, cartilage	later	side
chron	time	lumb	loin or lower back
cran, crani	skull, cranium	medi	middle
dist	away from a point of reference	path	disease, suffering
dors	back	pelv	pelvis, washbasin
eti	cause	physi	nature
femor	thigh	poster	back, behind
gastr	stomach	proxim	near to a point of reference
glut	buttock	spin	spine or thorn

WORD ROOT	DEFINITION	WORD ROOT	DEFINITION
stasis	standing still	tom	cut
super	above	umbilic	navel
thorac	chest	ventr	belly, front

SUFFIX	DEFINITION	SUFFIX	DEFINITION
-ad	toward	-ic	pertaining to
-al	pertaining to	-ior	pertaining to
-ar	pertaining to	-y	process of

SELF QUIZ 2.1

Review the word parts of the human body's terminology by working carefully through the exercises that follow. Soon, we will apply this new information to build medical terms.

> **Success Hint:**   Once you get to the crossword puzzle at the end of the chapter, remember to check back here for clues! Your clues are indicated by the puzzle icon.

A.   Provide the definition of the following prefixes and suffixes.

1. bi-   _____

2. -ior   _____

3. -ic   _____

4. -al   _____

5. ana-   _____

6. uni-   _____

2.1 7. hypo-   _____

B.   Provide the word root for each of the following terms.

2.2 1. front   _____

2. back   _____

3. back, behind   _____

4. head   _____

5. heart   _____

6. abdomen   _____

7. nature   _____

8. disease, suffering   _____

9. middle   _____

10. standing still   _____

11. chest   _____

12. belly   _____

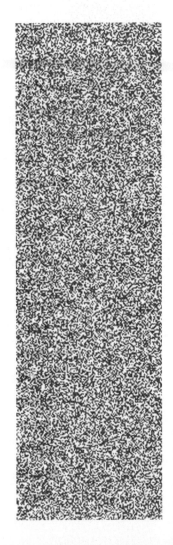

13. cut   _____

14. above   _____

15. flank, groin _____

16. to enter, invade _____

17. cause   _____

18. to heal   _____

[anatomy and physiology overview]

The study of body structure is known as **anatomy.** The term is constructed from three word parts:

ana/tom/y

The prefix ana- means *up, toward, apart,* the word root tom means *cut,* and the suffix -y refers to *process of.* When we put the meanings together, the term *anatomy* means *the process of cutting apart.*

The word *anatomy* was first used by the ancient Greeks, who used cadaver dissection to explore body structure. Today, we use the term to describe the study of body structure—a very appropriate name for this "cutting" science! Specifically, the study of anatomy involves the identification of body components and their locations relative to one another.

The study of body function is known as **physiology.** The term can be shown as:

physi/o/logy

The word root physi means *nature,* and the suffix -logy means *study of.* Combined, the term *physiology* literally means *study of nature.* Thus, physiology refers to the study of the nature of living things. It is concerned with body functions, and seeks answers to the question "how does it work?"

The functions of the human body work hand in hand to keep the body alive and as healthy as possible. Most body functions respond to a change, like a cold breeze or exposure to a virus, by making internal adjustments in the body. The goal of these functions is to keep the internal body at a constant, stable state despite changes in the world around us. Why keep the body stable? Because the molecules that form us work best under very stable conditions. The process of maintaining internal stability is a central concept of human physiology, and is called **homeostasis.** This word is constructed of three word parts:

home/o/stasis

The word root home means *sameness, or unchanging,* the combining vowel is the letter o, and stasis is a word root that means *standing still.* The term *homeostasis* thereby describes its meaning: *maintaining internal stability.*

Building Blocks of the Body

The increasingly complex parts that make up the body are its building blocks (Figure 2.1▦). From simple to complex, they include:

■ **Atoms and molecules:** nonliving particles that are capable of combining with one another to form more complex structures. Important molecules of the body include proteins, lipids (fats), carbohydrates, and nucleic acids.

enrichment module enrichment module enrichment module enrichment module enrichment module enrichment module enrichment module enrichment module

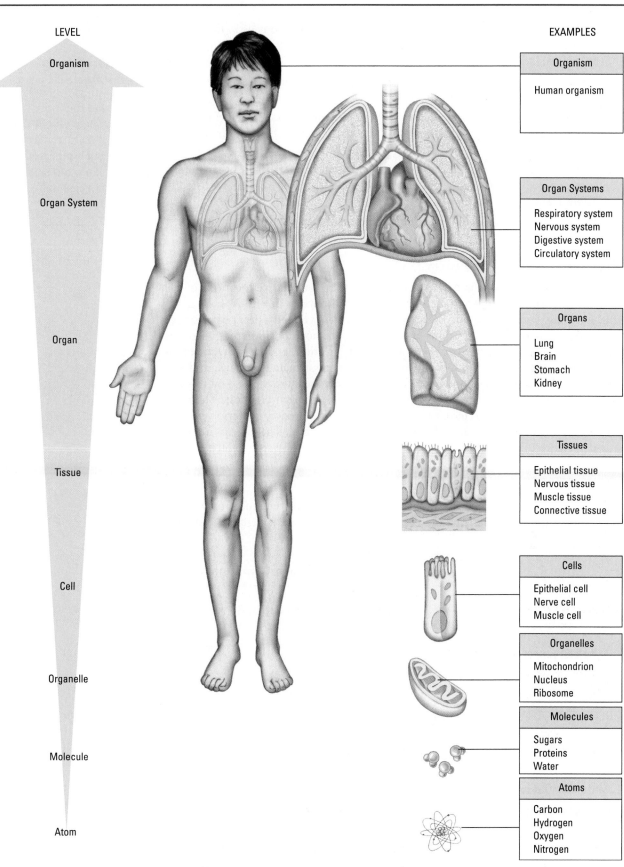

LEVEL

Organism

Organ System

Organ

Tissue

Cell

Organelle

Molecule

Atom

EXAMPLES

Organism

Human organism

Organ Systems

Respiratory system
Nervous system
Digestive system
Circulatory system

Organs

Lung
Brain
Stomach
Kidney

Tissues

Epithelial tissue
Nervous tissue
Muscle tissue
Connective tissue

Cells

Epithelial cell
Nerve cell
Muscle cell

Organelles

Mitochondrion
Nucleus
Ribosome

Molecules

Sugars
Proteins
Water

Atoms

Carbon
Hydrogen
Oxygen
Nitrogen

Figure 2.1 :::: **Building blocks of the body.**

Complexity increases in the direction of the arrow.

- **Cells:** the most basic living unit. There are about 30 trillion cells in the human body, and more than 200 different types that vary in size and shape according to their function.
- **Tissues:** a combination of similar cells that share a common goal, such as providing movement, protection, or secretion.
- **Organs:** a combination of two or more different types of tissues to form a structure that performs a general function. The brain, stomach, and pancreas are examples of organs.
- **Organ systems:** a combination of organs and associated structures that share a common goal. There are eleven organ systems in the body, which are listed in Table 2.1::::.
- **Organism:** the whole, complete human body that is capable of survival.

> **[thinking critically!]**
>
> Cells are the most basic unit of life. Are they, in turn, composed of living particles, or are the subcellular particles not living?

Directional Terms

Directional terms are words that are used to describe the relative locations of the body or its parts. Since the human body can move into many positions, such as sitting, standing, lying on one side, lying on the back, etc., we need a point of reference before we can describe the locations of body parts. The body position that is used as a reference is commonly known as the **anatomical position,** and is an erect (standing) posture with the arms at the side, palms of the hands facing forward, and legs together with feet pointing forward. Directional terms are always based on this reference position, even though the patient may be in a different position. The most commonly used directional terms are **superior, inferior, anterior, posterior, medial, lateral, proximal, distal, ventral, dorsal, cephalic,** and **caudal.** These terms are illustrated in Figure 2.2::::, and defined in the Getting to the Root of It section on p. 33–35.

Anatomical Planes

A plane is an imaginary flat field that is used as a point of reference for viewing three-dimensional objects. Anatomical planes are used to help describe the loca-

Table 2.1   :::   The Organ Systems and Their Organ Components

ORGAN SYSTEM	ORGANS
integumentary system	skin
skeletal system	bones, joints
muscular system	muscles
nervous system	brain, spinal cord, nerves
endocrine system	pituitary gland, thyroid gland, parathyroid glands, adrenal glands, pancreas, thymus, gonads
cardiovascular system	heart, blood vessels
lymphatic system	spleen, lymphatic vessels
respiratory system	nose, pharynx, larynx, trachea, bronchi, lungs
digestive system	tongue, pharynx, esophagus, stomach, liver, salivary glands, pancreas, small intestine, large intestine, rectum
urinary system	kidneys, ureters, urinary bladder, urethra
female reproductive system	ovaries, uterus, fallopian tubes, vagina, vestibular glands
male reproductive system	testes, epididymus, vas deferens, prostate gland, seminal vesicles, bulbourethral glands

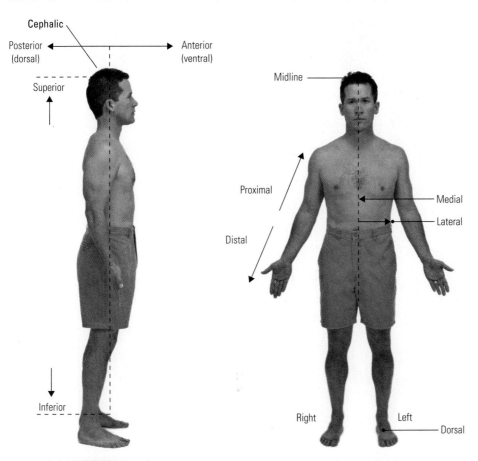

Figure 2.2
Directional terms.
(a) Anterior (front) view.
(b) Lateral (side) view.

tions of areas of the body relative to one another. They are much like viewing the results of imaginary knives that have segmented the body into sliced sections (Figure 2.3). There are three primary anatomical planes:

- **Frontal or coronal plane:** a vertical plane that passes through the body from side to side, dividing the body into anterior and posterior portions.
- **Sagittal plane:** a vertical plane that passes through the body from front to back, dividing the body into right and left portions. A midsagittal plane divides the body equally; it is also known as a median plane. A parasagittal plane divides the body unequally.
- **Transverse plane:** a horizontal plane that divides the body into superior (upper) and inferior (lower) portions.

Anatomical Regions

The regions of the body are external areas that have been named to give medical health workers the ability to communicate possible problems that may be revealed during a physical examination. The most commonly used body region terms are **cephalic, cervical, thoracic, brachial, abdominal, gluteal, inguinal, lumbar,** and **femoral.** They are shown in Figure 2.4 . In addition to the anatomical body region terms, there are also common terms for the body regions, such as head, neck, chest or thorax, arm, belly or abdomen, buttock, groin, loin or lower back and thigh regions. Patients may often use these common terms in describing their symptoms.

The abdominal region is further divided into smaller regions to assist medical health workers in locating and communicating medical problems with greater accuracy. The divisions of the abdomen are illustrated in Figure 2.5a , and include the **epigastric** (above the belly), **hypograstric** (below the belly), **hypochondriac** (just below the cartilage of the ribs), **iliac** (on either side of the hypogastric region), **lumbar**

[thinking critically!]

Which plane of section would be best to use in order to view a whole body organ in the abdomen, such as the stomach?

[FYI]

Hypochondriac
You may recognize the term *hypochondriac;* it is also used to indicate a person with an imaginary illness.

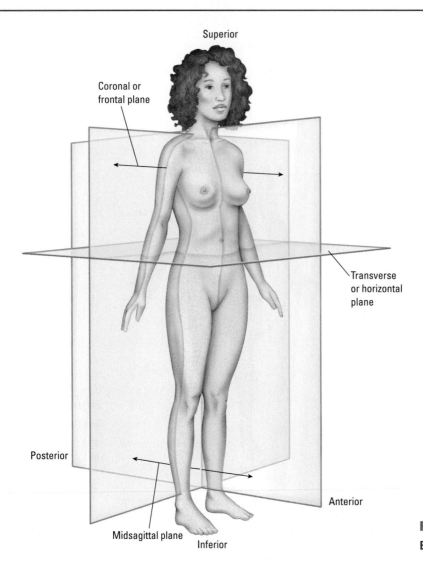

Superior

Coronal or
frontal plane

Transverse
or horizontal
plane

Posterior

Anterior

Midsagittal plane

Inferior

Figure 2.3 ::::

Body planes.

(on either side of the umbilical region), and **umbilical** (area containing the navel) regions. An alternative set of abdominal divisions are shown in Figure 2.5b, in which the abdomen is divided into four quadrants.

Body Cavities

The basic design of the human body consists of a central **trunk** or torso with attached **appendages.** The appendages are the head, arms, and legs. The trunk and head are not internally solid structures, but include spaces that are partially filled with organs, connecting structures, and fluids. The spaces are called **cavities** and their internal contents are known as **viscera.** There are two main cavities, the **dorsal cavity** and the **ventral cavity.** Each of these contains smaller cavities, which are illustrated in Figure 2.6::::.

The cavities are each surrounded by a moist membrane that helps control the spread of infections and keeps the internal organs moist and lubricated. The thoracic and abdominal cavities are separated by a sheet of muscle, called the **diaphragm.** However, the abdominal and pelvic cavities are not separated. Anatomists often refer to these two neighboring spaces using a combined term, **abdominopelvic cavity.**

[**thinking critically!**]

Terms associated with organs and disease are often built from word parts describing the body region where they are located. Can you think of a body part or disease that contains the word part *brach,* which means arm?

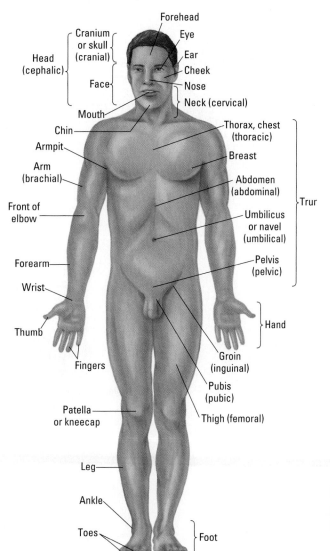

Forehead
Eye
Ear
Cheek
Nose
Neck (cervical)

Cranium
or skull
(cranial)

Head
(cephalic)

Face

Mouth

Chin

Armpit

Arm
(brachial)

Front of
elbow

Forearm

Wrist

Thumb

Fingers

Patella
or kneecap

Leg

Ankle

Toes

Thorax, chest
(thoracic)

Breast

Abdomen
(abdominal)

Umbilicus
or navel
(umbilical)

Pelvis
(pelvic)

Trur

Hand

Groin
(inguinal)

Pubis
(pubic)

Thigh (femoral)

Foot

Figure 2.4 ::::

Common anatomical regions of the body, anterior view.

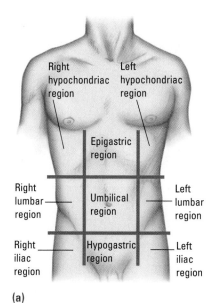

Right
hypochondriac
region

Left
hypochondriac
region

Epigastric
region

Right
lumbar
region

Umbilical
region

Left
lumbar
region

Right
iliac
region

Hypogastric
region

Left
iliac
region

(a)

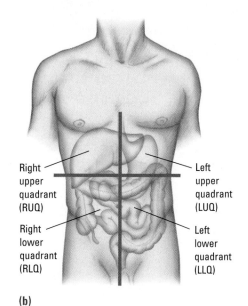

Right
upper
quadrant
(RUQ)

Left
upper
quadrant
(LUQ)

Right
lower
quadrant
(RLQ)

Left
lower
quadrant
(LLQ)

(b)

Figure 2.5 ::::

The abdomen and abdominal regions.

(a) Abdominal regions are mapped according to imaginary lines, as shown.
(b) The abdomen may also be divided into four quadrants. The organs are shown superimposed.

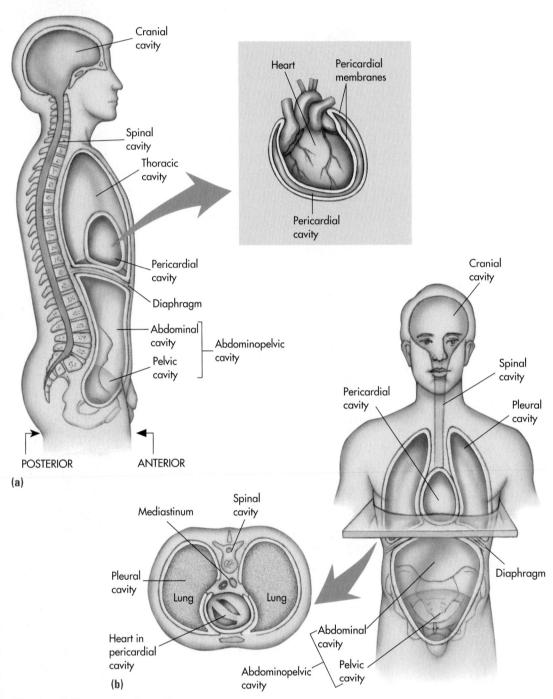

Figure 2.6 :::: **Body cavities.**

(a) Lateral view of a sagittal section through the body.
(b) Anterior view of a frontal section through the body.

getting to the root of it | anatomy and physiology terms

Many of the anatomy and physiology terms are formed from roots that are used to construct the more complex medical terms of the human body, including symptoms, diseases, and treatments. In this section, we will review the terms that describe the structure and function of the human body *in relation to their word roots*, which are shown in **bold.**

Study the word roots and terms in this list and complete the review exercises that follow.

Word Root (Meaning)	Terms Formed from the Word Root (Pronunciation)	Definition
abdomin (abdomen)	**abdomin**al cavity (ab DOM ih nal)	the space inside the belly or abdomen; viscera include the stomach, pancreas, spleen, liver, and most of the intestines
	abdominal region (ab DOM ih nal)	the belly region or abdomen, which contains several more specific regions including the epigastric, hypograstric, hypochondriac, iliac, lumbar, and umbilical regions
	abdominopelvic cavity (ab dom ih noh PELL vik KAV ih tee)	the body area encompassing both the abdominal and pelvic cavities
anter (front)	**anter**ior (an TEE ree or)	pertaining to the front
brach (arm)	**brach**ial region (BRAY kee-al)	the region of the body pertaining to the arm; also called the arm region
cardi (heart)	**cardi**ovascular system (kar dee oh VAS kyoo lahr)	the body system that circulates blood throughout the body via the heart and blood vessels
caud (tail)	**caud**al (KAWD al)	pertaining to the tail
cephal (head)	**cephal**ic region (seh FAL ik)	the region of the body pertaining to the head; also called the head region
cervic (neck)	**cervic**al region (SER vih kal)	the region of the body pertaining to the neck; also called the neck region
chondr (cartilage)	hypo**chondr**iac region (high poh KON dree ak)	part of the abdominal region specific to the area just below the cartilages of the ribs, which includes a right and left hypochondriac region on either side of the epigastric region; also called the infrachondral region
cran, crani (skull, cranium)	**crani**al (KRAY nee al)	pertaining to the head
	cranial cavity (KRAY nee al)	the space inside the cranium; viscera include the brain
dist (away from)	**dist**al (DISS tal)	pertaining away from a point of reference
dors (back)	**dors**al (DOR sal)	pertaining to the back
	dorsal cavity	contains the cranial and spinal cavities

Word Root (Meaning)	Terms Formed from the Word Root (Pronunciation)	Definition
femor (thigh)	**femor**al region (FEHM or al)	the region of the body pertaining to the thigh; also called the thigh region
gastr (stomach)	epi**gastr**ic region (ep ih GAS trik)	part of the abdominal region specific to the area above the belly (see Figure 2.4)
	hypo**gastr**ic region (high poh GAS trik)	part of the abdominal region specific to the area below the belly
glut (buttock)	**glut**eal region (GLOO tee al)	the region of the body pertaining to the buttock; also called the buttock region
hom, home (same)	**home**ostasis (hoh mee oh STAY siss)	the process of maintaining internal stability
ili (thigh, groin)	left **ili**ac region (ILL ee ak)	part of the abdominal region specific to the area located to the left of the hypogastric region
	right **ili**ac region (ILL ee ak)	part of the abdominal region specific to the area located to the right of the hypogastric region
infer (below)	**infer**ior (in FEE ree or)	pertaining to below a reference point
inguin (groin)	**inguin**al region (ING gwih nal)	the region of the body pertaining to the groin; also called the groin region
lumb (loin or lower back)	left **lumb**ar region (LUM bar)	part of the abdominal region specific to the area located to the left of the umbilical region
	right **lumb**ar region (LUM bar)	part of the abdominal region specific to the area located to the right of the umbilical region
medi (middle)	**medi**al (MEE dee al)	toward the middle
	mediolateral (mee dee oh LATT er al)	pertaining to the middle and to the side
pelv (washbasin, pelvis)	**pelv**ic cavity (PELL vik)	the space inside the pelvic area; viscera include urinary bladder, part of intestines, internal reproductive organs, rectum
physi (nature)	**physi**ologist (fiz ee ALL oh jist)	one who studies the nature of living things
	physiology (fiz ee ALL oh jee)	the study of the nature of living things
poster (back)	**poster**ior (poss TEE ree or)	pertaining to the back
	posterolateral (poss tee oh LATT er al)	pertaining to the back and to the side
	posteroanterior (poss ter oh an TEE ree or)	pertaining to the back and to the front
proxim (near to a reference point)	**proxim**al (PROK sim al)	pertaining near to a point of reference

Word Root (Meaning)	Terms Formed from the Word Root (Pronunciation)	Definition
spin (spine or thorn)	**spin**al cavity (SPY nal)	the space inside the spinal column (also called the vertebral canal); viscera include the spinal cord
super (above)	**super**ior (soo PEE ee or)	pertaining to above a reference point
	superolateral (soo PER roh LATT er al)	pertaining to above and to the side
thorac (chest)	**thorac**ic cavity (tho RASS ik)	the space inside the chest or thorax; viscera incluce heart, aorta, lungs, esophagus, bronchi
	thoracic region (tho RASS ik)	the region of the body pertaining to the chest; also called the chest region or thorax
tom (to cut)	ana**tom**ical position (an ah TOM ih kal)	the body position that is used as a reference for directional terms; it is an erect posture with the arms at the side, palms of the hands facing forward, and legs together with feet pointing forward
	ana**tom**y (ah NAH tom ee)	the science of body structure
umbilic (navel)	**umbilic**al region (um BILL ih kal)	the area of the abdomen that contains the navel
ventr (belly)	**ventr**al (VEHN tral)	adjective meaning pertaining to the belly
	ventral cavity (VEHN tral)	contains the thoracic, abdominal, and pelvic cavities

OTHER IMPORTANT TERMS

The terms in this table are related to the structure and function of the human body, but are not built from word roots.

appendage	the head, arms, and legs attached to the trunk of the body
atom (ATT om)	a nonliving particle that is capable of combining with other atoms to form more complex structures
cell	the most basic living unit
diaphragm (DYE ah fram)	a sheet of muscle that separates the thoracic and abdominal cavities
digestive system	the body system that converts food into a form the body can use for energy, growth, and repair; its organs include the tongue, pharynx, esophagus, stomach, liver, salivary glands, pancreas, small intestine, large intestine, and rectum
endocrine system (EHN doh krin)	the body system that regulates body function by secreting hormones; its organs include the pituitary gland, thyroid gland, parathyroid glands, adrenal glands, pancreas, thymus, and gonads

female reproductive system (REE proh DUCK tivv)	the female body system that enables reproduction by producing germ cells; its organs include the ovaries, uterus, fallopian tubes, vagina, and vestibular glands
frontal or **coronal plane** (kor ROHN al)	a vertical plane that passes through the body from side to side, dividing the body into anterior and posterior portions
integumentary system (in teg yoo MEN tah ree)	the body system that provides a barrier to protect against fluid loss, physical damage, and invasion by microorganisms; its major organ is the skin
lymphatic system (lim FATT ik)	organs include the spleen, lymphatic vessels
male reproductive system (REE proh DUCK tivv)	the male body system that enables reproduction by producing germ cells; its organs include the testes, epididymus, vas deferens, prostate gland, seminal vesicles, and bulbourethral glands
midsagittal plane (mid SAJ ih tal)	a sagittal plane that divides the body equally; also called a median plane
molecule (mall eh kyool)	a nonliving particle that is capable of combining with other molecules to form more complex structures
muscular system (MUSS kyoo lahr)	the body system that enables complex movement; its primary organs are the muscles
nervous system (NER vuss)	the body system that enables perception through the senses, integrates information to form thoughts and memories, and controls body movements and many internal functions; its organs include the brain, spinal cord, and nerves
organ	a structure made of two or more different types of tissue that performs a general function in the body
organ system	a combination of organs and associated structures that share a common goal; there are eleven organ systems in the body
organism (OR gah nizm)	the whole, complete human body that is capable of survival
parasagittal plane (pair ah SAJ ih tal)	a sagittal plane that divides the body unequally
respiratory system (RESS pih rah tor ee)	the body system responsible for bringing oxygen into the bloodstream; its organs include the nose, pharynx, larynx, trachea, bronchi, and lungs
sagittal plane (SAJ ih tal)	a vertical plane that passes through the body from front to back, dividing the body into right and left portions
skeletal system (SKELL eh tal)	the body system that provides structure and support for other systems and aids in movement; its organs include the bones and joints
tissue (TISH oo)	a group of similar cells that share a common goal or function

transverse plane (tranz VERS)	a horizontal plane that divides the body into superior and inferior sections
trunk	the torso of the body
urinary system (YOO rih nair ee)	the body system that performs waste excretion; its organs include the kidneys, ureters, urinary bladder, and urethra
viscera (VISS er ah)	the internal contents of body cavities, including organs, fluid, and connecting structures

SELF QUIZ 2.2

Success Hint: Use the audio glossary on the CD and CW for additional help with pronunciation of these terms.

SAY IT—SPELL IT!

Review the terms of the human body by speaking the phonetic pronunciation guides out loud, then writing in the correct spelling of the term.

2.3 1. ah NAH tom ee _____

2.4 2. an TEE ree or _____

3. poss TEE ree or _____

4. KAWD al _____

5. seh FAL ik _____

6. DISS tal _____

7. PROK sim al _____

8. DOR sal _____

9. VEHN tral _____

10. in FEE ree or _____

11. soo PEE ree or _____

12. LATT er al _____

13. MEE dee al _____

MATCH IT!

Match the term on the left with the correct definition on the right.

_____ 1. abdominal cavity   a. most inferior ventral cavity

_____ 2. pelvic cavity   b. contains heart and lungs

_____ 3. spinal cavity   c. contains the brain

_____ 4. thoracic cavity   d. just below the diaphragm

_____ 5. cranial cavity   e. pertains to posterior spaces

_____ 6. dorsal cavity   f. contains the spinal cord

_____ 7. abdominal region   g. head region

_____ 8. thoracic region   h. lower back region

_____ 9. gluteal region   i. thigh region

_____10. epigastric region   j. belly region

_____11. cephalic region   k. a division of the abdomen

_____12. lumbar region   l. buttocks region

_____13. femoral region   m. chest region

_____14. integumentary system   n. includes bones and joints

_____15. skeletal system   o. includes the skin

_____16. cardiovascular system   p. includes the kidneys

_____17. urinary system   q. includes the stomach

_____18. digestive system   r. includes the heart

BREAK IT DOWN!

Analyze and separate each term into its word parts by labeling each word part using p = prefix, r = root, cv = combining vowel, and s = suffix.

1. anterior   _____

2. posterior   _____

3. caudal   _____

4. cephalic   _____

2.5   5. distal   _____

6. proximal   _____

7. dorsal   _____

8. ventral   _____

9. inferior   _____

2.6   10. superior   _____

11. lateral   _____

12. medial   _____

13. posteroanterior   _____

14. unilateral   _____

15. mediolateral   _____

16. epigastric   _____

17. hypogastric   _____

18. hypochondriac   _____

19. iliac   _____

20. lumbar   _____

21. umbilical   _____

WORD BUILDING

Construct or recall medical terms from the following meanings.

1. pertaining to both sides   _____

2. toward the head   _____

3. pertaining to the belly   _____

4. pertaining to the back and to the front   _____

5. pertaining to away from   _____

6. pertaining to above and to the side   _____

7. toward the middle   _____

2.7   8. pertaining to the middle and to the side   _____

9. pertaining to the back and to the side   _____

10. a term that indicates that one body part is below another   _____

11. pertaining to the middle   _____

FILL IT IN!

Fill in the blanks with the correct terms.

1. An imaginary flat field that provides a reference point for the body is called an

   _____ _____

2. A vertical plane dividing the body into front and back portions is called

   a _____, or _____, plane.

3. A midsagittal plane is a _____ plane that divides the body

   into _____ portions.

4. A horizontal plane dividing the body into upper and lower portions is referred to

   as a _____ plane.

5. The body torso is not a solid structure, but contains a large space known as

   the _____ _____

6. The two primary cavities of the body are the _____ cavity and

   the _____ cavity.

7. The _____ _____ contains the brain and is

   located in the skull.

8. Structures located inside cavities are generally known as _____

9. The Latin origin of the word root dors is *dorsum*, and it means

   _____

10. The heart, lungs, and aorta are contained within the _____ cavity.

11. The stomach, pancreas, and most of the intestines are located within a

    membrane-lined space called the _____ cavity.

12. The dorsal cavity includes two cavities. They are the _____

    _____ and the _____ _____

13. A sheet of muscle divides the abominal and _____ cavities.

    It is called the _____

14. The abdominal and _____ cavities can be described as a single

    large space called the _____ cavity.

15. The dorsal cavity includes the cranial and _____ cavities.

16. The pituitary gland, thyroid gland, and adrenal glands are components of the

    _____ system.

17. The kidneys, ureters, urinary bladder, and urethra combine to form the

    _____ _____

18. The cardiovascular system includes the _____ and the blood

    vessels.

19. The head region is called the _____ region. It is attached to the

    trunk by the neck region, or _____ region.

20. The phonetic pronunciation for this term, _____, is written

    as *ING gwih nal.*

21. The anatomical term for the region of the lower back is the _____

    region, while that for the belly is the _____ region.

22. The common term for the thoracic region is _____ region.

23. The thigh region is also known as the _____ region.

24. The term hypogastric is constructed from the prefix _____ that

    means _____, the word root _____ that means

    belly, and the suffix -ic that means _____

2.12 25. The _____ region is located between the right and left lumbar

    regions and above the _____ region.

26. The hypogastric region is located between the right and left _____

2.13   regions and below the _____ region.

2.14 27. The term iliac is constructed from the word root _____, which

    means flank or groin, and the suffix -ac, which means _____

28. A word root and combining vowel that means *unchanging* or *sameness* is

2.15   _____

[medical terms of the

human body]

As discussed earlier in the chapter, the body's goal is to keep itself alive and healthy. Each system performs functions that endeavor to keep the body in a constant, stable state by adjusting to stimuli. This is the process of maintaining homeostasis. What happens when body functions fail to maintain homeostasis? A general condition of instability results, which we call **disease.** In general, the term disease refers to a state of the body in which homeostasis has faltered due to any cause.

The study of disease is a field known as **pathology.** This term can be shown as:

path/o/logy

where the word root, *path*, is derived from the Greek word for suffering or disease, *pathos*. Recall that the suffix, -logy, means *study of.* A **pathologist** is a physician who specializes in disease. In this word, the suffix is changed from -logy to -logist, which means *one who studies.* In hospitals and clinics, the pathology department is where patient specimens are analyzed and identified (Figure 2.7::::).

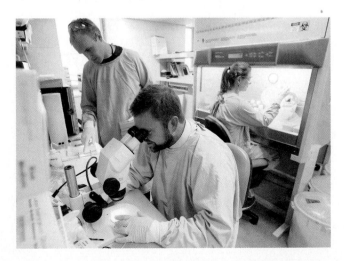

Figure 2.7 ::::

Pathology lab. A pathology lab within a clinic or hospital includes equipment that assists in the evaluation of patient specimens.

let's construct terms!

In this section, we will assemble all of the word parts to construct medical terminology related to the human body. Abbreviations are used to indicate each word part: **p** = prefix, **r** = root, **cv** = combining vowel, and **s** = suffix. Recall from Chapter 1 that the addition of a combining vowel to the word root creates the combining form for the term. Note that some terms are not constructed from word parts, but they are included here to expand your vocabulary.

The medical terms of the human body are listed in the following three sections:

- Symptoms and Signs
- Diseases and Disorders
- Treatments, Procedures, and Devices

Each section is followed by review exercises. Study the lists in these tables and complete the review exercises that follow.

Symptoms and Signs

WORD PARTS (WHEN APPLICABLE)			TERM	DEFINITION
Part	Type	Meaning		
			fever	a symptom in which body temperature rises above the normal 98.6°F
			pain	an unpleasant sensory and emotional experience that is associated with tissue damage
			sensation	a feeling or mental experience perceiving any stimulus
			sign	an abnormality that is discoverable by an objective examination
			symptom (SIMP tumm)	an appearance or sensation experienced by a patient that deviates from the normal, healthy state

---

SELF QUIZ 2.3

MATCH IT!

Match the term on the left with the correct definition on the right.

_____1. fever

_____2. pain

_____3. sensation

_____4. sign

_____5. symptom

a. an abnormality that is discoverable by an objective examination

b. an appearance or sensation experienced by a patient that deviates from the normal, healthy state

c. a symptom in which body temperature rises above the normal 98.6°F

d. an unpleasant sensory and emotional experience that is associated with tissue damage

e. a feeling or mental experience perceiving any stimulus

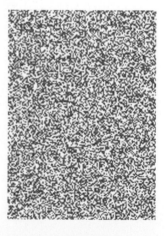

WORD BUILDING

Construct or recall medical terms from the following meanings.

1. a symptom in which body temperature rises above the normal 98.6°F

   _____

2. an unpleasant sensory and emotional experience that is associated with tissue damage

   _____

3. a feeling or mental experience perceiving any stimulus

   _____

4. an abnormality that is discoverable by an objective examination

   _____

5. an appearance or sensation experienced by a patient that deviates from the normal, healthy state

   _____

FILL IT IN!

Fill in the blanks with the correct terms.

1. During a physical examination, a physician found evidence of a lump in the right breast of a patient after the patient complained of local tenderness. The patient's experience is called a _____, while the evidence revealed by the exam is known as a _____

2. An elevated body temperature, or _____, is one example of a sign.

3. Injuries are often associated with an unpleasant sensory experience known as _____

4. Because pain is a mental experience as a result of a stimulus, it is also a _____

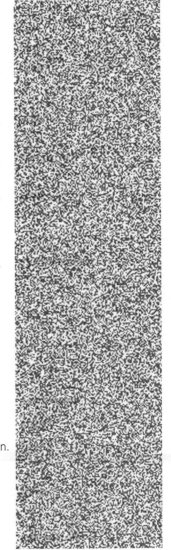

Diseases and Disorders

WORD PARTS (WHEN APPLICABLE)			TERM	DEFINITION
Part	Type	Meaning		
			acute (ah KYOOT)	adjective describing a disease of short duration and often with a sharp, or severe, effect

> [FYI]
>
> **Acute**
> The term *acute* is derived from the Latin word *acutus,* which means sharp. It describes a symptom or sign that strikes quickly, such as would result from a sharp stab.

chron	r	time	**chronic** (KRON ik)	adjective describing a disease of long duration, usually with a slow progression
-ic	s	pertaining to		

WORD PARTS (WHEN APPLICABLE)			TERM	DEFINITION
Part	Type	Meaning		
			disease (dih ZEEZ)	a state of the body in which homeostasis has faltered due to any cause
iatr/o gen -ic	r/cv r s	to heal producing pertaining to	**iatrogenic** (eye ah troh JEN ik)	adjective meaning a disease that is induced by medical treatment
idi/o path -ic	r/cv r s	person, self disease pertaining to	**idiopathic** (ID ee oh PATH ik)	adjective meaning a disease of unknown cause
infect -ion	r s	to enter, invade pertaining to	**infection** (in FEKK shun)	the multiplication of parasitic organisms within the body, such as bacteria, viruses, and fungi
			inflammation (in flah MAY shun)	a response to a trauma that is marked by the symptoms of redness, swelling, heat, and pain
			sequelae (SEE kwel ee)	conditions following and resulting from a disease
			trauma (TRAW mah)	a wound or injury

[FYI]

Inflammation

The Latin word *inflammation* is the origin of this term, which literally means to ignite or set ablaze. Because the symptoms of inflammation are heat, swelling, redness, and pain, this term is aptly named!

Sequelae

The term *sequelae* is a plural form of the word sequela. It is derived from the Latin word *sequo,* which means to follow.

Trauma

Trauma is the Greek word for a wound, and is used to describe any wound or injury that is accidental or inflicted on purpose.

disease focus | Diagnosis

Perhaps the greatest challenge in medicine is the reliable determination of a disease. A correct diagnosis is essential to treat any condition effectively. As a result of improving technologies, this important part of medicine has experienced many recent improvements. The five most important improvements to diagnostics include endoscopy, CAT scans, PET scans, magnetic resonance imaging, and ultrasound.

Endoscopy involves the use of a long, flexible tube that can be inserted into the patient (Figure 2.8::::). At the end of the tube, a camera may be inserted that enables the physician to view the patient's internal anatomy on a nearby monitor. The tube end may also contain surgical attachments, enabling a surgeon to manipulate internal body structures while viewing through the monitor. Endoscopes have become modified over recent years for specific uses. As you proceed through the chapters of this text, the various types of endoscopes will be described.

CAT scans are similar to x-rays, except they use computer imaging to produce a three-dimensional image of the body (Figure 2.9::::). Referred to by the acronym for *computed axial tomography,* a CAT scan is produced by beams of energized particles (or x-rays) that are focused on a specific plane of the body. The beam is projected from different positions to permit scanning from multiple angles while the patient remains stationary, and the information from the scan is relayed to a computer. A computer processes the information to produce cross-sectional images or "slices" of body regions. CAT scans are useful when cross-sectional images of organs in the chest or abdomen, muscles, and bone are needed. Speed and relatively low cost make CAT scans the standard for evaluation of trauma to most areas of the body.

PET scans employ computers and radioactive substances to examine the metabolic activity of various parts of the body (Figure 2.10::::). A radioactive substance is combined with a metabolically important material, such as glucose, to form a "cocktail" that is inhaled or injected into the patient. Once inside the patient, the cocktail is absorbed into a metabolically active organ and releases its charged particles. The charged particles are detected by the PET scan and interpreted by the computer to create color-coded images of the organ's metabolic activity. The term *PET* is an acronym for *positron emission tomography*.

Among all the diagnostic imaging techniques available, the **MRI** (the acronym for *magnetic resonance imaging*) has generated the most excitement in the medical community. It offers the clearest, most complete images of soft tissues that are currently possible (Figure 2.11::::). Although MRI is continually being improved

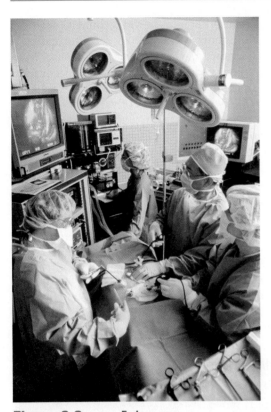

Figure 2.8 :::: **Endoscopy.**

A surgical procedure using an endoscope to view and remove an internal mass.

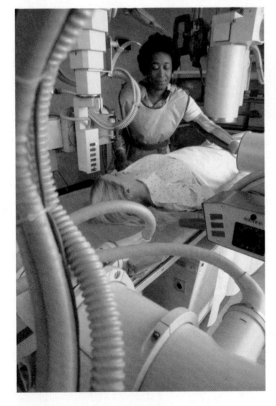

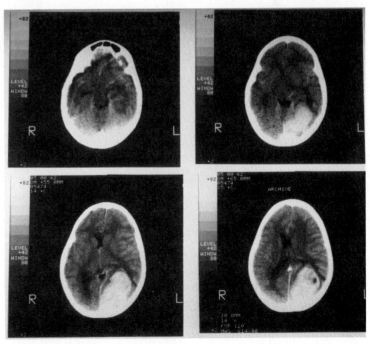

Figure 2.9 :::: **CAT scan.**

The image at left shows a CAT scan procedure. The four images at right show four CAT scans of the head region. The white mass in these images reveals a brain tumor.

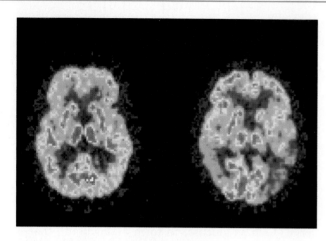

Figure 2.10 :::: **PET scan.** The two images of the brain highlight areas of metabolic activity.

and upgraded, in its present form it utilizes a powerful magnetic field generated within a chamber in which the patient lies. The magnetic field traces the element hydrogen, which is a component of water, in the patient's body. Since bones contain very little water compared to soft tissues, MRI can peer directly through them. In fact, MRI distinguishes between internal structures on the basis of their differences in water content. Once the hydrogen atoms have been detected, the information is analyzed by computer, which creates a 3-D image. Multiple colors may be added by computer enhancement to make the image look more realistic, or to distinguish more clearly between structures of varying water content.

Ultrasound imaging, or **sonography,** involves the pulsation of harmless sound waves through a body region. As the waves travel through tissues of varying density, they produce echoes that can be collected by the instrument. A computer analyzes the echoes and constructs a sectional image that outlines internal body structures (Figure 2.12::::). Because of its harmless nature, ultrasound imaging has proven useful in prenatal care by allowing an early view of a developing fetus (a child before birth) in the uterus. However, it is not effective for viewing structures surrounded by bone like the brain and spinal cord, because sound waves cannot penetrate dense objects.

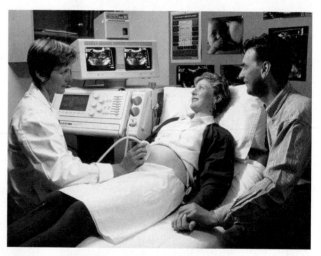

Figure 2.12 :::: **Ultrasound imaging.** The use of sound waves produces a computer-enhanced image of this couple's child on the monitor, allowing parents an exciting early view of their child and giving physicians a noninvasive way of viewing internal structures in the human body.

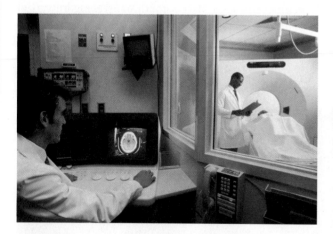

Figure 2.11 :::: **MRI.** An MRI procedure room.

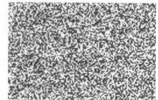

SELF QUIZ 2.4

SAY IT—SPELL IT!

Review the terms of the human body by speaking the phonetic pronunciation guides out loud, then writing in the correct spelling of the term.

1. eye ah troh JENN ik _____

2. ID ee oh PATH ik _____

3. in flah MAY shun _____

4. SEE kwel ee _____

5. ah KYOOT   _____

6. KRON ik   _____

7. dih ZEEZ   _____

8. in FEKK shun   _____

9. TRAW mah   _____

MATCH IT!

Match the term on the left with the correct definition on the right.

_____1. idiopathic

_____2. infection

_____3. inflammation

_____4. trauma

_____5. iatrogenic

_____6. sequelae

_____7. acute

_____8. chronic

_____9. disease

a. a wound or injury

b. redness, swelling, heat, and pain

c. a disease of unknown cause

d. multiplication of bacteria in the body

e. adjective describing a disease of short duration and often with a sharp, or severe, effect

f. a state of the body in which homeostasis has faltered due to any cause

g. a condition following and resulting from a disease

h. disease that is induced by medical treatment

i. adjective describing a disease of long duration, usually with a slow progression

BREAK IT DOWN!

Analyze and separate each term into its word parts by labeling each word part using p = prefix, r = root, cv = combining vowel, and s = suffix.

1. iatrogenic   _____

2. idiopathic   _____

3. infection   _____

4. chronic   _____

WORD BUILDING

Construct or recall medical terms from the following meanings.

1. adjective describing a disease of short duration and often with a sharp, or severe, effect   _____

2. adjective describing a disease of long duration, usually with a slow progression   _____

3. a state of the body in which homeostasis has faltered due to any cause   _____

4. adjective meaning a disease that is induced by medical treatment

    _____

5. adjective meaning a disease of unknown cause

    _____

6. the multiplication of parasitic organisms within the body, such as bacteria, viruses, and fungi

    _____

7. a response to a trauma that is marked by the symptoms of redness, swelling, heat, and pain

    _____

8. a condition following and resulting from a disease

    _____

9. a wound or injury

    _____

FILL IT IN!

Fill in the blanks with the correct terms.

1. The medical science concerned with all aspects of a disease is called

    _____.

2. When the cause for a disease cannot be identified, it is called an

    _____ disease.

3. A growing colony of bacteria is a frequent cause of _____.

    A common result is redness, swelling, heat, and pain, which are symptoms

    of _____.

4. The primary theme of a course in pathology is _____.

5. A frequent result of motorcycle accidents is a wound to the head of the rider,

    called head _____.

Treatments, Procedures, and Devices

WORD PARTS (WHEN APPLICABLE)			TERM	DEFINITION
Part	Type	Meaning		
			computed axial tomography scan (AX ee al toh MOG rah fee)	a diagnostic scan similar to x-ray, in which data from beams of energized particles (or x-rays) are computer interpreted to produce a three-dimensional, cross-sectional "slice" or image of the body (Figure 2.9); abbreviated **CAT scan**
			diagnosis (dye ahg NOH siss)	the determination of the nature of a disease
endo-	p	within	**endoscopy** (ehn DOSS koh pee)	a diagnostic procedure involving a visual examination using an **endoscope**, which includes a camera, fiber optics, and a long flexible tube that can be inserted into the patient (Figure 2.8)
-scope	s	viewing instrument		
-y	s	process of		
eti/o	r/cv	cause	**etiology** (ee tee ALL oh jee)	study of the causes of disease
-logy	s	study of		

WORD PARTS (WHEN APPLICABLE)			TERM	DEFINITION
Part	Type	Meaning		
			examination	an evaluation made for the purpose of diagnosis by identifying physical evidence of disease, such as signs and symptoms
			magnetic resonance imaging (mag NETT ik REZ oh nenns)	a diagnostic scan that uses a powerful magnetic field generated within a chamber in which a patient lies; the field traces the element hydrogen in the patient's body, the results of which are the clearest, most complete computer-generated three-dimensional images of soft tissues that are currently possible; abbreviated **MRI** (Figure 2.11)
path/o -logist	r/cv s	disease one who studies	**pathologist** (path ALL oh jist)	one who studies disease
path/o -logy	r/cv s	disease study of	**pathology** (path ALL oh jee)	the study of disease
			positron emission tomography scan (PAHZ ih tron ee MISH uhn toh MOG rah fee)	a diagnostic scan that employs computers and radioactive substances to examine the metabolic activity of various parts of the body and create color-coded images; abbreviated **PET scan** (Figure 2.10)
			prognosis (prog NOH siss)	a forecast of the probable cause or outcome of a disease
			ultrasound (ULL trah sound)	a diagnostic procedure in which harmless sound waves are pulsated through body tissues ; the pulse echoes are converted into images of internal body structures by computer; also called **sonography** (Figure 2.12)

SELF QUIZ 2.5

SAY IT—SPELL IT!

Review terms related to the treatments of the human body by saying the phonetic pronunciation out loud, then writing the correct spelling of the term.

1. prog NOH siss   _____

2. dye ahg NOH siss   _____

3. ee tee ALL oh jee   _____

4. ULL trah sound   _____

5. path ALL oh jee   _____

6. ehn DOSS koh pee   _____

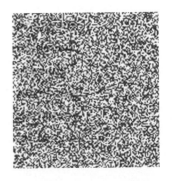

MATCH IT!

Match the term on the left with the correct definition on the right.

_____1. etiology

_____2. pathology

_____3. endoscopy

_____4. pathologist

_____5. prognosis

_____6. diagnosis

_____7. PET scan

_____8. CAT scan

_____9. MRI

a. a determination of the nature of a disease

b. one who studies disease

c. acronym for magnetic resonance imaging

d. study of the causes of disease

e. diagnostic imaging procedure that measures metabolic activity

f. the study of disease

g. forecast of the cause or outcome of a disease

h. diagnostic imaging that "slices" through the body without a knife

i. diagnostic procedure using a flexible probe and camera

BREAK IT DOWN!

Analyze and separate each term into its word parts by labeling each word part using p = prefix, r = root, cv = combining vowel, and s = suffix.

1. endoscopy   _____

2. etiology   _____

3. pathology   _____

4. pathologist   _____

WORD BUILDING

Construct or recall medical terms from the following meanings.

1. Prediction of the course of a disease   _____

2. Determination of the nature of a disease   _____

3. Acronym for computed axial tomography   _____

4. The study of disease   _____

5. Diagnostic use of sound waves   _____

6. Measures metabolic rate   _____

7. Study of the causes of disease   _____

FILL IT IN!

Fill in the blanks with the correct terms.

1. The study of the causes of disease is called _____. This term is composed of a word root and combining vowel, eti/o, which means *cause*, and the suffix -logy, which means _____.

2. A common goal of a physical examination is a _____.

3. A neurosurgeon has examined a patient and made a prediction of full recovery.

   The prediction is called a _____.

4. A diagnostic procedure that provides three-dimensional images of body regions

   with the use of high-powered magnets is called _____.

5. A diagnostic procedure that produces images on a computer screen that are similar

   to slices through the body is called _____ _____.

abbreviations of the human body

The abbreviations that are associated with introductory terms of the human body are
summarized here. Study these abbreviations, and review them in the exercise that
follows.

ABBREVIATION	DEFINITION	ABBREVIATION	DEFINITION
ant	anterior	MRI	magnetic resonance imaging
AP	anteroposterior	PA	posteroanterior
CAT scan	computed axial tomography scan	PET scan	positron emission tomography scan
inf	inferior	pos	posterior
lat	lateral	sup	superior
med	medial		

SELF QUIZ 2.6

Fill in the blanks with the abbreviation or the complete medical term.

Abbreviation	Medical Term
1. PET scan	_____
2. _____	computed axial tomography scan
3. MRI	_____
4. _____	anterior
5. pos	_____
6. _____	inferior
7. sup	_____
8. _____	medial
9. lat	_____
10. _____	anteroposterior
11. PA	_____

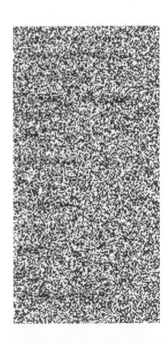

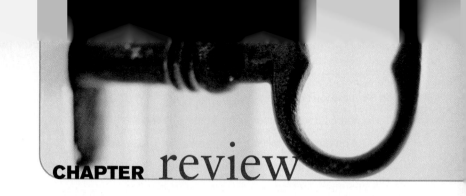

In this section, we will review all the word parts and medical terms from this chapter. As in earlier tables, the word roots are shown in **bold.**

Check each word part and medical term to be sure you understand the meaning. If any are not clear, please go back into the chapter and review that term. Then, complete the review exercises that follow.

[word parts **checklist**]

Prefixes

- ❏ ana-
- ❏ bi-
- ❏ epi-
- ❏ hypo-
- ❏ uni-

Word Roots/Combining Vowels

- ❏ **abdomin**/o
- ❏ **anter**/o
- ❏ **brach**/i
- ❏ **card**/i, **cardi**/o
- ❏ **caud**/o
- ❏ **cephal**/o
- ❏ **cervic**/o
- ❏ **chondr**/o
- ❏ **chron**/o
- ❏ **cran**/o, **crani**/o

- ❏ **dist**/o
- ❏ **dors**/o
- ❏ **eti**/o
- ❏ **femor**/o
- ❏ **gastr**/o
- ❏ **glut**/e
- ❏ **hom**/o, **home**/o
- ❏ **iatr**/o
- ❏ **idi**/o
- ❏ **ili**/o
- ❏ **infect**/o
- ❏ **infer**/o
- ❏ **inguin**/o
- ❏ **later**/o
- ❏ **lumb**/o
- ❏ **medi**/o
- ❏ **path**/o
- ❏ **pelv**/i

- ❏ **physi**/o
- ❏ **poster**/o
- ❏ **proxim**/o
- ❏ **spin**/o
- ❏ **stasis**
- ❏ **super**/o
- ❏ **thorac**/o
- ❏ **tom**/o
- ❏ **umbilic**/o
- ❏ **ventr**/o

Suffixes

- ❏ -ad
- ❏ -al
- ❏ -ar
- ❏ -ic
- ❏ -ior
- ❏ -y

[medical terminology **checklist**]

- ❏ **abdomin**al cavity
- ❏ **abdomin**al region
- ❏ **abdomin**o**pelv**ic cavity
- ❏ acute
- ❏ an**atom**ical position
- ❏ an**atom**y
- ❏ **anter**ior
- ❏ **anter**o**medi**al
- ❏ **anter**o**poster**ior
- ❏ appendage
- ❏ atom
- ❏ **brach**ial region
- ❏ **cardi**o**vascul**ar system
- ❏ **caud**al

- ❏ cell
- ❏ **cephal**ad
- ❏ **cephal**ic region
- ❏ **cervic**al region
- ❏ **chron**ic
- ❏ computed axial tomography (CAT scan)
- ❏ coronal plane
- ❏ **crani**ad
- ❏ **crani**al
- ❏ **crani**al cavity
- ❏ diagnosis
- ❏ diaphragm
- ❏ digestive system

- ❏ disease
- ❏ **dist**al
- ❏ **dors**al
- ❏ **dors**al cavity
- ❏ endocrine system
- ❏ endoscope
- ❏ endoscopy
- ❏ epi**gastr**ic region
- ❏ **eti**ology
- ❏ examination
- ❏ female reproductive system
- ❏ **femor**al region
- ❏ fever
- ❏ **front**al plane

❏ **glut**eal region
❏ **home**ostasis
❏ hypo**chondr**iac region
❏ hypo**gastr**ic region
❏ **iatrogen**ic
❏ **idiopath**ic
❏ **ili**ac region
❏ infection
❏ **infer**ior
❏ inflammation
❏ infra**chondr**al
❏ **inguin**al region
❏ integumentary system
❏ **later**al
❏ **lumb**ar region
❏ lymphatic system
❏ magnetic resonance imaging (MRI)
❏ male reproductive system
❏ **medi**al plane
❏ **medi**o**later**al
❏ midsagittal plane

❏ molecule
❏ muscular system
❏ nervous system
❏ organ
❏ organ systems
❏ organism
❏ pain
❏ parasagittal plane
❏ **path**ologist
❏ **path**ology
❏ **pelv**ic cavity
❏ **physi**ologist
❏ **physi**ology
❏ positron emission tomography (PET scan)
❏ **poster**ior
❏ **poster**o**anter**ior
❏ **poster**o**later**al
❏ prognosis
❏ **proxim**al
❏ respiratory system
❏ sagittal plane

❏ sensation
❏ sequelae
❏ sign
❏ skeletal system
❏ sonography
❏ **spin**al cavity
❏ **super**ior
❏ **super**o**later**al
❏ symptom
❏ **thorac**ic cavity
❏ **thorac**ic region
❏ tissue
❏ transverse plane
❏ trauma
❏ trunk
❏ ultrasound
❏ **umbilic**al region
❏ uni**later**al
❏ urinary system
❏ **ventr**al
❏ **ventr**al cavity
❏ viscera

[show what **you know!**]

BREAK IT DOWN!

Analyze and separate each term into its word parts by labeling each word part using p = prefix, r = root, cv = combining vowel, and s = suffix.

Example: 1.   anatomy   ana/tom/y

2.   physiology   _____

3.   cranial   _____

4.   unilateral   _____

5.   anteromedial   _____

6.   posterolateral   _____

7.   cephalic   _____

8.   abdominopelvic   _____

9.   epigastric   _____

10. hypochondriac   _____

11. homeostasis   _____

WORD BUILDING

Construct or recall medical terms from the following meanings.

Example:
1. the process of cutting   anatomy
2. toward the head   _____
3. away from a body part   _____
4. pertaining to two sides   _____
5. toward the middle   _____
6. a horizontal plane   _____
7. a vertical plane down the middle   _____
8. the cavity within the skull   _____
9. the chest cavity   _____
10. the cavity containing the stomach   _____
11. the arm region   _____
12. the belly region   _____
13. the region containing the navel   _____
14. to the front and to the back   _____

CASE STUDY

Fill in the blanks with the correct terms.

1. A patient was given a physical examination following complaints of headache and dizziness. The complaints were possible

   (a) _____ of a (b) _____ of the brain, located within the

   (c) _____ cavity. The examination revealed a physical (d) _____ in the form of a

   vascular leak. Additional complications arose when the patient added the symptom of nausea and pain in the belly, or

   (e) _____ region. A physical exam indicated the pain source was in the area to the right of the navel,

   or the (f) _____ _____ _____. The cause was not identifi-

   able, so the condition was described as (g) _____, but it was concluded that the abdominal pain was

   not associated with the earlier complaints. Clearly, the patient's ability to maintain internal stability, or

   (h) _____, had been lost. The patient was referred to a neurosurgeon, who described an exploratory

   operation that would cut through the (i) _____, or back side, of the skull to enter the

   (j) _____ _____. The connections between the brain and the

   (k) _____ _____ would not be disturbed by the operation. The operation would be

   followed up with visits to the clinic's (l) _____ department, which specializes in the treatment of disease.

[piece it all **together!**]

CROSSWORD

From the chapter material, fill in the crossword puzzle with answers to the following clues.

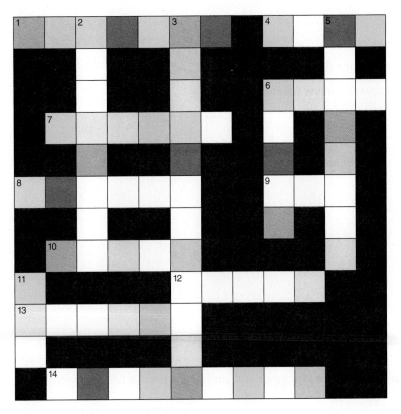

ACROSS

1. This term literally means the *process of cutting*. (Find puzzle piece 2.3)
4. The word root of *pertaining away from*. (Find puzzle piece 2.5)
6. Prefix that means *beneath*. (Find puzzle piece 2.1)
7. The most inferior of the major body cavities. (Find puzzle piece 2.9)
8. The body cavity that contains an organ attached to the brain. (Find puzzle piece 2.10)
9. The prefix that means *above* or *on top of*. (Find puzzle piece 2.12)
10. The definition of the opposite to posterior. (Find puzzle piece 2.2)
12. A midsagittal plane divides the body into right and left portions. (Find puzzle piece 2.8)
13. An abdominal region on both sides of the lower back. (Find puzzle piece 2.11)
14. The abdominal region that contains the navel. (Find puzzle piece 2.13)

DOWN

2. A term that means *front*. (Find puzzle piece 2.4)
3. The term meaning *pertaining to the middle and to the side*. (Find puzzle piece 2.7)
5. The head is located _____ to the neck. (Find puzzle piece 2.6)
6. The combining form that means *unchanging* or *sameness*. (Find puzzle piece 2.15)
11. The word root that means *flank* or *groin*. (Find puzzle piece 2.14)

WORD UNSCRAMBLE

From the completed crossword puzzle, unscramble:

1. All of the letters that appear in **green** squares

   ☐ _ _ _ ☐ _ _ _ _ _

   Clue: a disease that raises many questions

2. All of the letters that appear in **red** squares

   ☐ _ _ _ _ _ _

   Clue: a reported experience that aids in a diagnosis

3. All of the letters that appear in **yellow** squares

   _ _ _ _ _ ☐

   Clue: a term that means *back*

4. All of the letters that appear in **blue** squares

   ☐ ☐ ☐ _ _ _ ☐

   Clue: a term that means *belly*

5. All of the letters that appear in **pink** squares

   _ ☐ _ _ ☐ _ _

   Clue: pertaining to the thigh

6. All of the letters that appear in **peach** squares

   _ ☐ _ _ _

   Clue: definition of the anterior side

Now write down each of the letters that are boxed and unscramble them to find the hidden medical terms that complete the sentence:

_ _ _ _ _ _ and _ _ _ _ _ _ are visceral organs in the abdominal cavity.

MEDmedia wrap-up

www.prenhall.com/wingerd

Before you go on to the next chapter, take advantage of the free CD-ROM and study guide website that accompany this book. Simply load the CD-ROM for additional activities, games, animations, videos, and quizzes linked to this chapter. Then visit www.prenhall.com/wingerd for even more!

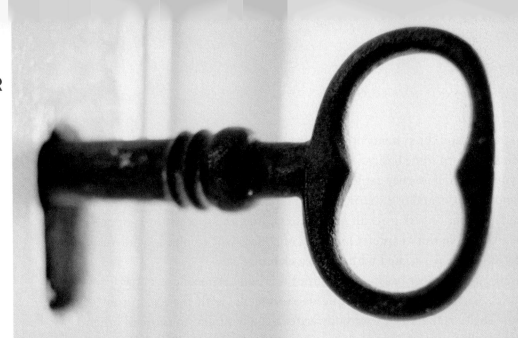

CHAPTER 3

Cells, Tissues, and Cancer

LEARNING OBJECTIVES

After completing this chapter, you will be able to:

- Define and spell the word parts used to create medical terms for cells, tissues, and cancer

- Identify the organs of cells, tissues, and cancer and describe their structure and function

- Define common medical terms used for cells, tissues, and cancer

- Break down and define common medical terms used for symptoms, diseases, disorders, procedures, treatments, and devices for cells, tissues, and cancer

MEDmedia

www.prenhall.com/wingerd

Enhance your study with the power of multimedia! Each chapter of this book links to activities, games, animations, videos, and quizzes that you'll find on your CD-ROM. Plus, you can click on www.prenhall.com/wingerd, to find a free chapter-specific companion website that's loaded with additional practice and resources.

 CD-ROM

- Audio Glossary
- Exercises & Activities
- Flashcard Generator
- Animations
- Videos

 Companion Website

- Exercises & Activities
- Audio Glossary
- Drug Updates
- Current News Updates

A secure distance learning course is available at www.prenhall.com/onekey.

To understand the systems of the body and their medical terminology, we must explore some basic concepts of the human body. This chapter will take you on a brief journey exploring these concepts, which include cell structure and function, and tissue structure and function. Because cancer is caused by mutations in cells that result in diseased tissue, the special topic of cancer is included in this chapter. Our study of cancer will emphasize the medical terminology associated with this dreaded disease.

Cells are the most basic living unit of the body. Amazingly, every form of life on earth is composed of one or more cells, with the exception of viruses. The cells that form your body are extremely similar to those of other humans, and even to those of other animals. The study of cells is called *cytology*. This is a constructed word that can be shown as:

cyt/o/logy

The word root cyt means *cell,* and as you have learned earlier, the suffix -logy means *study of.* One who studies cytology is called a cytologist. In this word, the suffix is changed from -logy to -logist, which means *one who studies.*

Tissue is composed of cells. It is defined as a combination of similar cells that share a common goal, such as providing movement, protection, or secretion. The word *tissue* is a term that comes from the French word *tissu,* which means *woven.* Early scientists used this term because, under the microscope, it appeared that similar cells were "woven" together to form interconnected groups, much like textiles were woven together to form clothing. They also used the Greek term for textile or loom, *histos,* by calling the study of tissues *histology.* Similarly, one who studies tissues is called a *histologist.*

[FYI]

Cell
The word *cell* was first used in the 16th century by Robert Hooke when he observed plant cork under his newly invented microscope. The cork caverns reminded him of rooms used by monks, which were called cells at the time.

word parts focus

PREFIX	DEFINITION	PREFIX	DEFINITION
ana-	up, toward, apart	hyper-	excessive, above normal
dys-	bad, abnormal	meta-	after, change
epi-	upon	neo-	new

WORD ROOT	DEFINITION	WORD ROOT	DEFINITION
aden	gland	melan	darkness of color, black
carcin	cancer	my	muscle
chrom	color	neur	nerve, nervous system
cyt	cell	nucl, nucle	kernel, nucleus
fibr	fiber	onc	tumor
gen, gene	formation, cause, produce	organ	tool
hist	tissue	oste	bone
lei	smooth	rhabd	rod, rod-shaped
lip	lipid, fat	sarc	flesh, muscle
mal	bad	thel	nipple

SUFFIX	DEFINITION	SUFFIX	DEFINITION
-al	pertaining to	-osis	process or condition that is usually abnormal
-elle	small		
-gen	formation, cause, produce	-plasia	a shape, formation (may also be used as a word root)
-genesis	origin, cause		
-genic	pertaining to formation, causing, producing	-plasm	something shaped (may also be used as a word root)
-ic	pertaining to	-sis	state of
-logy	study of	-some	body
-logist	one who studies	-stasis	standing still (may also be used as a word root)
-oid	resemblance to		
-oma	abnormal swelling, tumor	-um	pertaining to

[FYI]

Constructed Suffixes

Some suffixes are actually constructed from multiple word parts themselves. In the case of the suffixes -genesis and -genic, the suffixes actually consist of the word root, *gen* and *gene;* the suffixes -sis, which means state of, and -ic, which means pertaining to. Over time the usage of these combinations has spurred their evolution into suffixes unto themselves.

SELF QUIZ 3.1

Review the word parts of cells, tissues, and cancer terminology by working carefully through the exercises that follow. Soon, we will apply this new information to build medical terms.

Success Hint: Once you get to the crossword puzzle at the end of the chapter, remember to check back here for clues! Your clues are indicated by the puzzle icon.

A. Provide the prefix or suffix for the following definitions.

1. new   _____

2. upon   _____

3. abnormal process or
   condition   _____

4. state of   _____

5. bad, abnormal   _____

6. origin, cause   _____

3.1   7. standing still   _____

8. shape, formation   _____

9. abnormal swelling   _____

10. body   _____

11. pertaining to   _____

B. Provide the word root for each of the following terms.

1. lipid, fat   _____

2. cancer   _____

3.2   3. flesh, muscle   _____

4. fiber   _____

5. dark, black   _____

6. nerve   _____

7. smooth   _____

3.3   8. tumor   _____

9. rod or rod-shaped   _____

10. muscle   _____

11. nipple   _____

12. tissue   _____

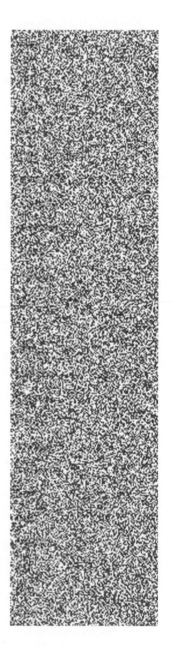

[anatomy and physiology overview]

The structural organization of the human body is much like that of a building: Both are composed of small, simple particles that are combined to form larger, more complex parts (see Figure 2.1 in Chapter 2). The larger parts are then organized to form a structure that is capable of functioning as a whole, living organism. In the body, cells are the most basic living building block. They are assembled to build the more complex structures, such as tissues, organs, and systems.

Cells

As discussed in Chapter 2, cells are composed of atoms and molecules. These non-living particles combine in an organized manner to form the various parts of a cell. Cells are divided into three general parts: **cell membrane, cytoplasm,** and **nucleus.** These structures are shown in Figure 3.1 ⬚⬚⬚.

The cell membrane is the outer boundary of the cell. It is composed mostly of protein and lipids (fats). The cell membrane regulates the movement of materials in and out of the cell.

The cytoplasm forms the main substance of the cell. It consists of a thick fluid that contains functional packets known as **organelles.** The organelles perform most cell functions, including the construction of molecules, the release of energy, and the storage of energy.

The nucleus is the part of the cell that contains the genetic material called **DNA.** DNA is the universal acronym for the chemical term *deoxyribonucleic acid.* DNA is a very large molecule that contains more than 30,000 **genes,** units which contain hereditary information. During cell division, each molecule of DNA becomes packed

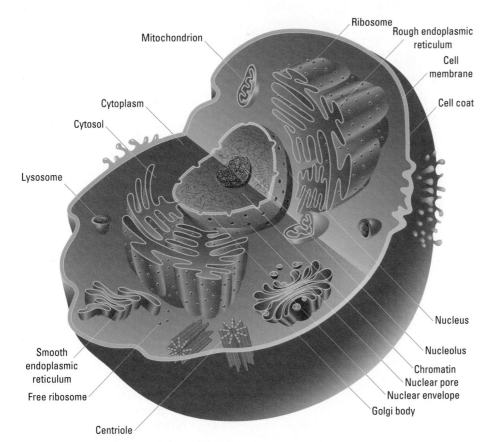

Figure 3.1 ⬚⬚⬚

The parts of a cell.
Mitochondrion, ribosomes, endoplastic reticulum, and centrioles are organelles of a cell.

Labels on figure:
Mitochondrion
Ribosome
Rough endoplasmic reticulum
Cell membrane
Cell coat
Cytoplasm
Cytosol
Lysosome
Nucleus
Nucleolus
Chromatin
Nuclear pore
Nuclear envelope
Golgi body
Smooth endoplasmic reticulum
Free ribosome
Centriole

into a structure that usually bears an X-shape, called a **chromosome**. The nuclei of all human cells each contain 46 chromosomes, except mature sex cells, which contain 23 chromosomes.

Tissues

A tissue is a group of similar cells that form a particular function, such as providing movement, protecting other parts of the body, or secreting substances. Since about 1860, scientists have categorized all known tissues into four main types. The four general types of tissues are **epithelial tissue, connective tissue, muscle tissue,** and **nervous tissue.**

Epithelial tissue consists of cells that are arranged closely together (Figure 3.2::::). It is also known as **epithelium.** The cells of epithelial tissue may be flat, cube-shaped, or columnar, and may form a single layer to create a thin barrier, or multiple layers to establish a thick, protective barrier. Most epithelial tissues cover body surfaces and line body cavities, forming a protective sheet over other tissues. Some epithelial cells specialize in releasing a substance they produce. This process is called **secretion.** Secretory cells are often supported by other cells, forming structures known as **glands.**

Connective tissue consists of widely scattered cells that are surrounded by extracellular material (Figure 3.3::::). The term *connective* describes the tissue's general function. In addition to forming a connection between organs, the tissue provides support for softer parts of the body and protects them from physical in-

[**FYI**]

Epithelial Tissue
The term *epithelial* was first used by the Greek father of medicine, Aristotle, to describe the skin around the nipples.

[**thinking critically!**]

How would you distinguish epithelial tissue from connective tissue when viewing them under a microscope?

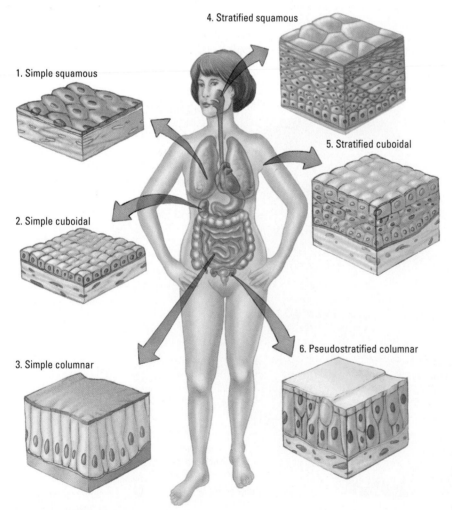

1. Simple squamous
2. Simple cuboidal
3. Simple columnar
4. Stratified squamous
5. Stratified cuboidal
6. Pseudostratified columnar

Figure 3.2 ::::

Epithelial tissues. Notice that each type of epithelium consists of tightly packed cells.

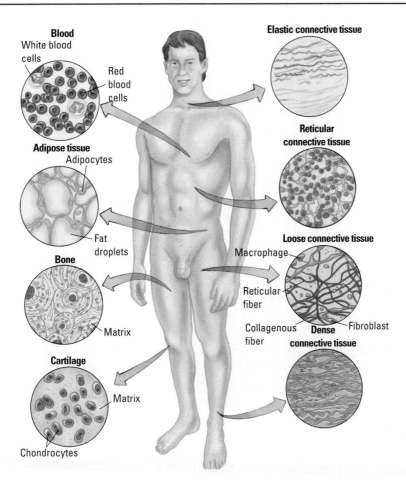

Figure 3.3 ::::

Connective tissues. Each type of connective tissue consists of widely scattered cells that produce their own surroundings.

jury. The abundant extracellular material in connective tissue consists of protein fibers and a fluid that is thickened with carbohydrate molecules. The protein fibers and carbohydrate molecules are secreted by connective tissue cells. Connective tissue forms the bones, joints, and material between other organs. In addition to bone and cartilage, connective tissue includes fat and blood.

Muscle tissue consists of cells that are specialized to contract (Figure 3.4::::). When muscle cells become smaller by contracting, they produce movement. There are three types of muscle tissue: **skeletal muscle, smooth muscle,** and **cardiac muscle.** Skeletal muscle tissue forms the muscles attached to bones. Its contraction produces the movements of the arms, legs, head, and other moving parts. Skeletal muscle also generates heat, which warms your body when it is cold outside. Smooth muscle is located in the walls of hollow organs, such as the stomach, small intestine, and blood vessels. Its contraction propels material through the hollow organs. Smooth muscle is named after its smooth appearance under a microscope. Cardiac muscle forms the wall of the heart, and produces the heart's contractions that keep blood flowing.

Nervous tissue consists of specialized cells called **neurons,** which carry information in the form of electrochemical impulses (Figure 3.5::::). Together with supportive cells called **neuroglial cells,** they form the brain, spinal cord, and nerves.

[FYI]

Muscle
The term *muscle* was coined by the ancient Romans, who observed the similarity between the contracting muscles beneath the skin and little mice. Flex and relax your biceps to find your "little mice."

[FYI]

Nerves
The term *nerve* is a vocabulary word from the Latin word *nervus,* which means *sinew or cord.* The term *neuron* also means *sinew or cord,* but comes from the Greek language. During a surgery, nerves look like thin white strings or cords.

[thinking critically!]

What specialized function distinguishes muscle tissue from all other tissues?

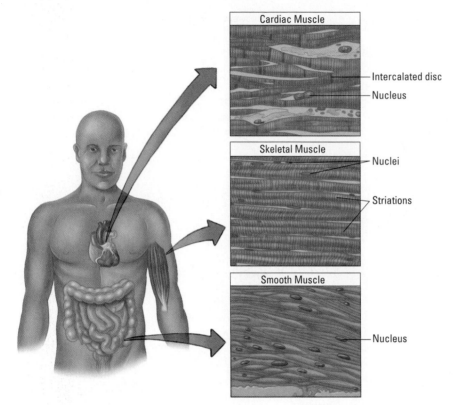

Figure 3.4 :::: **Muscle tissue.**

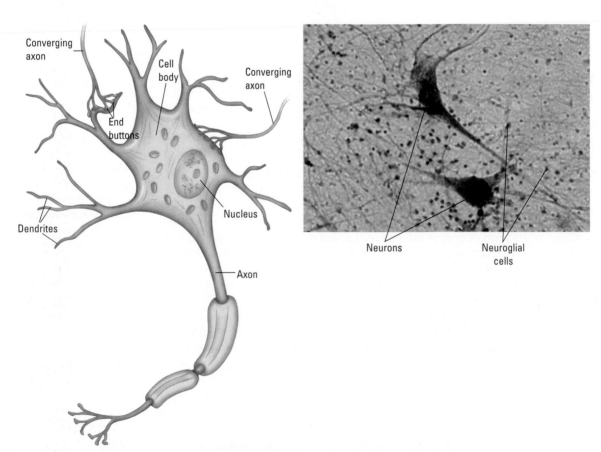

Figure 3.5 :::: **Nervous tissue.** The image on the left is a photograph of nervous tissue taken through a microscope.

getting to the root of it | anatomy and physiology terms

Many of the anatomy and physiology terms are formed from roots that are used to construct the more complex medical terms of cells, tissues, and cancer, including symptoms, diseases, and treatments. In this section, we will review the terms that describe the structure and function of cells and tissues *in relation to their word roots,* which are shown in **bold.**

Study the word roots and terms in this list and complete the review exercises that follow.

Word Root (Meaning)	Terms Formed from the Word Root (Pronunciation)	Definition
chrom (color)	**chrom**osome (KROH moh sohm)	an X-shaped structure in a cell's nucleus that bears DNA; all human cells contain 46 chromosomes, except mature sex cells, which contain 23
cyt (cell)	**cyt**oplasm (SIGH toh plazm)	a thick fluid that contains organelles and forms the main substance of the cell
neur (nerve)	**neur**oglial cells (noo ROH glee all)	supportive cells within nervous tissue
	neuron (NOO ron)	a specialized cell of nervous tissue
nucl, nucle (kernel, nucleus)	**nucle**us (NOO klee uss)	the part of the cell that contains DNA
organ (tool)	**organ** (OR gahn)	a structure made of two or more different types of tissue that performs a general function in the body
	organelle (OR gahn ell)	small structures within the cytoplasm that perform most cell functions, such as the construction of molecules and the release and storage of energy
	organism (OR gahn izm)	the complete human body that is capable of survival
thel (nipple)	epi**thel**ial tissue (ep ih THEE lee al)	tissue consisting of closely arranged cells that are flat, cube-shaped, or columnar
	epi**thel**ium (ep ih THEE lee umm)	tissue consisting of closely arranged cells that are flat, cube-shaped, or columnar

OTHER IMPORTANT TERMS
The terms in this table are related to the structure and function of cells and tissues, but are not built from word roots that are presented in this chapter.

cardiac muscle (KAR dee ak)	muscle tissue that forms the wall of the heart and pushes blood through the circulatory system
cell membrane	the outer boundary of the cell, composed of mostly protein and lipids (fats), which regulates the movement of materials in and out of the cell
cell	the most basic living unit

connective tissue	tissue consisting of widely scattered cells surrounded by extracellular material rich in protein fibers and fluid that connects, supports, and protects; it is found in bones, joints, and in between organs
DNA	the universal acronym for deoxyribonucleic acid
genes	components of DNA that carry hereditary information
gland	a structure made of one or more cells with the primary function of secretion
muscle tissue	tissue consisting of cells that are specialized to contract
nervous tissue	tissue consisting of cells that are specialized to carry information in the form of electrochemical impulses
skeletal muscle (SKELL eh tal)	muscle tissue that connects to bones and whose contraction causes bones to move
smooth muscle	muscle tissue within the walls of hollow organs whose contractions propel materials through them
tissue (TISH oo)	a group of similar cells that share a common goal or function

SELF QUIZ 3.2

SAY IT—SPELL IT!

Review the terms of cells and tissues by speaking the phonetic pronunciation guides out loud, then writing in the correct spelling of the term.

Success Hint: Use the audio glossary on the CD and CW for additional help with pronunciation of these terms.

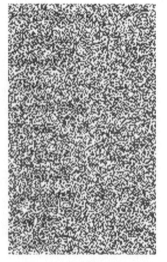

1. KROH moh sohm   _____

2. SIGH toh plazm   _____

3. ep ih THEE lee al   _____

4. TISH oo   _____

5. ep ih THEE lee umm   _____

6. OR gahn   _____

7. OR gahn ell   _____

8. OR gah nizm   _____

9. noo ROH glee all   _____

10. NOO ron   _____

11. NOO klee uss   _____

MATCH IT!

Match the term on the left with the correct definition on the right.

_____1. tissue   a. the most basic unit of life

_____2. cells   b. the whole, functional being

_____3. atoms and molecules   c. nonliving particles

_____4. organism   d. a combination of similar cells

_____5. cytologist   e. means *kernel*

_____6. cell membrane   f. means *colored body*

_____7. the most basic living unit   g. functional packets in a cell

_____8. organelles   h. cell

_____9. muscle   i. carry hereditary information

_____10. nucleus   j. one who studies cells

_____11. chromosome   k. outer boundary of a cell

_____12. gene   l. tissue consisting of specialized cells that contract

BREAK IT DOWN!

Analyze and separate each term into its word parts by labeling each word part using p = prefix, r = root, cv = combining vowel, and s = suffix.

Constructed Word   **Word Construction**

1. cytoplasm   _____

3.4   2. organelle   _____

3. chromosome   _____

4. epithelium   _____

5. organism   _____

WORD BUILDING

Construct or recall medical terms from the following meanings.

3.5   1. cell's outer boundary   _____

2. part of the cell containing DNA   _____

3. acronym for deoxyribonucleic acid   _____

4. contain the hereditary information   _____

5. group of similar cells   _____

6. tissue that connects and supports   _____

3.6   7. muscle that moves bones   _____

8. tissue specialized to carry information   _____

9. main cell of nervous tissue   _____

10. tissue with cells close together   _____

11. cardiac muscle   _____

12. supportive cells of nervous tissue   _____

FILL IT IN!

Fill in the blanks with the correct terms.

1. The simplest building block level in the human body includes nonliving particles known as _____ and _____.

3.7 2. The most basic unit of life is the _____. When a group of similar cells is combined to perform a common goal, it is called _____.

3. The smallest living unit that forms the brain is called a _____.

3.8 4. The three parts of a cell are the cell membrane, the _____, and the nucleus.

5. The Greek word that means *a thing formed* is _____.

6. The cell membrane is the outer _____ of a cell. It serves to _____ the movement of materials in and out of the cell.

7. The term *organelle* literally means _____.

8. The parts of a cell that perform many of its functions, such as construction of molecules and release of energy, are called _____.

9. The _____, or kernel of a cell contains the genetic material.

10. The acronym for the molecule composed of many genes is

3.9   _____.

11. The word root in the term chromosome means _____, and the suffix means _____.

3.10 12. A _____ is a group of similar cells that combine to perform a common function. One who studies tissues is called a _____.

13. The type of tissue that consists of cells arranged closely together is

3.11   _____. It includes cells that are specialized in the release of products, or _____, and which form _____.

14. A tissue that consists of widely scattered cells that are surrounded by proteins and a thickened fluid is _____ tissue. The three functions of this tissue are connecting organs together, _____, and protection.

15. A tissue that is named after the Latin word for *little mouse* is _____ tissue. Its cells are specialized to produce movement by _____.

16. The type of _____ tissue that moves bones to produce body movement is called _____ muscle. The tissue that contracts to move swallowed food through the stomach is _____ muscle. The tissue that contracts to move blood through the heart and the body is _____ muscle.

17. A combination of similar cells specialized to carry information through the body by way of electrochemical impulses is known as _____ _____. It includes specialized cells called _____ and supportive cells known as _____ cells.

3.12

[medical terms of

[cells, tissue, and cancer]

Cancer is one of the most life-threatening diseases of adults in our time. According to the American Cancer Society, it is the cause for nearly 40 percent of all deaths annually in the United States. Cancer is characterized by an abnormal growth of cells. The disease begins when the DNA within a cell undergoes a change, or **mutation,** that results in the loss of regulated cell division (Figure 3.6a::::). The mutated cell may then undergo a physical change, known as **dysplasia.** In some cases, the changed cell may take on a more permanent physical change, known as **anaplasia,** in many cases forming a cluster of nonfunctional cells called a **tumor** or **neoplasm.** The development of a tumor is shown in Figure 3.6. If the cells grow slowly into a mass without spreading to other body tissues, the tumor is usually not life-threatening and is called **benign.** The word *benign* means *quiet, peaceful.* (Notice that the *g* is silent, as in the word *sign.*) If, on the hand, the tumor cells grow quickly and spread, the tumor is **malignant** and the condition of cancer can be diagnosed. The word *malignant* is derived from the Latin word root *mal,* which means *bad.* Cells spread from a malignant tumor along blood and lymphatic pathways during the process called **metastasis,** which leads to the establishment of secondary tumors in other areas of the body.

The study of cancer is the constructed word **oncology.** It can be written as:

onc/o/logy

where onc is a word root that means *tumor* and -logy, as you should recall, is the suffix that means *study of.* A physician who specializes in the treatment of this deadly disease is an **oncologist.** An oncology ward is the area of a hospital where cancer patients receive treatment.

Cancers may arise from epithelial tissue, connective tissue, muscle tissue, or even nervous tissue. They are named primarily from the tissue of origin. A cancer type may also be named by color characteristics or certain other distinguishing features.

The constructed terms of cancer are formed from the word parts listed at the beginning of this chapter, and are assembled according to some basic rules. As a general rule, benign tumors that arise from connective tissue or muscle tissue are usually named by adding the suffix -oma. Malignant tumors (cancers) of connective or muscle tissue origin are often named by adding the term sarcoma because sarcomas are almost always malignant. For example, a **myoma** is a benign tumor of muscle, whereas a **myosarcoma** is a malignant tumor of muscle. A **lipoma** is a benign tumor of fat, while a **liposarcoma** is a malignant tumor of fat. For tumors that arise from epithelial and nervous tissue, the suffix -oma is used to describe both benign and malignant tumors. The use of the word root *carcin,* however, indicates the tumor is malignant. Thus, a **neuroma** is a tumor of nervous tissue, but it might be benign or malignant. However, a **neurocarcinoma** is a *malignant* tumor, or cancer, of nervous tissue.

[FYI]

Cancer
The term *cancer* literally means *crab* in Latin. It was first named by the ancient Romans, whose surgeons tried to remove certain tumors. The tumor shapes reminded these early surgeons of shore crabs.

[thinking critically!]

How is a malignant tumor, or cancer, different from a benign tumor?

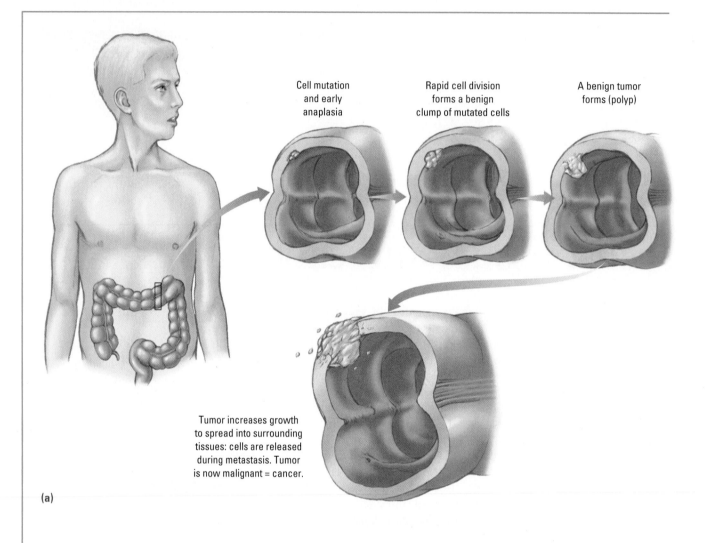

Cell mutation
and early
anaplasia

Rapid cell division
forms a benign
clump of mutated cells

A benign tumor
forms (polyp)

Tumor increases growth
to spread into surrounding
tissues: cells are released
during metastasis. Tumor
is now malignant = cancer.

(a)

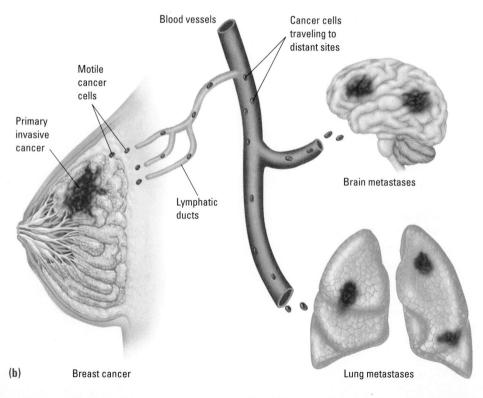

Blood vessels

Cancer cells
traveling to
distant sites

Motile
cancer
cells

Primary
invasive
cancer

Brain metastases

Lymphatic
ducts

(b)   Breast cancer

Lung metastases

Figure 3.6 ::::

Development of cancer.
(a) Cancer of the large intestine,
or colorectal cancer, arises from
mutations that cause a normal
cell to become dysplasic, then
anaplasic, forming a tumor.
(b) Metastasis. A primary tumor
may shed mutated cells to other
organs during metastasis, which
are carried by blood and lymphatic
vessels.

let's construct terms!

In this section, we will assemble all of the word parts to construct medical terminology related to cells, tissues, and cancer. Abbreviations are used to indicate each word part: **p** = prefix, **r** = root, **cv** = combining vowel, and **s** = suffix. Note that some terms are not constructed from word parts, but they are included here to expand your vocabulary.

The medical terms of cells, tissues, and cancer are listed in the following three sections:

- Symptoms and Signs
- Diseases and Disorders
- Treatments, Procedures, and Devices

Each section is followed by review exercises. Study the lists in these tables and complete the review exercises that follow.

Symptoms and Signs

WORD PARTS (WHEN APPLICABLE)			TERM	DEFINITION
Part	Type	Meaning		
ana- plasia	p r	up, toward, apart shape, formation	**anaplasia** (an ah PLAY zee ah)	a loss of structural organization in a tissue that is permanent
dys- plasia	p r	bad, abnormal shape, formation	**dysplasia** (diss PLAY zee ah)	abnormal tissue development
hyper- plasia	p r	excessive shape, formation	**hyperplasia** (high per PLAY zee ah)	an increase in the number of cells in a tissue, other than by tumor development
meta- stasis	p r	after, change standing still	**metastasis** (meh TASS tah siss)	the spreading of cancer cells from the primary tumor
			remission (ree MISH unn)	improvement or absence of signs of disease

---

SELF QUIZ 3.3

SAY IT—SPELL IT!

Review the terms of cells and tissues by speaking the phonetic pronunciation guides out loud, then writing in the correct spelling of the term.

1. an ah PLAY zee ah   _____

2. diss PLAY zee ah   _____

3. high per PLAY zee ah   _____

4. meh TASS tah siss   _____

5. ree MISH unn   _____

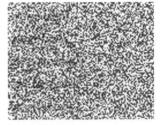

MATCH IT!

Match the term on the left with the correct definition on the right.

_____1. anaplasia

a. an increase in the number of cells in a tissue, other than by tumor development

_____2. dysplasia

b. improvement or absence of signs of disease

_____3. hyperplasia

c. a loss of structural organization in a tissue

_____4. metastasis

d. abnormal tissue development

_____5. remission

e. the spreading of cancer cells from the primary tumor

BREAK IT DOWN!

Analyze and separate each term into its word parts by labeling each word part using p = prefix, r = root, cv = combining vowel, and s = suffix.

1. dysplasia   _____

2. anaplasia   _____

3. hyperplasia   _____

4. metastasis   _____

WORD BUILDING

Construct or recall medical terms from the following meanings.

1. improvement or absence of signs of disease   _____

2. the spreading of cancer cells from the primary tumor   _____

3. abnormal tissue development   _____

4. loss of tissue organization   _____

5. increase in the number of cells within a tissue   _____

FILL IT IN!

Fill in the blanks with the correct terms.

1. A change in the DNA of a cell is called a _____. A mutated cell may undergo an abnormal physical change, called _____. A permanent physical change is known as _____. In some cases, the permanently changed cells form a cluster of abnormal cells known as a tumor, or neoplasm.

2. The spreading of cancer cells from the primary tumor is a process known as

_____.

3. Successful treatment of cancer results in the death of cancer cells and a cessation of metastasis. This treatment goal is known as _____.

Diseases and Disorders

WORD PARTS (WHEN APPLICABLE)			TERM	DEFINITION
Part	Type	Meaning		
aden/o	r/cv	gland	**adenocarcinoma** (ADD eh noh kar sih NOH mah)	a malignant tumor of glandular epithelial tissue; abbreviated **Adeno-Ca**
carcin	r	cancer		
-oma	s	tumor		
aden	r	gland	**adenoma** (add eh NOH mah)	a benign tumor of glandular epithelial tissue
-oma	s	tumor		
			benign (bee NINE)	adjective describing a noninvasive, slow growing tumor; nonmalignant
			cancer in situ (KANN ser in SIH tyoo)	cancer in the early stages prior to metastasis (*in situ* generally means *confined to a place of origin*)
			cancer (KANN ser)	a disease characterized by the aggressive, unregulated growth of abnormal cells and their spreading to other tissues
carcin	r	cancer	**carcinoma** (kar sih NOH mah)	a cancer, or malignant tumor
-oma	s	tumor		
carcin/o	r/cv	cancer	**carcinogen** (kar SIN oh jenn)	a substance that causes cancer
-gen	s	formation, cause, producer		
epi-	p	upon	**epithelioma** (ep ih THEE lee OH mah)	a tumor that originates from epithelium, usually from the skin
thel/i	r/cv	nipple		
-oma	s	tumor		
fibr	r	fiber	**fibroma** (fye BROH mah)	a benign tumor of fibrous connective tissue
-oma	s	tumor		
fibr/o	r/cv	fiber	**fibrosarcoma** (FYE broh sahr KOH mah)	a malignant tumor originating from fibrous connective tissue
sarc	r	flesh, muscle		
-oma	s	tumor		
lei/o	r/cv	smooth	**leiomyoma** (LYE oh my OH mah)	a benign tumor of smooth muscle
my	r	muscle		
-oma	s	tumor		
lei/o	r/cv	smooth	**leiomyosarcoma** (LYE oh my OH sahr KOH mah)	a carcinoma that originates from smooth muscle
my/o	r/cv	muscle		
sarc	r	flesh, muscle		
-oma	s	tumor		
lip	r	fat, lipid	**lipoma** (lip OH mah)	a benign tumor of fat tissue
-oma	s	tumor		
lymph	r	clear water or fluid, lymphatic	**lymphoma** (limm FOH mah)	a malignant solid tumor of lymphoid tissue
-oma	s	tumor		
			malignant (mah LIG nant)	an adjective describing an aggressive, life-threatening, invasive tumor

WORD PARTS (WHEN APPLICABLE)			TERM	DEFINITION
Part	Type	Meaning		
melan	r	dark, black	**melanoma**	a cancer that bears a dark pigment, usually arising
-oma	s	tumor	(mell ah NOH mah)	from pigment-producing cells of the skin
my	r	muscle	**myoma**	a benign tumor of muscle tissue
-oma	s	tumor	(my OH mah)	
neo	p	new	**neoplasm**	a new growth of abnormal cells; a tumor
plasm	r	something shaped	(NEE oh plazm)	
neur	r	nerve	**neuroma**	a tumor that originates from nervous tissue
-oma	s	tumor	(noo ROH mah)	
onc/o	r/cv	tumor	**oncogenic**	adjective meaning causing tumors
-genic	s	pertaining to formation, causing, producing	(ong koh JENN ik)	
oste/o	r/cv	bone	**osteosarcoma**	a malignant cancer of bone
sarc	r	flesh, muscle	(OSS tee oh sahr	
-oma	s	tumor	KOH mah)	
rhabd/o	r/cv	rod, rod-shape	**rhabdomyoma**	a benign tumor that originates from skeletal muscle,
my	r	muscle	(RABB doh my OH mah)	which consists of rod-shaped cells
-oma	s	tumor		
rhabd/o	r/cv	rod, rod-shape	**rhabdomyosarcoma**	a malignant tumor that originates from skeletal
my/o	r/cv	muscle	(RABB doh my OH	muscle, which consists of rod-shaped cells
sarc	r	flesh, muscle	sahr KOH mah)	
-oma	s	tumor		
sarc	r	flesh, muscle	**sarcoma**	a tumor arising from connective tissue that is almost
-oma	s	tumor	(sahr KOH mah)	always malignant

disease focus | The Genetics of Cancer

According to the American Cancer Society, cancer kills more than 500,000 Americans each year, making it one of the two leading causes of death among adults in the United States (the other leading cause is heart disease). Cancer is a dynamic process that is caused by mutations to DNA (Figure 3.6). A mutation changes the sequence of the building blocks of DNA in a cell, which leads to serious genetic changes in the normal cell cycle. During the past two decades, researchers have identified several different genetic mechanisms that produce cancer. There are two gene types that we will focus on here: oncogenes and suppressor genes.

Oncogenes

Oncogenes are mutated genes that cause the reproduction of mutated cells. Oncogenes can result from exposure to certain substances that cause DNA damage.

These substances are called carcinogens, and they include:

- Environmental sources of radiation like ultraviolet light and x-rays
- Chemicals such as benzene and formaldehyde
- Several types of viruses

When some oncogenes cause overproduction of cell growth factors, the result is uncontrolled growth and division among the cells that produce them. Cancers called **sarcomas** and **gliomas** often originate in this manner.

Suppressor Genes

In addition to stimulating cell growth and division, a mutation may also lead to the loss of mechanisms controlling cell growth that are present in normal cells. In all healthy cells, genes are present in the DNA that slow or stop cell growth and division. These genes are called *suppressor genes*. When suppressor genes receive a mutation, the machinery that normally guides the cell slowly through the cell cycle is lost, resulting in uncontrolled growth. As the abnormal cell grows and divides without control, individual cells that carry the mutation may leave the colony and enter the bloodstream or lymph flow. In this situation, the abnormal cells may travel to other sites in the body, where they create new cancer sites. This process is called metastasis (see Figure 3.6). Cancers resulting from mutations of suppressor genes include **melanoma** and many types of **neoplasms** arising from visceral organs.

SELF QUIZ 3.4

SAY IT—SPELL IT!

Review the terms of cancer by speaking the phonetic pronunciation guides out loud, then writing in the correct spelling of the term.

1. ADD eh noh kar sih NOH mah _____
2. add eh NOH mah _____
3. kar sih NOH mah _____
4. kar SIN oh jenn _____
5. ep ih THEE lee OH mah _____
6. fye BROH mah _____
7. FYE broh sahr KOH mah _____
8. LYE oh my OH mah _____
9. LYE oh my OH sahr KOH mah _____
10. lip OH mah _____
11. limm FOH mah _____
12. mell ah NOH mah _____
13. my OH ma _____
14. NEE oh plazm _____
15. noo ROH mah _____
16. ong koh JENN ik _____
17. OSS tee oh sahr KOH mah _____
18. RABB doh my OH mah _____
19. RABB doh my OH sahr KOH mah _____
20. sahr KOH mah _____
21. bee NINE _____
22. KANN ser _____
23. KANN ser in SIH tyoo _____
24. mah LIG nant _____

MATCH IT!

Match the term on the left with the correct definition on the right.

_____ 1. malignant tumor   a. disease characterized by a malignant tumor

_____ 2. benign tumor   b. cancer in early stages prior to metastasis

_____ 3. cancer in situ   c. a noninvasive, slow growing tumor

_____ 4. cancer   d. a life threatening, invasive tumor

_____ 5. neoplasm   e. a cancer that bears a dark pigment, usually of the skin

_____ 6. lipoma   f. adjective meaning causing tumors

_____ 7. lymphoma   g. a benign tumor of muscle tissue

_____ 8. melanoma   h. a benign tumor that originated from skeletal muscle

_____ 9. myoma   i. a malignant cancer of bone

_____ 10. neuroma   j. a new growth of abnormal cells; a tumor

_____ 11. oncogenic   k. a tumor that originated from nervous tissue

_____ 12. osteosarcoma   l. a benign tumor of fat tissue

_____ 13. rhabdomyoma   m. a malignant solid tumor of lymphoid tissue

BREAK IT DOWN!

Analyze and separate each term into its word parts by labeling each word part using p = prefix, r = root, cv = combining vowel, and s = suffix.

Constructed Word	Word Construction
1. fibroma	_____
2. carcinoma	_____
3. carcinogen	_____
4. epithelioma	_____
3.13 5. fibrosarcoma	_____
6. leiomyoma	_____
3.14 7. lipoma	_____
8. melanoma	_____
9. leiomyosarcoma	_____
10. myoma	_____
3.15 11. neoplasm	_____

3.16 12. neuroma _____

13. oncogenic _____

14. rhabdomyoma _____

15. rhabdomyosarcoma _____

16. sarcoma _____

WORD BUILDING

Construct or recall medical terms from the following meanings.

1. a tumor arising from nervous tissue _____

2. a tumor arising from connective tissue
   that is almost always malignant _____

3. a malignant tumor of fat _____

4. a benign tumor originating from
   skeletal muscle _____

5. a noninvasive, slow growing tumor _____

6. cancer in the early stages prior to
   metastasis _____

7. a cancer originating from fibrous
   connective tissue _____

8. a substance that causes cancer _____

9. a tumor originating from epithelial
   tissue _____

FILL IT IN!

Fill in the blanks with the correct terms.

1. If a tumor grows relatively slowly and does not spread to other parts of the body,
   the tumor is _____. However, a tumor that grows rapidly and
   infiltrates other parts of the body is a _____ tumor. In this
   aggressive form, the cells spread through blood and lymphatic pathways in the
   process known as metastasis.

2. A tumor that arises from connective tissue is known as a _____,
   whereas a tumor arising from epithelial tissue is called an _____.

3. A rhabdosarcoma is a cancer that originates from _____
   _____ tissue.

4. A tumor that arises from nervous tissue is termed a _____.

5. A liposarcoma is a malignant tumor of _____, while a
   _____ is a fat tumor that is not malignant.

Treatments, Procedures, and Devices

WORD PARTS (WHEN APPLICABLE)			TERM	DEFINITION
Part	**Type**	**Meaning**		
chem/o	r/cv	chemistry	**chemotherapy**	treatment using drugs; abbreviated
therapy	r	treatment	(KEE moh THAIR ah pee)	**chemo** (Figure 3.7 ::::)
cyt/o	r/cv	cell	**cytology**	the field of study concerned with the structure and
-logy	s	study of	(sigh TALL oh jee)	function of cells
cyt/o	r/cv	cell	**cytologist**	a scientist or technician who studies cell structure
-logist	s	one who studies	(sigh TALL oh jist)	and function
hist/o	r/cv	tissue	**histologist**	a scientist or technician who studies or identifies
-logist	s	one who studies	(hiss TALL oh jist)	tissues
hist/o	r/cv	tissue	**histology**	the study of tissue
-logy	s	study of	(hiss TALL oh jee)	
onc/o	r/cv	tumor	**oncology**	the study of tumors
-logy	s	study of	(ong KALL oh jee)	
radi/o	r/cv	light energy, radiation	**radiotherapy**	treatment of cancer using radioactive materials
therapy	r	treatment	(ray dee oh THAIR ah pee)	

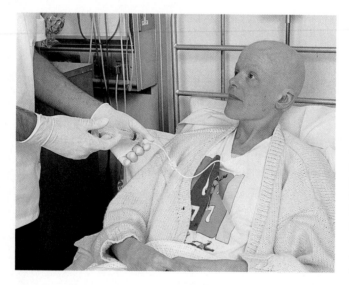

Figure 3.7 ::::

Cancer treatment. A patient with cancer undergoing a blood test in preparation for additional chemotherapy and radiotherapy. Hair loss is a common side effect of chemotherapy.
Source: Simon Fraser/Royal Victoria Infirmary, Newcastle/Science Photo Library/Photo Researchers, Inc.

SELF QUIZ 3.5

SAY IT—SPELL IT!

Review the terms of cancer by speaking the phonetic pronunciation guides out loud, then writing in the correct spelling of the term.

1. KEE moh THAIR ah pee _____

2. sigh TALL oh jee _____

3. hiss TALL oh jist _____

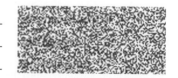

4. ong KALL oh jee _____

5. ray dee oh THAIR ah pee _____

6. sigh TALL oh jist _____

7. hiss TALL oh jee _____

BREAK IT DOWN!

Analyze and separate each term into its word parts by labeling each word part using p = prefix, r = root, cv = combining vowel, and s = suffix.

1. oncology _____

2. oncologist _____

3. cytology _____

4. cytologist _____

WORD BUILDING

Construct or recall medical terms from the following meanings.

1. treatment using drugs _____

2. the study of cancer _____

3. study of tissues _____

4. one who studies cells _____

5. treatment using radioactive materials _____

FILL IT IN!

Fill in the blanks with the correct terms.

1. One of the most life-threatening diseases among U.S. adults is cancer. The study of this disease is known as _____, and one who studies or practices in this field is called an _____.

2. The study of the cell is called _____, and one who performs this study is a _____.

3. The study of tissues is known as _____, and one who studies tissues is a _____.

4. A common treatment for cancer that utilizes drugs to destroy the cancer cells is _____. Another treatment exposes cancer cells to radioactive material, and is called _____.

abbreviations of cells, tissues, and cancer

The abbreviations that are associated with cells, tissues, and cancer are summarized here. Study these abbreviations, and review them in the exercise that follows.

ABBREVIATION	DEFINITION	ABBREVIATION	DEFINITION
Adeno-Ca	adenocarcinoma	Mets	metastasis
CA	cancer	St	stage (of cancer development)
chemo	chemotherapy	TNM	tumor, node, metastasis

SELF QUIZ 3.6

Fill in the blanks with the abbreviation or the complete medical term.

Abbreviation

1. _____

2. Adeno-Ca

3. _____

4. CA

5. _____

6. Mets

Medical Term

chemotherapy

_____

stage (of cancer development)

_____

tumor, node, metastasis

_____

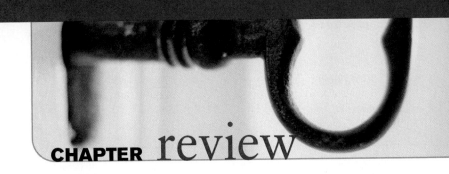

CHAPTER review

In this section, we will review all the word parts and medical terms from this chapter. As in earlier tables, the word roots are shown in **bold.**

Check each word part and medical term to be sure you understand the meaning. If any are not clear, please go back into the chapter and review that term. Then, complete the review exercises that follow.

[word parts **checklist**]

Prefixes

- [ ] ana-
- [ ] dys-
- [ ] epi-
- [ ] hyper-
- [ ] meta-
- [ ] neo-

Word Roots/Combining Vowels

- [ ] **aden**/o
- [ ] **carcin**/o
- [ ] **chrom**/o
- [ ] **cyt**/o
- [ ] **fibr**/o
- [ ] **gen**/o, **gene**/o
- [ ] **hist**/o
- [ ] **lei**/o

- [ ] **lip**/o
- [ ] **lei**/o
- [ ] **mal**/o
- [ ] **melan**/o
- [ ] **my**/o
- [ ] **neur**/o
- [ ] **nucl**/o, **nucle**/o
- [ ] **onc**/o
- [ ] **organ**/o
- [ ] **oste**/o
- [ ] **rhabd**/o
- [ ] **sarc**/o
- [ ] **thel**/i

Suffixes

- [ ] -al
- [ ] -elle

- [ ] -gen
- [ ] -genesis
- [ ] -genic
- [ ] -ic
- [ ] -logy
- [ ] -logist
- [ ] -oid
- [ ] -oma
- [ ] -osis
- [ ] -plasia
- [ ] -plasm
- [ ] -sis
- [ ] -some
- [ ] -stasis
- [ ] -um

[medical terminology **checklist**]

- [ ] **aden**o**carcin**oma (Adeno-Ca)
- [ ] ana**plasia**
- [ ] atoms
- [ ] benign
- [ ] cancer (CA)
- [ ] cancer in situ
- [ ] **carcin**ogen
- [ ] **carcin**oma
- [ ] **cardi**ac muscle
- [ ] cell membrane
- [ ] cells
- [ ] **chem**otherapy (chemo)
- [ ] **chrom**osomes
- [ ] connective tissue
- [ ] **cyt**ology
- [ ] dys**plasia**

- [ ] epi**thel**ial tissue
- [ ] epi**thel**ioma
- [ ] epi**thel**ium
- [ ] **fibr**oma
- [ ] **fibr**o**sarc**oma
- [ ] genes
- [ ] **hist**ology
- [ ] hyper**plasia**
- [ ] **lei**o**my**oma
- [ ] **lei**o**my**o**sarc**oma
- [ ] **lip**oma
- [ ] **mal**ignant
- [ ] **melan**oma
- [ ] metastasis (Mets)
- [ ] molecules
- [ ] muscle tissue

- [ ] **my**oma
- [ ] neo**plasm**
- [ ] nervous tissue
- [ ] **neur**oglia
- [ ] **neur**oma
- [ ] **neur**on
- [ ] **nucle**us
- [ ] **onc**ogenic
- [ ] **onc**ologist
- [ ] **onc**ology
- [ ] **organ** systems
- [ ] **organ**elles
- [ ] **organ**s
- [ ] **oste**o**sarc**oma
- [ ] **radi**otherapy
- [ ] remission

☐ **rhabdomy**oma	☐ smooth muscle
☐ **rhabdomyosarc**oma	☐ stage (of cancer development)
☐ **sarc**oma	(St)
☐ skeletal muscle	

☐ tissues	
☐ tumor, node, metastasis (TNM)	

[show what **you know!**]

BREAK IT DOWN!

Analyze and separate each term into its word parts by labeling each word part using p = prefix, r = root, cv = combining vowel, and s = suffix.

Constructed Word	Word Construction
	r cv s
Example: 1. cytology	cyt/o/logy
2. cytologist	_____
3. cytoplasm	_____
4. chromosome	_____
5. organelle	_____
6. histology	_____
7. epithelium	_____
8. cardiac	_____
9. neuroglial	_____
10. anaplasia	_____
11. carcinoma	_____
12. carcinogen	_____
13. dysplasia	_____
14. epithelioma	_____
15. fibrosarcoma	_____
16. hyperplasia	_____
17. leiomyosarcoma	_____
18. metastasis	_____
19. melanoma	_____
20. neoplasm	_____
21. oncogenic	_____
22. oncologist	_____
23. rhabdomyosarcoma	_____

WORD BUILDING

Construct or recall medical terms from the following meanings.

Example:	1.	the most basic unit of life	_____ cells _____
	2.	a combination of similar cells	_____
	3.	a term meaning *small tool*	_____
	4.	a term that means *kernel*	_____
	5.	a tissue that covers and lines	_____
	6.	epithelium that secretes	_____
	7.	a tissue that connects structures	_____
	8.	a tissue with cells that contract	_____
	9.	muscle tissue of the heart	_____
	10.	muscle tissue that moves bones	_____
	11.	a tissue specialized in communication	_____
	12.	a tumor that grows slowly and does not spread	_____
	13.	a tumor that grows rapidly and spreads	_____
	14.	the disease resulting from a malignancy	_____
	15.	one who studies cancer	_____
	16.	improvement or absence of signs of disease	_____
	17.	a benign tumor of fibrous connective tissue	_____
	18.	a carcinoma of smooth muscle	_____
	19.	a benign tumor of fat tissue	_____
	20.	spreading of cells from a primary tumor	_____
	21.	a cancer with a dark pigment	_____
	22.	a new growth; a tumor	_____
	23.	adjective meaning causing tumors	_____

CASE STUDY

Fill in the blanks with the correct terms.

1. A patient checked in to the clinic with complaints of muscle and joint pain, abdominal pain, and lethargy. A physical exam showed soft tissue lumps of unknown origin at the shoulder, abdomen, and back. The patient was immediately referred to

    (a) _____ for further testing for possible tumors. Samples of similar cell groups, or

    (b) _____, were analyzed in the pathology lab using (c) _____ techniques,

    and cells with altered genetic molecules, or (d) _____, were identified. The cell's DNA was found to

    be (e) _____, and the cells showed advanced changes, or (f) _____. The

    most mutated cells were found in large numbers in (g) _____ muscle tissue specimens taken from the abdominal wall. (h) _____ tissue specimens from the brain, (i) _____ tissue

specimens from abdominal skin, and (j) _____ tissue specimens from bone were also evaluated, but

were found negative. The patient was then scheduled for surgery. During surgery, (k) _____, or

clusters of mutated cells, were found in abdominal skeletal muscle, nearby lymph nodes, and smooth muscle in the

stomach, small intestine, and other visceral (l) _____. The specialist, or

(m) _____, concluded that the tumor originated in skeletal muscle of the abdominal wall, calling the

cancer a (n) _____. From the primary site, the mutated cells (o) _____ to

abdominal organs, bone tissue, and joints by way of lymphatic channels. The treatment prescribed focused on arresting

(p) _____ activity of the tumors by applying chemicals in (q) _____

and radiation in (r) _____ in multiple doses over a three-month period. The specialist indicated a

(s) _____ of 50 percent survival during the first six months following treatment.

[piece it all **together!**]

CROSSWORD

From the chapter material, fill in the crossword puzzle with answers to the following clues.

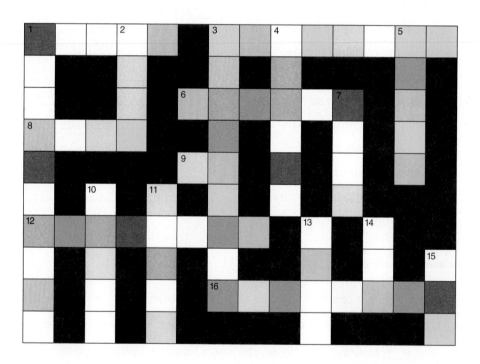

ACROSS

1. What are the most basic units of life? (Find puzzle piece 3.7)
3. A study of the cell. (Find the puzzle piece 3.17)
6. A suffix; what a soldier does when at attention. (Find puzzle piece 3.1)
8. A word root and combining vowel for the word *tumor.* (Find puzzle piece 3.3)
9. Abbreviation for anteroposterior. (Review from Chapter 2)
12. The muscle tissue that is attached to bones. (Find puzzle piece 3.6)
16. The part of a cell that regulates materials going in and out. (Find puzzle piece 3.5)

DOWN

1. An X-shaped structure that contains DNA. (Find puzzle piece 3.4)
2. Word root and combining vowel for a tumor that arose from fat tissue. (Find puzzle piece 3.14)
3. Literally, *a thing formed within a cell.* (Find puzzle piece 3.8)
4. A combination of similar cells. (Find puzzle piece 3.10)
5. Epithelium specialized in secretion. (Find puzzle piece 3.11)
7. A word root for *flesh* or *muscle.* (Find puzzle piece 3.2)
10. A tissue with cells specialized to carry information. (Find puzzle piece 3.12)
11. A word root and combining vowel for the word *nerve.* (Find puzzle piece 3.16)
13. The word root for the word *fiber.* (Find puzzle piece 3.13)
14. An acronym for the molecule-containing genes. (Find puzzle piece 3.9)
15. A prefix for the word *new.* (Find puzzle piece 3.15)

WORD UNSCRAMBLE

From the completed crossword puzzle, unscramble:

1. All of the letters that appear in **green** squares

   __ ☐ __ __ __ __ __ __

   Clue: the study of one of the United States' most deadly diseases

2. All of the letters that appear in **red** squares

   __ __ __ __ __ ☐

   Clue: the tissue that enables you to run and jump

3. All of the letters that appear in **yellow** squares

   __ __ __/☐

   Clue: a word root and combining vowel for a substance often avoided by dieters

4. All of the letters that appear in **blue** squares

   __ __ __ ☐ __ __ __ __ __

   Clue: a constructed word meaning *bad form*

5. All of the letters in **pink** squares

   __ __ ☐ __ __ __ __ __

   Clue: a constructed word meaning dark cancer

6. All of the letters in **peach** squares

   __ ☐ __ __ __ __

   Clue: a malignant neoplasm

7. All of the letters in **orange** squares

   — — ☐ — — —

   Clue: a word that means "woven" in French

8. All of the letters in **gray** squares

   ☐ — / —

   Clue: the word root and combining vowel for the movers in your body

Now write down each of the letters that are boxed and unscramble them to find the hidden medical term of cancer:

— — — — — — — — .

MEDmedia wrap-up

www.prenhall.com/wingerd

Before you go on to the next chapter, take advantage of the free CD-ROM and study guide website that accompany this book. Simply load the CD-ROM for additional activities, games, animations, videos, and quizzes linked to this chapter. Then visit www.prenhall.com/wingerd for even more!

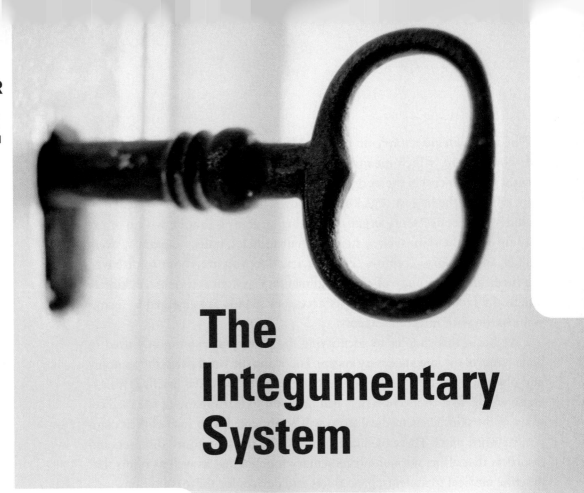

CHAPTER

4

The Integumentary System

LEARNING OBJECTIVES

After completing this chapter, you will be able to:

- Define and spell the word parts used to create terms for the integumentary system

- Identify the major organs of the integumentary system and describe their structure and function

- Break down and define common medical terms used for symptoms, diseases, disorders, procedures, treatments, and devices associated with the integumentary system

- Build medical terms from the word parts associated with the integumentary system

- Pronounce and spell common medical terms associated with the integumentary system

MEDmedia

www.prenhall.com/wingerd

Enhance your study with the power of multimedia! Each chapter of this book links to activities, games, animations, videos, and quizzes that you'll find on your CD-ROM. Plus, you can click on www.prenhall.com/wingerd, to find a free chapter-specific companion website that's loaded with additional practice and resources.

 CD-ROM

- Audio Glossary
- Exercises & Activities
- Flashcard Generator
- Animations
- Videos

 Companion Website

- Exercises & Activities
- Audio Glossary
- Drug Updates
- Current News Updates

A secure distance learning course is available at www.prenhall.com/onekey.

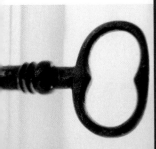

The word *integumentary* (in teg you MEN tah ree) comes from the Latin word *tegere*, which means *to cover*. And indeed it does: The integumentary system covers the body like a giftwrap. Its largest component is the skin, which is the largest organ of the body. The integumentary system also includes smaller accessory organs and other structures that lie within or extend through the skin, such as hair and hair follicles, nails, oil glands, sweat glands, and sensory receptors (Figure 4.1::::). As you are about to discover, the medical terminology of the integumentary system is extensive, largely due to the fact that the skin and its accessory glands are engaged in a constant battle with infectious agents.

We begin this chapter by identifying the word parts commonly used to build terms of the integumentary system. Following the word parts, the anatomy and physiology of the integumentary system will be explored briefly. This exercise will form a connection that will help you to learn many of the medical terms of the skin. Then, medical terms will be presented with each of their component word parts. These medical terms include the symptoms, diseases, and disorders that afflict normal integumentary functioning, as well as terms that describe medical treatments, procedures and devices for these conditions.

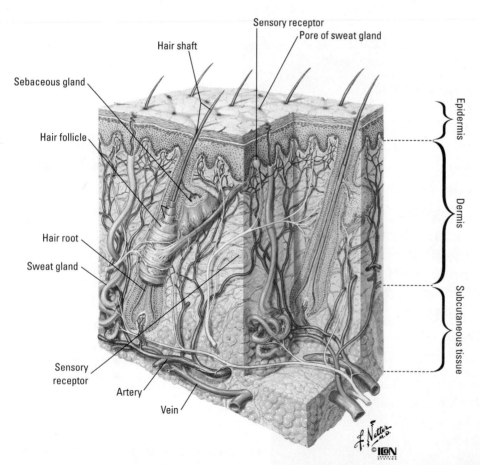

Figure 4.1 ::::
Anatomy of the skin.
Illustration of a section of skin showing key structures.
Source: Icon Learning Systems.

word parts focus

Let's look at word parts. The following table contains a list of word parts that when combined build many of the terms of the integumentary system.

PREFIX	DEFINITION	PREFIX	DEFINITION
a-	without	intra-	within
an-	without	per-	through
ep-	upon, on, over	sub-	beneath
epi-	upon, on, over		

WORD ROOT	DEFINITION	WORD ROOT	DEFINITION
aden	gland	leuk	white
auto	self	myc	fungus
bi	life (the prefix bi- means two, but the root word *bi* means life)	necr	death
		onych	nail
crypt	hidden	pachy	thick
cutane	skin	rhytid	wrinkles
derm, derma, dermat	skin	scler	thick
eryth, erythr	red	seb	sebum, or oil
heter	other	trich	hair
hidr	sweat	xer	dry
kerat	horny tissue, outer hard layer		

SUFFIX	DEFINITION	SUFFIX	DEFINITION
-ectomy	surgical removal, or excision	-osis	condition of
-ia	condition of a diseased or abnormal state	-ous	pertaining to
		-phagia	eating or swallowing
-is	pertaining to	-plasty	surgical repair
-itis	inflammation	-rrhea	excessive discharge
-malacia	softening	-tome	instrument used to cut material
-opsy	view of		

SELF QUIZ 4.1

Review the word parts of integumentary system terminology by working carefully through the exercises that follow. Soon, we will apply this new information to build medical terms.

Success Hint: Once you get to the crossword puzzle at the end of the chapter, remember to check back here for clues! Your clues are indicated by the puzzle icon.

A.   Provide the definition of the following prefixes and suffixes.

4.1   1. epi-   _____

       2. intra-   _____

       3. per-   _____

       4. sub-   _____

       5. -ectomy   _____

       6. -ia   _____

       7. -is   _____

       8. -itis   _____

       9. -malacia   _____

      10. -opsy   _____

      11. -rrhea   _____

      12. -osis   _____

      13. -ous   _____

      14. -phagia   _____

      15. -plasty   _____

      16. -tome   _____

B.   Provide the word root for each of the following terms.

4.2   1. gland   _____

       2. self   _____

4.3   3. life   _____

       4. skin   _____

       5. hidden   _____

       6. red   _____

       7. sweat   _____

       8. other   _____

       9. outer hard layer   _____

      10. white   _____

      11. fungus   _____

      12. death   _____

      13. nail   _____

14. thick   _____

15. wrinkles   _____

16. oil   _____

17. hair   _____

[anatomy and physiology overview]

The most important function of the integumentary system is protection. The skin establishes a physical barrier that protects against the loss of body fluids, damage due to physical injury or ultraviolet light, and invasion by microorganisms. The skin also helps regulate body temperature by forming an insulating blanket around the body, and the blood vessels it contains help the body maintain homeostasis with changing outside temperatures by regulating blood flow. Your sweat glands also assist in temperature regulation when it's hot outside, as well as help remove waste materials. Meanwhile, sensory receptors in the skin provide you with valuable information about the outside environment, such as heat, cold, touch, pressure, and pain.

The Skin

You have just learned that your skin covers your body to protect it from the outside environment. As a protective and insulating cover, it helps your body to maintain homeostasis. Anatomically, the skin consists of two distinct layers that are bound tightly together. The outer, superficial layer is called the _epidermis_, and the inner, deep layer is the _dermis_.

EPIDERMIS

The outermost layer of the skin is a relatively thin region called the **epidermis**. The term epidermis is derived from the Greek word for _outer skin_. The term is composed of the prefix epi- that means _upon, on, over_ and the word root, derm that means _skin_. The epidermis is composed of epithelial tissue. Under the microscope (Figure 4.2), you can see that it includes many layers of cells. These layers are composed of tightly packed cells, which do not permit any blood vessels to penetrate. New cells are produced from the deepest layer of cells only. As new cells are produced, the older cell layers are pushed upward, allowing the epidermis to be completely replaced every 7–10 days.

As cells approach the surface of the skin, they become filled with the tough, waterproof protein, **keratin,** and eventually die. As a result, the superficial layers of

[FYI]

Epidermis
Although your skin is a dynamic organ, the outer layer of the epidermis is not alive. This outermost, horny layer is continuously sloughed off and replaced to maintain a shield from microorganisms and dehydration.

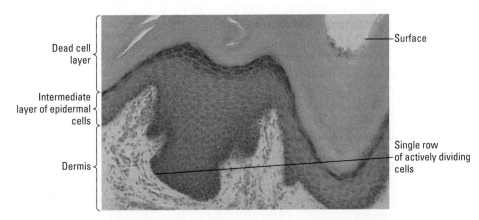

Dead cell layer

Intermediate layer of epidermal cells

Dermis

Surface

Single row of actively dividing cells

Figure 4.2 ::::
Layers of the epidermis.

the skin are composed of dead cells that are mostly keratin. The term *keratin* is a vocabulary term derived from the Greek word for horn, *keras*. Keratin is also a major component of hair and nails.

The color of skin is determined by the genes within the DNA of specialized skin cells located deep within the epidermis. The genes regulate the amount of pigment proteins that are produced by these skin cells. The protein is a brown color and is called **melanin,** named after the Greek word *melan* that means *black* or *dark*. The more melanin that is produced, the darker the skin becomes. The melanin protects your skin from ultraviolet light, which can damage DNA and lead to skin cancer. Exposure to ultraviolet light stimulates the production of melanin to increase the protective shield that it forms. In people with light-colored skin, this effect is called *tanning*.

DERMIS

The deep layer of the skin is much thicker than the epidermis, and is called the **dermis** (Figure 4.1). In contrast to the epithelium of the epidermis, the dermis is composed of connective tissue. It contains lots of blood vessels and is rich in the tough protein, **collagen.** The term *collagen* is a word constructed from the Greek *kolla*, which means *glue,* and the suffix -gen, which you learned from the previous chapter to mean *producing*. As its name suggests, collagen glues the dermis into a cohesive unit with thick, tough fibers that weave throughout. Collagen also glues the dermis to the underlying layer of tissue known as the **subcutaneous layer,** which is mostly fat. The dermis also contains another protein, **elastin,** which is named for its property of elasticity. Elastin behaves like a rubber band, giving your skin its ability to stretch and retract. As you grow older, your skin will produce decreased amounts of elastin, causing the skin to lose its elasticity with increasing age.

In addition to blood vessels and proteins, numerous accessory organs and structures are embedded within the dermis, and some extend through it. Remember that they include hair and hair follicles, nails, oil glands, sweat glands, and sensory receptors. They are described next.

Hair, Hair Follicles, and Nails

The skin covering your body is filled with **hair,** although you probably cannot see most of it. The only body areas lacking hair are the palms of the hands, soles of the feet, and eyelid surfaces. Hair provides some protection from ultraviolet light, and often assists in the sensation of touch.

A hair consists of a portion embedded in the skin, called the **hair root,** and a portion above the skin surface, called the **hair shaft** (Figure 4.3▒▒). A supportive sheath of epithelial cells, known as the hair follicle, surrounds most of the hair root. The term *follicle* is derived from the Latin word for a small sac, *folliculus*. The hair follicle is actually a downward growth of the epidermis into the dermis, which surrounds the hair root like a small sac. The deepest part of the hair follicle contains several layers of cells that divide to produce new hair cells. Like the lower layers of the epidermis, the hair cells are pushed up by younger hair cells. As they move toward the skin surface, the cells gradually undergo changes that eventually result in their death and replacement by keratin. As a result, the hair shaft is completely composed of keratin, and is therefore nonliving. Also like the epidermis, hair receives its color by the production of melanin near the dividing cells.

A **nail,** such as a fingernail or toenail, is formed much the same way (Figure 4.4▒▒). It begins as a part of the epidermis, then the cells compress, fill with keratin, and die as they are pushed upward and forward. The white area at the base of a nail is near its formation site. Since it is in the shape of a crescent moon, it is called the **lunula,** from *luna,* the Latin word for moon. The visible pink area of the nail is the **nail body,** and the **cuticle** is a flap of dead epidermal cells at the proximal edge of the nail. The term *cuticle* is derived from *cutis,* the Latin word for skin. The word root for skin, *cutane,* is also derived from *cutis.* An alternate word for cuticle is

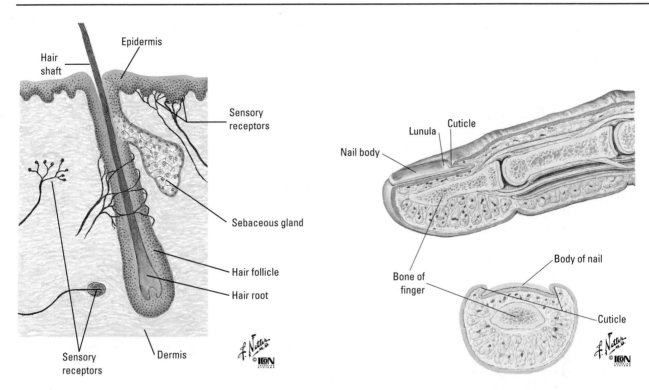

Figure 4.3 :::: **The hair and hair follicle, and associated structures.**
Source: Icon Learning Systems.

Figure 4.4 :::: **Nail structure, side view and cross sectional view.**
Source: Icon Learning Systems.

eponychium, which is a constructed term composed of the prefix ep-, which means upon or around, and the word root *onych* which is derived from the Greek word for *nail*. Because the formation of keratin requires calcium, a deficiency in your diet of this important mineral is often expressed by the development of thin, brittle nails.

Sebaceous (Oil) Glands

Oil glands are also known as **sebaceous glands.** The term *sebaceous* is derived from the Latin word *sebum,* which means an *oily fluid.* The fluid released from these glands is indeed an oily fluid, serving to lubricate the skin and hair by forming an oily film. **Sebum** is a mixture of lipids (fats), salts, water, and cholesterol. Sebaceous glands are usually connected to a nearby hair follicle by a short duct, which carries sebum from the gland to the hair and surface of the skin (Figure 4.3).

Occasionally, the ducts that carry sebum may become plugged by large amounts of sebum or dead cells, especially during puberty, when sebaceous gland activity is accelerated by sex hormones. The sebum and dead cells are a source of nourishment to bacteria that normally populate the skin surface. Increased amounts of sebum can thereby lead to a local skin infection. A plugged duct or swollen gland is called a blackhead, and may lead to the formation of a pimple or boil if the bacteria become established. Cleansing the skin frequently helps to minimize growth of bacteria.

Sweat Glands

Sweat glands are widely distributed throughout the skin in great numbers. They secrete a watery substance simply called sweat or perspiration, which consists of water, salts, and small amounts of the metabolic waste material, urea. The secretion of sweat helps maintain body temperature by cooling the body off as it evaporates, and to a lesser extent, aids the kidneys in the elimination of metabolic wastes. Each gland originates as a single tube that is tightly coiled into a ball in the dermis (Figure 4.1). As sweat is secreted, it passes from the coil into a winding duct that opens onto the skin surface by way of a pore.

Sensory Receptors

The skin contains millions of microscopic structures known as **sensory receptors.** Each receptor is a specialized ending to a neuron, and is capable of initiating a nerve impulse when stimulated (Figure 4.3). A stimulus may be in the form of a change in temperature, a pressure change, a movement of nearby tissues, or damage to nearby cells. The receptors are physically connected to the brain by way of sensory nerves. Once the impulse is received and interpreted by the brain, the sensations of heat or cold, pressure and fine touch, and pain may be brought to your awareness. The presence of sensory receptors in your skin enables you to detect changes in the outside world, and gives your body the ability to respond to these changes in order to maintain homeostasis, or a stable internal environment.

getting to the root of it | anatomy and physiology terms

Many of the anatomy and physiology terms are formed from roots that are also used to construct the medical terms of the integumentary system, including symptoms, diseases, and treatments. In this section, we will review the terms that describe the structure and function of the integumentary system in relation to their word roots, which are shown in **bold.**

The suffixes and prefixes that are used in these terms are also provided as a review. As you review the list, note how the change of a prefix or a suffix alters the meanings of the terms.

Study the word roots and terms in this list and complete the review exercises that follow.

Word Root (Meaning)	Terms Formed from the Word Root (Pronunciation)	Definition
colla (glue)	**colla**gen (KALL ah jenn)	a tough protein forming the white fibers of connective tissue
cutane (skin)	sub**cutane**ous (sub kyoo TAY nee us)	pertaining to under the skin; abbreviated **sc**
	dermis (DER miss)	the lower vascular layer of skin composed of connective tissue
derm, derma, dermat (skin)	epi**derm**is (ep ih DER miss)	the upper layer of skin, composed of epithelial tissue
	hypo**derm**ic (high poh DER mik)	pertaining to under the skin
	intra**derm**al (in trah DER mal)	pertaining to within the skin
elast (change shape)	**elast**in (ee LASS tin)	an elastic protein of connective tissue

Word Root (Meaning)	Terms Formed from the Word Root (Pronunciation)	Definition
kerat (horn)	keratin (KAIR ah tin)	water-proofing protein of the epidermis and hair
	keratogenic (KAIR ah toh JENN ik)	originating from the outer epidermal layers
melan (black, dark)	melanin (MELL an in)	protein of the skin that provides a brownish pigment
onych (nail)	eponychium (ep oh NIK ee um)	a flap of dead epithelial cells at the edge of a nail; also called cuticle
seb (oily fluid)	sebaceous glands (see BAY shuss)	oil glands embedded within the skin
	sebum (SEE bum)	a mixture of oil, salts, water, and cholesterol secreted by sebaceous glands

OTHER IMPORTANT TERMS
The terms in this table are related to the structure and function of the integumentary system, but are not built from word roots.

cuticle (KYOO ti kl)	a flap of dead epithelial cells at the edge of a nail
hair	composed of a hair root that is formed from living cells below the skin surface, and a hair shaft that extends above the skin surface
hair follicle (fall ih kl)	a sheath of epithelium that surrounds the hair root
hair root	the part of a hair that is located beneath the skin surface
hair shaft	the part of a hair located above the skin surface
lunula (LOO nyoo lah)	the pale area at the proximal end of the nail
nail	a flattened disk at the distal ends of the fingers and toes composed of compressed, dead epithelial cells
sensory receptor (SEN soh ree ree SEP tor)	a specialized ending of a sensory neuron that responds to a particular stimulus
sweat glands	coiled, tubular glands in the dermis that secrete sweat onto the skin surface

SELF QUIZ 4.2

SAY IT—SPELL IT!

> **Success Hint:** Use the audio glossary on the CD and CW for additional help with pronunciation of these terms.

Review the terms of the integumentary system by speaking the phonetic pronunciations out loud, then writing the correct spelling of the term.

1. in teg you MEN tah ree   _____
2. ep ih DER miss   _____
3. DER miss   _____
4. KAIR ah tin   _____
5. MELL an in   _____
6. KALL ah jenn   _____
7. ee LASS tin   _____
8. FALL ih kl   _____
9. LOO nyoo lah   _____
10. ep oh NIK ee um   _____
11. KYOO ti kl   _____
12. see BAY shuss   _____
13. SEE bum   _____

FILL IT IN!

Fill in the blanks with the correct terms.

4.4 1. The term *integumentary* is derived from the Latin word *tegere,* which means

_____ _____. The major functions of the

integumentary system include _____ from invasion by micro-

organisms and ultraviolet light, temperature regulation, and reception of sensations.

4.5 2. The skin is composed of two layers, an outer _____ and a thicker,

deep layer called the dermis. The epidermis is composed of _____

tissue, and the dermis is composed of _____ tissue. The upper

layers of the epidermis consist of dead cells filled with the tough waterproofing

protein _____.

3. Near the deep, mitotically active cell layer are specialized cells that produce the brown

pigment protein known as _____, which provides skin color.

4. The connective tissue of the dermis is filled with a tough protein,

_____ and an elastic protein, _____.

5. A hair consists of a hair _____ embedded within the dermis and a hair shaft above the skin surface. The root is sheathed by a downward extension of the epidermis, known as the hair _____. The hair shaft is composed of the protein _____, and is nonliving material. Nails are also composed of this hard protein.

4.6   6. Sebaceous glands and sweat glands are both located within the dermis. They communicate to the skin surface by way of ducts. Sebaceous glands secrete an oily fluid called _____, which lubricates hair and skin. Sweat glands secrete a watery, salty liquid. Also located within the dermis are numerous sensory _____, which respond to stimuli including heat, cold, pressure, fine touch, and pain.

MATCH IT!

Match the term on the left with the correct definition on the right.

_____ 1. follicle   a. originating from the outer epidermal layers

_____ 2. sebaceous   b. means *production of glue*

_____ 3. epidermis   c. word root for skin

_____ 4. collagen   d. a lubricating fluid

_____ 5. elastin   e. means *small sac*

_____ 6. derm or cutane   f. an elastic protein in the dermis

_____ 7. melanin   g. word root for nail

4.7 _____ 8. keratogenic   h. the superficial layer of skin

_____ 9. onych   i. a brown protein pigment

_____10. lunula   j. oil gland

_____11. sebum   k. means *moon*

[medical terms of the

integumentary system]

The integumentary system can experience many types of challenges to its homeostasis. As the outermost organ of the body, the skin is more subject to extremes in temperature, damage by injury, and damage by infections than any other organ. Many types of inherited and acquired diseases may also afflict the skin. In many cases, it is the first part of the body to display symptoms of an internal condition, since it is the body part with which we are most familiar—we often see, feel, and touch our skin throughout the day. The protection that it provides to your overall health is significant: a loss of skin, such as occurs from a serious burn, can lead to death due to dehydration and infection.

The medical field that specializes in the health and disease of the integumentary system is known as **dermatology.** It is a constructed word that can be shown as

dermat/o/logy

where *dermat* is another word root that means skin, o is the combining vowel, and -logy is a suffix that means *study of.* Three other word roots that mean skin are *derm, derma* and *cutane* (see the preceding section). A physician specializing in dermatology is commonly known as a dermatologist.

In "Getting to the Root of It" in the previous section, you saw how learning just one word root helps you to understand many of the anatomy and physiology terms. Now, we will take you a step further and show you that, by adding a combining vowel to those word roots to make a combining form, then using a prefix and suffix, you can form many of the medical terms related to the integumentary system. You are on your way to mastery of the medical terms related to the integumentary system!

let's construct terms!

In this section, we will assemble all of the word parts to construct medical terminology related to the integumentary system. Abbreviations are used to indicate each word part: **p** = prefix, **r** = root, **cv** = combining vowel, and **s** = suffix. Note that some terms are not constructed from word parts, but they are included here to expand your vocabulary.

The medical terms of the integumentary system are listed in the following three sections:

- Symptoms and Signs
- Diseases and Disorders
- Treatments, Procedures, and Devices

Each section is followed by review exercises. Study the lists in these tables and complete the review exercises that follow.

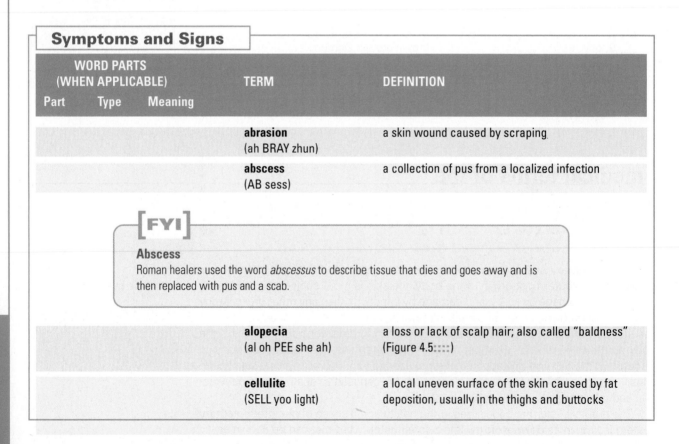

Symptoms and Signs

WORD PARTS (WHEN APPLICABLE)			TERM	DEFINITION
Part	Type	Meaning		
			abrasion (ah BRAY zhun)	a skin wound caused by scraping
			abscess (AB sess)	a collection of pus from a localized infection

> **[FYI]**
>
> **Abscess**
> Roman healers used the word *abscessus* to describe tissue that dies and goes away and is then replaced with pus and a scab.

| | | | **alopecia** (al oh PEE she ah) | a loss or lack of scalp hair; also called "baldness" (Figure 4.5⁞⁞⁞⁞) |
| | | | **cellulite** (SELL yoo light) | a local uneven surface of the skin caused by fat deposition, usually in the thighs and buttocks |

WORD PARTS (WHEN APPLICABLE)			TERM	DEFINITION
Part	Type	Meaning		

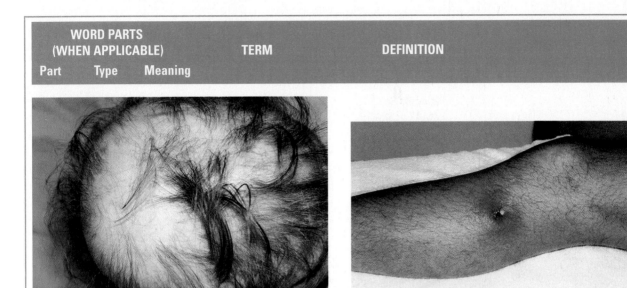

Figure 4.5 :::: **Alopecia, or balding.**
Source: BioPhoto Associates/Photo Researchers, Inc.

Figure 4.6 :::: **Furuncle.**
Courtesy of Jason L. Smith, MD.

			cicatrix (SIK ah trix)	a scar
			comedo (KOM ee doh)	an elevated lesion formed from the buildup of sebum and keratin; also called a pimple
			contusion (kon TOO zhun)	an injury to the skin causing discoloration and swelling without breaking the skin surface; also called a bruise
			cyst (sist)	a closed sac or pouch containing fluid
			diaphoresis (DYE ah for REE sis)	profuse (not necessarily excessive) sweating
			edema (eh DEE mah)	swelling caused by accumulation of fluid
eryth/e -ma	r/cv s	red singular	**erythema** (er ih THEE mah)	general term for redness of the skin
			fissure (FISH er)	a narrow break or slit in the skin (Figure 4.10)
			furuncle (FOO rung kl)	a localized skin infection originating from a hair follicle (Figure 4.6::::)
			induration (in doo RAY shun)	the formation of local hard areas on the skin or elsewhere
			jaundice (JAWN diss)	an abnormal yellow coloring of the skin; also called xanthoderma
			keloid (KEE loyd)	an overgrowth of scar tissue (Figure 4.7::::)
			laceration (LASS er AY shun)	a torn or jagged wound
			lesion (LEE zhun)	a change in tissues due to disease or injury

WORD PARTS (WHEN APPLICABLE)			TERM	DEFINITION
Part	Type	Meaning		
			macule (MAK yool)	a discolored flat spot, such as a freckle (Figure 4.10)
			nevus (NEE vus)	a circumscribed pigmented area, a mole, or a birthmark; plural form is nevi (NEE vye) (Figure 4.8)

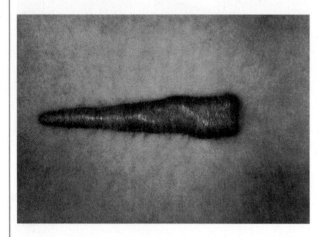

Figure 4.7 :::: **Keloid.**
Courtesy of Jason L. Smith, MD.

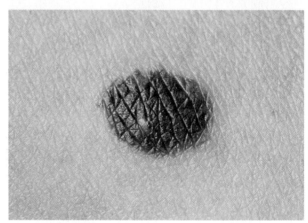

Figure 4.8 :::: **Nevus.**
Courtesy of Jason L. Smith, MD.

WORD PARTS			TERM	DEFINITION
			pallor (PALL or)	abnormal lack of skin color; paleness
			papule (PAP yool)	a small, solid, circumscribed skin elevation (Figure 4.10)
			petechia (peh TEE kee ah)	a pinpoint skin hemorrhage (a hemorrhage is a break in blood vessels); the plural form is petechiae (peh TEE kee ee)
			pruritus (proo RYE tuss)	a symptom of itching
			purpura (PER pew rah)	a purple-red discoloration resulting from hemorrhage into the skin (Figure 4.9)

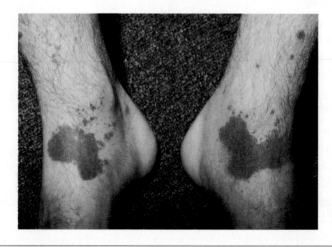

Figure 4.9 ::::
Purpura.
Courtesy of Jason L. Smith, MD.

WORD PARTS (WHEN APPLICABLE)			TERM	DEFINITION
Part	Type	Meaning		
			pustule (PUS tyool)	a small circumscribed skin elevation that contains pus (Figure 4.10⸬)
			ulcer (ULL ser)	an eroded lesion of the skin or mucous membrane (Figure 4.10)
			urticaria (er tih KARE ree ah)	skin eruption usually caused by an allergic reaction to foods, infection, or injury; also called hives
			verruca (ver ROO kah)	a small circumscribed skin elevation caused by a virus; also called a wart
			vesicle (VESS ih kl)	a small elevation of the epidermis that contains fluid; also called a blister (Figure 4.10)
			wheal (WEEL)	a temporary, itchy elevation of the skin, usually with a white center and red perimeter; also called a welt (Figure 4.10)

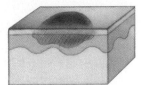

A macule is a discolored spot on the skin; freckle

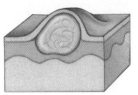

A pustule is a small, elevated, circumscribed lesion of the skin that is filled with pus; varicella (chickenpox)

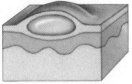

A wheal is a localized, evanescent elevation of the skin that is often accompanied by itching; urticaria

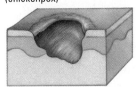

An erosion or ulcer is an eating or gnawing away of tissue; decubitus ulcer

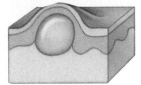

A papule is a solid, circumscribed, elevated area on the skin; pimple

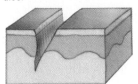

A fissure is a crack-like sore or slit that extends through the epidermis into the dermis; athlete's foot

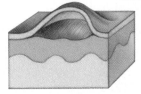

A vesicle is a small fluid filled sac; blister. A bulla is a large vesicle.

Figure 4.10 ⸬

Common skin signs. Each of the illustrations depict a section through skin.
Source: Pearson Education.

SELF QUIZ 4.3

SAY IT—SPELL IT!

Review the terms of the integumentary system by speaking the phonetic pronunciations out loud, then writing the correct spelling of the term.

1. ver ROO kah   _____

2. er tih KARE ree ah   _____

3. eh DEE mah   _____

4. in doo RAY shun   _____

5. NEE vus   _____

6. sist   _____

7. al oh PEE she ah   _____

8. PAP yool   _____

9. kon TOO zhun   _____

10. DYE ah for REE sis   _____

MATCH IT!

Match the term on the left with the correct definition on the right.

_____ 1. abscess   a. an abnormal yellow coloring of the skin

_____ 2. cicatrix   b. an elevated lesion caused by buildup of sebum

_____ 3. comedo   c. an overgrowth of scar tissue

_____ 4. cyst   d. a scar

_____ 5. furuncle   e. a wart

_____ 6. jaundice   f. a fluid-containing closed sac or pouch

_____ 7. keloid   g. a skin eruption caused by an allergic reaction

_____ 8. lesion   h. a small pus-filled skin elevation

4.8 _____ 9. macule   i. a tissue change due to injury or disease

_____10. nevus   j. a collection of pus from a localized infection

_____11. papule   k. a temporary itchy elevation, or welt

_____12. purpura   l. a discolored flat spot, like a freckle

_____13. pustule   m. a small, solid, circumscribed skin elevation

_____14. wheal   n. a mole or birthmark

_____15. urticaria   o. a skin infection originating from a hair follicle

_____16. verruca   p. a condition caused by hemorrhage into the skin

WORD BUILDING

Construct or recall medical terms from the following meanings.

1. a skin wound caused by scraping   _____

4.9 2. a benign tumor or mole   _____

3. also known as "baldness" _____

4. the medical term for "pimple" _____

5. a discolored wound beneath the epidermis _____

6. an infected hair follicle _____

7. profuse sweating _____

8. the formation of local hard areas on the skin _____

9. a narrow slit or break in the skin _____

4.10 10. a torn or jagged wound or cut _____

11. abnormal lack of skin color _____

12. a small pus-filled circumscribed elevation _____

13. small pinpoint hemorrhages on the skin _____

14. a blister _____

FILL IT IN!

Fill in the blanks with the correct terms.

1. A child's fall caused a 10 cm wide _____ on the thigh.

2. Due to a lack of cleanliness, an _____ formed on the wound.

3. Approximately 40 percent of men older than 40 years of age experience male pattern baldness, a form of _____.

4. The deep cut healed after several weeks, leaving a _____ in its place.

5. A _____ is a skin blemish common to most individuals of all ages.

6. Certain individuals experience _____ with relatively low levels of stress, requiring water replacement and frequent showers.

7. The formation of local hard areas on the skin is diagnosed as _____.

8. The blow to the thigh failed to break the skin, but caused a painful _____.

9. The elevation on the skin of the face was found to be filled with fluid, giving it the classification of _____.

10. The patient had signs of abnormal local redness, or _____, and local inflammation, or _____, suggesting an allergic reaction to the drugs.

11. The tear in the skin produced a jagged opening, or _____.

12. The symptom of itching, or _____, combined with abnormal lack of skin color, or _____, and pinpoint skin hemorrhages along the arm known as _____, suggested a circulatory disorder.

13. Fever and the sudden development of blisters, or _____, leading to their conversion to pus-filled skin elevations, or _____, led the physician to diagnose chicken pox with possible secondary skin infection.

Diseases and Disorders

WORD PARTS (WHEN APPLICABLE)			TERM	DEFINITION
Part	Type	Meaning		
			acne (AK nee)	an inflammatory eruption of the skin caused by bacterial infection of sebaceous glands and ducts (Figure 4.11::::)
kerat -osis	r s	horny tissue condition of	**actinic keratosis** (ak TIN ik kair ah TOH siss)	a precancerous skin condition caused by exposure to sunlight. It is marked by overgrowths of the outer epidermal layer
			albinism (AL bin izm)	a genetic condition characterized by the lack or reduction of melanin; an individual with this condition is referred to as albino
carcin -oma	r s	cancer tumor	**basal cell carcinoma** (BAY sal sell kar sin NOH mah)	a tumor arising from the epithelium of the epidermis; it can spread locally if not treated, but seldom metastasizes (Figure 4.12::::)

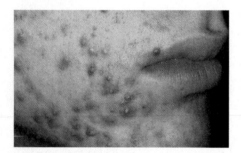

Figure 4.11 :::: Acne.
Courtesy of Jason L. Smith, MD.

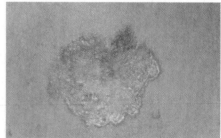

Figure 4.12 :::: Basal cell carcinoma.
Courtesy of Jason L. Smith, MD.

			carbuncle (KAR bung kl)	a skin infection composed of a cluster of boils caused by staphylococci bacteria (Figure 4.13::::)
cellul -itis	r s	little cell inflammation	**cellulitis** (sell you LYE tiss)	inflammation of connective tissue (in the dermis) caused by infection (Figure 4.14::::)

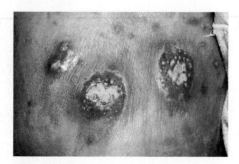

Figure 4.13 :::: Carbuncle.
Courtesy of Jason L. Smith, MD.

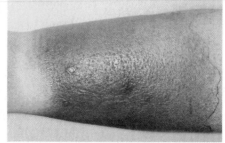

Figure 4.14 :::: Cellulitis.
Source: Camera M.D. Studios. Carroll H. Weiss, Director. 8290 N.W. 26th Place, Sunrise, FL 33322.

WORD PARTS (WHEN APPLICABLE)			TERM	DEFINITION
Part	Type	Meaning		
			decubitus ulcer (dee KYOO bih tus ULL ser)	a skin sore caused by pressure or immobility while lying down; also called bed sore (Figure 4.15::::)
dermat	r	skin	**dermatitis** (der mah TYE tiss)	inflammation of the skin (Figure 4.16::::)
-itis	s	inflammation		

[FYI]

Dermatitis

There are many forms of dermatitis, which are named according to the cause. For example, actinic dermatitis is caused by sunlight (actinic is derived from the Greek word for ray of light), and contact dermatitis is caused by physical contact with an allergen. Each case results in a skin rash, producing local pain, redness, and swelling.

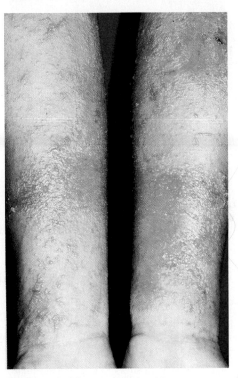

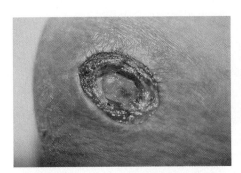

Figure 4.15 :::: **Decubitus ulcer.**
Courtesy of Karen Lou Kennedy, Pressure Ulcers in Adults: Prediction and Prevention by the Agency for Health Care Policy and Research, 1992. Rockville, MD: Department of Health and Human Services.

Figure 4.16 :::: **Dermatitis.**
Source: BioPhoto Associates/Photo Researchers, Inc.

dermat/o	r/cv	skin	**dermatofibroma** (DER mah toh fye BROH mah)	fibrous tumor of the skin
fibr	r	fiber		
-oma	s	tumor		
			ecchymosis (ek ih MOH siss)	a purplish patch on the skin caused by leaking blood vessels (Figure 4.17::::)
			eczema (EK zeh mah)	an inflammatory skin disease characterized by redness, blisters, scaling, and sensations of itching and burning

WORD PARTS (WHEN APPLICABLE)			TERM	DEFINITION
Part	**Type**	**Meaning**		
erythr/o	r/cv	red	**erythroderma** (eh rith roh DER mah)	abnormal redness of the skin
derm	r	skin		
a	s	singular		
			gangrene (GANG green)	tissue death and decay caused by loss or reduction in blood supply
			herpes (HER peez)	a skin eruption characterized by clusters of deep blisters that appear periodically; there are many variations, all of which are caused by members of the virus family Herpesvirus (Figure 4.18::::)

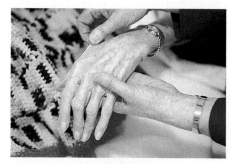

Figure 4.17 :::: **Ecchymosis.**
Source: DeGrazia/Custom Medical Stock Photo.

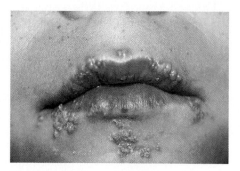

Figure 4.18 :::: **Herpes.**

The blisters often last for several days to one week, and form in response to periodic outbreaks of the virus.
Courtesy of Jason L. Smith, MD.

hidr	r	sweat	**hidradenitis** (high drad en EYE tiss)	inflammation of a sweat gland
aden	r	gland		
-itis	s	inflammation		
hyper-	p	excessive	**hyperhidrosis** (high per high DROH siss)	excessive perspiration
hidr	r	sweat		
-osis	s	condition of		
			impetigo (im peh TYE goh)	contagious skin infection characterized by blisters that later erupt to form a yellowish crust (Figure 4.19::::)
sarc	r	muscle, flesh	**Kaposi's sarcoma** (KAP oh seez sar KOH mah)	a form of skin cancer characterized by the formation of purple or brown patches on the skin that spread by way of lymphatics; used as a sign of AIDS (Figure 4.20::::)
-oma	s	tumor		
lei/o	r/cv	smooth	**leiodermia** (lye oh DER mee ah)	abnormally smooth skin
derm	r	skin		
-ia	s	condition		
leuk/o	r/cv	white	**leukoderma** (loo koh DER mah)	abnormally light-colored skin
derm	r	skin		
-a	s	singular		

WORD PARTS (WHEN APPLICABLE)			TERM	DEFINITION
Part	Type	Meaning		

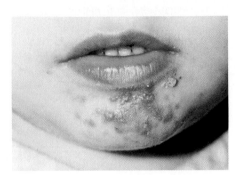

Figure 4.19 :::: Impetigo.
Courtesy of Jason L. Smith, MD.

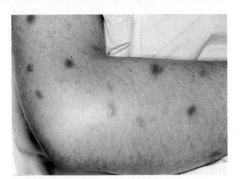

Figure 4.20 :::: Kaposi's sarcoma.
Courtesy of Jason L. Smith, MD.

Part	Type	Meaning	Term	Definition
melan	r	black	**melanoma** (mell ah NOH mah)	malignant skin tumor that arises from melanocytes (pigmented cells) (Figure 4.21::::)
-oma	s	tumor		
necr	r	death	**necrosis** (neh KROH siss)	disease-related death of tissue
-osis	s	condition of		
onych/o	r/cv	nail	**onychocryptosis** (ON ih koh krip TOH siss)	ingrown nail (abnormally buried in skin)
crypt	r	hidden		
-osis	s	condition of		
onych/o	r/cv	nail	**onychomalacia** (ON ih koh mah LAY she ah)	softening of the nails
-malacia	s	softening		
onych/o	r/cv	nail	**onychomycosis** (ON ih koh my KOH siss)	fungal infection of the nails (Figure 4.22::::)
myc	r	fungus		
-osis	s	condition of		

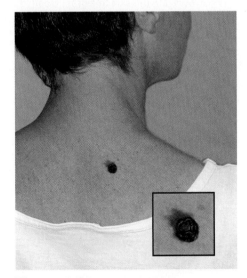

Figure 4.21 :::: Melanoma.
Source: Pearson Education.

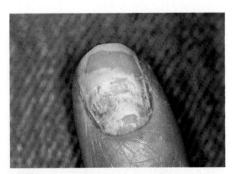

Figure 4.22 :::: Onychomycosis.
Courtesy of Jason L. Smith, MD.

WORD PARTS (WHEN APPLICABLE)			TERM	DEFINITION
Part	Type	Meaning		
onych/o	r/cv	nail	**onychophagia**	abnormal behavior of nail biting or eating
-phagia	s	to eat	(ON ih koh FAY jee ah)	
pachy	r	thick	**pachyderma**	abnormal thickening of the skin
derm	r	skin	(pak ee DER mah)	
-a	s	singular		
par-	p	around	**paronychia**	infection around the nail (Figure 4.23::::)
onych	r	nail	(pair oh NIK ee ah)	
-ia	s	condition		
pedicul	r	body louse	**pediculosis**	infestation of the hair and skin with lice (Figure
-osis	s	condition of	(peh dik yoo LOH sis)	4.24::::)

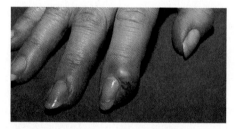

Figure 4.23 :::: **Paronychia.**
Source: Leonard Morse, Medical Images, Inc.

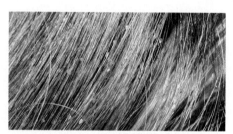

Figure 4.24 :::: **Pediculosis.**
Courtesy of Jason L. Smith, MD.

			psoriasis	a chronic skin condition characterized by red
			(soh RYE ah siss)	lesions covered with silvery scales (Figure 4.25::::)
			scabies	skin eruption caused by the female itch mite, which
			(SKAY bees)	burrows into the skin to extract blood; this disorder causes mild dermatitis (redness, swelling, and itching)
scler/o	r/cv	hard	**scleroderma**	thickening of the skin caused by swelling and
derm	r	skin	(sklair oh DER mah)	thickening of fibrous connective tissue (Figure 4.26::::)
-a	s	singular		

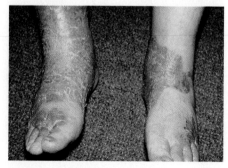

Figure 4.25 :::: **Psoriasis.**
Courtesy of Jason L. Smith, MD.

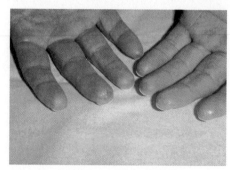

Figure 4.26 :::: **Scleroderma.**
Source: Logical Images/Custom Medical Stock Photo.

WORD PARTS (WHEN APPLICABLE)			TERM	DEFINITION
Part	Type	Meaning		
seb/o -rrhea	r/cv s	oil excessive discharge	**seborrhea** (SEB or EE ah)	sebaceous gland hyperactivity, resulting in excessive discharge of sebum
carcin -oma	r s	cancer tumor	**squamous cell carcinoma** (SKWAY muss sell kar sih NOH mah)	a skin cancer arising from the epidermis, it usually appears as a firm, red elevation with scales; it grows relatively slowly but is capable of metastasis in its later stages (Figure 4.27▦); abbreviated **SqCCa**
			systemic lupus erythematosus (sis TEM ik LOO pus air ih them ah TOH siss)	a chronic inflammatory disease of connective tissue affecting the skin and many other organs; its early stages are characterized by red patches on the face and joint pain; abbreviated **SLE** and commonly called lupus
			tinea (TIN ee ah)	a fungal infection of the skin; also called ringworm (Figure 4.28▦)

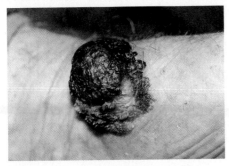

Figure 4.27 ▦ Squamous cell carcinoma.
Courtesy of Jason L. Smith, MD.

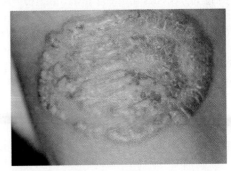

Figure 4.28 ▦ Tinea.
Although it is a fungal infection, tinea is often called ringworm.
Courtesy of Jason L. Smith, MD.

trich/o myc -osis	r/cv r s	hair fungus condition of	**trichomycosis** (TRIK oh my KOH siss)	fungus on the hair surface
			vitiligo (vit ill EYE goh)	a condition in which a loss of pigment-producing cells results in whitish areas of skin
xer/o derm -a	r/cv r s	dry skin singular	**xeroderma** (zee roh DER mah)	abnormally dry skin

disease focus | Wound Repair

The skin provides remarkable protection from physical injury, chemical hazards, and bacterial invasion. Its protective barrier is formed by the epidermis, which is relatively thick with many layers of cells and is covered with the waxy, tough protein, keratin. However, the skin has its protective limits, since it can experience damage from cuts, scrapes, bites, burns, and other challenges. In the event of an injury that damages the skin's protective barrier, the body triggers a response called **inflammation,** which sends fluids carrying phagocytic white blood cells to the injury site. Once the invading microorganisms have been brought under control, the skin proceeds to heal itself. The remarkable ability of the skin to heal even after considerable damage has occurred is largely due to the presence of stem cells in the dermis and cells in the deepest layer of the epidermis, all of which can generate new tissue.

When an injury extends through the epidermis into the dermis, bleeding occurs and the inflammatory response begins. Clotting mechanisms in the blood are soon activated, and a clot or **scab** forms within several hours or less. The scab temporarily restores the integrity of the epidermis and restricts the entry of microorganisms. Soon after the scab is formed, cells of the deep epidermal layer begin to divide by mitosis and migrate to the edges of the scab. About one week after the injury, the edges of the wound are pulled together by contraction. Although the mechanism of contraction is uncertain, it is an important part of the healing process when damage has been extensive. In a major injury, if epithelial cell migration and tissue contraction cannot cover the wound, suturing the edges of the injured skin together, or even replacement of lost skin with skin grafts, may be required to restore the skin.

As epithelial cells continue to migrate around the scab, the dermis is repaired by the activity of stem cells. These active cells produce collagen fibers and ground substance. Blood vessels soon grow into the dermis, restoring circulation. If the injury is very minor, the epithelial cells will eventually restore the epidermis once the dermis has been regenerated.

In injuries that are not very minor, the repair mechanisms are unable to restore the skin to its original condition. The repaired region will contain an abnormally large number of collagen fibers, and relatively few blood vessels. Damaged sweat and sebaceous glands, hair follicles, muscle cells, and nerves are seldom repaired. They are usually replaced by the fibrous tissue. The result is the formation of an inflexible, fibrous **scar tissue.**

Major injuries such as wounds from surgery or extensive burns often need intensive medical intervention. If epithelial cell migration and tissue contraction cannot cover the wound, death from infection, temperature instability, or fluid loss can occur. In the case of a surgical wound, the edges of the injured skin must be sutured together to protect the wound and give the skin an opportunity to heal itself. If the injury involves extensive burns, replacement of lost skin with skin grafts may be necessary to restore the skin. If the graft is successful the edges of the graft will functionally integrate with existing skin and the body will heal.

SELF QUIZ 4.4

SAY IT—SPELL IT!

Review the terms of the integumentary system by speaking the phonetic pronunciation guides out loud, then writing in the correct spelling of the term.

1. sklair oh DER mah _____

2. ON ih koh FAY jee ah _____

3. neh KROH siss _____

4. im peh TYE goh _____

5. dee KYOO bih tus ULL ser _____

6. TRIK oh my KOH siss _____

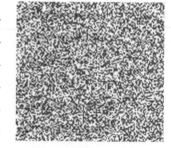

FILL IT IN!

Fill in the blanks with the correct terms.

1. The patient was not properly turned during prolonged bed rest, resulting in the
4.11   development of numerous _____ _____.

2. The cluster of boils was diagnosed as a _____.

3. After several recurrent bouts of redness, blisters, and scaling that were accompanied
   by pruritus and burning, the patient was diagnosed with _____.

4. A slow-growing epidermal tumor is classified as a _____

   _____ _____.

5. An infection of sebaceous glands that often strikes with the onset of puberty is
4.12   known as _____.

6. The reduction of circulation to the right leg resulted in tissue death and decay,
   or _____, and required amputation to avoid systemic infection.

7. The patient exhibited several skin infections, including the fungal infection
   _____, the mite infection resulting in _____,
   and infestation of the hair and skin with lice, or _____.

MATCH IT!

Match the term on the left with the correct definition on the right.

_____1. albinism   a. a loss of pigment-producing cells

_____2. herpes   b. a chronic skin condition with silvery scales

_____3. impetigo   c. abbreviation for systemic lupus erythematosus

_____4. Kaposi's sarcoma   d. a contagious skin infection with blisters and
                                        yellow crust

_____5. psoriasis   e. abbreviation for a slow growing form of skin
                                        cancer

_____6. SqCCa   f. a recurrent skin eruption caused by viral infection

4.13 _____7. SLE   g. a form of skin cancer used as a sign for AIDS

_____8. vitiligo   h. genetic condition resulting in reduction of melanin

BREAK IT DOWN!

**Analyze and separate each term into its word parts by labeling each word
part using p = prefix, r = root, cv = combining vowel, and s = suffix.**

1. dermatitis   _____

2. dermatofibroma   _____

3. erythroderma   _____

4.14 4. seborrhea   _____

5. onychomalacia   _____

6. pachyderma   _____

7. onychokryptosis   _____

WORD BUILDING

Construct or recall medical terms from the following meanings.

1. inflammation of dermal
   connective tissue   _____

2. a skin infection composed of a
   cluster of boils   _____

3. forms blisters that later erupt to
   form a yellowish crust   _____

4. a skin eruption caused by mites   _____

5. inflammation of the skin   _____

4.15   6. abnormal redness of the skin   _____

7. excessive perspiration   _____

4.16   8. condition of death   _____

9. softening of the nails   _____

10. abnormal nail biting or eating   _____

11. condition of fungus on the hair   _____

12. abnormally dry skin   _____

Treatments, Procedures, and Devices

WORD PARTS (WHEN APPLICABLE)			TERM	DEFINITION
Part	**Type**	**Meaning**		
			biopsy (BYE op see)	surgical removal of tissue for evaluation; abbreviated **bx**
			debridement (day breed MON)	removal of diseased or dead tissue and foreign matter from a wound (Figure 4.29░░░)
derm	r	skin	**dermabrasion** (DERM ah BRAY zhun)	removal of skin scars with abrasives, such as sandpaper
abras	r	to rub away		
-ion	s	process		
dermat/o	r/cv	skin	**dermatoautoplasty** (DER mah toh AW toh PLASS tee)	surgical repair using the patient's skin for a skin graft; also called an autograft (AW toh graft)
auto	r	self, same		
-plasty	s	surgical repair		
dermat/o	r/cv	skin	**dermatoheteroplasty** (DER mah toh HETT er oh PLASS tee)	surgical repair using skin from a source other than the patient for a skin graft; also called allograft (ALL oh graft)
heter/o	r/cv	different		
-plasty	s	surgical repair		

WORD PARTS (WHEN APPLICABLE)			TERM	DEFINITION
Part	Type	Meaning		

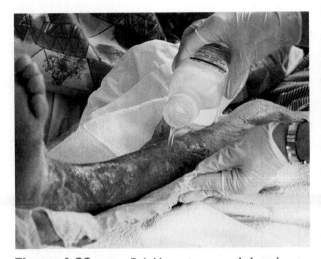

Figure 4.29 :::: **Debridement, or wound cleansing.**
In this photograph, the patient is suffering from a second degree burn on the leg.

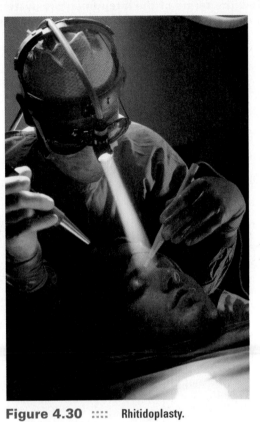

Figure 4.30 :::: **Rhitidoplasty.**
This is a common form of plastic surgery in which the skin is pulled and sutured to decrease skin wrinkles.

Part	Type	Meaning	TERM	DEFINITION
derma -tome	s	skin cutting device	**dermatome** (DER mah tohm)	an instrument used to cut skin
dermat/o -plasty	r/cv s	skin surgical repair	**dermatoplasty** (DER mah toh plass tee)	surgical repair of the skin
			emollient (ee MALL ee ent)	an agent that softens or smoothes the skin
onych -ectomy	r s	nail excision	**onychectomy** (on ee KEK toh mee)	excision (surgical removal) of a nail
per- cutane -ous	p r s	through skin pertaining to	**percutaneous** (per kyoo TAY nee uss)	pertaining to through the skin
rhytid -ectomy	r s	wrinkle excision	**rhytidectomy** (rit ih DEK toh mee)	excision of wrinkles
rhytid/o -plasty	r/cv s	wrinkle surgical repair	**rhytidoplasty** (RIT ih doh PLASS tee)	surgical repair of wrinkles (Figure 4.30::::)

SELF QUIZ 4.5

SAY IT—SPELL IT!

Review the terms of the integumentary system by speaking the phonetic pronunciation guides out loud, then writing in the correct spelling of the term.

1. BYE op see   _____

2. day breed MON   _____

3. DERM ah BRAY zhun   _____

4. DER mah toh AW toh PLASS tee   _____

5. DER mah toh HETT er oh PLASS tee   _____

6. DER mah tohm   _____

7. DER mah toh plass tee   _____

8. ee MALL ee ent   _____

9. on ee KEK toh mee   _____

10. per kyoo TAY nee uss   _____

11. rit ih DEK toh mee   _____

12. RIT ih doh PLASS tee   _____

MATCH IT!

Match the term on the left with the correct definition on the right.

_____1. dermatome   a. excision (surgical removal) of a nail

_____2. onychectomy   b. surgical repair of wrinkles

_____3. dermatoplasty   c. an agent that smoothes the skin

_____4. emollient   d. pertaining to through the skin

_____5. rhytidectomy   e. an instrument used to cut skin

_____6. percutaneous   f. surgical removal of tissue for evaluation

_____7. dermabrasion   g. surgical repair of the skin

_____8. debridement   h. excision of wrinkles

_____9. dermatoheteroplasty   i. removal of diseased or dead tissue from a wound

_____10. rhytidoplasty   j. surgical repair using a patient's skin for a skin graft

_____11. dermatoautoplasty   k. removal of skin scars with abrasives

_____12. biopsy   l. surgical repair using skin from a source other than the patient for a skin graft

BREAK IT DOWN!

Analyze and separate each term into its word parts by labeling each word part using p = prefix, r = root, cv = combining vowel, and s = suffix.

1. dermatoplasty   _____

2. dermatome   _____

3. rhitidoplasty _____

4. dermatoautoplasty _____

4.17 5. onychectomy _____

WORD BUILDING

Construct or recall medical terms from the following meanings.

4.18 1. a skin specialist _____

2. surgical removal of live tissue _____

3. surgical repair of the skin _____

4. excision of skin wrinkles _____

5. surgical repair of skin wrinkles _____

abbreviations of the integumentary system

The abbreviations that are associated with the integumentary system are summarized here. Study these abbreviations, and review them in the exercise that follows.

ABBREVIATION	DEFINITION	ABBREVIATION	DEFINITION
BCC	basal cell carcinoma	SLE	systemic lupus erythematosus
bx	biopsy	SqCCa	squamous cell carcinoma
sc	subcutaneous		

SELF QUIZ 4.6

Fill in the blanks with the abbreviation or the complete medical term.

Abbreviation	Medical Term
1. _____	biopsy
2. BCC	_____
3. _____	subcutaneous
4. SLE	_____
5. _____	squamous cell carcinoma

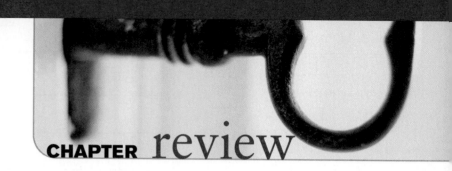

In this section, we will review all the word parts and medical terms from this chapter. As in earlier tables, the word roots are shown in **bold.**

Check each word part and medical term to be sure you understand the meaning. If any are not clear, please go back into the chapter and review that term. Then, complete the review exercises that follow.

[word parts **checklist**]

Prefixes

- ❑ a-
- ❑ an-
- ❑ dys-
- ❑ ep-
- ❑ epi-
- ❑ intra-
- ❑ per-
- ❑ sub-

Word Roots/Combining Vowels

- ❑ **aden**/o
- ❑ **auto**
- ❑ **bi**/o
- ❑ **crypt**/o

- ❑ **cutane**/o
- ❑ **derm**/o, **derma, dermat**/o
- ❑ **eryth**/e, **erythr**/o
- ❑ **heter**/o
- ❑ **hidr**/o
- ❑ **kerat**/o
- ❑ **leuk**/o
- ❑ **myc**/o
- ❑ **necr**/o
- ❑ **onych**/o
- ❑ **pachy**/o
- ❑ **rhytid**/o
- ❑ **scler**/o
- ❑ **seb**/o
- ❑ **trich**/o
- ❑ **xer**/o

Suffixes

- ❑ -ectomy
- ❑ -ia
- ❑ -is
- ❑ -itis
- ❑ -malacia
- ❑ -opsy
- ❑ -osis
- ❑ -ous
- ❑ -phagia
- ❑ -plasty
- ❑ -rrhea
- ❑ -tome

[medical terminology **checklist**]

- ❑ abrasion
- ❑ abscess
- ❑ acne
- ❑ actinic **kerat**osis
- ❑ albinism
- ❑ alopecia
- ❑ basal cell **carcin**oma (BCC)
- ❑ biopsy (bx)
- ❑ carbuncle
- ❑ **cellul**itis
- ❑ cicatrix
- ❑ collagen
- ❑ comedo
- ❑ contusion
- ❑ cuticle

- ❑ cyst
- ❑ debridement
- ❑ decubitus ulcer
- ❑ **derm**abrasion
- ❑ **dermat**itis
- ❑ **dermat**o**auto**plasty
- ❑ **dermat**o**fibr**oma
- ❑ **dermat**o**heter**oplasty
- ❑ **dermat**ome
- ❑ **dermat**oplasty
- ❑ **derm**is
- ❑ diaphoresis
- ❑ ecchymosis
- ❑ eczema
- ❑ edema

- ❑ elastin
- ❑ emollient
- ❑ epi**derm**is
- ❑ ep**onych**ium
- ❑ **eryth**ema
- ❑ **erythr**o**derm**a
- ❑ fissure
- ❑ furuncle
- ❑ gangrene
- ❑ hair
- ❑ hair follicle
- ❑ hair root
- ❑ hair shaft
- ❑ herpes
- ❑ **hidr**aden**itis**

❏ hyper**hidr**osis
❏ hypo**derm**ic
❏ impetigo
❏ induration
❏ intra**derm**al
❏ jaundice
❏ Kaposi's **sarc**oma
❏ keloid
❏ **kerat**in
❏ **kerat**ogenic
❏ laceration
❏ **leioderm**ia
❏ lesion
❏ **leukoderm**a
❏ lunula
❏ macule
❏ melanin
❏ nail
❏ **necr**osis
❏ nevus

❏ **onych**ectomy
❏ **onych**o**crypt**osis
❏ **onych**omalacia
❏ **onych**o**myc**osis
❏ **onych**ophagia
❏ **pachyderm**a
❏ pallor
❏ papule
❏ par**onych**ia
❏ **pedicul**osis
❏ per**cutane**ous
❏ petechia
❏ pruritus
❏ psoriasis
❏ purpura
❏ pustule
❏ **rhytid**ectomy
❏ **rhytid**oplasty
❏ scabies
❏ **scleroderm**a

❏ **seb**aceous glands
❏ **seb**orrhea
❏ **seb**um
❏ sensory receptors
❏ squamous cell **carcin**oma (SqCCa)
❏ sub**cutane**ous (sc)
❏ sweat glands
❏ systemic lupus **eryth**ematosus (SLE)
❏ tinea
❏ **trich**o**myc**osis
❏ ulcer
❏ urticaria
❏ verruca
❏ vesicle
❏ vitiligo
❏ wheal
❏ **xeroderm**a

[show what **you know!**]

BREAK IT DOWN!

Analyze and separate each term into its word parts by labeling each word part using p = prefix, r = root, cv = combining vowel, and s = suffix.

			p r s
Example:	1.	epidermis	epi/derm/is
	2.	dermatitis	
	3.	ecchymosis	
	4.	onychomalacia	
	5.	leioderma	
	6.	hidradenitis	
	7.	scleroderma	
	8.	dermatofibroma	
	9.	trichomycosis	
	10.	percutaneous	
	11.	dermatome	
	12.	onychokryptosis	
	13.	paronychia	
	14.	rhytidoplasty	
	15.	keratogenic	
	16.	leukoderma	

17. dermatoplasty _____

18. hypodermic _____

19. erythroderma _____

20. pachyderma _____

21. onychophagia _____

22. leioderma _____

23. onychomycosis _____

WORD BUILDING

Construct or recall medical terms from the following meanings.

Example:

1. surgical removal of tissue for testing _____ biopsy _____

2. a collection of pus from a local infection _____

3. inflammation of connective tissue _____

4. abnormal redness of the skin _____

5. fungal infection of a nail _____

6. a cluster of boils _____

7. abnormally dry skin _____

8. disease-related death of tissue _____

9. tissue type of the epidermis _____

10. a skin wound caused by scraping _____

11. an infection arising from a follicle _____

12. blisters that later form a yellowish crust _____

13. a small, solid circumscribed skin elevation _____

14. a discolored flat spot _____

15. derived from the Latin word "to soften" _____

16. one who specializes in skin ailments _____

17. an over growth of scar tissue _____

18. an ingrown nail _____

19. abnormal nail eating (or biting) _____

20. a precancerous condition caused by sunlight _____

21. another term for jaundice _____

22. abnormally smooth skin _____

23. excessive perspiration _____

24. abnormal thickening of the skin _____

25. hyperactivity of sebaceous glands _____

26. abnormally light skin _____

CASE STUDY

Fill in the blanks with the correct terms.

1. At the (a) _____ clinic where patients with skin ailments are referred, a patient with an unusual skin

condition was observed. The skin condition included a generalized inflammation, or (b) _____, which

included abnormal redness, or (c) _____, swelling, and pain. It was concluded that the inflammation

originated in the outer layers of the skin, and was thereby (d) _____. Skin damage caused by

sunlight, a precancerous condition known as (e) _____, was ruled out as a diagnosis, along with all

known forms of skin cancer. Rather, an infectious agent was the likely cause. After several days of general inflammation,

fluid-filled skin elevations, or (f) _____, appeared. The elevations gave the patient symptoms of

itching or (g) _____. Scratching the elevations produced open sores, or

(h) _____, which upon healing left scars, or (i) _____. In some areas, the

scar tissue became overgrown, forming (j) _____. An evaluation of the scar tissue included surgical

removal of the surrounding skin, or (k) _____, using a (l) _____. The

procedure revealed an infection that extended through the skin, or was (m) _____, and persistent.

Treatment included the removal of diseased tissue, or (n) _____, and antibiotic treatments were

prescribed. Since some scar tissue affected the face, abrasives were used during the (o) _____

procedure. However, when this treatment failed, an autograft was applied in the (p) _____ procedure,

with improved results.

[piece it all **together!** 🧩]

CROSSWORD

From the chapter material, fill in the crossword puzzle with answers to the following clues.

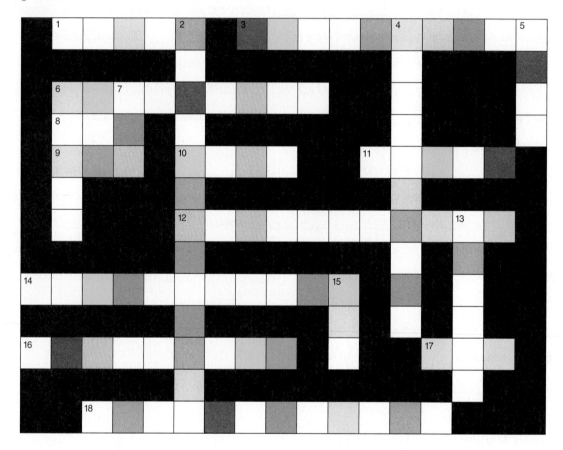

ACROSS

1. The meaning of the word root *aden*. (Find puzzle piece 4.2)
3. The primary function of the integumentary system. (Find puzzle piece 4.4)
6. When sebaceous glands work too hard. (Find puzzle piece 4.14)
8. The prefix that means *upon*. (Find puzzle piece 4.1)
9. The meaning of life; word root and combining vowel. (Find puzzle piece 4.3)
10. A bacterial party in sebaceous glands and ducts. (Find puzzle piece 4.12)
11. A benign skin tumor, usually a mole. (Find puzzle piece 4.9)
12. Excision of a nail. (Find puzzle piece 4.17)
14. Anything that originates from the outer epidermal layers. (Find puzzle piece 4.7)
16. A term that literally means *lying down*. (Find puzzle piece 4.11)
17. Abbreviation for a chronic inflammatory disease of connective tissue. (Find puzzle piece 4.13)
18. Light-skinned people may suffer from this after a day in the sun without sun block. (Find puzzle piece 4.15)

DOWN

2. A skin specialist. (Find puzzle piece 4.18)

4. The dermis is composed of this tissue. (Find puzzle piece 4.5)

5. A word root meaning *dead.* (Find puzzle piece 4.16)

6. A fluid that lubricates skin and hair. (Find puzzle piece 4.6)

7. The same as 9 Across. (Find puzzle piece 4.3)

13. Kids with freckles have plenty of these. (Find puzzle piece 4.8)

15. This type of wound creates a skin fissure. (Find puzzle piece 4.10)

WORD UNSCRAMBLE

From the completed crossword puzzle, unscramble:

1. All of the letters that appear in **green** squares

   □ _ _ _ _ _ _

   Clue: a thousand years ago many believed these were given by toads

2. All of the letters that appear in **red** squares

   _ □ _ _ _ _

   Clue: a viral disease that can give you the "creeps"

3. All of the letters that appear in **yellow** squares

   _ _ □ _

   Clue: a closed sac filled with fluid

4. All of the letters in **orange** squares

   _ _ _ _ _ _ □ _ _ _

   Clue: any swelling, redness, and itching of the skin

5. All of the letters that appear in **gray** squares

   _ _ _ □ _ / _

   Clue: the combining form for the word "nail"

6. All of the letters in **pink** squares

   _ _ _ _ □ _ _ _

   Clue: a pigment condition that shows most in dark-skinned people

7. All of the letters in **peach** squares

   _ □ _ _ _ _ _ _ _

   Clue: an integumentary gland that works like an oil can

Now write down each of the letters that are boxed and unscramble them to find the hidden medical term of the integumentary system: _ _ _ _ _ _ _.

MEDmedia wrap-up

www.prenhall.com/wingerd

Before you go on to the next chapter, take advantage of the free CD-ROM and study guide website that accompany this book. Simply load the CD-ROM for additional activities, games, animations, videos, and quizzes linked to this chapter. Then visit www.prenhall.com/wingerd for even more!

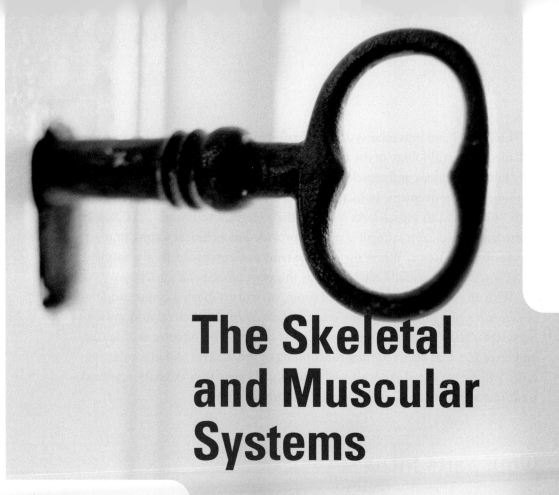

CHAPTER

5

The Skeletal and Muscular Systems

MEDmedia

www.prenhall.com/wingerd

Enhance your study with the power of multimedia! Each chapter of this book links to activities, games, animations, videos, and quizzes that you'll find on your CD-ROM. Plus, you can click on www.prenhall.com/wingerd, to find a free chapter-specific companion website that's loaded with additional practice and resources.

 CD-ROM

- Audio Glossary
- Exercises & Activities
- Flashcard Generator
- Animations
- Videos

 Companion Website

- Exercises & Activities
- Audio Glossary
- Drug Updates
- Current News Updates

A secure distance learning course is available at www.prenhall.com/onekey.

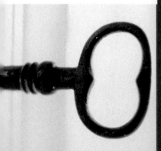

The skeletal and muscular systems are combined in this chapter because the medical terminology of the two systems is associated very closely. As you may know, the bones and muscles work hand in hand to support the body and produce body movement. In fact, nearly every one of the 206 bones in your body is attached to muscles. As a result, their medical terminology is closely related, and medical treatment is usually provided in a clinical setting that addresses both systems. When the two systems are combined in a treatment program, they are usually referred to as the *musculoskeletal system*.

With an emphasis on using word roots, we will establish a connection between the terms for the anatomy and physiology of the skeletal and muscular systems and related medical terms in this chapter. The symptoms, diseases, and disorders that afflict normal functioning of the skeletal and muscular systems will be explored, and we will also study terms that describe medical treatments, procedures, and devices for these conditions.

word parts focus

Let's look at word parts. The following table contains a list of word parts that when combined build the terms of the skeletal and muscular systems.

PREFIX	DEFINITION	PREFIX	DEFINITION
a-	without	para-	near, alongside
an-	without	peri-	around
dia-	around, passing through	poly-	many
dys-	bad, abnormal	quad-	four
end-, endo-	within	sym-	together, joined
epi-	upon	syn-	together, joined
ortho-	straight, normal		

WORD ROOT	DEFINITION	WORD ROOT	DEFINITION
ankyl	crooked, not straight	clon	spasm, twitching
arthr, articul	joint	condyl	knuckle of a joint
burs	purse or sac, bursa	cost	rib
carp	wrist	cran, crani	skull, cranium
cartil	gristle, cartilage	duct	lead, move
cel	hernia, protrusion	fasci	fascia
chir	hand	femor, femur	thigh, femur
chondr	gristle, cartilage	fibul	clasp of buckle, fibula

WORD ROOT	DEFINITION	WORD ROOT	DEFINITION
ili	flank, groin, ilium	phalang, phalanx	row of soldiers, phalanges
ischi	haunch, hip joint, ischium	pod	foot
kinesi	motion	physis	growth
kyph	hump	pub	grown up
lamin	thin	rachi	spine, or vertebral column
lord	bent forward	radi	spoke of a wheel, radius
menisc	crescent-shaped moon, meniscus	sacr	sacred, sacrum
myel, myelon	bone marrow	scoli	curved
my, myos	muscle	skelet	dried up, skeleton
neur	sinew or cord (usually applied to nerves, but in the muscular system it refers to fascia)	spondyl	vertebra
		stern	chest, sternum
		synov, synovi	binding of eggs, synovial
orth	straight	tars	flat surface
oste	bone	taxi	reaction to a stimulus
pariet	wall	ten, tend, tendin	to stretch out, tendon
patell	small pan, patella	vers	turn
ped	child	vertebr	a joint, vertebra
petr	stone		

SUFFIX	DEFINITION	SUFFIX	DEFINITION
-algia	pain	-pathy	disease
-asthenia	weakness	-plasia	shape, formation
-cele	hernia, protrusion	-plegia	paralysis
-centesis	puncture; a surgical puncture to aspirate fluids	-practic	one who practices
		-ptosis	falling downward
-clasia, -clasis, -clast	break apart	-physis	growth
-desis	surgical fixation, fusion	-schisis	split, fissure
-dynia	pain	-tic	pertaining to
-iatry	treatment, specialty	-tomy	cutting into; incision
-ist	one who practices	-trophy	development
-otomy	cutting into; surgical removal or excision	-um	pertaining to
		-y	process of

SELF QUIZ 5.1

Review the word parts of skeletal and muscular systems terminology by working carefully through the exercises that follow. Soon, we will apply this new information to build medical terms.

> **Success Hint:** Once you get to the crossword puzzle at the end of the chapter, remember to check back here for clues! Your clues are indicated by the puzzle icon.

A. Provide the definition of the following prefixes and suffixes.

1. a- _____
2. dys- _____
3. ortho- _____
4. para- _____
5. poly- _____
6. quad- _____
7. syn- _____
8. -algia _____
9. -asthenia _____
10. -centesis _____
11. -clast _____
12. -desis _____
13. -dynia _____
14. -pathy _____
15. -tomy _____
16. -plegia _____
17. -physis _____
18. -ptosis _____
19. -schisis _____

B. Provide the word root for each of the following terms.

1. crooked, not straight _____
2. joint _____
3. hand _____
4. twitching, spasm _____
5. rib _____
6. cranium _____
7. motion _____
8. hump _____
9. bent forward _____
10. curved _____

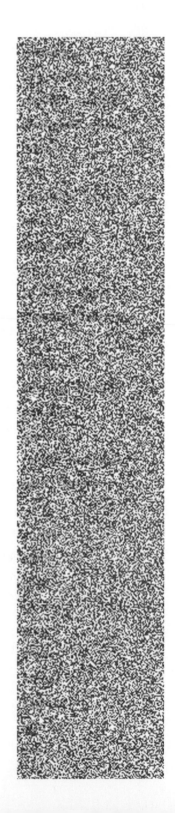

11. bone marrow _____

5.3 12. muscle _____

13. bone _____

14. child _____

15. stone _____

16. foot _____

17. the spine _____

18. vertebra _____

19. synovial _____

20. reaction to a stimulus _____

5.4 21. tendon _____

[anatomy and physiology overview]

The skeletal and muscular systems provide for the structure and movement of the body. They comprise the bones, joints, and muscles, and supporting structures including fascia, tendons, and ligaments. In the sections that follow you will read about the structures of both systems individually, and learn how these two systems work together to enable you to support and move your body.

Structure and Function of the Skeletal System

The skeletal system consists of the bones and joints of the body. The study of bones is known as **osteology,** and the study of joints is **arthrology.** The term osteology can be shown as

oste/o/logy

where oste is the root word for *bone,* and –logy is the suffix for *study of.* An **osteologist** is a professional who studies bones. The term arthrology can be shown as

arthr/o/logy

where arthr is the root word for *joint,* which is also called an *articulation.* A professional who studies joints is called an **arthrologist.** Together, the bones and joints are the organs that form the **skeleton.** The term skeleton is derived from the Greek word *skeletos* that means *withered, dried up,* giving us a mental image of a dead bone quite well. But the skeleton in a living person is a somewhat flexible, dynamic structure that performs several important functions:

■ **Support:** the strong, rigid skeleton forms a structural frame that offers other body structures a sturdy place for support.

■ **Protection:** some bones physically surround internal body organs, like the cranial bones around the brain and the ribcage around the heart and lungs. The hardness of bone provides a partial shield from injury to these and other organs.

■ **Aid in movement:** bones provide a place of attachment for skeletal muscles, enabling coordinated movements to occur. The rigid nature of bones provides leverage for attached muscles, giving them something firm to pull against during contraction.

■ **Blood cell formation:** blood cells are manufactured by a blood-forming connective tissue called red bone marrow that is located within certain bones.

■ **Storage:** bone tissue is the storehouse and main reserve for two important minerals, calcium and phosphate, which are needed for muscle contraction, nerve cell function, and movement of materials across cell membranes.

Bones come in a variety of shapes and sizes, including long and slender, short and wide, flat, and irregular. Despite these differences, all bones have a similar internal organization. Using a long bone as an example (Figure 5.1::::), study the internal components of bones; they are listed and described with other terms in the Getting to the Root of It—Anatomy and Physiology Terms table (following our discussion of the muscular system).

A hard, durable structure is a bone's most characteristic feature. The hardness is provided by minerals, which are produced by bone cells. Bone cells also produce the strong, tough protein collagen that interweaves throughout bone to strengthen it further. Together, the minerals and collagen form the **bone matrix.**

Your body functions best in a state of homeostasis, which we talked about in Chapter 2. Each organ in your body must make adjustments and undergo change in order to maintain this stability, including your bones. Each one of your bones is a living, dynamic organ that participates in this process. For example, exercise causes muscles to pull on your bones, and in response, the bones change by becoming thicker and stronger. A lack of exercise has the opposite effect.

What enables bones to change in response to body needs? The living component of your bones, the cells, produce change by secreting new matrix or dissolving old matrix. The primary type of bone cell is an **osteocyte,** which can produce new bone matrix by secreting mineral salts and collagen. The term *osteocyte* literally means *bone cell,* since the word root, *oste,* means bone and the suffix, -cyte, means *cell.*

Two other types of bone cells are also present in a living bone. **Osteoblasts** are bone cells that move throughout a bone to secrete new bone matrix. The suffix, -blast, means *bud* or *sprout,* and is used to identify a precursor, active cell. **Osteo-**

[thinking critically!]

What important function of bone becomes altered when the red bone marrow becomes afflicted with disease?

[thinking critically!]

What two types of bone cells do you suppose are called into action following an accident resulting in a bone fracture?

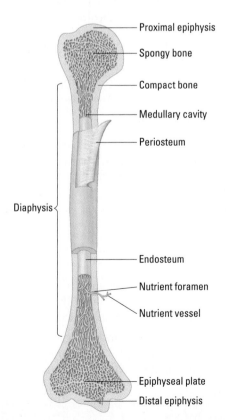

- Proximal epiphysis
- Spongy bone
- Compact bone
- Medullary cavity
- Periosteum

Diaphysis

- Endosteum
- Nutrient foramen
- Nutrient vessel

- Epiphyseal plate
- Distal epiphysis

Figure 5.1 ::::

Parts of a bone.

clasts, which also move around bone, perform the opposite function—they dissolve bone matrix. The suffix, -clast, means *broken into pieces,* which accurately describes the function of osteoclasts. The interactions of the three bone cell types are regulated by hormones, providing you with homeostasis of bone that allows for change in response to changes in body demands.

BONES OF THE SKELETON

The terminology of the skeleton and the bones that form it includes the names of each of the bones. The bones are listed and described in the Getting to the Root of It—Anatomy and Physiology Terms table (following our discussion of the muscular system) and illustrated in Figure 5.2::::.

[FYI]

Latin Words
Many of the terms you are learning that name body parts are the original Latin or Greek words that were used in ancient times. The word maxilla is Latin for jaw-bone, mandible is Latin for a chewer or jaw, humerus is Latin for shoulder, and ulna is Latin for elbow or arm.

[FYI]

Clavicle
Clavicle is Latin for *small key.* Early Roman physicians compared the shape of a clavicle with the S-shape of old Roman keys.

Coccyx
The word coccyx is Greek for the cuckoo bird. The Greeks must have thought that the bone they were naming looked like the beak of the cuckoo.

The Phalanges
The term phalanges is Latin for *row of soldiers*—very reminiscent of fingers and toes!

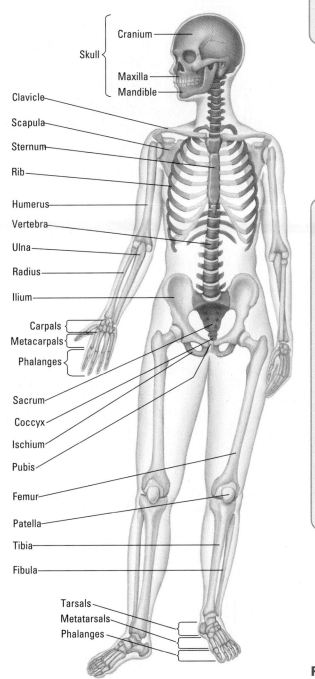

Skull
Cranium
Maxilla
Mandible
Clavicle
Scapula
Sternum
Rib
Humerus
Vertebra
Ulna
Radius
Ilium
Carpals
Metacarpals
Phalanges
Sacrum
Coccyx
Ischium
Pubis
Femur
Patella
Tibia
Fibula
Tarsals
Metatarsals
Phalanges

(a) ▮ Appendicular skeleton   ▯ Axial skeleton

Figure 5.2 ::::

The bones of the skeleton.
(a) The skeleton, anterior view.

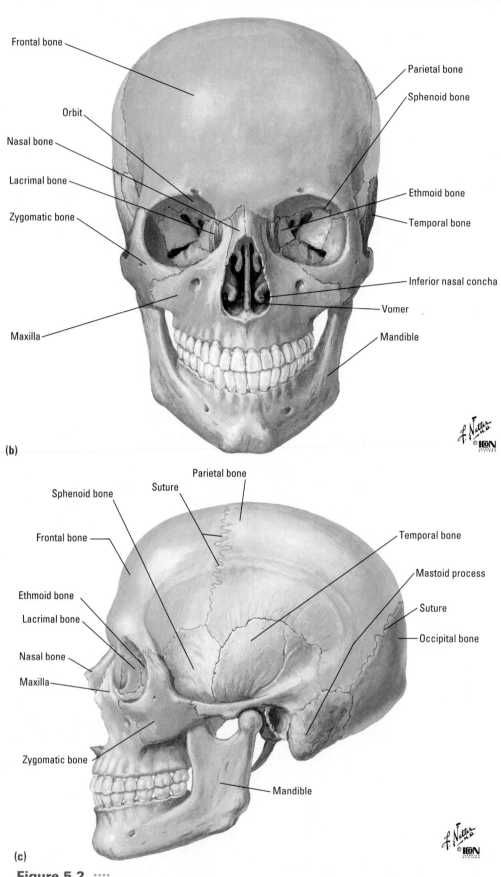

Figure 5.2 ::::

(b) The skull, anterior view.
(c) The skull, lateral view.
Source: Icon Learning Systems.

THE JOINTS

In addition to bones, the joints, or articulations, are organs of the skeletal system. Joints help to hold your bones together, and in many cases, stabilize the union between two bones to permit movement of the body. Often, joints are stabilized themselves by tough bands of fibrous connective tissue that connect one bone to another, which are called **ligaments.**

Three types of joints are present in the body, which are distinguishable by the nature of the material that connects two bones together. They are **synovial joints, cartilaginous joints,** and **fibrous joints.**

Many of your body's joints, such as the knee, shoulder, and elbow, are synovial joints. They permit more movement between bones than any other joints of the body. Synovial joints consist of a sac of connective tissue surrounding the joint space that contains a clear, slightly yellow fluid called **synovial fluid** (Figure 5.3::::).The fluid provides lubrication and a shock-absorbing liquid cushion. Synovial joints are usually strengthened by ligaments, and may include stabilizing plates of cartilage called **menisci** and shock-absorbing sacs of fluid called **bursae.**

Cartilaginous joints are more rigid than synovial joints, allowing less movement between opposing bones. As the name suggests, the material between the bones is cartilage, which is a slightly flexible, soft type of connective tissue. Cartilaginous joints include the **costal cartilages** between ribs and the sternum, the **intervertebral discs** between vertebrae, and the **symphysis pubis** where the pubic bones fuse together. A temporary cartilaginous joint occurs on most growing bones, and is called the **epiphyseal plate.** It is the site of lengthwise bone growth during childhood.

Fibrous joints consist of a tough, fibrous connective tissue between opposing bones. Because this material is not flexible, they allow very little or no movement between bones. For example, the tight, immoveable sutures of the cranium are fibrous joints.

The terms associated with joints are listed and defined in the Getting to the Root of It—Anatomy and Physiology Terms table (following our discussion of the muscular system), and are illustrated in Figure 5.3.

Synovial
The term synovial was first named by Roman physicians, who noticed an egg yolk-like fluid leaking from injured knee joints. They combined the prefix syn- that means *together* with the root word *ovi* that means *egg* to describe the fluid within the knee. The combined term, synovial, was later used to describe any joint of the body that contains a fluid-filled compartment.

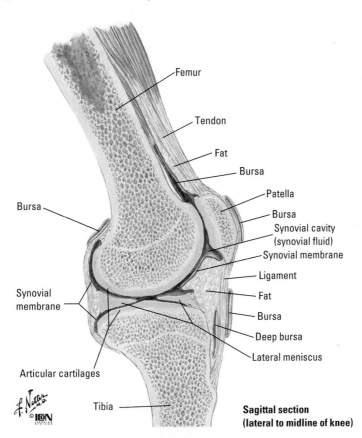

Figure 5.3 ::::

Anatomy of joints. The knee joint, a complex synovial joint.
Source: Icon Learning Systems.

Structure and Function of the Muscular System

The muscular system consists of more than 500 muscles. Many of these are illustrated in Figure 5.4⸬. The primary function of muscles is to produce movement. Nearly every muscle in your body attaches to one or more bones by way of a **tendon**. As the muscle contracts (shortens), it pulls on the tendon, which draws the bone closer, producing movement. When the muscle is relaxed, it returns the bone to its previous position. Because your bones contain attachments to many muscles that can contract independently, you are capable of making complex movements.

In addition to producing movement, the muscular system generates heat, which is a byproduct of the energy used during contraction. This heat comes in very handy—on cold days you may shiver and goose bumps may appear on your skin; this is your body's way of generating heat to keep you warm inside.

Muscle Terms
Many of the terms associated with muscles include the word root *my*. It is derived from the Greek word *mys* or *myos,* which means *muscle*. You might recall from Chapter 2 that the word muscle means *little mouse* in Latin.

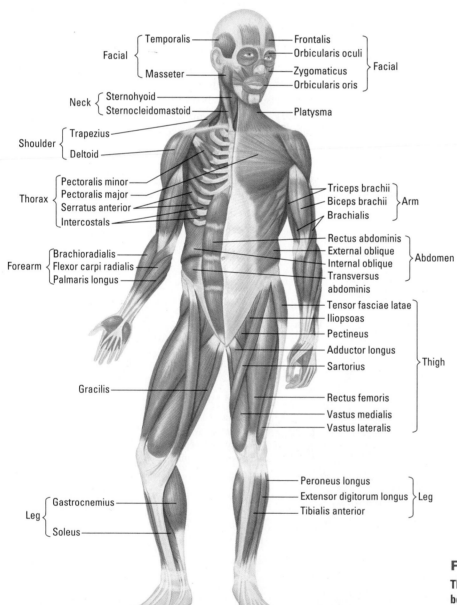

Figure 5.4 ⸬

The major muscles of the human body.
(a) Anterior view;
(b) Posterior view.

(a)

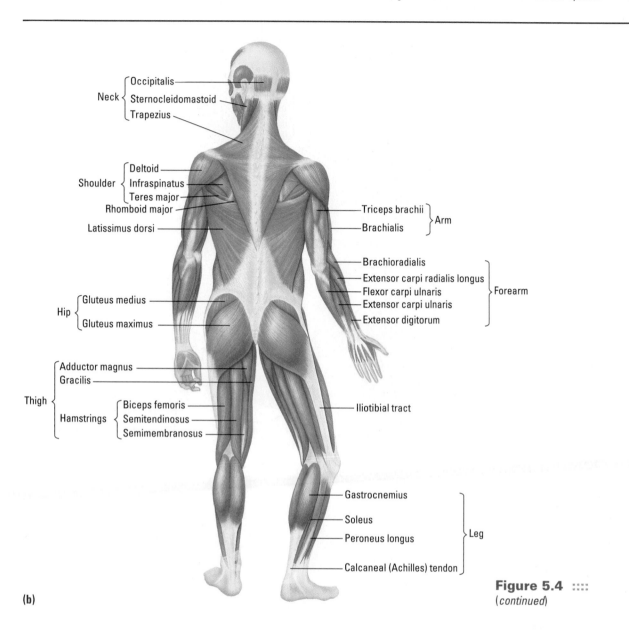

Figure 5.4 ::::
(*continued*)

(b)

MUSCLE STRUCTURE

The primary component of a muscle is skeletal muscle tissue. In this tissue, the muscle cells are long and rod-like, and are bundled together to form the *meat* of a muscle (Figure 5.5::::). Other types of muscle tissue include cardiac muscle, which forms the heart wall, and smooth muscle, found in hollow organs like the stomach and blood vessels.

Muscles are closely associated with connective tissue (Figure 5.6::::). The connective tissue is a tough, fibrous material known as **fascia.** The fascia surrounds individual muscle cells, groups of cells known as muscle bundles, and the whole muscle. In most cases, the fascia extends beyond the length of the muscle to form a tendon. This arrangement establishes an extremely strong connection between the tendon and the muscle. As a result, when an injury to a tendon occurs, the tendon may be torn at its center or at its attachment to a bone, but very rarely at its attachment to the muscle.

MUSCLE ACTIONS

The close relationship between muscle and bone is what makes it possible for you to move. Muscle contraction occurs when all of the muscle fibers in a muscle shorten at the same time, causing the muscle to shorten in its overall length. Because the

[thinking critically!]

Why would injury or illness to a tendon affect the ability of the attached muscle to move a bone?

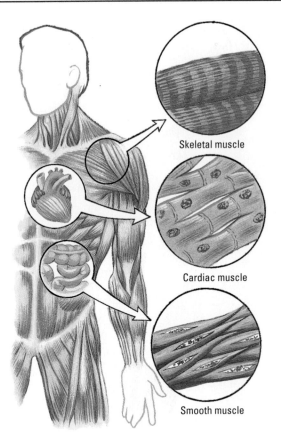

Skeletal muscle

Cardiac muscle

Smooth muscle

Figure 5.5 ::::

The three types of muscle tissues and their locations.

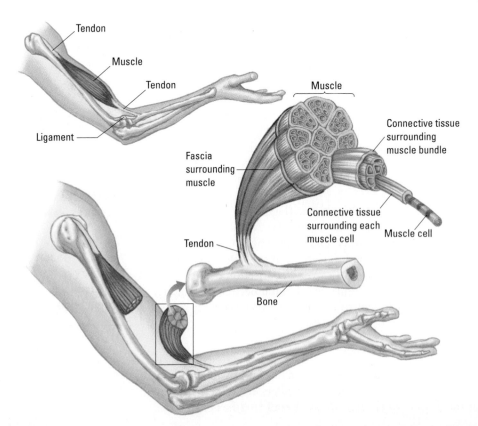

Tendon

Muscle

Tendon

Ligament

Muscle

Connective tissue surrounding muscle bundle

Fascia surrounding muscle

Connective tissue surrounding each muscle cell

Muscle cell

Tendon

Bone

Figure 5.6 ::::

Muscle structure.

fascia of a muscle is continuous with a tendon, contraction of the muscle causes the muscle to pull on the tendon, increasing its tension. As a result, the tendon pulls on the bone to which it is attached. If the bone is not held rigid by the contraction of other muscles, the bone will move in response, producing body movement.

Most body movements involve the contractions of several muscles at once. As a result of this coordinated activity, a number of motions, or actions, are possible. The primary muscle actions are listed and defined in the Getting to the Root of It— Anatomy and Physiology Terms table and illustrated in Figure 5.7::::. As you review the illustration, practice each muscle action by moving an arm or leg in the direction depicted.

NAMING BONES, JOINTS, AND MUSCLES

The 206 bones in your body are named using Latin or Greek derivatives that describe something about that bone. Joints are named in a similar manner. For example, part of the name for the inferior nasal conchae is derived from the Latin word *concha* for shell. This is very descriptive of those bones because they are shaped like a scroll and resemble a conch shell. A meniscus is a crescent-shaped cartilage in the knee. It derives its name from the Greek work *meniskos,* which means crescent-shaped moon and is descriptive of the shape of a meniscus.

Many bone or joint names may be combined to form new names or terms. For example, humeroradial is a combined name that describes a joint between the humerus and radius of the arm. Also, you may recognize the combined term sacroiliac, which is the name of a joint between the sacrum and the ilium.

The same formula holds true for the naming of all of the 500 or so muscles of your body. You may recall from Chapter 3 that the term muscle is derived from the

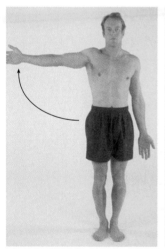
Abduction

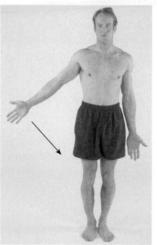
Adduction

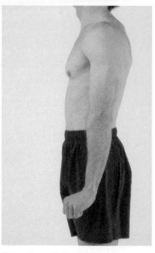
Extension of left arm

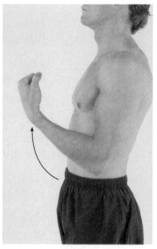
Flexion of left forearm

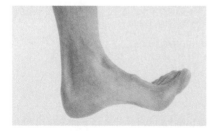
Dorsiflexion of toes

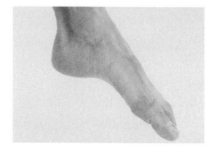
Plantar flexion of foot

Figure 5.7 :::: **The primary muscle actions.** *Source: Pearson Education.*

Latin term *musculus*, which means *little mouse*. In using this word, the Romans were comparing the appearance of muscles to that of little mice. The most common descriptors used in naming muscles are muscle location, attachments, and muscle shape. For example, the biceps brachii is the muscle responsible for moving the forearm when you flex your arm at the elbow. Notice that this muscle's name is composed of two Latin words. *Biceps* means two heads and refers to its two attachment sites at the shoulder, and *brachii* (the plural form of the word brachium) means arm. Nearly all of the muscles of the body are named in a similar manner, using Latin or Greek derivatives that describe something about the muscle.

getting to the root of it | anatomy and physiology terms

Many of the anatomy and physiology terms are formed from roots that are also used to construct the more complex medical terms of the skeletal and muscular systems, including symptoms, diseases, and treatments. In this section, we will review the terms that describe the structure and function of the skeletal and muscular systems in relation to their word roots, which are shown in **bold.**

Study the word roots and terms in this list and complete the review exercises that follow.

Word Root (Meaning)	Terms Formed from the Word Root (Pronunciation)	Definition
articul (joint)	**articul**ar cartilage (ahr TIK yoo lahr KAR tih lij)	a smooth layer of cartilage covering the epiphyses of bones and found only in synovial joints
burs (purse or sac)	**burs**a (BER sah)	a small fluid-filled sac in the shoulder, elbow, and knee joints that provides a cushioning effect during movement
carp (wrist)	**carp**als (KAR pals)	the small bones of the wrist
	meta**carp**als (mett ah KAR pals)	the small narrow bones of the hand
cartil (gristle, cartilage)	**cartil**aginous joint (kar tih LAJ ih nuss)	a joint where the material between bones consists of cartilage that allows some movement between bones.
cran, crani (skull, cranium)	**cran**ium (KRAY nee um)	part of the skull, the bones that surround the brain
duct (lead, move)	ab**duct**ion (ahb DUK shun)	movement away from the body midline
	ad**duct**ion (add DUK shun)	movement toward the body midline
	circum**duct**ion (sir kum DUK shun)	turning the distal end of a bone in a circle
fasci (fascia)	**fasci**a (FAH shee uh)	a tough, fibrous connective tissue
femur, femor (thigh bone)	**femur** (FEE mer)	the bone of the upper leg or thigh
fibr (fiber)	**fibr**ous joint (FYE bruss)	a joint where the material between bones consists of fibrous connective tissue that allows very little or no movement between them

Word Root (Meaning)	Terms Formed from the Word Root (Pronunciation)	Definition
fibul (clasp or buckle)	**fibul**a (FIB yoo lah)	the smaller of the two bones of the lower leg
flex (bend)	dorsi**flex**ion (dor see FLEK shun)	bending the foot or toes upward
	flexion (FLEK shun)	decreasing the angle between bones (bending a joint)
	plantar **flex**ion (PLAN tar FLEK shun)	bending of the sole of the foot by curling the toes downward toward the ground
ili (flank, groin)	**ili**um (ILL ee um)	the upper, wing-shaped bone of the pelvic girdle
ischi (haunch, hip joint)	**ischi**um (ISS kee um)	the inferior bone of the pelvic girdle
menisc (crescent-shaped moon)	**menisc**us (men ISS kuss)	a crescent-shaped cartilage that helps to stabilize joint movements; plural form is menisci
neur (cord or sinew)	apo**neur**osis (APP oh noo ROH siss)	a flattened tendon, it functions as a fascia that joins muscles together or joins muscle to bone
oste (bone)	end**oste**um (ehn DOSS tee um)	a thin layer of connective tissue that lines the marrow cavity
	osteoblast (OSS tee oh blast)	a bone cell that is mobile and secretes bone matrix
	osteoclast (OSS tee oh klast)	a bone cell that dissolves bone matrix
	osteocyte (OSS tee oh sight)	a bone cell that is stationary, locked within bone matrix
	peri**oste**um (pair ee OSS tee um)	a thin layer of fibrous connective tissue that forms the outermost layer of a bone
pariet (wall)	**pariet**al bones (pah RYE eh tal)	part of the skull, two bones at the top of the head
patell (small pan)	**patell**a (pah TELL ah)	the bone that forms the kneecap
phalang (row of soldiers)	**phalang**es of the fingers (fah LAN jeez)	the small narrow bones of the fingers; singular form is phalanx (FA lanks)
	phalanges of the toes (fah LAN jeez)	the small narrow bones of the toes
physis (growth)	dia**physis** (dye AFF ih siss)	the long, narrow shaft portion of long bones
	epi**physis** (eh PIFF ih siss)	the end of a long bone
pub (grown up)	**pub**is (PYOO biss)	the anterior part of the pelvic girdle
	symphysis **pub**is (SIM fih siss PYOO biss)	a cartilaginous joint that is the point of fusion for two pubic bones

Word Root (Meaning)	Terms Formed from the Word Root (Pronunciation)	Definition
radi (spoke of a wheel)	**radi**us (RAY dee us)	the bone of the forearm (lower arm) that is in line with the thumb
sacr (sacred, sacrum)	**sacr**um (SAK rum)	four vertebrae that fuse in early childhood into a single bone forming the dorsal wall of the pelvis
skelet (dried up)	appendicular **skelet**on (app en DIK yoo lahr SKELL eh ton)	a division of the skeleton that includes the bones of the appendages and pectoral and pelvic girdles
	axial **skelet**on (AK see al SKELL eh ton)	a division of the skeleton that includes the bones that are located along or near the central vertical axis of the body; it includes the bones of the skull and the bones of the thoracic cage
	skeletal muscle (SKELL eh tal)	the muscle tissue that forms the muscles attached to bones
stern (chest)	**stern**um (STER num)	the breastplate
synov, synovi (binding of eggs; synovial)	**synovi**al joint (sin OH vee al)	a joint containing synovial fluid within a sac of connective tissue allowing for the most movement between bones relative to fibrous joints and cartilaginous joints
	synovial fluid (sin OH vee al)	the fluid produced by the synovial membrane, which provides lubrication and a shock-absorbing cushion in synovial joints
tars (flat surface)	meta**tars**us (mett ah TAR suss)	the bones of the foot; also called the metatarsal bones
	tarsus (TAR suss)	the bones of the ankle; also called the tarsal bones
ten, tend, tendin (to stretch out, tendon)	**tend**on (TEN dunn)	a band of fibrous tissue that connects muscle to bone
vers (turn)	e**vers**ion (ee VER zhun)	turning a body part outward
	in**vers**ion (in VER zhun)	turning a body part inward
vertebr (a joint, vertebra)	cervical **vertebr**ae (SER vih kal VER teh bray)	the first seven bones of the vertebral column, numbered C1 to C7 from superior to inferior
	inter**vertebr**al disc (in ter VER teh bral)	fibrocartilaginous disc located between vertebrae
	lumbar **vertebr**ae (LUM bar VER teh bray)	five vertebrae of the lower spine, numbered L1 to L5
	thoracic **vertebr**ae (tho RASS ik VER teh bray)	12 vertebrae of the thorax, numbered T1 to T12; each one articulates with a pair of ribs
	vertebral column (VER teh bral)	the spinal column; 31 vertebrae in a linear formation

OTHER IMPORTANT TERMS

The terms in this table are related to the structure and function of the skeletal and muscular systems, but are not built from word roots covered in this chapter.

clavicles (KLAV ih klz)	the two collarbones
coccyx (KOK six)	three to five fused vertebrae that form the tailbone; plural form is **coccyges** (KOK si jes)
compact bone	bone tissue (connective tissue) consisting of compacted, hardened mineral salts and collagen arranged in circular layers around a central canal
depression (dee PREH shun)	lowering a body part
elevation (ell eh VAY shun)	raising a body part
extension (eks TEN shun)	increasing the angle between bones (straightening a joint)
frontal bone	part of the skull, the bone of the forehead
humerus (HYOO mer uss)	the bone of the brachium (upper arm)
lacrimal bones	two facial bones between each orbit and the nose
ligament (LIGG ah ment)	tough bands of fibrous connective tissue that stabilize joints
lower limbs	the two legs, left and right
mandible (MAN dih bl)	the lower jaw bone
marrow cavity (MAIR oh)	an internal chamber within the diaphysis; also called the medullary (MED yoo lar ee) cavity
maxilla (mak SIH lah)	the upper jaw bone of the face
nasal bones (NAY zl)	two facial bones forming the bridge of the nose
pronation (proh NAY shun)	turning the palm downward
red bone marrow (MAIR oh)	soft, gel-like connective tissue within spongy bone where blood cells are manufactured
rotation (roh TAY shun)	turning a bone on its own axis
scapula (SKAP yoo lah)	the bone forming the shoulder blade
spongy bone	bone tissue consisting of thin plates of hardened bone forming an interlocking meshwork, with blood-rich, red bone marrow in between the plates; under a microscope, spongy bone looks like a sponge
supination (soo pin AY shun)	turning the palm upward

tibia (TIBB ee ah)	the larger of the two bones of the lower leg
ulna (ULL nah)	the lateral bone of the forearm, which is not in line with the thumb
upper limbs	the two arms, right and left
vomer (VOH mer)	a facial bone forming part of the nasal septum
xiphoid process (ZIGH foyd)	cartilage located at the lower end of the sternum, which attaches to the diaphragm
yellow bone marrow (MAIR oh)	connective tissue rich in fat, which occupies the marrow cavity of bones
zygomatic bones (zigh goh MATT ik)	two facial bones forming part of each cheek

SELF QUIZ 5.2

SAY IT—SPELL IT!

Success Hint: Use the audio glossary on the CD and CW for additional help with pronunciation of these terms.

Review the terms of the skeletal system by speaking the phonetic pronunciation out loud, then writing in the correct spelling of the term.

1. dye AFF ih siss   _____

2. eh PIFF ih siss   _____

3. pair ee OSS tee um   _____

4. ehn DOSS tee um   _____

5. KRAY nee um   _____

6. SFEE noyd   _____

7. zigh goh MATT ik   _____

8. app en DIK yoo lahr   _____

9. KLAV ih klz   _____

10. SKAP yoo lah   _____

11. fah LAN jeez   _____

12. ISS kee um   _____

13. sin OH vee al   _____

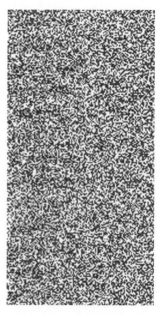

MATCH IT!

Match the term on the left with the correct definition on the right.

_____ 1. eversion

_____ 2. muscle

_____ 3. fascia

_____ 4. lumbar vertebrae

_____ 5. flexion

_____ 6. skeletal

_____ 7. skeletal muscle

_____ 8. muscle fiber

_____ 9. extension

_____10. pronation

_____11. adduction

_____12. tendon

_____13. xiphoid process

_____14. rotation

a. straightening the arm or leg

b. tissue that forms the "meat" of a muscle

c. Greek for withered, dried up

d. turning the palms downward

e. turning a body part outward

f. a skeletal muscle cell

g. connective tissue covering of muscle

h. moving your arm to your side

i. a tough connection between muscle and bone

j. an organ that moves bones

k. L1 to L5

l. turning a bone on its axis

m. bending the arm at the elbow

n. cartilage located at the lower end of the sternum

BREAK IT DOWN!

Analyze and separate each term into its word parts by labeling each word part using p = prefix, r = root, cv = combining vowel, and s = suffix.

1. endosteum   _____

2. periosteum   _____

3. diaphysis   _____

4. epiphysis   _____

5. osteocyte   _____

WORD BUILDING

Construct or recall medical terms from the following meanings.

1. cartilage found only in synovial joints   _____

2. fluid-filled sac that provides a cushion   _____

3. bones of the ankle   _____

4. bones of the wrist   _____

5. allows some movement between bones   _____

6. turning the distal end of a bone in a circle   _____

7. the bones of the face   _____

8. allows very little or no movement between bones

    _____

9. the smaller of the two bones of the lower leg

    _____

10. bending of foot or toes upward   _____

11. bending of the sole of the foot by curling the toes downward

    _____

12. facial bones between each orbit and the nose

    _____

13. the lower jaw facial bone   _____

14. crescent-shaped cartilage within the knee

    _____

15. the bone at the back of the cranium   _____

16. bones of the shoulder area   _____

17. three, fused bones that together form the pelvis

    _____

18. anterior part of the pelvic girdle   _____

19. a bone in line with the thumb   _____

20. T1 to T12   _____

21. the spinal column   _____

22. the tailbone   _____

23. bone tissue made of compacted, hardened mineral salts and collagen

    _____

24. the bone of the forehead   _____

25. the bridge of the nose   _____

FILL IT IN!

Fill in the blanks with the correct terms.

1. When skeletal and muscular systems are combined into a common treatment

    program, they are jointly referred to as the _____ system.

2. The skeletal system functions in _____ of body structures,

    protection of organs, assistance in moving, blood cell formation, and mineral

    _____.

3. A movement turning the palm upward is called _____.

4. The _____ is the kneecap named for its resemblance to a small pan.

5. A bone consists of two types of bone tissue, compact bone and

    _____ bone.

6. Bone matrix is composed of mineral salts and _____, produced

    by _____ and osteoblasts. A third type of bone cell dissolves the

    bone matrix. These cells are called _____.

7. _____ bone marrow is a soft, gel-like connective tissue within

    spongy bone where blood cells are manufactured.

8. A tendon attaches a bone to a _____, whereas a band of connective tissue that connects a bone to another bone is a _____.

9. The muscular system performs two important functions: _____, and the generation of _____.

5.5 10. In addition to skeletal muscle fibers, a muscle is composed of connective tissue coverings known as _____. These coverings converge at the end of a muscle to form a tough _____, which attaches to bone.

5.6 11. Bone has a very _____ quality, giving it a rock-like strength.

12. Moving your arm away from your body's side is an action called _____.

13. When you lower a body part it is called _____, but when you raise a body part it is called _____.

medical terms of the

skeletal and muscular systems

The diseases of the skeletal and muscular systems are often the result of physical injury, but may also be caused by infections, tumor development, and inherited disorders. The branch of medicine that focuses on these diseases is known as **orthopedics,** which is commonly abbreviated to **ortho.** The term "orthopedic" is a constructed word that can be shown as

orth/o/ped/ic

where the root word orth is derived from the Greek word, *orthos,* which means *straight.* The root word ped is also from the Greek, and means *child.* The suffix, -ic, as we learned earlier, means *pertaining to.* A physician specializing in orthopedics is known as an **orthopedist.**

In "Getting to the Root of It" in the previous section, you saw how learning just one word root helps you to understand some of the anatomy and physiology terms. Now, we will take you a step further, and show you that, by adding a combining vowel to those word roots to make a combining form, then using a prefix and suffix, you can form many of the medical terms related to the skeletal and muscular systems. You are on your way to mastery of the medical terms related to the skeletal and muscular systems!

[FYI]

Orthopedic
Orthopedic is a term first used by French physician Dr. Nicholas Andry in 1791 while addressing the childhood diseases polio, rickets, and osteomyelitis, each of which left children with skeletal deformities. Literally, the term means *to straighten a child.*

let's construct terms!

In this section, we will assemble all of the word parts to construct medical terminology related to the skeletal and muscular systems. Abbreviations are used to indicate each word part: **p** = prefix, **r** = root, **cv** = combining vowel, and **s** = suffix. Note that some terms are not constructed from word parts, but they are included here to expand your vocabulary.

The medical terms of the skeletal and muscular systems are listed in the following three sections:

- Symptoms and Signs
- Diseases and Disorders
- Treatments, Procedures, and Devices

Each section is followed by review exercises. Study the lists in these tables and complete the review exercises that follow.

Symptoms and Signs

WORD PARTS (WHEN APPLICABLE)			TERM	DEFINITION
Part	**Type**	**Meaning**		
arthr	r	joint	**arthralgia**	pain in a joint
-algia	s	pain	(ahr THRAL jee ah)	
a-	p	without	**ataxia**	an inability to coordinate muscles while executing
taxi	r	reaction to a stimulus	(ah TAK see ah)	a voluntary movement
-a	s	singular		
a-	p	without	**atrophy**	lacking development, or wasting
-trophy	s	development	(AT roh fee)	
brady-	p	slow	**bradykinesia**	abnormally slow movement
kinesi	r	motion	(BRAD ee kih NEE see ah)	
-a	s	singular		
dys-	p	bad, abnormal	**dyskinesia**	difficulty in movement
kinesi	r	motion	(dis kih NEE see ah)	
-a	s	singular		
dys-	p	bad, abnormal	**dystrophy**	deformities arising during development
-trophy	s	development	(DISS troh fee)	
hyper-	p	excessive	**hypertrophy**	excessive development
-trophy	s	development	(high PER troh fee)	
my	r	muscle	**myalgia**	muscle tenderness or pain
-algia	s	pain	(my AL jee ah)	
ten/o	r/cv	tendon	**tenodynia**	pain in a tendon
-dynia	s	pain	(TEN oh DINN ee ah)	

SELF QUIZ 5.3

SAY IT—SPELL IT!

5.7 1. my AL jee ah

  2. BRAD ee kih NEE see ah

  3. dis kih NEE see ah

  4. ahr THRAL jee ah

  5. high PER troh fee

  6. AT roh fee

  7. ah TAK see ah

  8. TEN oh DINN ee ah

BREAK IT DOWN!

Analyze and separate each term into its word parts by labeling each word part using p = prefix, r = root, cv = combining vowel, and s = suffix.

  1. arthralgia

  2. ataxia

  3. atrophy

  4. bradykinesia

  5. dyskinesia

  6. dystrophy

  7. hypertrophy

  8. myalgia

  9. tenodynia

FILL IT IN!

Fill in the blanks with the correct terms.

5.8 1. The inability to coordinate voluntary muscle movements is _____.

  2. A pain in a joint is generally referred to as _____.

  3. An abnormally slow movement is called _____.

  4. Difficulty in movement is known as _____.

  5. A deformity arising during development is called a _____.

  6. A pain that arises from a tendon is called _____.

  7. A muscle tenderness or pain is a _____.

Diseases and Disorders

Part	Type	Meaning	TERM	DEFINITION
a- chondr/o -plasia	p r/cv s	without cartilage shape, formation	**achondroplasia** (ah kon droh PLAY zee ah)	abnormal, slow growth of long bones resulting in unusually short, stocky limbs (Figure 5.8▦)
ankyl -osis	r s	crooked condition of	**ankylosis** (an kill OH siss)	abnormal condition of joint stiffness
arthr -itis	r s	joint inflammation	**arthritis** (ahr THRYE tiss)	inflammation and degeneration of a joint
athr/o chondr -itis	r/cv r s	joint cartilage inflammation	**arthrochondritis** (AHR throh kon DRY tiss)	inflammation of cartilages within joints
			bunion (BUN yun)	abnormal enlargement of the joint at the base of the big toe

[FYI]

Bunion

The term, *bunion,* is derived from the Old French word, *buigne,* which means a swelling caused by a blow to the head. However, the modern meaning is limited to a swelling of the big toe. It is often caused by wearing shoes that are too tight, producing friction on the big toe causing the joint to swell.

Part	Type	Meaning	TERM	DEFINITION
burs -itis	r s	purse or sac inflammation	**bursitis** (ber SIGH tiss)	inflammation of a bursa
burs/o -lith	r/cv r	purse or sac stone	**bursolith** (BER soh lith)	a calcium deposit (or stone) within a bursa
carp -al	r s	wrist pertaining to	**carpal tunnel syndrome** (KAR pal TUNN el SIN drohm)	repetitive stress injury in which the nerves of the wrist generate pain impulses due to inflammation of synovial sheaths; abbreviated **CTS** (Figure 5.9▦)
carp/o -ptosis	r/cv s	wrist falling down	**carpoptosis** (KAR poh TOH siss)	drooping of the wrist; also called wrist drop
chondr/o -malacia	r/cv s	cartilage softening	**chondromalacia** (kon droh mah LAY she ah)	deterioration or softening of cartilage
			cramps	prolonged, involuntary muscular contractions
crani/o -schisis	r/cv s	skull, cranium split, fissure	**cranioschisis** (KRAY nee OSS kih siss)	a congenital fissure of the skull
disk -itis	r s	disk inflammation	**diskitis** (diss KYE tiss)	inflammation of an intervertebral disk
dys- -trophy	p s	bad, abnormal development	**Duchenne's muscular dystrophy** (doo SHENZ)	a congenital condition resulting in progressive muscular weakness and deterioration; abbreviated **DMD**
epi- condyl -itis	p r s	upon knuckle of a joint inflammation	**epicondylitis** (ep ih kon dih LYE tiss)	inflammation of the cartilages of the elbow

WORD PARTS (WHEN APPLICABLE)			TERM	DEFINITION
Part	**Type**	**Meaning**		

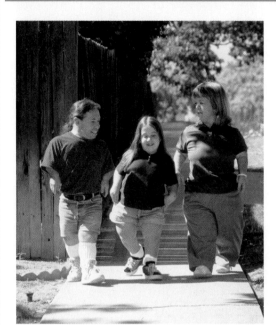

Figure 5.8 :::: **Achondroplasia.** Three achondroplastic dwarfs are shown in this photograph, the condition of which is characterized by reduced height and short limbs.

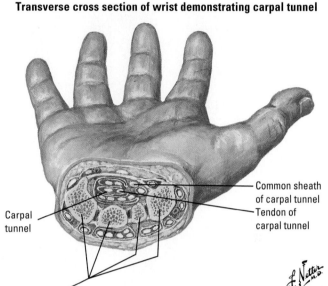

Transverse cross section of wrist demonstrating carpal tunnel

Common sheath of carpal tunnel

Tendon of carpal tunnel

Carpal tunnel

Bones of the wrist (carpal bones)

Figure 5.9 :::: **Carpal tunnel syndrome.** The inflammation and pain in the wrist that characterize CTS is produced when the synovial sheaths surrounding the tendons of the hand muscles, shown in this illustration of a section through a wrist, swell due to repetitive use. The swelling presses on the median nerve, which passes through the tunnel, to cause local pain. *Source: Icon Learning Systems.*

			fracture (FRAK sher)	a break in a bone (see Figure 5.19)
			gout (GOWT)	abnormal deposition of uric acid crystals in the joints (usually the big toe joints), causing localized pain (Figure 5.10::::); also called gouty arthritis

[FYI]

Gout

The term, *gout,* is derived from the Latin word *gutta,* which means *a drop.* The foot pain that characterizes gout was thought to be caused by a body fluid dripping internally onto the joint. It was a malady common to European aristocracy prior to the 20th century, made worse by poor dietary habits that included salty foods.

			herniated disk (HER nee ay ted)	a rupture of an intervertebral disk, resulting in the protrusion of tissue against spinal nerves, which generates pain (Figure 5.11::::)
kyph -osis	r s	hump condition of	**kyphosis** (kih FOH siss)	a deformity of the spine characterized by the presence of a hump; also called hunchback (Figure 5.12::::)

WORD PARTS (WHEN APPLICABLE)			TERM	DEFINITION
Part	Type	Meaning		

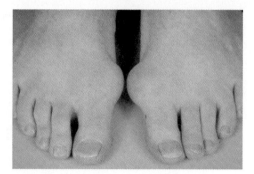

Figure 5.10 ::::

Gout. Also known as gouty arthritis, it often strikes the big toe, as seen in this photograph.
Source: Reprinted from the Clinical Slide Collection on the Rheumatic Diseases, © 1991, 1995. Used by permission of the American College of Rheumatology.

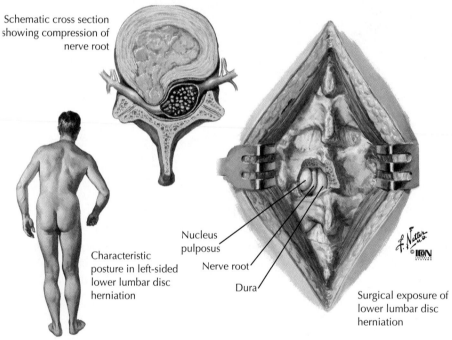

Schematic cross section showing compression of nerve root

Characteristic posture in left-sided lower lumbar disc herniation

Nucleus pulposus

Nerve root

Dura

Surgical exposure of lower lumbar disc herniation

Figure 5.11 ::::

Herniated disk. A herniated disk is a protrusion of the disk's liquid center, called the nucleus pulposus, which often pushes into the spinal cord to cause pain and loss of movement (upper left). In the diagram on the right, a surgeon must cut through the skin and muscles of the back, and often into the vertebra, in order to access the lesion. *Source: Icon Learning Systems.*

Part	Type	Meaning	TERM	DEFINITION
later	r	side	**lateral epicondylitis** (LAT er al ep ih kon dih LYE tiss)	inflammation of the lateral tendon of the elbow; also called tennis elbow
-al	s	pertaining to		
epi-	p	upon		
condyl	r	knuckle of a joint		
-itis	s	inflammation		
lord	r	bent forward	**lordosis** (lor DOH siss)	a deformity of the spine characterized by an anterior curve of the lumbar area (Figure 5.12)
-osis	s	condition of		
			Marfan's syndrome (mahr FAHNZ SIN drohm)	inherited condition resulting in excessive cartilage formation at the epiphyseal plates, forming long arms and legs

WORD PARTS (WHEN APPLICABLE)			TERM	DEFINITION
Part	Type	Meaning		

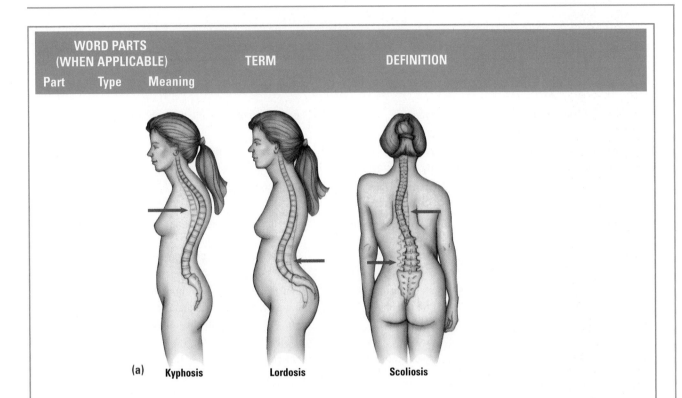

(a) Kyphosis   Lordosis   Scoliosis

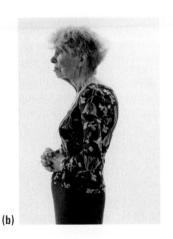

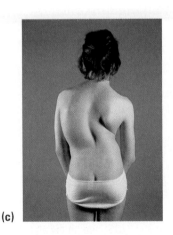

(b)   (c)

Figure 5.12 ::::

Spinal disfigurements.
(a) Spinal disfigurements compared to normal spinal curves.
(b) Kyphosis. A woman with kyphosis (back hump), which has formed as a result of osteoporosis.
(c) Scoliosis. A lateral curvature of the spine; this example is a relatively severe case that requires treatment by immobilization and surgery.

Part	Type	Meaning	TERM	DEFINITION
maxill	r	upper jaw	**maxillitis**	inflammation of the maxilla
-itis	s	inflammation	(mak sill EYE tiss)	
menisc	r	crescent-shaped moon	**meniscitis** (MEN iss EYE tiss)	inflammation of a meniscus
-itis	s	inflammation		
my	r	muscle	**myasthenia gravis**	weakness in the muscles
-asthenia	s	weakness	(my ass THEE nee ah)	
myel	r	bone marrow	**myeloma**	a malignant tumor of bone marrow
-oma	s	tumor	(my ah LOH mah)	
my/o	r/cv	muscle	**myoclonus**	a spasm or twitching of a muscle or muscle group
clon	r	spasm	(my oh KLOH nus)	
-us	s	in motion		

WORD PARTS (WHEN APPLICABLE)			TERM	DEFINITION
Part	**Type**	**Meaning**		
my/o	r/cv	muscle	**myocele**	protrusion of a muscle through its fascia
-cele	s	protrusion	(my oh SELL)	
myos	r	muscle	**myositis**	inflammation of muscle tissue
-itis	s	inflammation	(my oh SYE tiss)	
oste	r	bone	**osteitis**	inflammation of a bone
-itis	s	inflammation	(OSS tee EYE tiss)	
oste	r	bone	**osteitis deformans**	viral infection of bone that causes deformities of the
-itis	s	inflammation	(OSS tee EYE tiss	skeleton resulting from the acceleration of bone
deformans		deformity (French)	day for MANZ)	loss; also called Paget's disease
oste/o	r/cv	bone	**osteoarthritis**	a form of arthritis characterized by an age-related
athr	r	joint	(OSS tee oh ahr THRYE tiss)	deterioration of joints that is accompanied by
-itis	s	inflammation		erosion of cartilage and painful inflammation (Figure 5.13▒)
oste/o	r/cv	bone	**osteocarcinoma**	cancer of bone
carcin	r	cancer	(OSS tee oh kar sih OH mah)	
-oma	s	tumor		
oste/o	r/cv	bone	**osteochondritis**	inflammation of bone and associated cartilage
chondr	r	cartilage	(OSS tee oh kon DRY tiss)	
-itis	s	inflammation		
oste/o	r/cv	bone	**osteofibroma**	a benign tumor of bone, in which the tumor contains
fibr	r	fiber	(OSS tee oh fye BROH mah)	fibrous connective tissue that surrounds bone
-oma	s	tumor		
oste/o	r/cv	bone	**osteogenesis**	an inherited condition resulting in impaired growth
-genesis	s	origin, cause	**imperfecta**	and fragile bones, leading to progressive skeletal
im-	p	opposite of	(OSS tee oh JENN eh siss	deformation and frequent fractures
perfect	r	perfect	im per FEK tah)	
-a	s	singular		
oste/o	r/cv	bone	**osteomalacia**	a gradual and painful softening of bones
-malacia	s	softening	(OSS tee oh mah LAY she ah)	
oste/o	r/cv	bone	**osteomyelitis**	a painful bone infection caused by bacteria,
myel	r	bone marrow	(OSS tee oh my eh LYE tiss)	characterized by inflammation of the red bone
-itis	s	inflammation		marrow
oste/o	r/cv	bone	**osteonecrosis**	death of bone tissue
necr	r	death	(OSS tee oh neh KROH siss)	
-osis	s	condition of		
oste/o	r/cv	bone	**osteopetrosis**	excessive formation of dense bone, which crowds
petr	r	stone	(OSS tee oh peh TROH siss)	out marrow cavities and leads to cutting off blood
-osis	s	condition of		supply to bone; also known as marble bone
oste/o	r/cv	bone	**osteoporosis**	abnormal loss of bone density (Figure 5.14▒)
por	r	small hole	(OSS tee oh por ROH siss)	
-osis	s	condition of		
oste/o	r/cv	bone	**osteosarcoma**	cancer of bone (Figure 5.15▒)
sarc	r	flesh, meat	(OSS tee oh sar KOH mah)	
-oma	s	tumor		

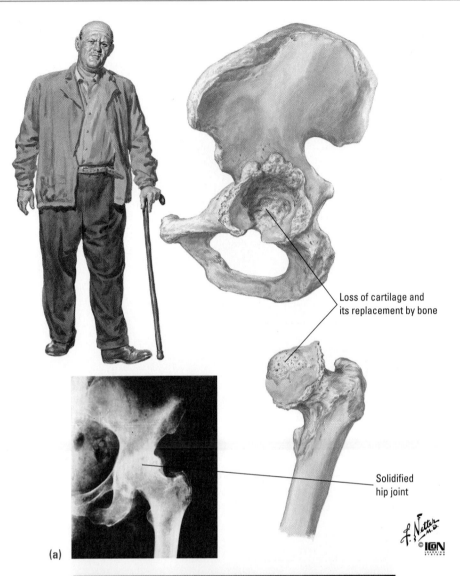

Loss of cartilage and
its replacement by bone

Solidified
hip joint

(a)

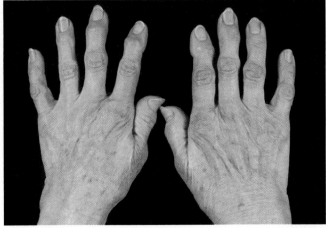

(b)

Figure 5.13

Osteoarthritis.

(a) Osteoarthritis is a common disease of old age, resulting from the deterioration of cartilage within synovial joints. In this illustration, the elderly patient has difficulty walking because the cartilage of the hip joint has been replaced by bone.
Source: Icon Learning Systems
(b) Photograph of osteoarthritis within the joints of the hand.
Source: L. Samsuri/Custom Medical Stock Photo.

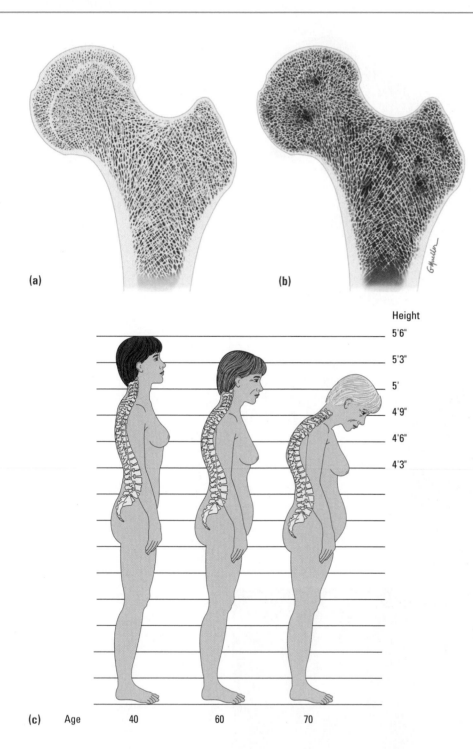

(a)

(b)

(c)   Age   40   60   70

Height
5'6"
5'3"
5'
4'9"
4'6"
4'3"

Figure 5.14 ::::
Osteoporosis.
(a) Normal spongy bone.
(b) Spongy bone with osteoporosis, which is characterized by a loss of bone material.
(c) Spinal curvatures resulting from osteoporosis of the vertebral column.
Source: Pearson Education.

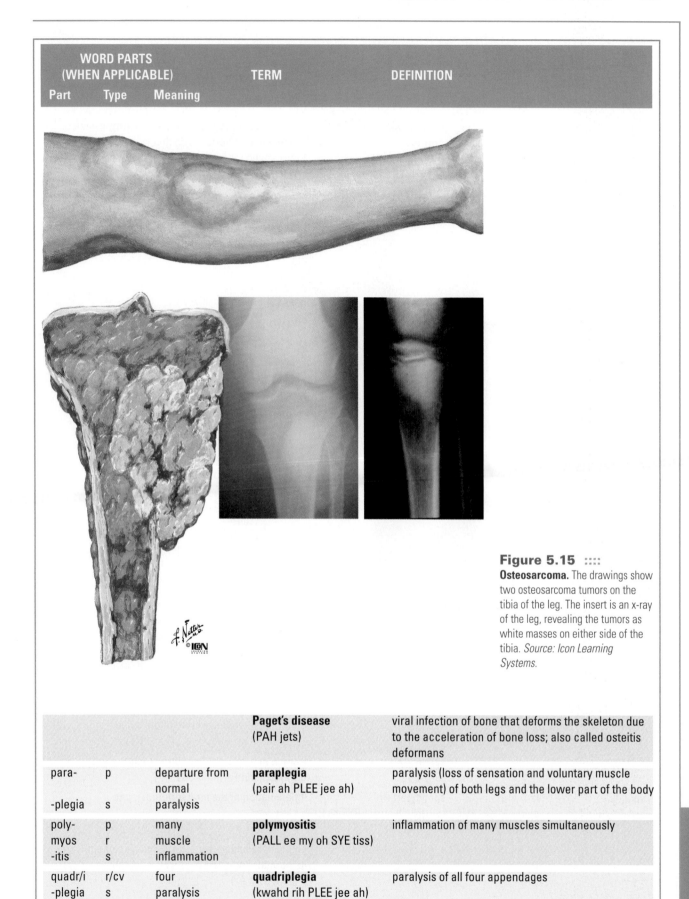

WORD PARTS (WHEN APPLICABLE)			TERM	DEFINITION
Part	Type	Meaning		
			Paget's disease (PAH jets)	viral infection of bone that deforms the skeleton due to the acceleration of bone loss; also called osteitis deformans
para-	p	departure from normal	**paraplegia** (pair ah PLEE jee ah)	paralysis (loss of sensation and voluntary muscle movement) of both legs and the lower part of the body
-plegia	s	paralysis		
poly-	p	many	**polymyositis** (PALL ee my oh SYE tiss)	inflammation of many muscles simultaneously
myos	r	muscle		
-itis	s	inflammation		
quadr/i	r/cv	four	**quadriplegia** (kwahd rih PLEE jee ah)	paralysis of all four appendages
-plegia	s	paralysis		

Figure 5.15 ::::
Osteosarcoma. The drawings show two osteosarcoma tumors on the tibia of the leg. The insert is an x-ray of the leg, revealing the tumors as white masses on either side of the tibia. *Source: Icon Learning Systems.*

WORD PARTS (WHEN APPLICABLE)			TERM	DEFINITION
Part	Type	Meaning		
rheumat	r	discharge	**rheumatoid**	a form of arthritis characterized by progressive,
-oid	s	resemblance to	**arthritis**	gradual joint deterioriation that is caused by an
arthr	r	joint	(ROO mah toyd	autoimmune response; abbreviated **RA** (Figure 5.16::::)
-itis	s	inflammation	ahr THRYE tiss)	

Joint Pathology in Rheumatoid Arthritis

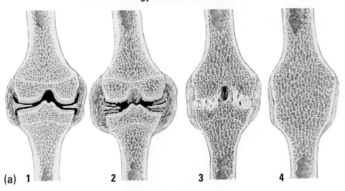

(a) 1   2   3   4

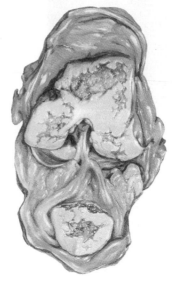

(b)

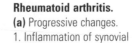

Figure 5.16 ::::

Rheumatoid arthritis.
(a) Progressive changes.
1. Inflammation of synovial membrane
2. Progression of inflammation and beginning of cartilage destruction.
3. Complete loss of synovial membrane, which leads to fibrous tissue.
4. Advanced stage of complete joint loss and osteoporosis.
(b) A knee joint opened at the front reveals a large erosion of articular cartilage of the femur and patella.
Source: Icon Learning Systems.

scoli	r	curved	**scoliosis**	abnormal lateral curvature of the spine (Figure 5.12)
-osis	s	condition of	(SKOH lee OH siss)	
			spinal cord injury	trauma to the spinal cord often resulting in
			(SPY nal)	paralysis; abbreviated **SCI**
spondyl	r	vertebra	**spondylarthritis**	inflammation of the intervertebral joints
arthr	r	joint	(SPON dill ahr THRYE tiss)	
-itis	s	inflammation		
			sprain	an injury resulting from stretching a ligament beyond its normal range, tearing its collagen fibers (Figure 5.17::::)

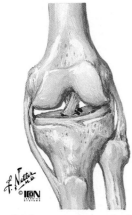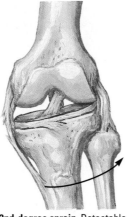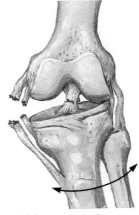

1st-degree sprain. Localized joint pain and tenderness but no joint laxity

2nd-degree sprain. Detectable joint laxity plus localized pain and tenderness

3rd-degree sprain. Complete disruption of ligaments and gross joint instability

Figure 5.17 ::::

Sprain. A sprain involves damage to one or more ligaments, which are categorized into three degrees of injury as shown. *Source: Icon Learning Systems.*

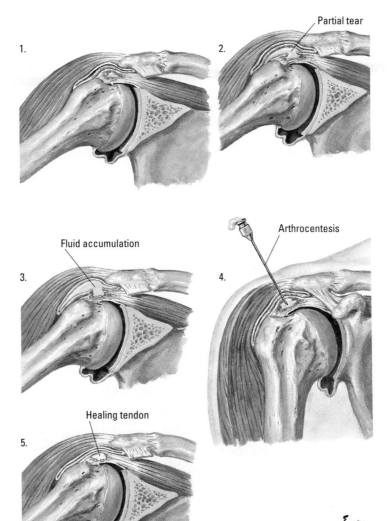

Partial tear

Fluid accumulation

Arthrocentesis

Healing tendon

Figure 5.18 ::::

Rotator cuff tendonitis. A normal rotator cuff can become injured by overuse or the physical tear of tendons. In this series of illustrations, the rotator cuff has torn, resulting in fluid accumulation within the tendon (upper two figures). Athrocentesis reduces the inflammation. *Source: Icon Learning Systems.*

WORD PARTS (WHEN APPLICABLE)			TERM	DEFINITION
Part	Type	Meaning		
			strain	an injury resulting from stretching a muscle beyond its normal range, tearing muscle tissue
synovi/o	r/cv	synovial	**synoviosarcoma** (sin OH vee oh sark KOH mah)	cancer of a synovial membrane in a joint
sarc	r	flesh, meat		
-oma	s	tumor		
tendon	r	tendon	**tendonitis** (TEN dunn EYE tiss)	inflammation of a tendon, such as rotator cuff tendonitis (pitcher's shoulder) (Figure 5.18::::)
-itis	s	inflammation		
ten/o	r/cv	tendon	**tenosynovitis** (TEN oh sin oh VYE tiss)	inflammation of a tendon and the synovial membrane that surrounds it
synov	r	synovial		
-itis	s	inflammation		

disease focus | Fractures

A fracture is a break in a bone. Because bones have a variety of shapes and densities and breaks can occur from a variety of circumstances, fractures may take on a wide range of forms. Overall, orthopedists describe fractures by their location or site, general qualities, and the external look of the break. Orthopedists use these characteristics to group fractures into primary and secondary categories. The two primary categories of fractures are:

■ **Closed,** also called **simple,** fractures are completely internal to the body.

■ **Open,** also called **compound,** fractures project through the skin, outside the body.

The terms that describe secondary categories of fractures are listed in Table 5.1::: and illustrated in Figure 5.19::::.

Many fractures fall into more than one category. For example, a closed or simple Colles fracture is an internal break in the distal part of the radius, and an open or compound Colles fracture is a break in the distal radius that penetrates through the skin. What other fractures do you think may fall into multiple groups?

Table 5.1 ::: **Secondary Categories of Fractures**

CATEGORY	DEFINITION
Colles (KOH leez)	a break in the distal part of the radius
comminuted (KOM ih noo ted)	a break resulting in fragmentation of the bone
compression (kom PREH shun)	a crushed break, often due to weight or pressure applied to a bone during a fall
displaced	a break causing an abnormal alignment of bone pieces
epiphyseal (eh PIFF ih see al)	a break at the location of the growth plate, which can affect growth of the bone
greenstick	a slight break in a bone that appears as a slight fissure in an x-ray
nondisplaced	a break in which the broken bones retain their alignment
Pott's	a break at the ankle that affects both bones of the leg
spiral	a spiral-shaped break often caused by twisting stresses along a long bone

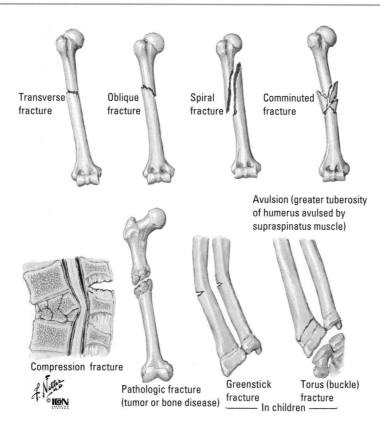

Transverse fracture

Oblique fracture

Spiral fracture

Comminuted fracture

Avulsion (greater tuberosity of humerus avulsed by supraspinatus muscle)

Compression fracture

Pathologic fracture (tumor or bone disease)

Greenstick fracture

Torus (buckle) fracture

——— In children ———

Figure 5.19 ::::
Bone fractures. *Source: Icon Learning Systems*

SELF QUIZ 5.4

SAY IT—SPELL IT!

Review the terms of the skeletal and muscular systems by speaking the phonetic pronunciation out loud, then writing the correct spelling of the term.

5.9   1.   ah kon droh PLAY zee ah   _____

5.10 2.   AHR throh kon DRY tiss   _____

3.   KAR poh TOH siss   _____

4.   KRAY nee OSS kih siss   _____

5.   ep ih kon dih LYE tiss   _____

6.   kih FOH siss   _____

7.   MEN iss EYE tiss   _____

8.   my oh co SEEL   _____

9.   OSS tee oh ahr THRYE tiss   _____

10.   OSS tee oh kon DRY tiss   _____

11.   OSS tee oh mah LAY she ah   _____

5.11 12.   PALL ee my oh SYE tiss   _____

13.   kwahd rih PLEE jee ah   _____

14.   SKOH lee OH siss   _____

15.   sin OH vee oh sark KOH mah   _____

16.   PAH jets   _____

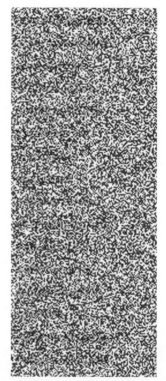

BREAK IT DOWN!

Analyze and separate each term into its word parts by labeling each word part using p = prefix, r = root, cv = combining vowel, and s = suffix.

1. arthrotomy   _____

2. cranioschisis   _____

3. myasthenia   _____

4. osteofibroma   _____

5. polymyositis   _____

6. lordosis   _____

FILL IT IN!

Fill in the blanks with the correct terms.

1. A calcium deposit or stone within a bursa is called a _____.

2. A serious infection within the joint cavity of the knee can result in a deterioration of the joint cartilage, called _____.

3. A child is occasionally born with a _____, or skull fissure.

4. A chronic inflammation of an intervertebral disk, or _____, can lead to a hunchback, or _____.

5. Inflammation of the cartilages of the elbow, or _____, is often accompanied with difficulty in moving the arm, or _____ of the arm.

6. Inflammation of muscle, or _____, is usually associated with muscle pain or _____.

7. A blow to the face can cause an inflammation of bone, or _____, and if the maxilla is involved, the condition known as _____.

8. _____ is a form of arthritis that is relatively common among senior patients.

9. Although the term _____ is derived from a word that means "swelling of the head," it is a painful swelling at the base of the big toe.

10. A fracture of the distal part of the radius is known as a _____ fracture, while a break at the ankle that involves the tibia and fibula is a _____ fracture.

11. An x-ray is required to confirm a _____ or closed fracture, while an open or _____ fracture is easy to identify during a physical exam.

12. A _____ fracture is a difficult type of fracture to stabilize.

5.12 13. A _____ fracture results from a twisting movement that exceeds the strength of the bone.

14. A fracture type that only affects children is the _____ fracture.

15. A congenital condition that results in progressive myasthenia and deterioration is called DMD, or _____ muscular dystrophy.

16. A laminectomy is sometimes prescribed in severe cases of a _____ disk.

17. Some historians believe Abraham Lincoln may have suffered from _____ syndrome, due to his abnormally long arms and legs and other possible signs.

18. Also known as osteitis deformans, _____ disease is an infection of bone that inhibits the activity of _____, or mobile bone producing cells.

5.13 19. A _____ is an injury to muscle tissue, whereas a

5.14 _____ is an injury resulting in the tear of collagen fibers within a ligament.

5.15 20. People who suffer from _____ experience _____ in the big toe.

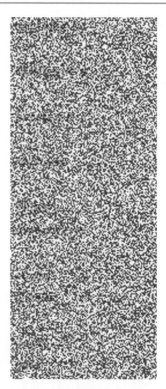

Treatments, Procedures, and Devices

WORD PARTS (WHEN APPLICABLE)			TERM	DEFINITION
Part	Type	Meaning		
arthr/o -centesis	r/cv s	joint puncture	**arthrocentesis** (AHR throh sen TEE siss)	surgical puncture of a joint to aspirate (suction) fluids from the synovial cavity (Figure 5.20 ::::)
arthr/o -clasia	r/cv s	joint break apart	**arthroclasia** (ahr throh KLAY zee ah)	breaking of an abnormally stiff joint during surgery to increase range of motion
arthr/o -desis	r/cv s	joint surgical fixation	**arthrodesis** (AHR throh DEE siss)	surgical fixation (stabilization) of a joint
arthr/o gram	r/cv s	joint recording	**arthrogram** (AHR throh gram)	x-ray film of a joint after injection of air, contrast media, or both

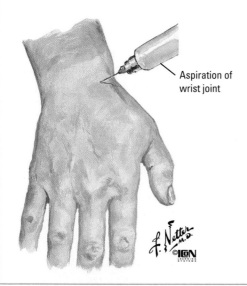

Aspiration of wrist joint

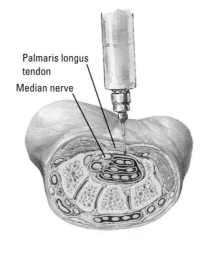

Palmaris longus tendon
Median nerve

Figure 5.20 ::::
Arthrocentesis. The aspiration of fluid is a common treatment for joint injuries resulting in inflammation, such as carpal tunnel syndrome in this illustration. *Source: Icon Learning Systems.*

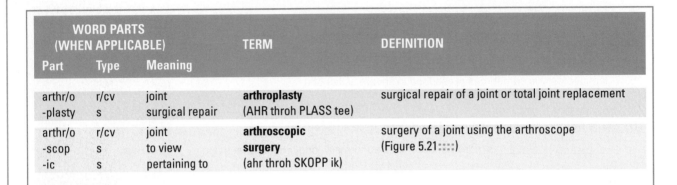

WORD PARTS (WHEN APPLICABLE)			TERM	DEFINITION
Part	**Type**	**Meaning**		
arthr/o	r/cv	joint	**arthroplasty**	surgical repair of a joint or total joint replacement
-plasty	s	surgical repair	(AHR throh PLASS tee)	
arthr/o	r/cv	joint	**arthroscopic**	surgery of a joint using the arthroscope
-scop	s	to view	**surgery**	(Figure 5.21 ::::)
-ic	s	pertaining to	(ahr throh SKOPP ik)	

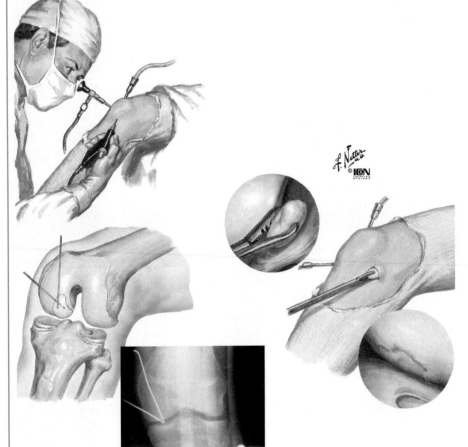

Figure 5.21 ::::

Arthroscopic surgery.
Arthroscopic surgery involves the surgery of a joint with the use of a flexible arthroscope and other surgical tools. In this example, the surgeon inserts the arthroscope to evaluate the damage, then uses instruments to excise a tumor from the knee joint. *Source: Icon Learning Systems.*

arthr/o	r/cv	joint	**arthroscopy**	endoscopic visual examination of a joint cavity
-scopy	s	process of viewing	(ahr THROSS koh pee)	using a fiber optic instrument, called the arthroscope
athr/o	r/cv	joint	**arthrotomy**	surgical incision into a joint
-tomy	s	incision	(ahr THROTT oh mee)	
burs	r	purse or sac	**bursectomy**	excision (surgical removal) of a bursa
-ectomy	s	excision	(ber SEK toh mee)	
burs/o	r/cv	purse or sac	**bursotomy**	surgical incision into a bursa
-tomy	s	incision	(ber SOTT oh mee)	
chir/o	r/cv	hand	**chiropractic**	a field of therapy that mainly involves manipulation of
-practic	s	practice	(KIGH roh PRAK tik)	the vertebral column
chir/o	r/cv	hand	**chiropractor**	a specialist in chiropractic
-practor	s	one who practices	(KIGH roh PRAK tor)	

WORD PARTS (WHEN APPLICABLE)			TERM	DEFINITION
Part	Type	Meaning		
chondr	r	cartilage	**chondrectomy**	excision of a joint cartilage
-ectomy	s	excision	(kon DREK toh mee)	
chondr/o	r/cv	cartilage	**chondroplasty**	surgical repair of a joint cartilage
-plasty	s	surgical repair	(KON droh plass tee)	
cost	r	rib	**costectomy**	excision of a rib
-ectomy	s	excision	(koss TEK toh mee)	
crani/o	r/cv	skull, cranium	**cranioplasty**	surgical repair of a defect in the cranium
-plasty	s	surgical repair	(KRAY nee oh plass tee)	
crani/o	r/cv	skull, cranium	**craniotomy**	surgical entry into the cranium
-tomy	s	incision	(KRAY nee OTT oh mee)	
disk	r	intervertebral disk	**diskectomy**	excision of an intervertebral disk
-ectomy	s	excision	(disk EK toh mee)	
electr/o	r/cv	electricity	**electromyography**	a diagnostic procedure that records the strength of muscle contraction; abbreviated **EMG** (Figure 5.22)
my/o	r/cv	muscle	(ee LEK troh my OG	
-graphy	s	recording process	rah fee)	

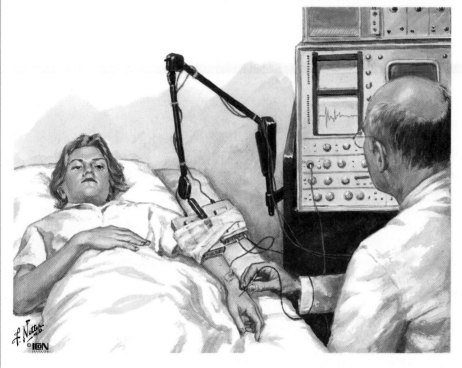

Figure 5.22

Electromyography. The procedure involves the application of electrical stimuli to muscles, which causes muscle contraction. As shown in this illustration, the data can be recorded onto a monitor and printed.
Source: Icon Learning Systems.

fasci/o	r/cv	fascia	**fasciotomy**	surgical incision into fascia
-tomy	s	incision	(FASH ee OTT oh mee)	
lamin	r	thin	**laminectomy**	excision of part of a vertebra known as the lamina, often as part of a treatment for a herniated (ruptured) disk
-ectomy	s	excision	(LAHM ih NEK toh mee)	
menisc	r	meniscus	**meniscectomy**	surgical removal of a meniscus
-ectomy	s	excision	(MEN ih SEK toh mee)	
my/o	r/cv	muscle	**myoplasty**	surgical repair of muscle tissue
-plasty	s	surgical repair	(MY oh plass tee)	

WORD PARTS (WHEN APPLICABLE)			TERM	DEFINITION
Part	**Type**	**Meaning**		
my/o	r/cv	muscle	**myorrhaphy**	closing a muscle with sutures
-rrhaphy	s	suturing	(my OR ah fee)	
orth/o	r/cv	straight	**orthotics**	construction and fitting of orthopedic appliances to
-tic	s	pertaining to	(or THOTT iks)	assist in patient movement, such as lifts, prosthetic
-s	s	plural		devices, etc.
orth/o	r/cv	straight	**orthotist**	a physician specializing in orthotics
-ist	s	one who practices	(OR thott ist)	
oste	r	bone	**ostectomy**	excision of bone
-ectomy	s	excision	(oss TEK toh mee)	
oste/o	r/cv	bone	**osteoclasis**	surgical breaking of a bone to correct a defect
-clasis	s	break apart	(OSS tee oh KLAY siss)	
oste/o	r/cv	bone	**osteopath**	a physician trained in osteopathy; abbreviated **OD**
-path	s	disease	(OSS tee oh path)	and also called an osteopathic surgeon
oste/o	r/cv	bone	**osteopathy**	a medical field that emphasizes the relationship
-pathy	s	disease	(OSS tee OPP ah thee)	between the musculoskeletal system and overall
				health with an emphasis on preventative medicine
oste/o	r/cv	bone	**osteoplasty**	surgical repair of bone
-plasty	s	surgical repair	(OSS tee oh plass tee)	
pod	r	foot	**podiatrist**	a physician trained in podiatry; also called a
-iatrist	s	one who practices in the field of	(poh DYE ah trist)	chiropodist
pod	r	foot	**podiatry**	medical field specializing in treating the foot
-iatry	s	field of	(poh DYE ah tree)	
			prosthesis	an artificial substitute for a missing body part such
			(pross THEE siss)	as a leg or hand
rachi/o	r/cv	vertebral column	**rachiotomy**	surgical incision into the vertebral column
-tomy	s	incision	(RAY kee OTT oh mee)	
			spinal fusion	surgical connection of adjacent vertebrae, usually
			(SPY nal	as a treatment for a herniated disk; also called
			FYOO zhun)	spondylosyndesis
spondyl/o	r/cv	vertebra	**spondylosyndesis**	surgically connecting adjacent vertebrae, commonly
syn	r	connect	(SPON dih loh sin DEE siss)	called spinal fusion
-desis	s	surgical fixation		
synov	r	synovial	**synovectomy**	excision of a joint's synovial membrane
-ectomy	s	excision	(sin oh VEK toh mee)	
ten/o	r/cv	tendon	**tenomyoplasty**	surgical repair of a muscle and its tendon
my/o	r/cv	muscle	(TEN oh MY oh plass tee)	
-plasty	s	surgical repair		
ten/o	r/cv	tendon	**tenorrhaphy**	closing a tendon with sutures
-rrhaphy	s	suturing	(ten OR ah fee)	
ten/o	r/cv	tendon	**tenotomy**	incision into a tendon
-tomy	s	incision	(ten OTT oh mee)	

SELF QUIZ 5.5

SAY IT—SPELL IT!

Review the terms of the skeletal and muscular systems by speaking the phonetic pronunciation out loud, then writing in the correct spelling of the term.

1. AHR throh sen TEE siss _____
2. ahr throh KLAY zee ah _____
3. AHR throh DEE siss _____
4. AHR throh PLASS tee _____
5. ahr THROSS koh pee _____
6. ber SEK toh mee _____
5.16 7. KIGH roh PRAK tik _____
8. kon DREK toh mee _____
9. koss TEK toh mee _____
10. KRAY nee oh plass tee _____
11. KRAY nee OTT oh mee _____
12. ee LEK troh my OG rah fee _____
13. FASH ee OTT oh mee _____
14. LAHM ih NEK toh mee _____
15. MEN ih SEK toh mee _____
16. my OR ah fee _____
5.17 17. OSS tee oh KLAY siss _____
18. OSS tee OPP ah thee _____
5.18 19. RAY kee OTT oh mee _____
20. SPON dih loh sin DEE siss _____
21. sin oh VEK toh mee _____
22. TEN oh MY oh plass tee _____
23. ten OR ah fee _____
24. poh DYE ah tree _____

MATCH IT!

Match the term on the left with the correct definition on the right.

_____1. arthrocentesis

_____2. arthrodesis

_____3. arthroplasty

_____4. arthroscopic surgery

_____5. bursectomy

_____6. chondroplasty

_____7. costectomy

_____8. craniotomy

_____9. electromyography

_____10. fasciotomy

_____11. laminectomy

_____12. meniscectomy

_____13. myorrhaphy

_____14. orthotics

_____15. osteoclasis

_____16. spondylosyndesis

_____17. synovectomy

_____18. tenomyoplasty

_____19. tenotomy

a. a spinal fusion

b. surgical removal of a bursa

c. excision of a rib

d. surgical puncture into a joint for aspiraton

e. incision into a tendon

f. surgical stabilization of a joint

g. closing a muscle with sutures

h. surgical breakage of a bone

i. surgical repair of a joint

j. excision of a meniscus

k. surgical repair of a muscle and its tendon

l. surgery of a joint using an arthroscope

m. surgical repair of a joint cartilage

n. incision into the cranium

o. surgical incision into fascia

p. abbreviated EMG

q. construction and fitting of orthopedic appliances

r. excision of a synovial membrane

s. excision of part of a vertebra

FILL IT IN!

Fill in the blanks with the correct terms.

5.19 1. A _____ is a specialist in manipulation of the vertebral column, while a physician specializing in treatments of the foot is a _____. The medical specialty focused on diseases of the skeletal and muscular systems is called _____, which literally means to straighten a child. A condition in a synovial joint may lead to bursitis, which can be diagnosed by an incision into the bursa, called a _____. If necessary, the bursa can be removed during a _____.

2. An injury to the knee can be observed using an endoscope during the _____ procedure. If the meniscus is found to be torn, it may be removed during a _____ procedure.

3. A severe injury to the head may require a _____ in an effort to relieve intracranial hemorrhage. If cranial bones require surgical correction, a _____ may become necessary.

4. In patients suffering from chronic muscle weakness or _____, an EMG or _____ may be used to determine the extent of the weakness.

5. During surgical intervention to stabilize a joint, called _____, breaking the damaged joint to increase range of motion, or _____, is sometimes necessary.

5.20 6. The surgical removal of a rib, or a _____, is necessary with severe thoracic injuries.

5.21 7. A _____, the excision of part of a vertebra, is often used to relieve pain that is caused by a _____ intervertebral disk. The procedure removes the _____ of the vertebra.

5.22 8. Spondylosyndesis includes the prefix _____, which means to join or come together.

9. Individuals who have lost body parts may obtain artificial _____.

10. The study of bones is known as _____, and the study of joints is called _____.

abbreviations of the skeletal and muscular systems

The abbreviations that are associated with the skeletal and muscular systems are summarized here. Study these abbreviations, and review them in the exercise that follows.

ABBREVIATION	DEFINITION	ABBREVIATION	DEFINITION
ACL	anterior cruciate ligament; a ligament that stabilizes the knee joint	ortho	orthopedics
		RA	rheumatoid arthritis
		ROM	range of motion
CTS	carpal tunnel syndrome	SCI	spinal cord injury
EMG	electromyogram	THR	total hip replacement
HNP	herniated nucleus pulposus; a herniated intervertebral disk	TKA	total knee arthroplasty
		TKR	total knee replacement
MG	myasthenia gravis	Vertebrae	
OA	osteoarthritis	C1 through C7	the seven cervical vertebrae
OD	physician specializing in osteopathy	T1 through T12	the twelve thoracic vertebrae
		L1 through L5	the five lumbar vertebrae

SELF QUIZ 5.6

Fill in the blanks with the abbreviation or the complete medical term.

Abbreviation   **Medical Term**

1. _____   spinal cord injury

2. TKA   _____

3. _____   rheumatoid arthritis

4. MG   _____

5. _____   herniated nucleus pulposus

6. EMG   _____

5.23   7. _____   anterior cruciate ligament

8. THR   _____

9. _____   the five lumbar vertebrae

10. CTS   _____

11. _____   range of motion

12. OA   _____

5.24   13. _____   total knee replacement

5.25   14. T1–T12   _____

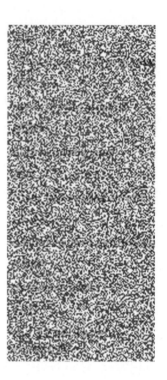

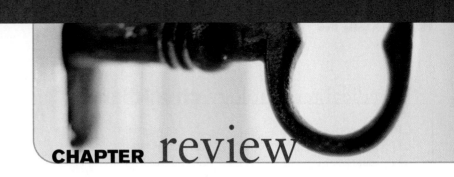

CHAPTER review

In this section, we will review all the word parts and medical terms from this chapter. As in earlier tables, the word roots are shown in **bold.**

Check each word part and medical term to be sure you understand the meaning. If any are not clear, please go back into the chapter and review that term. Then, complete the review exercises that follow.

[word parts **checklist**]

Prefixes

- ❏ a-
- ❏ an-
- ❏ dia-
- ❏ dys-
- ❏ end-, endo-
- ❏ epi-
- ❏ para-
- ❏ peri-
- ❏ poly-
- ❏ quad-
- ❏ sym-
- ❏ syn-

Word Roots/Combining Vowels

- ❏ **ankyl**/o
- ❏ **arthr**/o, **articul**/o
- ❏ **burs**/o
- ❏ **carp**/o
- ❏ **cartil**/o
- ❏ **cel**/o
- ❏ **chir**/o
- ❏ **chondr**/o
- ❏ **clon**/o
- ❏ **condyl**
- ❏ **cost**/o
- ❏ **cran**/o, **crani**/o
- ❏ **duct**/o
- ❏ **fasci**/o
- ❏ **femor**/o, **femur**/o

- ❏ **fibul**/o
- ❏ **ili**/o
- ❏ **ischi**/o
- ❏ **kinesi**/o
- ❏ **kyph**/o
- ❏ **lamin**/o
- ❏ **lord**/o
- ❏ **menisc**/o
- ❏ **myel**/o, **myelon**/o
- ❏ **my**/o, **myos**/o
- ❏ **neur**/o
- ❏ **orth**/o
- ❏ **oste**/o
- ❏ **pariet**/o
- ❏ **patell**/o
- ❏ **ped**/o
- ❏ **petr**/o
- ❏ **phalang**/o, **phalanx**
- ❏ **physis**
- ❏ **pod**/o
- ❏ **pub**/o
- ❏ **rachi**/o
- ❏ **rad**/i
- ❏ **sacr**/o
- ❏ **scoli**/o
- ❏ **skelet**/o
- ❏ **spondyl**/o
- ❏ **stern**/o
- ❏ **synov**/o, **synovi**/o
- ❏ **tars**/o

- ❏ **taxi**/o
- ❏ **ten**/o, **tend**/o, **tendin**/o
- ❏ **vers**/o
- ❏ **vertebr**/o

Suffixes

- ❏ -algia
- ❏ -asthenia
- ❏ -cele
- ❏ -centesis
- ❏ -clasia, -clasis, -clast
- ❏ -desis
- ❏ -dynia
- ❏ -iatry
- ❏ -ist
- ❏ -otomy
- ❏ -pathy
- ❏ -plasia
- ❏ -plegia
- ❏ -practic
- ❏ -ptosis
- ❏ -physis
- ❏ -schisis
- ❏ -tic
- ❏ -tomy
- ❏ -trophy
- ❏ -um
- ❏ -y

[medical terminology **checklist**]

- abduction
- achondroplasia
- adduction
- ankylosis
- aponeurosis
- appendicular skeleton
- arthralgia
- arthritis
- arthrocentesis
- arthrochondritis
- arthroclasia
- arthrodesis
- arthrogram
- arthrologist
- arthrology
- arthroplasty
- arthroscopic
- arthroscopy
- arthrotomy
- articular cartilage
- ataxia
- atrophy
- axial skeleton
- bradykinesia
- bunion
- bursa
- bursectomy
- bursitis
- bursolith
- bursotomy
- carpal
- carpal tunnel syndrome
- carpoptosis
- cartilaginous joint
- cervical vertebra
- chiropractic
- chiropractor
- chondrectomy
- chondromalacia
- chondroplasty
- circumduction
- clavicle
- Colles' fracture
- comminuted fracture
- compound (closed) fracture
- compression fracture
- costal cartilage
- costectomy
- cramps
- cranioplasty
- cranioschisis
- craniotomy
- cranium

- depression
- diaphysis
- diskectomy
- diskitis
- displaced fracture
- Duchenne's muscular dystrophy
- dyskinesia
- dystrophy
- electromyography
- elevation
- endosteum
- epicondylitis
- epiphyseal fracture
- epiphyseal plate
- epiphysis
- eversion
- facial bones
- fascia
- fasciotomy
- femur
- fibrous joint
- fibula
- fissure
- flexion
- gout
- greenstick fracture
- herniated disk
- humerus
- hypertrophy
- ilium
- inferior nasal concha
- intervertebral disc
- inversion
- ischium
- kyphosis
- lacrimal bone
- laminectomy
- ligament
- lordosis
- lumbar vertebra
- mandible
- Marfan's syndrome
- marrow cavity
- matrix
- maxilla
- maxillitis
- meniscitis
- meniscus
- meniscectomy
- metacarpal
- metatarsal
- muscle fiber
- musculoskeletal

- myalgia
- myasthenia
- myeloma
- myoclonus
- myocoele
- myoplasty
- myositis
- nasal bone
- nondisplaced fracture
- orthopedics
- orthopedist
- orthotics
- ostectomy
- osteitis
- osteoarthritis
- osteoblast
- osteocarcinoma
- osteochondritis
- osteoclasis
- osteoclast
- osteocyte
- osteofibroma
- osteogenesis imperfecta
- osteologist
- osteology
- osteomalacia
- osteomyelitis
- osteonecrosis
- osteopathy
- osteopetrosis
- osteoplasty
- osteoporosis
- osteosarcoma
- Paget's disease
- paraplegia
- parietal bone
- periosteum
- phalange
- podiatry
- polymyositis
- Pott's fracture
- pronation
- prosthesis
- quadriplegia
- rachiotomy
- radius
- red marrow
- rib
- rotation
- sacrum
- scapula
- scoliosis
- skeletal muscle

❑ **skelet**on	❑ **synov**ectomy	❑ **ten**omyoplasty
❑ spiral fracture	❑ **synov**ial fluid	❑ **ten**orraphy
❑ **spondylarthr**itis	❑ **synov**ial joint	❑ **ten**osynovitis
❑ **spondyl**osyndesis	❑ **synov**iosarcoma	❑ **ten**otomy
❑ sprain	❑ **tars**al	❑ thoracic **vertebr**a
❑ strain	❑ **tendin**itis	❑ ulna
❑ supination	❑ **tend**on	❑ zygomatic bone
❑ sym**physis** pubis	❑ **ten**odynia	

[show what **you know!**]

WORD BUILDING

Construct or recall medical terms from the following meanings.

Example: 1. a gradual and painful softening of bone — osteomalacia

2. abnormal loss of bone density

3. paralysis of lower body, including both legs

4. abnormal lateral curve of the spine

5. inflammation of a tendon and synovial membrane

6. x-ray film of a joint

7. inflammation of a meniscus

8. surgical incision into a joint

9. muscular weakness

10. protrusion of muscle through its fascia

11. a repetitive stress injury of the wrist

12. a fracture caused by crushing

13. a viral infection of bone that accelerates bone loss

14. a rupture of an intervertebral disk

15. surgical repair of a joint

16. pain in a tendon

17. a calcium deposit within a bursa

18. abnormal condition of joint stiffness

19. abnormally slow movements

20. cancer of a synovial membrane in a joint

21. surgical stabilization of a joint

22. inflammation of the maxilla

23. a spasm of a muscle or muscle group

24. excessive formation of compact bone   _____

25. a congenital fissure of the skull   _____

26. lacking development, or wasting   _____

CASE STUDIES

Fill in the blanks with the correct terms.

1. A 35-year-old patient received injuries during a weekend touch football game in the park. Upon his arrival at emergency, he

    presented an open, or (a) _____ fracture of the tibia, pain and discoloration of the ankle that

    suggested damage to a tendon, or (b) _____, and muscle tenderness or

    (c) _____ that suggested damaged muscle fibers or (d) _____, and

    inflammation of all muscles of the right lower extremity, or (e) _____. An x-ray examination revealed

    a fracture at the ankle, called a (f) _____ fracture, with associated inflammation of the Achilles

    tendon, or generalized (g) _____. After several weeks of stabilization, death of bone tissue, or

    (h) _____, had occurred in place of the expected healing. Tissue samples exhibited evidence of

    staphylococcus bacteria, indicating a diagnosis of (i) _____. The infection had spread to cartilages

    in the foot, establishing a condition of bone and cartilage inflammation, or (j) _____. Synovial fluid

    from the knee of the same leg was withdrawn during a (k) _____ procedure to determine the spread

    of the bacteria, since the thigh bone, or (l) _____, was experiencing inflammation, or

    (m) _____. Unfortunately, the results were positive and an endoscopic visual examination, or

    (n) _____, of the knee joint was made to determine damage levels. Treatment of the knee was

    confined to multiple antibiotic therapy. A foot specialist, or (o) _____, was consulted for treatment

    protocol for the foot and ankle. When antibiotic treatments failed, advanced infection resulted in a gangrenous condition,

    and amputation was required. An (p) _____ was contacted to fit with an artificial foot, or

    (q) _____.

2. A 75-year-old female was initially seen by her personal general practitioner when she complained of difficulty in movement,

    or (r) _____. The GP referred her to (s) _____ when her bent-over posture, or

    (t) _____, and x-ray exams indicated a loss of bone density, or (u) _____.

    The orthopedist recommended hormone therapy with calcium supplements and mild exercise for the bone loss, and also

    reported advanced joint degeneration in her carpometacarpal and metacarpophalangeal joints that was diagnosed as

    (v) _____ due to her advanced age. Upon closer examination, additional bone formations were

    present, and upon biopsy, were found to be malignant tumors that originated from the #5 metacarpal bone. The diagnosis of

    (w) _____ or (x) _____ was given, and irradiation treatments prescribed.

[piece it all **together!**]

CROSSWORD

From the chapter material, fill in the crossword puzzle with answers to the following clues.

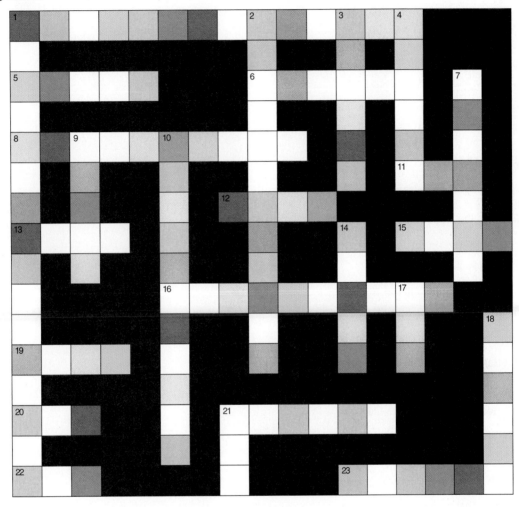

ACROSS

1. Growth abnormality resulting in short, stocky limbs. (Find puzzle piece 5.9)
5. A word root and combining vowel for tendon. (Find puzzle piece 5.4)
6. The part of a vertebra removed during a laminectomy. (Find puzzle piece 5.21)
8. A necessary component of vertebral column surgery. (Find puzzle piece 5.18)
11. Abbreviation for anterior cruciate ligament. (Find puzzle piece 5.23)
12. This disease makes sufferers *drop*. (Find puzzle piece 5.15)
13. The nature of bone due to its mineral salts. (Find puzzle piece 5.6)
15. Meaning of the suffix *-algia*. (Find puzzle piece 5.1)
16. Surgical removal of a rib. (Find puzzle piece 5.20)
19. Bones with the word root *cost*. (Find puzzle piece 5.2)
20. Abbreviation for total knee replacement. (Find puzzle piece 5.24)
21. The connective tissue associated with a muscle. (Find puzzle piece 5.5)
22. A prefix for together or joined. (Find puzzle piece 5.22)
23. A weekend athlete suffers often from this muscle injury. (Find puzzle piece 5.13)

DOWN

1. Inflammation of cartilage within a joint. (Find puzzle piece 5.10)
2. Inflammation of many muscles at once. (Find puzzle piece 5.11)
3. A fracture caused by twisting stresses. (Find puzzle piece 5.12)
4. The inability to coordinate voluntary movements. (Find puzzle piece 5.8)
7. A real pain in the neck, if a neck muscle is injured. (Find puzzle piece 5.7)
9. A word root and combining vowel, which together is pronounced just like the name of the largest city in Egypt. (Find puzzle piece 5.16)
10. A frequent procedure if you suffer from osteogenesis imperfecta. (Find puzzle piece 5.17)
14. This prefix has the opposite meaning of *crooked*. (Find puzzle piece 5.19)
17. A word root for muscle. (Find puzzle piece 5.3)
18. A common sports injury to a ligament. (Find puzzle piece 5.14)
21. What you have when the answers to a test come easily.

WORD UNSCRAMBLE

From the completed crossword puzzle, unscramble:

1. All of the letters that appear in **green** squares

   ☐_ _ _ _ _ _ _

   Clue: Inflammation of bone tissue

2. All of the letters that appear in **red** squares

   _ ☐_ _ _ _ _ _ _

   Clue: A common complaint on cold mornings before stretching

3. All of the letters that appear in **yellow** squares

   _ ☐_ _ _ _ _

   Clue: What muscle builders may fear the most

4. All of the letters in **orange** squares

   _ _ _☐_ _ _ _ _ _ _

   Clue: Orthopedists and football players are very familiar with this procedure

5. All of the letters that appear in **blue** squares

   _ _ _ _☐_ _ _ _ _ _ _

   Clue: A disease that leaves your bones weak and brittle, often causing kyphosis

6. All of the letters in **purple** squares

   ☐_ _ _ _ _ _ _ _

   Clue: Often a symptom of tennis elbow or pitcher's shoulder

7. All of the letters in **peach** squares

   _ _ _ _☐_ _ _

   Clue: A common diagnosis if raising your arm causes pain

8. All of the letters in **pink** squares

▢_ __ __ __ __

Clue: A common type of fracture to the wrist

9. All of the letters in **gray** squares

__ __ __ __ __ __ ▢__ __

Clue: An abnormal lateral curvature of the spine

Now write down each of the letters that are boxed and unscramble them to find the hidden medical term of the musculoskeletal system: __ __ __ __ __ __ __ __ __

Clue: If old Gepetto had an MD, he would have specialized in this field

MEDmedia wrap-up

www.prenhall.com/wingerd

Before you go on to the next chapter, take advantage of the free CD-ROM and study guide website that accompany this book. Simply load the CD-ROM for additional activities, games, animations, videos, and quizzes linked to this chapter. Then visit www.prenhall.com/wingerd for even more!

CHAPTER 6

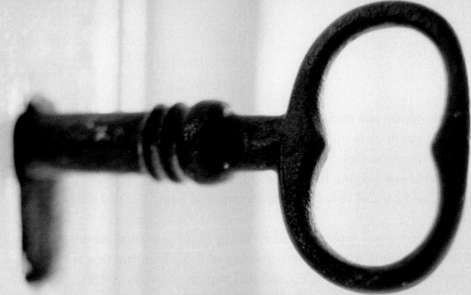

The Nervous System and Mental Health

LEARNING OBJECTIVES

After completing this chapter, you will be able to:

- Define and spell the word parts used to create terms for the nervous system

- Identify the major organs of the nervous system and describe their structure and function

- Break down and define common medical terms used for symptoms, diseases, disorders, procedures, treatments, and devices associated with the nervous system

- Build medical terms from the word parts associated with the nervous system

- Pronounce and spell common medical terms associated with the nervous system

 MEDmedia

www.prenhall.com/wingerd

Enhance your study with the power of multimedia! Each chapter of this book links to activities, games, animations, videos, and quizzes that you'll find on your CD-ROM. Plus, you can click on www.prenhall.com/wingerd, to find a free chapter-specific companion website that's loaded with additional practice and resources.

CD-ROM

- Audio Glossary
- Exercises & Activities
- Flashcard Generator
- Animations
- Videos

 Companion Website

- Exercises & Activities
- Audio Glossary
- Drug Updates
- Current News Updates

A secure distance learning course is available at www.prenhall.com/onekey.

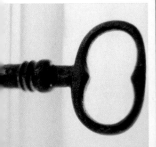

The nervous system is a complex part of the body that has been studied extensively, yet there is still much more to learn. It is composed of the brain, spinal cord, and nerves. Together, these important organs enable you to sense the world around you, integrate this information to form thoughts and memories, and control your body movements and many internal functions.

In this chapter, we will explore the terms of the healthy, normal nervous system before proceeding with the medical terms of neurology. But first we will examine the word parts that are associated with the nervous system.

word parts focus

Let's look at word parts. The following table contains a list of word parts that when combined build many of the terms of the nervous system.

PREFIX	DEFINITION	PREFIX	DEFINITION
a-	without	mono-	single
di-	two	pan-	all, entire
dys-	bad, abnormal	para-	near, alongside
hemi-	one-half	poly-	many
hydro-	water	pre-	before
hyper-	excessive	tetra-	four

WORD ROOT	DEFINITION	WORD ROOT	DEFINITION
alges	pain	lys	break apart, dissolution
astheni	weakness	mening	membrane, meninges
cephal	head	ment	the mind
cerebell	little brain, cerebellum	myel	spinal cord, or bone marrow, or
cerebr	brain, cerebrum		medulla, or myelin sheath
cran, crani	skull, cranium	neur	sinew or cord, nerve
dur	hard	phas	speech
embol	a throwing in	plegi	paralysis
encephal	brain	psych	the mind
esthes	sensation, perception	quad, quadri	four
gangli / ganglion	knot, swelling	radic, radicul	nerve root
gli	glue, neuroglia	somat	the body
gnos	knowledge	thalam	inner chamber, thalamus

SUFFIX	DEFINITION	SUFFIX	DEFINITION
-algia	pain	-oid	resemblance to
-asthenia	weakness	-paresis	slight paralysis
-cele	a swelling or hernia	-phagia	eating or swallowing
-gram	recording	-phasia	speaking (may also be used as a root, as phas)
-iatry	treatment, specialty		
-itis	inflammation	-plegia	paralysis
-lepsy	seizure		

SELF QUIZ 6.1

Review the word parts of nervous system terminology by working carefully through the exercises that follow. Soon, we will apply this new information to build medical terms.

A. Provide the definition of the following prefixes and suffixes.

1. a- _____

2. di- _____

3. dys- _____

4. hemi- _____

5. hydro- _____

6. mono- _____

7. pan- _____

8. tetra- _____

9. -algia _____

10. -cele _____

11. -iatry _____

12. -itis _____

13. -oid _____

14. -paresis _____

15. -phasia _____

16. -plegia _____

17. -lepsy _____

B. Provide the word root for each of the following terms.

1. weakness _____

2. head _____

3. little brain _____

4. cerebrum _____

5. hard _____

6. sensation _____

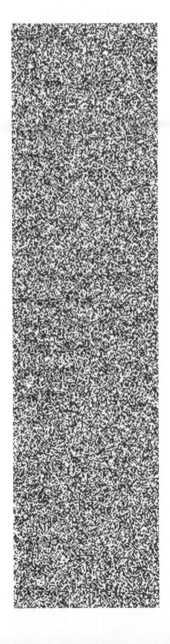

7. knot, swelling _____

8. break apart _____

9. membrane _____

10. mind _____

11. spinal cord, myelin _____

12. nerve _____

13. speech _____

14. paralysis _____

15. four _____

16. nerve root _____

17. the body _____

18. inner chamber _____

19. cranium _____

20. brain _____

21. glue _____

[anatomy and physiology overview]

enrichment module enrichment module enrichment module enrichment module enrichment module

The nervous system provides a system of communication between its primary organ, the **brain,** and the distant parts of the body. Its goal is to monitor changes in the environment inside and outside the body, interpret the changes, and initiate a response in an effort to maintain homeostasis. It does all of this by way of electrochemical messages called **nerve impulses.** Nerve impulses race through your body every moment, traveling along special routes, or **nerves,** at high speeds.

As a whole, the nervous system is a complex series of organs and structures that extend throughout your body. In addition to the brain, its organs include the spinal cord and many miles of nerves. The nervous system is divided into two main groups: the **central nervous system (CNS),** which includes the brain and spinal cord, and the **peripheral nervous system (PNS),** which includes the nerves and sensory receptors. The organizational scheme is further detailed in Figure 6.1▦.

Nervous Tissue

As you recall from Chapter 3, the nervous system contains specialized tissue that conducts nerve impulses. The functional cells of nervous tissue are called **neurons,** which receive support from nearby **neuroglial cells** (Figure 6.2▦). Each neuron consists of a **cell body** and numerous branches. The cell body contains the nucleus and most of the cytoplasm, and the branches include many **dendrites,** which carry impulses toward the cell body, and a single **axon,** which carries impulses away. The term *dendrite* is from the Greek word for *tree,* and *axon* means *axis* or *central point* in Greek.

In many neurons, the axon is covered with numerous neuroglial cells known as **Schwann cells,** which provide a white-colored protective sheath that is mostly fat. Known as the **myelin sheath,** it enables an axon to extend great distances through the body by offering it protection and insulation (some axons are nearly one meter—about three feet—in length!).

[FYI]

Schwann Cells
The German anatomist Theodor Schwann discovered Schwann cells in 1875 when he teased apart the fatty white covering of axons and was surprised to find they were living cells.

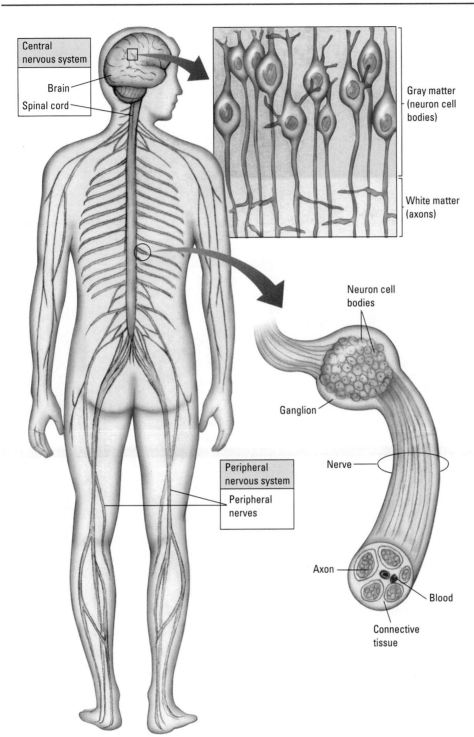

Figure 6.1

Organization of the nervous system.

Neurons have the ability to conduct nerve impulses very quickly, providing an excellent method of communication. But how does one cell communicate with another? Adjacent neurons communicate by releasing chemicals across tiny gaps that separate them, called **synapses.** The term *synapse* is derived from *synapsis,* the Greek word for *junction.* The chemicals, known as **neurotransmitters,** are released by a neuron when a nerve impulse reaches its distal end. The neurotransmitters then diffuse across the synapse to contact the adjacent cell. Contact with the next neuron may stimulate it to trigger a nerve impulse, or in some cases, may inhibit it.

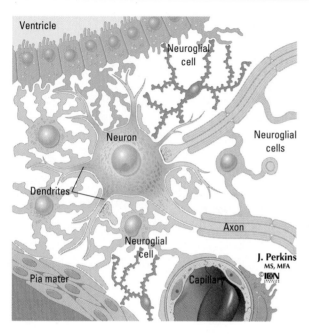

Ventricle

Neuroglial cell

Neuroglial cells

Neuron

Dendrites

Axon

Neuroglial cell

J. Perkins
MS, MFA
©ICON

Pia mater

Capillary

Figure 6.2 ::::

Neurons and nervous tissue organization. The neuron is shown in yellow, and three types of neuroglial cells are shown in various colors.
Source: Icon Learning Systems.

Central Nervous System

The central nervous system is the "central station" for incoming and outgoing nerve impulses. As you have just learned, it includes the brain and spinal cord. Both organs are protected by bones, including the cranium and the vertebral column, and by a thick set of membranes called the **meninges.** The meninges are located between the soft nervous tissue of the brain and spinal cord and the hard bones, forming a protective cover that is several layers in thickness (Figure 6.3::::). The layers include an outer tough fibrous **dura mater,** a middle **arachnoid,** and an inner thin **pia mater.** A narrow space exists between the arachnoid and pia mater, called the **subarachnoid space.**

> [**FYI**]
>
> **The Meninges**
> The term *dura mater* is from the Arabic word for *hard mother* and *pia mater* means *soft mother.* Perhaps the person who first coined these terms was thinking of mother quite often! You might recognize the meaning of arachnoid if you suffer from arachnophobia, or fear of spiders. Both words are derived from the Greek word for spider or cobweb, *arachne.* Apparently, the thin interlacing fibers that form the arachnoid reminded its discoverers of a spider's cobweb.

THE BRAIN

The brain receives sensory information, interprets and integrates this information, and controls muscle and glandular responses. Its nerve impulse activity also provides you with your memory, thoughts, dreams, and personality. It receives a large blood supply to fuel its constant activity. The blood flow is critical; if it is restricted for more than a few minutes, neurons begin to expire. The brain is located in the cranial cavity, and weighs about 1.4 kg (3 pounds). Extending from the brain are 12 pairs of nerves, called **cranial nerves.**

In general, the brain is composed of nervous tissue that includes both gray matter and white matter. Gray matter consists mainly of neuron cell bodies and dendrites, whereas white matter consists of axons that are covered with the white insulative myelin sheath. The axons carry nerve impulses to adjacent neurons. Thus, white matter carries nerve impulses, while gray matter serves as integrative centers.

[**thinking critically!**]

Some drugs cause neurotransmitters to be released more readily, while other drugs inhibit the release of neurotransmitters. Do you think an inhibitory drug would be likely to cause a state of mental depression, or mental attentiveness? Why?

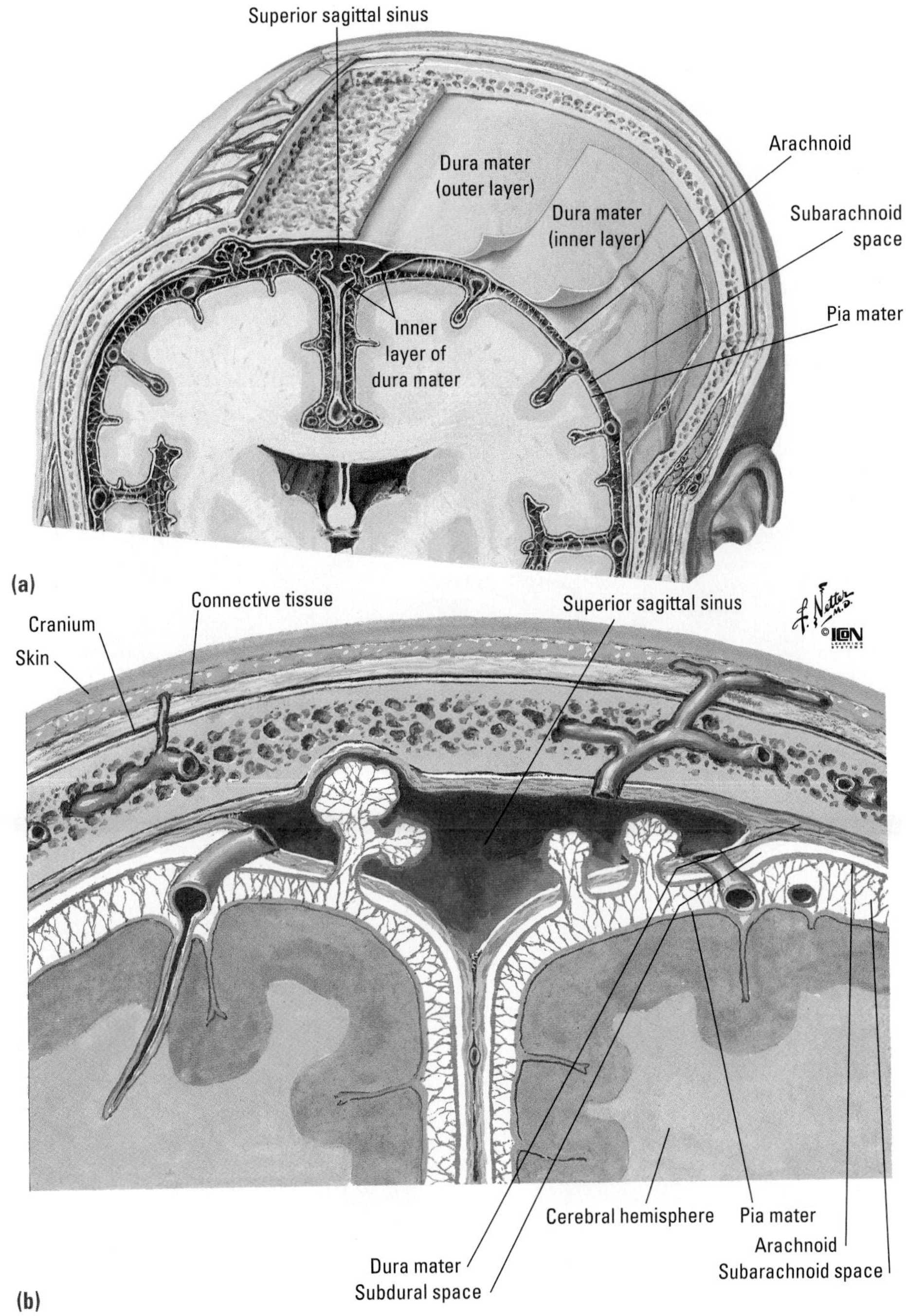

(a)

(b)

Figure 6.3 ::::

The meninges surround the brain and spinal cord.

(a) Section through the head with the cranium partially removed. The thick, parchment-like dura mater is shown pulled upward to reveal the subarachnoid space and the pia mater attached to the brain surface. **(b)** A sectional view through the top of the brain, frontal view. The large blue space is the superior sagittal sinus, an enlarged vein where CSF is reabsorbed upon its return after circulating around the brain and spinal cord within the subarachnoid space.
Source: Icon Learning Systems.

The brain includes four main parts: the **cerebrum,** the **cerebellum,** the **diencephalon,** and the **brain stem** (Figure 6.4::::).The cerebrum is the largest, most significant part of the brain filling most of the cranial cavity with its convoluted (wrinkled) mass. Indeed, the term *cerebrum* is the Latin word for *brain.* It is the center of thought, personality, emotions, memory, and sensory perception, and it initiates muscle contractions. Structurally, it is divided into the right and left **cerebral hemispheres.** A large fissure separates the two cerebral hemispheres, which is bridged by a band of nervous tissue called the **corpus callosum.** The most important functional part of the cerebrum is the **cerebral cortex,** which is an outer fringe of gray matter. The cerebral cortex is divided into functional zones known as **lobes.** Each lobe houses a cluster of neurons that perform a particular function in common,

[FYI]

Cerebrum
Erasistratus of Greece named the term *cerebrum* in the third century BC, to mean *brain.* The term *cerebellum* was also named, which is the diminutive of cerebrum and means *little brain.*

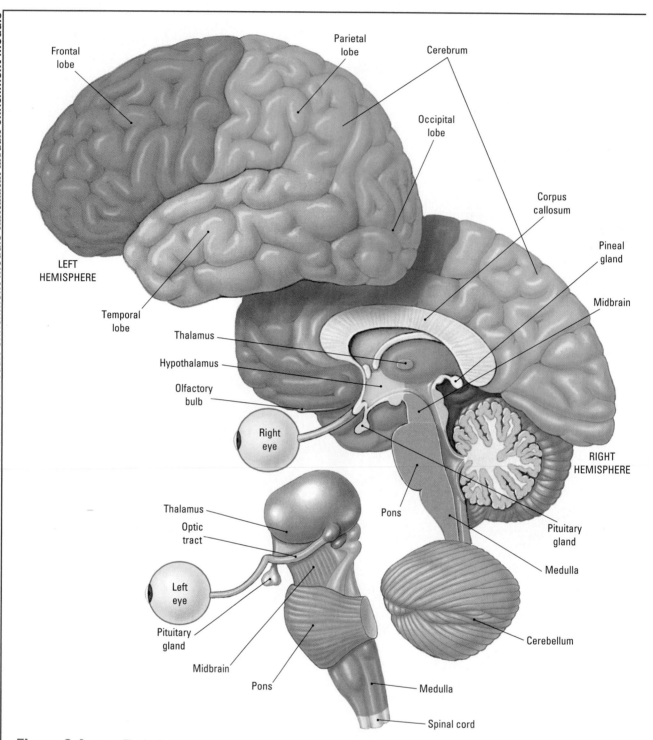

Figure 6.4 :::: **The brain.**

The brain is shown sectioned down its midline, separating it into right and left portions, with the diencephalon, cerebellum, and brain stem separated. The colored areas of the cerebrum illustrate the cerebral lobes. *Source: Pearson Education.*

such as the interpretation of sound, the control of voluntary muscles, the perception of sensory information from the skin, or the formation of personality traits.

Below and posterior to the cerebrum is a smaller convoluted mass, known as the cerebellum (which means *little brain*). The cerebellum coordinates muscle responses and manages equilibrium.

Beneath the cerebrum and anterior to the cerebellum is the diencephalon. The term *diencephalon* literally means *double brain*, appropriate because it contains two important areas, the **thalamus** and **hypothalamus.** The term *thalamus* is from a Latin word for *inner chamber,* which describes its location in the approximate center of the brain. The thalamus is a relay station, redirecting nerve impulses to and from the cerebrum. The hypothalamus is located below the thalamus, as the prefix *hypo-* suggests. It is the center for involuntary activities, such as regulation of heartbeat, thirst, blood pressure, and glandular functions.

Extending below the diencephalon to form the *stem* of the cauliflower-like brain is the brain stem, which includes the **medulla** and **pons.** The medulla transmits nerve impulses between the spinal cord and brain, and regulates breathing rhythms. The pons, which literally means *bridge,* provides a connection between the medulla and cerebellum.

Within the brain's center are several small spaces, known as **ventricles.** The term *ventricle* is derived from the Latin word for *little belly,* owing to their resemblance to little empty stomachs within the brain. The ventricles are each filled with a slightly yellowish fluid, known as **cerebrospinal fluid (CSF),** which is continuously produced from the blood supply. CSF circulates through the ventricles and around the brain and spinal cord by way of interconnecting channels. In a procedure called a **lumbar puncture (LP),** or spinal tap, CSF is withdrawn from a narrow space around the spinal cord for diagnostic purposes.

[FYI]

The Blood-Brain Barrier
Cerebrospinal fluid is produced as blood is pushed through small capillaries that are located inside the brain ventricles. As the blood flows, plasma escapes through tiny openings in the capillary walls. The plasma is called CSF as soon as it collects within the ventricles. The actual blood-brain barrier is created by specialized cells that border the ventricles, which permit only plasma, dissolved electrolytes, glucose, and other tiny molecules to enter into the ventricles but prevent the entry of bacteria and other unwanted cells.

THE SPINAL CORD

The spinal cord extends from its union with the medulla of the brain about 45 cm (18 inches) down the back. It passes through the spinal canal to terminate between L1 and L2. Lengthwise, the spinal cord is divided into 31 segments. Each segment includes a pair of **spinal roots,** which form spinal nerves as they leave the spinal cord. Thus, there are 31 pairs of **spinal nerves** along the length of the spinal cord (Figure 6.5::::).

Similar to the brain, the spinal cord consists of nervous tissue that includes both gray and white matter. The gray matter is in the center of the cord. The white matter is in the outer portions of the cord, and consists of long nerves that carry impulses up and down the spinal cord.

The Peripheral Nervous System

The peripheral nervous system, or PNS, consists of the nerves that course throughout the body carrying nerve impulses to and from the CNS. It also includes the ganglia and sensory receptors.

THE NERVES

The nerves of the body are branches from the 12 cranial nerves that communicate with the brain, and branches from the 31 pairs of spinal nerves that communicate with the spinal cord. Each nerve is composed of a combination of nervous tissue, blood vessels, and supportive connective tissue. The nervous tissue consists of the axons of neurons, which are bundled together and wrapped with layers of connective tissue (Figure 6.6::::). Axons carry nerve impulses at very high speeds, up to

[thinking critically!]

Can you determine the possible health threats that a tumor pressing against the hypothalamus would pose?

enrichment module enrichment module **enrichment module** enrichment module **enrichment module** enrichment module **enrichment module** enrichment module **enrichment module**

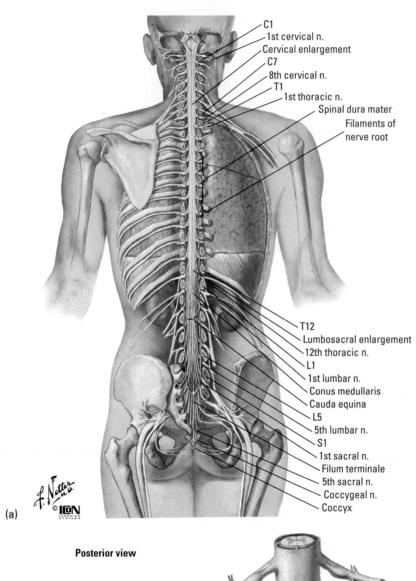

C1
1st cervical n.
Cervical enlargement
C7
8th cervical n.
T1
1st thoracic n.
Spinal dura mater
Filaments of nerve root

T12
Lumbosacral enlargement
12th thoracic n.
L1
1st lumbar n.
Conus medullaris
Cauda equina
L5
5th lumbar n.
S1
1st sacral n.
Filum terminale
5th sacral n.
Coccygeal n.
Coccyx

(a)

Posterior view

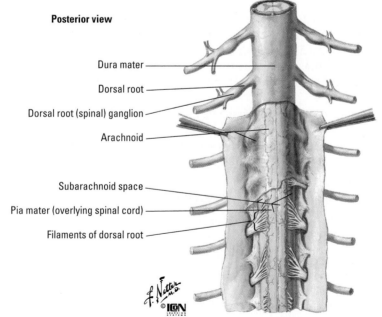

Dura mater
Dorsal root
Dorsal root (spinal) ganglion
Arachnoid
Subarachnoid space
Pia mater (overlying spinal cord)
Filaments of dorsal root

(b)

Figure 6.5 ::::

The spinal cord and its nerve roots.

(a) Posterior view of the body with the vertebral column removed, revealing the spinal cord and nerve roots.

(b) The spinal cord is shown dissected in this illustration to reveal the meninges and nerve roots. Note the cross section at the top of the figure, where the gray matter in the center of the cord is distinct from the white matter surrounding it.

Source: Icon Learning Systems.

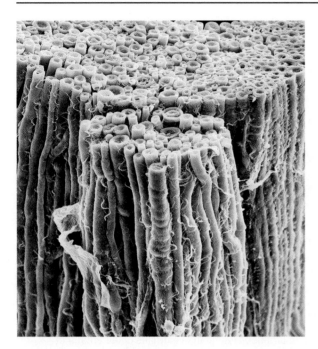

Figure 6.6 :::

Nerve fibers. Scanning electron photograph of a single, cut nerve reveals its composition of many individual nerve fibers, each supported by sheaths of connective tissue.

300 mph! The longest nerves extend from the base of your spinal cord to your feet, a distance of up to one meter (about three feet).

Your body's nerves transmit sensory or motor impulses; some can transmit both. **Sensory nerves** are also called **afferent nerves.** They carry nerve impulses from the sensory receptors (described later) to the brain or spinal cord. **Motor nerves** are also known as **efferent nerves,** and carry impulses from the brain or spinal cord to muscles and glands. Certain motor nerves carry impulses that are under your conscious control, known as **somatic,** while other motor nerves are unconsciously controlled, and are called **autonomic.**

GANGLIA

The **ganglia** are clusters of neuron cell bodies that lie outside the brain and spinal cord (the singular form is ganglion). The term *ganglion* means a *swelling* or *knot,* and describes its appearance as a swelling along the path of a spinal nerve route. Ganglia are centers where nerve impulses are passed from one neuron to another across synapses.

SENSORY RECEPTORS

The **sensory receptors** are nervous structures that respond to changes in the environment. A change may be in the form of a change in temperature, pressure, touch, or pain. Once the change occurs, it stimulates a sensory receptor to initiate a nerve impulse. The nerve impulse then travels along a sensory nerve to the spinal cord or brain.

As we learned in Chapter 4, sensory receptors are embedded within the skin. Smaller numbers are also found within the walls of visceral organs like the stomach and small intestine. Sensory receptors may also be combined within more complex structures, like the eye and ear, to form special sensory organs (special sensory organs are the topic of Chapter 7 and Chapter 8).

[thinking critically!]

Muscle contraction requires a stimulus from a nerve, in the form of a nerve impulse. Do you suppose the nerve stimulus is provided by a sensory nerve or a motor nerve?

getting to the root of it | anatomy and physiology terms

Many of the anatomy and physiology terms are formed from roots that are used to construct the more complex medical terms of the nervous system, including symptoms, diseases, and treatments. In this section, we will review the terms that describe the structure and function of the nervous system *in relation to their word roots,* which are shown in **bold**.

Study the word roots and terms in this list and complete the review exercises that follow.

Word Root (Meaning)	Terms Formed from the Word Root (Pronunciation)	Definition
arachn spider	**arachn**oid (ah RAK noyd)	the middle meninx, it surrounds a space filled with CSF known as the subarachnoid space
	sub**arachn**oid space (sub ah RAK noyd)	the space within the arachnoid, which is filled with CSF
cerebell little brain	**cerebell**um (ser eh BELL um)	the lower posterior part of the brain that is the center of muscle coordination and equilibrium
cerebr brain, cerebrum	**cerebr**ospinal fluid (ser eh broh SPY nal FLOO id)	a colorless fluid produced within the ventricles of the brain that provides liquid shock absorption and a source of nourishment for the brain and spinal cord; abbreviated CSF
	cerebrum (SER eh brum)	the largest part of the brain, it includes the right and left cerebral hemispheres, the corpus callosum, the cerebral cortex, and the lobes
	cerebral hemispheres (seh REE bral HEM iss feerz)	the right and left portions of the cerebrum, separated by the longitudinal fissure
	cerebral cortex (seh REE bral KOR teks)	the outer fringe of the cerebrum, which is composed of gray matter and is the site of nerve pathway termination and origin
	cerebral lobes	functional regions of the cerebral cortex
crani skull, cranium	**crani**um (KRAY nee um)	the dome-shaped part of the skull, which houses the cranial cavity
	cranial nerves (KRAY nee al)	12 pairs of nerves that unite with the brain
encephal brain	di**encephal**on (dye en SEFF ah lon)	the central part of the brain located beneath the cerebrum, which contains the thalamus and the hypothalamus
gangli / ganglion swelling, knot	**gangli**a (GANG lee ah)	clusters of neuron cell bodies that lie outside the CNS
mening membrane	**mening**es (men IN jeez)	the dura mater, arachnoid, and pia mater membranes surrounding the brain and spinal cord; the singular form is *meninx*
myel spinal cord, bone marrow, medulla, myelin sheath	**myel**in sheath (MY eh lin)	a white, fatty membrane that partially wraps the axons of certain neurons
neur sinew or cord, nerve	**neur**oglia (noo ROH glee ah)	supportive cells of nervous tissue
	neuron (NOO ron)	a functional cell of nervous tissue, which generates and transmits nerve impulses; each neuron consists of numerous dendrites, a centralized cell body, and a single axon
	neurotransmitter (noo roh TRANS mit ter)	a chemical that is released into a synapse from one neuron to cause a change in another neuron

Word Root (Meaning)	Terms Formed from the Word Root (Pronunciation)	Definition
spin spine	**spin**al cord	the cylindrical cord of nervous tissue extending through the spinal canal from its union with the medulla of the brain to the lumbar vertebral region
	spinal nerves	31 pairs of nerves that unite with the spinal cord
thalam inner chamber	**thalam**us (THAL ah mus)	area in the diencephalon that serves as a relay station of impulses
	hypo**thalam**us (high poh THAL ah mus)	located just below the thalamus, this area in the diencephalon is the center for involuntary functions

OTHER IMPORTANT TERMS

The terms in this table are related to the structure and function of the nervous system, but are not built from multiple word roots.

afferent nerves (AFF er ent)	nerves that carry impulses toward the CNS; also known as sensory nerves
brain	the prominent organ located within the cranial cavity; it is the center of conscious thought, memory, emotions, and muscle stimulus and is divided into the cerebellum, the cerebrum, the diencephalon, and the brain stem
brain stem	the lowermost part of the brain, it includes the medulla and the pons, which transmit impulses between the spinal cord and other parts of the brain
central nervous system	a main division of the nervous system that contains the brain and spinal cord; abbreviated CNS
corpus callosum (KOR pus kah LOH sum)	a band of white matter connecting the right and left hemispheres
dura mater (DOO ra MAY ter)	the outer meninx, it is composed of tough fibrous connective tissue
efferent nerves (EFF er ent)	nerves that carry impulses away from the CNS; also called motor nerves
medulla (meh DULL lah)	the lower part of the brain stem, which transmits nerve impulses between the spinal cord and brain and regulates breathing rhythms
peripheral nervous system	a main division of the nervous system that contains the peripheral nerves and ganglia
pia mater (PEE ah MAY ter)	the innermost meninx, it is a very thin membrane that adheres to the surface of the brain and spinal cord
pons	the upper part of the brain stem, which connects the medulla and cerebellum
synapse (SIN naps)	a tiny gap between an axon of one neuron and a dendrite or cell body of another neuron, across which information travels by way of neurotransmitters
ventricles (VEN trik lz)	membrane-enclosed cavities within the brain through which flows cerebrospinal fluid

SELF QUIZ 6.2

Success Hint: Once you get to the crossword puzzle at the end of the chapter, remember to check back here for clues! Your clues are indicated by the puzzle icon.

SAY IT—SPELL IT!

Review the terms of the nervous system by speaking the phonetic pronunciations out loud, then writing the correct spelling of the term.

1. NOO ron _____

2. noo ROH glee uh _____

3. DEN drights _____

6.1   4. AK sonz _____

6.2   5. MY eh lin _____

6. noo roh TRANS mit ter _____

6.3   7. men IN jeez _____

8. DOO ra MAY ter _____

6.4   9. PEE ah MAY ter _____

10. SER eh brum _____

11. seh REE bral   HEM is feerz _____

12. KOR pus   kah LOH sum _____

13. seh REE bral   KOR teks _____

14. ser eh BELL um _____

15. dye en SEFF ah lon _____

16. THAL ah mus _____

17. high poh THAL ah mus _____

18. meh DULL lah _____

19. ser eh broh SPY nal _____

20. AFF er ent _____

21. EFF er ent _____

22. GANG lee uh _____

FILL IT IN!

Fill in the blanks with the correct terms.

1. The brain is a part of the _____ nervous system, while the nerves are part of the _____ nervous system.

2. The _____ nervous system is a functional division that plays a major role in regulating involuntary activities.

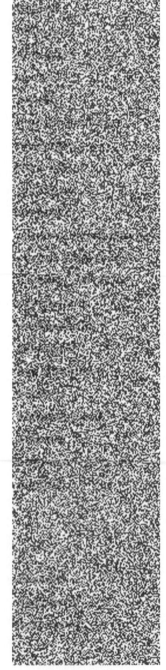

3. The prominent portion of the brain that is the central integration center for incoming and outgoing impulses is the _____. This structure consists of right and left cerebral _____. The outer part that is composed of gray matter is the cerebral _____.

4. The part of the brain that coordinates skeletal muscle and manages equilibrium is the _____, which means *little brain*.

6.5 5. The meninges include the pia mater, the _____, and the dura mater. The term *pia* means *delicate or soft,* and the term _____ means *hard*.

6. The part of the brain that conveys nerve impulses between the spinal cord and higher parts of the brain is the _____.

7. The diencephalon includes the thalamus and the _____.

6.6 8. Cerebrospinal fluid is a _____ fluid that fills the volume of the small spaces in the brain, called the _____.

9. The spinal cord contains _____ segments, each of which connects with a pair of spinal _____.

6.7 10. The peripheral nervous system consists of sensory nerves, _____ nerves, and nerves that carry both sensory and motor information. A _____ is a region where numerous neurons form synapses.

MATCH IT!

Match the term on the left with the correct definition on the right.

_____ 1. synapse

a. part of the diencephalon

_____ 2. neurotransmitter

b. contacts the spinal cord

_____ 3. neuron

c. carries impulses to the cell body

_____ 4. axon

d. right and left parts of the cerebrum

_____ 5. dendrite

e. supportive cells of nervous tissue

_____ 6. spinal nerve

f. cluster of neuron cell bodies in the PNS

_____ 7. afferent nerve

g. connects the cerebral hemispheres

_____ 8. cerebral cortex

h. coordinates muscle activities

_____ 9. cerebellum

i. consists of gray matter

_____10. medulla

j. the junction between adjacent neurons

_____11. cerebral hemispheres

k. carries impulses away from the cell body

_____12. neuroglia

l. chemicals that cross the synapse

_____13. ganglia

m. carries impulses toward the CNS

_____14. corpus callosum

n. may be motor, sensory or both

_____15. hypothalamus

o. functional cell of nervous tissue

[medical terminology of the

nervous system]

The study of the nervous system is a relatively young branch of science known as **neuroscience.** One who focuses their study in this field is a **neuroscientist.** The medical application within this field is called **neurology** and a physician specializing in general disorders of the nervous system is a neurologist. Specialists within the field of neurology include:

■ **Neurosurgeons,** whose medical practice focuses on brain or spinal cord surgery

■ **Psychiatrists,** physicians whose focus is mental illness

■ **Psychologists,** practitioners (not physicians) whose focus is on behavioral disorders.

Notice that four of the bold-faced terms in the preceding paragraph have something in common: Each begins with the word root *neur.* Recall from Chapter 3 that *neur* is a word root for many medical terms of the nervous system. It means *a cord or sinew,* and describes the appearance of long, string-like nerves that course throughout your body. The two remaining bold-faced terms begin with the word root *psych,* which means *the mind.* Many more interesting word origins occur among terms of the nervous system, as you are about to discover.

The health of the nervous system can experience many types of challenges. Nervous tissue is quite delicate and easily damaged. Therefore, it requires special protective features. You have already learned that protection from injury is provided not only by bones, but also by the meninges and CSF. Protection from pathogens circulating in the bloodstream is further assisted by a **blood-brain barrier,** which keeps most bacteria, harmful cells, and toxins from entering. Usually, the unwanted substances that successfully penetrate the blood-brain barrier are eliminated by special neuroglial cells, called microglia.

Despite the measures protecting the brain and spinal cord, they are susceptible to infectious diseases and injury, in addition to inherited conditions. For example, the most common affliction of the nervous system is **stroke.** Also known as a **cerebrovascular accident (CVA)**, it is a disruption of the normal flow of blood to the brain, causing brain damage (Figure 6.7::::). According to the Centers for Disease Control (CDC), in 2002 stroke claimed about 200,000 lives in the United States, making it the third most common cause of death (behind cancer and heart disease).

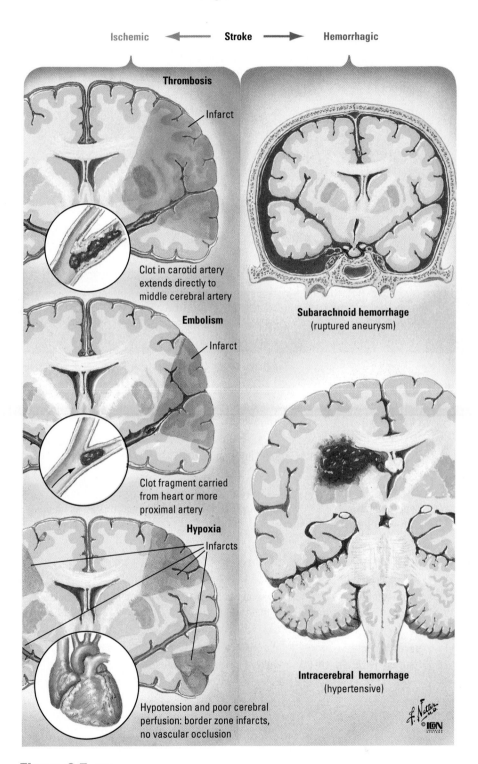

Diagnosis of Stroke

Ischemic ⟵ **Stroke** ⟶ Hemorrhagic

Thrombosis

Infarct

Clot in carotid artery extends directly to middle cerebral artery

Embolism

Infarct

Clot fragment carried from heart or more proximal artery

Hypoxia

Infarcts

Hypotension and poor cerebral perfusion: border zone infarcts, no vascular occlusion

Subarachnoid hemorrhage (ruptured aneurysm)

Intracerebral hemorrhage (hypertensive)

Figure 6.7 ::::

Cerebrovascular accident (CVA) or stroke. A stroke may result from two primary causes: a reduced blood flow to the brain (ischemic) or a sudden release of blood into brain tissue (hemorrhagic). Reduced blood flow can be caused by a thrombosis (top left), an embolism (middle left), or the result of a heart attack (lower left). A sudden release of blood can be caused by a ruptured aneurysm (upper right) or the breakage of blood vessels due to high blood pressure (lower right). *Source: Icon Learning Systems.*

let's construct terms!

In this section, we will assemble all of the word parts to construct medical terminology related to the nervous system. Abbreviations are used to indicate each word part: **p** = prefix, **r** = root, **cv** = combining vowel, and **s** = suffix. Recall from chapter one that the addition of a combining vowel to the word root creates the combining form for the term. Note that some terms are not constructed from word parts, but they are included here to expand your vocabulary.

The medical terms of the nervous system are listed in the following three sections:

- Symptoms and Signs
- Diseases and Disorders
- Treatments, Procedures, and Devices

Each section is followed by review exercises. Study the lists in these tables and complete the review exercises that follow.

Symptoms and Signs

Part	Type	Meaning	TERM	DEFINITION
a-	p	without	**aphasia**	inability to speak
phas	r	to speak	(ah FAY zee ah)	
-ia	s	condition of		
cephal	r	head	**cephalalgia**	a headache, or general pain to the head
-algia	s	pain	(seff al AL jee ah)	
dys-	p	difficult, pain	**dysphasia**	difficulty speaking
phas	r	to speak	(dis FAY zee ah)	
-ia	s	condition of		
hyper-	p	excessive	**hyperesthesia**	increased sensitivity to stimulation such as touch or pain
esthes	r	sensation	(HIGH per ess THEE zee ah)	
-ia	s	condition of		
neur	r	nerve	**neuralgia**	pain in a nerve
-algia	s	pain	(noo RAL jee ah)	
neur	r	nerve	**neurasthenia**	a vague condition of body fatigue often associated with depression
astheni	r	weakness	(noo ras THEE nee ah)	
-a	s	condition of		
par-	p	beside, around	**paresthesia**	abnormal sensation of numbness and tingling without an objective cause
esthes	r	sensation	(par ess THEE zee ah)	
-ia	s	condition of		

SELF QUIZ 6.3

SAY IT—SPELL IT!

Review the terms of the nervous system by speaking the phonetic pronunciation out loud, then writing the correct spelling of the term.

Success Hint: Use the audio glossary on the CD and CW for additional help with pronunciation of these terms.

1. seff al AL jee ah   _____

2. high per ess THEE zee ah   _____

3. ah FAY zee ah   _____

4. dis FAY zee ah   _____

5. noo RAL jee ah   _____

6. noo ras THEE nee ah   _____

7. par es THEE zee ah   _____

MATCH IT!

Match the term on the left with the correct definition on the right.

_____1. aphasia   a. difficulty with speech

_____2. cephalalgia   b. a vague condition of fatigue

_____3. paresthesia   c. increased sensitivity to a stimulus

_____4. neuralgia   d. a headache

_____5. hyperesthesia   e. inability to speak

_____6. neurasthenia   f. pain in a nerve

_____7. dysplasia   g. abnormal sensation of numbness

BREAK IT DOWN!

Analyze and separate each term into its word parts by labeling each word part using p = prefix, r = root, cv = combining vowel, and s = suffix.

1. cephalalgia   _____

2. hyperesthesia   _____

3. aphasia   _____

4. neuralgia   _____

5. neurasthenia   _____

WORD BUILDING

Construct or recall medical terms from the following meanings.

1. a headache   _____
2. excessive sensitivity to a stimulus _____
3. nerve pain   _____
4. literally, nerve weakness   _____
5. difficulty speaking   _____
6. abnormal sensation of weakness   _____

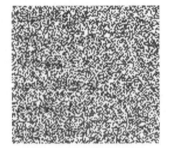

Diseases and Disorders

WORD PARTS (WHEN APPLICABLE)			TERM	DEFINITION
Part	Type	Meaning		
a-	p	without	**agnosia** (ahg NOH see ah)	a loss of the ability to interpret sensory information
gnos	r	knowledge		
-ia	s	condition of		
			Alzheimer's disease (ALTS high merz)	deterioration of brain function characterized by confusion, short term memory loss, and restlessness; abbreviated **AD** (Figure 6.8::::)

[FYI]

Alzheimer's Disease

Alzheimer's disease (AD) is a progressive, degenerative disease of the brain. It is characterized by short term memory loss, disorientation, and confusion. It is the most common cause of the general brain disorder, dementia, among people aged 60 years and older. It is named after the German physician Dr. Alois Alzheimer, who in 1906 was the first to draw the connection between the symptoms and the presence of abnormal clumps that form in the brain of patients who died of the disease. The clumps are now called amyloid plaques and neurofibrillary tangles in the cerebrum, and are irreversible changes without a known cause or cure.

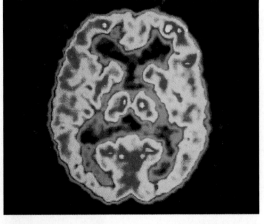
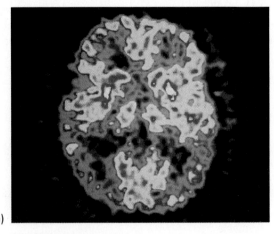

(a)   (b)

Figure 6.8 ::::   **Alzheimer's disease and PET scan images.**

(a) PET scan of a normal brain. The red and yellow areas represent normal metabolic activity of healthy neurons, and the blue and black areas represent low activity due to the presence of ventricles with CSF. *Source: Pearson Education.*

(b) PET scan of an Alzhemier patient's brain. Notice the reduction of activity in this scan relative to the normal brain scan. *Source: Pearson Education.*

WORD PARTS (WHEN APPLICABLE)			TERM	DEFINITION
Part	Type	Meaning		
a-	p	without	**amyotrophic**	progressive atrophy (loss of) muscle caused by
my/o	r/cv	muscle	**lateral sclerosis**	hardening of nervous tissue on the lateral columns of
-troph	s	development	(ah mih oh TROF ik	the spinal cord. It is also known as **Lou Gehrig's**
-ic	s	pertaining to	LAT er al	**disease** after the professional baseball player whose
later	r	side	skleh ROH sis)	experience with this disease brought it to national
-al	s	pertaining to		attention; abbreviated **ALS**
scler	r	hardening		
-osis	s	condition of		
cerebell	r	little brain	**cerebellitis**	inflammation of the cerebellum
-itis	s	inflammation	(ser eh bell EYE tiss)	
cerebr	r	brain	**cerebral aneurysm**	a type of cerebral vascular disease where a blood
-al	s	pertaining to	(seh REE bral	vessel supplying the brain becomes dilated
aneurysm		dilation	AN yoo rizm)	
cerebr	r	brain	**cerebral arteriosclerosis**	a type of cerebral vascular disease characterized by
-al	s	pertaining to	(seh REE bral	hardening of the arteries of the brain
arteri/o	r/cv	artery	ar tee ree oh skleh ROH sis)	
scler	r	hardening		
-osis	s	condition of		
cerebr	r	brain	**cerebral atherosclerosis**	a type of cerebral vascular disease where a buildup
-al	s	pertaining to	(seh REE bral	of fatty plaque on the inside wall of a vessel
ather/o	r/cv	fatty substance	ath er oh skleh ROH sis)	supplying the brain results in reduced blood flow
scler	r	hardening		
-osis	s	condition of		
cerebr	r	brain	**cerebral embolism**	presence of an embolism (floating blood clot) in a
-al	s	pertaining to	(seh REE bral	blood vessel supplying the brain
embol	r	a throwing in	EM boh lizm)	
-ism	s	condition of		
cerebr	r	brain	**cerebral palsy**	a condition revealed by partial muscle paralysis that
-al	s	pertaining to	(seh REE bral	is caused by a brain defect or lesion present at birth
			PAWL zee)	or shortly after; abbreviated **CP**
cerebr	r	brain	**cerebral thrombosis**	a thrombosis (lodged blood clot) within vessels
-al	s	pertaining to	(seh REE bral	supplying the brain
thromb	r	clot	throm BOH sis)	
-osis	s	condition of		
cerebr/o	r/cv	brain	**cerebrovascular accident**	caused by a thrombosis, embolism, or hemorrage
vascul	r	small vessel	(ser eh broh VASS	(blood loss), this disruption of the blood supply to
-ar	s	pertaining to	kyoo lar)	the brain results in functional losses or death; also
				called stroke and abbreviated **CVA** (Figure 6.7)
cerebr/o	r/cv	brain	**cerebrovascular disease**	a general disorder resulting from a change within
vascul	r	small vessel	(ser eh broh VASS	one or more blood vessels supplying the brain
-ar	s	pertaining to	kyoo lar)	
			coma	a general term describing several levels of
			(KOH mah)	decreased consciousness; also known as deep sleep
			dementia	literally *not in the mind,* impairment of mental
			(de MEN she ah)	function that is characterized by memory loss,
				disorientation, and confusion
dur	r	hard	**duritis**	inflammation of the dura mater
-itis	s	inflammation	(doo RYE tiss)	

WORD PARTS (WHEN APPLICABLE)			TERM	DEFINITION
Part	Type	Meaning		
encephal	r	brain	**encephalitis**	inflammation of the brain, usually caused by
-itis	s	inflammation	(en seff ah LYE tiss)	bacterial or viral infection (Figure 6.9▓)

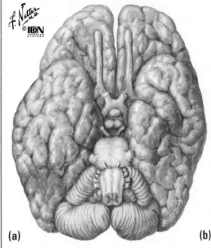

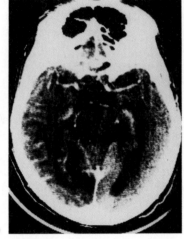

Figure 6.9 ▓ **Encephalitis.**
(a) Illustration of the ventral side of a brain with encephalitis. Notice the inflammation of the right and left temporal lobes and frontal lobes, shown in pink. It is usually caused by a release of bacterial toxins that penetrate the blood-brain barrier.
(b) CAT scan of a brain with encephalitis, which is represented by the abnormal presence of fluids along the edges of the brain (fluid appears white).
Source: Icon Learning Systems.

(a)   **(b)**

encephal/o	r/cv	brain	**encephalomalacia**	softening of brain tissue, usually caused by deficient
			(en seff ah loh mah	blood flow
-malacia	s	softening	LAY she ah)	
epi-	p	upon	**epilepsy**	a brain disorder characterized by recurrent seizures
-lepsy	s	seizure	(EP ih lep see)	

[FYI]

Epilepsy
Epileptic seizures have been written about since 400 BC, when they were first described by Hippocrates in his book *Sacred Disease*. His Greek culture believed it was a punishment for offending the gods. The term *epilepsia* literally means *seized upon by the gods*. The misconception that epilepsy is divine punishment or a form of evil persisted until the late 19th century.

gangli	r	knot, swelling,	**gangliitis**	inflammation of a ganglion
-itis	s	inflammation	(gang lee EYE tiss)	
gli	r	glue	**glioma**	a tumor of neuroglial cells (Figure 6.10▓)
-oma	s	tumor	(glee OH mah)	
hemi-	p	half	**hemiplegia**	paralysis on one side of the body
-plegia	s	paralysis	(hem ee PLEE jee ah)	
hydro-	p	water	**hydrocephalus**	increased volume of CSF in the brain ventricles of a
cephal	r	head	(high droh SEFF ah lus)	child before the cranial sutures have sealed, causing
-us	s	pertaining to		enlargement of the cranium
mening/i	r	membrane	**meningioma**	benign tumor of the meninges (Figure 6.11▓)
-oma	s	tumor	(meh nin jee OH mah)	

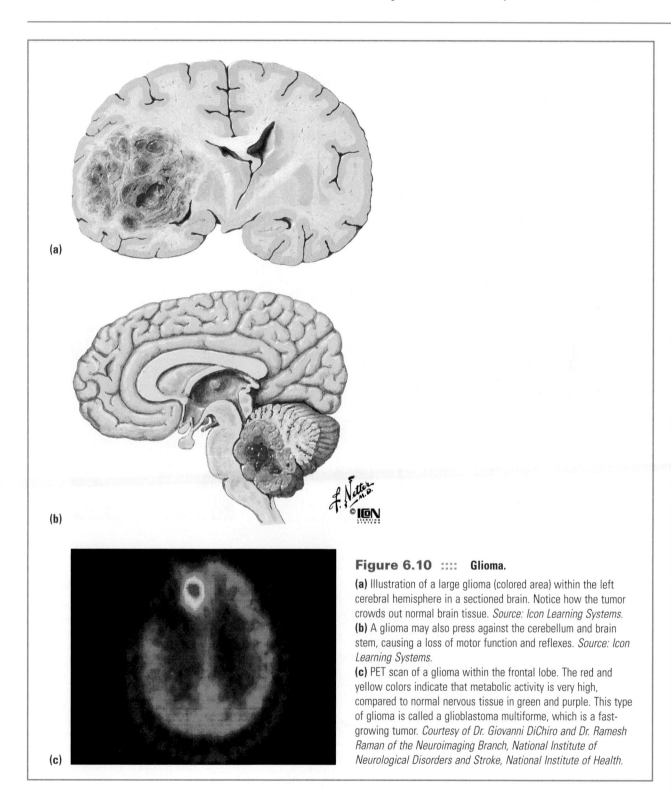

(a)

(b)

(c)

Figure 6.10 :::: Glioma.

(a) Illustration of a large glioma (colored area) within the left cerebral hemisphere in a sectioned brain. Notice how the tumor crowds out normal brain tissue. *Source: Icon Learning Systems.*
(b) A glioma may also press against the cerebellum and brain stem, causing a loss of motor function and reflexes. *Source: Icon Learning Systems.*
(c) PET scan of a glioma within the frontal lobe. The red and yellow colors indicate that metabolic activity is very high, compared to normal nervous tissue in green and purple. This type of glioma is called a glioblastoma multiforme, which is a fast-growing tumor. *Courtesy of Dr. Giovanni DiChiro and Dr. Ramesh Raman of the Neuroimaging Branch, National Institute of Neurological Disorders and Stroke, National Institute of Health.*

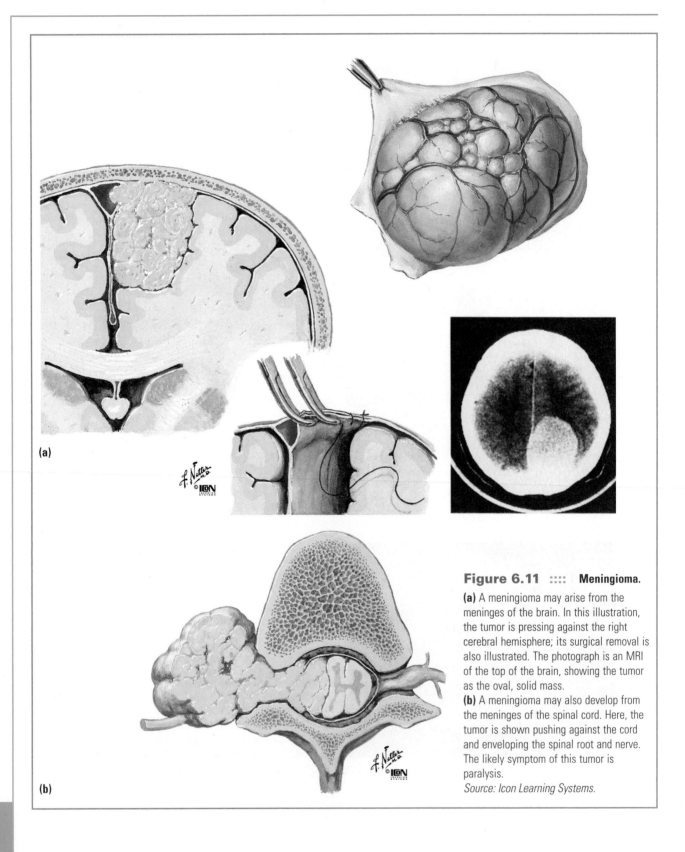

Figure 6.11 :::: **Meningioma.**

(a) A meningioma may arise from the meninges of the brain. In this illustration, the tumor is pressing against the right cerebral hemisphere; its surgical removal is also illustrated. The photograph is an MRI of the top of the brain, showing the tumor as the oval, solid mass.

(b) A meningioma may also develop from the meninges of the spinal cord. Here, the tumor is shown pushing against the cord and enveloping the spinal root and nerve. The likely symptom of this tumor is paralysis.

Source: Icon Learning Systems.

WORD PARTS (WHEN APPLICABLE)			TERM	DEFINITION
Part	Type	Meaning		
mening -itis	r s	membrane inflammation	**meningitis** (men in JYE tiss)	inflammation of the meninges, usually caused by bacterial or viral infection (Figure 6.12::::)
mening/o -cele	r/cv s	membrane hernia	**meningocele** (men IN goh seel)	protrusion of the meninges through an opening caused by a defect in the skull or spinal column (Figure 6.13::::)

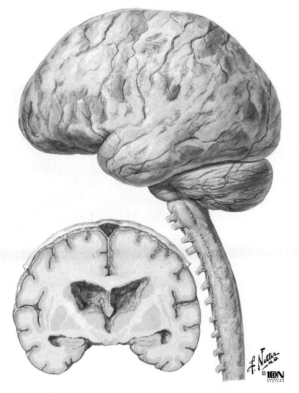

Figure 6.12 ::::

Meningitis. Caused by either bacterial or viral infection, it usually strikes the meninges of the spinal cord. If the infection spreads to the meninges of the brain, it may develop into encephalitis, a condition with more life-threatening consequences. The illustrations show a lateral view of the spinal cord and brain meningitis, and a cross section of brain meningitis. There is also involvement within the ventricles of the brain in this example.
Source: Icon Learning Systems.

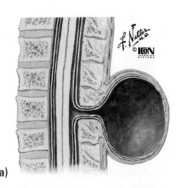

(a)

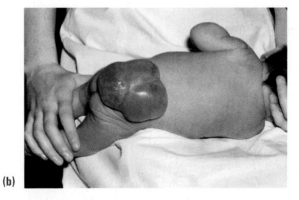

(b)

Figure 6.13 :::: Meningocele.

(a) A meningocele is a herniation of the meninges, usually associated with the spinal cord. It is illustrated in this cross-sectional view of a portion of the vertebral column as the large swelling. When it occurs in a newborn, it is a congenital defect known as *spina bifida. Source: Icon Learning Systems.*
(b) Photograph of a child born with spina bifida, with a large meningocele.

WORD PARTS (WHEN APPLICABLE)			TERM	DEFINITION
Part	**Type**	**Meaning**		
mening/o myel/o -cele	r/cv r/cv s	membrane spinal cord hernia	**meningomyelocele** (men IN goh MY eh loh seel)	protrusion of the meninges and spinal cord through the spinal column
mono- -plegia	p s	single paralysis	**monoplegia** (mon oh PLEE jee ah)	paralysis of one limb
scler -osis	r s	hardening condition of	**multiple sclerosis** (MULL tih pl skleh ROH sis)	the deterioration of the myelin sheath covering axons within the brain, exhibited by episodes of localized functional losses; abbreviated **MS** (Figure 6.14::::)

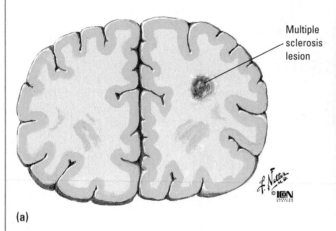

Multiple sclerosis lesion

(a)

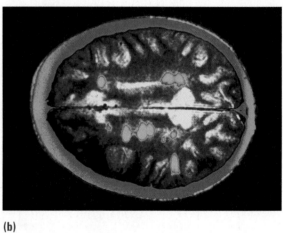

(b)

Figure 6.14 :::: **Multiple sclerosis (MS).**

(a) A disease characterized by the gradual development of small areas of hardened (sclerotic) tissue in the cerebrum, it results in a gradual loss of brain function. The illustration shows a single sclerotic lesion within the right cerebral hemisphere. *Source: Icon Learning Systems.*
(b) MRI of sclerotic lesions within the brain, which are characteristic of MS.

myel -itis	r s	spinal cord inflammation	**myelitis** (my eh LYE tiss)	inflammation of the spinal cord
narc/o -lepsy	r/cv s	numbness seizure	**narcolepsy** (NAR koh lep see)	a sleep disorder characterized by sudden uncontrollable attacks of sleep, attacks of paralysis, and hypnagogic hallucinations (dreams intruding wakefulness)
neur -itis	r s	nerve inflammation	**neuritis** (noo RYE tiss)	inflammation of a nerve
neur/o arthr/o -pathy	r/cv r/cv s	nerve joint disease	**neuroarthropathy** (NOOR oh ar THROP ah thee)	a disease of the nervous system resulting in pain within one or more joints
neur -oma	r s	nerve tumor	**neuroma** (noo ROH mah)	a general term for any tumor originating from nervous tissue
neur -osis	r s	nerve condition of	**neurosis** (noo ROH sis)	an emotional disorder involving a counterproductive way of dealing with stress

WORD PARTS (WHEN APPLICABLE)			TERM	DEFINITION
Part	Type	Meaning		
			palsy (PAWL zee)	paralysis of localized areas; the most common is Bell's palsy, in which facial muscles are paralyzed on one side of the head
para- -plegia	p s	beside, around paralysis	**paraplegia** (pair ah PLEE jee ah)	paralysis from the waist down
			Parkinson's disease	chronic degenerative disease of the brain indicated by hand tremors, rigidity, expressionless face, and shuffling gait; also called Parkinsonism and abbreviated **PD**
poli/o myel -itis	r/cv r s	gray spinal cord inflammation	**poliomyelitis** (poh lee oh my eh LYE tiss)	inflammation of gray matter of the spinal cord caused by one of several polioviruses that often leads to paralysis; also called **polio**
poly- neur -itis	p r s	many nerve inflammation	**polyneuritis** (pol ee noo RYE tiss)	inflammation of many nerves at one time
psych/o -pathy	r/cv s	mind disease	**psychopathy** (sigh KOP ah thee)	a disease of the mind
psych -osis	r s	mind condition of	**psychosis** (sigh KOH siss)	an incapacitating mental disorder indicated by a gross distortion of emotions, incapacity to recognize reality and relate to others, and cope with ordinary demands of daily life
psych/o somat -ic	r/cv r s	mind body pertaining to	**psychosomatic** (SIGH koh soh MAHT ik)	pertaining to both the mind and body
quadri- -plegic	r s	four paralysis	**quadriplegia** (kwod rih PLEE jee ah)	paralysis of all four limbs; also known as tetraplegia (tet rah PLEE jee ah)
radicul -itis	r s	nerve root inflammation	**radiculitis** (rah dik yoo LYE tiss)	inflammation of the spinal nerve roots
radicul/o -pathy	r/cv s	nerve root disease	**radiculopathy** (rah dik yoo LOP ah thee)	a disease of spinal nerve roots
			sciatica (sigh AT ih kah)	inflammation of the sciatic nerve, producing pain that extends from the thigh to the toes
			seizure (SEE zyoor)	a sudden attack of spasms or convulsions; seizures are classified as grand mal (also called tonic-clonic) which involves all muscle groups, petit mal (also called absence) which involves brief losses of consciousness without motor involvement, or partial, which involves only limited areas of the brain with local symptoms
			shingles	viral infection of the peripheral nerves that erupts as painful skin blisters along nerve tracts; also called herpes zoster
			syncope (SIN koh pee)	fainting, usually caused by a sudden loss of blood flow to the brain
			transient ischemic attack (iss KEM ik)	a brief episode of loss of blood flow to the brain that results in a temporary neurologic impairment, and often precedes a CVA; abbreviated **TIA**

disease focus | Accumulation of Fluids in the Brain

Two types of fluids circulate throughout the cranial cavity: blood in blood vessels, and cerebrospinal fluid (CSF) in ventricles and in the narrow channels that interconnect them. If either of these fluids escapes the boundaries of their containment, the pressure within the cranium, or intracranial pressure, will rise because of the rigid walls formed by the skull bones. Severe health problems occur when intracranial pressure rises.

Blood may escape from blood vessels coursing through the brain as a result of a severe head injury, or a congenital weakness in the wall of an artery known as an **aneurysm** (an aneurysm is a common cause of stroke, or CVA). In either case, blood vessels rupture, allowing blood to flow from the bloodstream into brain tissue and surrounding spaces. As a result, the pressure within the cranial cavity rises. A rise in intracranial pressure compresses the soft brain tissue by forcefully pushing against it. If medical intervention is not available and the extent of brain compression becomes severe, neural damage and dysfunction will result and often lead to unconsciousness and death. Medical intervention often includes surgical insertion of a draining tube to remove the excess blood, and if possible, surgical repair of the damaged vessels.

Cerebrospinal fluid is normally produced by a continual leakage of blood plasma through special capillary walls in the ventricles of the brain. The result is a constant, internal flow of CSF that begins in the ventricles and continues through channels that connect the ventricles to each other and to the subarachnoid space that surrounds the brain and spinal cord. At the top of the brain, the CSF is absorbed back into the bloodstream at the same rate at which it is produced.

Any disturbance of CSF production, circulation, or reabsorption may result in an increased fluid volume, causing a potentially dangerous increase in intracranial pressure. Such a disturbance can be caused by head injuries, masses such as tumors or abscesses blocking one of the flow channels, or congenital defects that restrict normal CSF circulation. During a disturbance, the ventricles gradually increase in volume as they fill with incoming CSF, much like filling a water balloon. As a result, brain tissue becomes compressed against the rigid cranial walls, leading to brain damage and functional deterioration.

In infants born with the congenital defect, the brain tissue is pushed against the flexible cranium that has not yet sutured, expanding the cranium to form an enlarged head. This condition is called **hydrocephalus**, or *water on the brain*. If a blockage in CSF circulation occurs in an adult brain, brain damage is often the result unless medical intervention is rapid. In either case, successful treatment usually involves the surgical installation of a shunt, which serves as a bypass to drain the excess CSF and reduce intracranial pressure.

SELF QUIZ 6.4

SAY IT—SPELL IT!

Review the terms of the nervous system by speaking the phonetic pronunciations out loud, then writing the correct spelling of the term.

1. seh REE bral   AN yoo rizm _____
2. en seff ah LYE tiss _____
6.8 3. gang lee EYE tiss _____
6.9 4. glee OH mah _____
5. ser eh bell EYE tiss _____
6.10 6. men IN goh seel _____
7. MULL tih pl   skleh ROH sis _____
8. my eh LYE tiss _____
6.11 9. noo RYE tiss _____
10. hem ee PLEE jee ah _____
11. poh lee oh my eh LYE tiss _____
6.12 12. pol ee noo RYE tiss _____
13. rah dik yoo LYE tiss _____

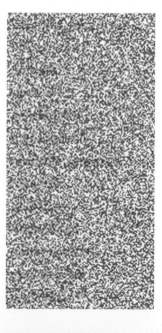

MATCH IT!

Match the term on the left with the correct definition on the right.

_____ 1. agnosia

_____ 2. cerebral palsy

_____ 3. coma

_____ 4. dementia

_____ 5. epilepsy

_____ 6. neurosis

_____ 7. Parkinsonism

_____ 8. psychosis

_____ 9. palsy

_____10. narcolepsy

_____11. sciatica

_____12. shingles

_____13. syncope

_____14. transient ischemic attack

a. recurrent seizures

b. incapacity to recognize reality

c. partial muscle paralysis caused by a brain defect

d. paralysis of localized areas

e. a sleep disorder

f. herpes zoster

g. decreased consciousness

h. inflammation of the sciatic nerve

i. *not in the mind*

j. brief episode of blood loss to the brain

k. fainting

l. inability to interpret sensory information

m. tremors and rigidity

n. having trouble dealing with stress

BREAK IT DOWN!

Analyze and separate each term into its word parts by labeling each word part using p = prefix, r = root, cv = combining vowel, and s = suffix.

1. cerebral arteriosclerosis   _____

2. encephalitis   _____

3. encephalomalacia   _____

4. gangliitis   _____

5. hydrocephaly   _____

6. meningitis   _____

7. meningomyelocele   _____

8. neuroarthropathy   _____

9. quadriplegia   _____

10. polyneuritis   _____

11. psychosomatic   _____

WORD BUILDING

Construct or recall medical terms from the following meanings.

1. blood vessel dilation supplying the brain   _____

2. disruption of blood supply to the brain   _____

3. inflammation of the dura mater   _____

4. inflammation of the brain   _____

5. a tumor of neuroglial cells   _____

6. inflammation of the meninges   _____

7. protrusion of the meninges and spinal cord   _____

8. viral infection of peripheral nerves   _____

9. a sleep disorder with sudden sleep attacks   _____

10. a brain defect causing partial muscle paralysis   _____

6.13 11. levels of unconsciousness; deep sleep   _____

12. abbreviation for Alzheimer's disease   _____

13. grand mal, petit mal, or partial seizures   _____

FILL IT IN!

Fill in the blanks with the correct terms.

1. The inability to interpret sensory information is known as _____,
which can be determined with EP studies and reflex testing.

6.14 2. Although the cause of _____ disease (AD) is not yet known, evidence
indicates the condition has been on the rise in recent years. One of its symptoms in
advanced stages is _____, which literally means *not in the mind*.

3. A brain disorder characterized by recurrent seizures is known
as _____.

4. The paralysis of facial muscles on one side is known as Bell's _____.

5. A chronic degenerative brain disorder characterized by hand tremors and rigidity is
called _____ disease.

6. Inflammation of the sciatic nerve, or _____, is often caused by a
herniated disk.

7. _____ is caused by a family of viruses that also cause chicken
pox, and is characterized by painful skin blisters that erupt along nerve tracts.

8. A sleep disorder characterized by sudden attacks of sleep is known as
_____.

9. An early sign of _____ ischemic attack, or TIA, is frequent spells
of fainting, or _____.

10. A brain defect during fetal development can result in the loss of muscle control
throughout life, a condition known as _____
_____ (CP).

6.15 11. A cerebrovascular accident is caused by a disruption in blood flow to the brain. This
condition is also called a _____.

Treatments, Procedures, and Devices

WORD PARTS (WHEN APPLICABLE)			TERM	DEFINITION
Part	**Type**	**Meaning**		
an-	p	without	**analgesic**	an agent that relieves pain
-alges	r	pain	(an al JEE zik)	
-ic	s	pertaining to		
an-	p	without	**anesthesia**	without feeling or sensation
esthes	r	sensation	(an ess THEE zee ah)	
-ia	s	condition of		
cerebr	r	brain	**cerebral angiography**	x-ray photograph of the blood vessels in the brain
-al	s	pertaining to	(seh REE bral	following injection of a contrast medium
angi/o	r/cv	vessel	an jee OG rah fee)	(Figure 6.15 :::::)
-graphy	s	recording		

[FYI]

-graphy or -gram
Remember that the suffix -graphy means *a procedure involving a recording instrument,* while the suffix -gram means *a written record.* In each of these procedures, switching the suffix from -graphy to -gram creates the term used for the written record.

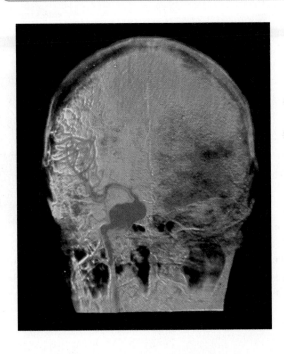

Figure 6.15 :::::
Cerebral angiography.

tom/o	r/cv	to cut	**computed tomography**	also called a **CT scan**, this procedure involves the use of a computer to interpret a series of images and construct from them a 3-dimensional view of the brain; this is particularly useful in diagnosing tumors
-graphy	s	recording	(toh MOG rah fee)	

WORD PARTS (WHEN APPLICABLE)			TERM	DEFINITION
Part	Type	Meaning		
crani	r	skull, cranium	**craniectomy**	excision (surgical removal) of part of the skull to
-ectomy	s	excision	(KRAY nee EK toh mee)	approach the brain (Figure 6.16 ::::)
crani	r	skull, cranium	**craniotomy**	incision (surgical entry) into the skull to approach
-otomy	s	incision	(kray nee OTT oh mee)	the brain
echo	r	to bounce	**echoencephalography**	use of **ultrasonography** (ull trah sun OG rah fee) or
encephal/o	r/cv	brain	(ek oh en SEFF ah	ultrasound (sound waves) to record brain
-graphy	s	recording	LOG rah fee)	structures; abbreviated **EchoEG**
electr/o	r/cv	electricity	**electroencephalography**	a procedure recording the electrical impulses of the
encephal/o	r/cv	brain	(ee lek troh en SEFF	brain (or brain waves); abbreviated **EEG** (Figure
-graphy	s	recording	ah LOG rah fee)	6.17 ::::)

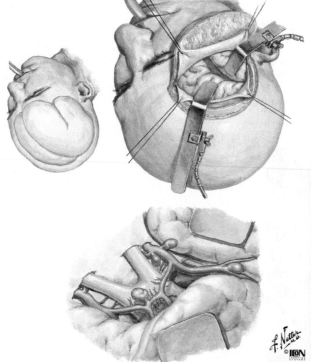

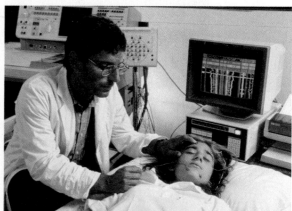

Figure 6.16 :::: **Cerebral aneurysm and craniectomy.**

As the lower illustration reveals, cerebral aneurysm is the abnormal dilation of arteries, which is caused by a weakening of the arterial walls. The upper illustration demonstrates a treatment for this condition, which includes a craniectomy followed by excision of the dilations.
Source: Icon Learning Systems.

Figure 6.17 :::: **Electroencephalogram (EEG).**

To obtain the EEG, electrodes attached to the patient's head pick up electrical signals and convey them to a computer for analysis and printing.

			evoked potential studies	also called **EP studies,** this group of diagnostic tests measures changes in brain waves during particular stimuli to determine brain function, providing a test for sight, hearing, and other senses
ganglion	r	swelling	**ganglionectomy**	excision of a ganglion; also called gangliectomy
-ectomy	s	excision	(GANG lee on EK toh mee)	(GANG lee EK toh mee)

WORD PARTS (WHEN APPLICABLE)			TERM	DEFINITION
Part	**Type**	**Meaning**		
			lumbar puncture (LUM bar)	aspiration (fluid withdrawal with a syringe) of CSF from the subarachnoid space in the lumbar region of the spinal cord (Figure 6.18▦); abbreviated **LP**

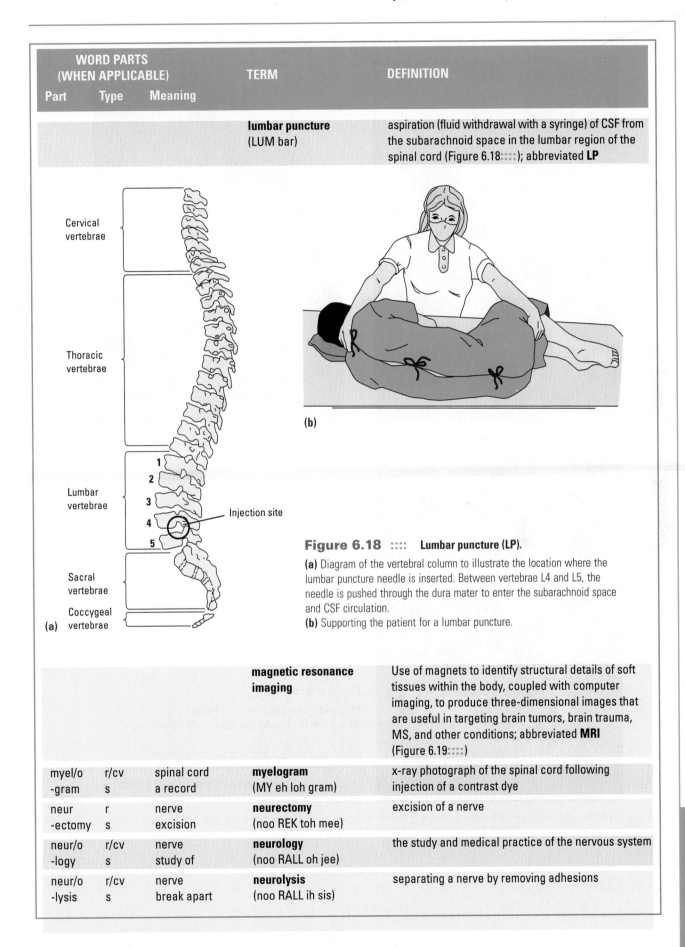

Cervical vertebrae

Thoracic vertebrae

Lumbar vertebrae

1
2
3
4
5

Injection site

Sacral vertebrae

Coccygeal vertebrae

(a)

(b)

Figure 6.18 ▦ **Lumbar puncture (LP).**

(a) Diagram of the vertebral column to illustrate the location where the lumbar puncture needle is inserted. Between vertebrae L4 and L5, the needle is pushed through the dura mater to enter the subarachnoid space and CSF circulation.
(b) Supporting the patient for a lumbar puncture.

WORD PARTS (WHEN APPLICABLE)			TERM	DEFINITION
			magnetic resonance imaging	Use of magnets to identify structural details of soft tissues within the body, coupled with computer imaging, to produce three-dimensional images that are useful in targeting brain tumors, brain trauma, MS, and other conditions; abbreviated **MRI** (Figure 6.19▦)
myel/o	r/cv	spinal cord	**myelogram** (MY eh loh gram)	x-ray photograph of the spinal cord following injection of a contrast dye
-gram	s	a record		
neur	r	nerve	**neurectomy** (noo REK toh mee)	excision of a nerve
-ectomy	s	excision		
neur/o	r/cv	nerve	**neurology** (noo RALL oh jee)	the study and medical practice of the nervous system
-logy	s	study of		
neur/o	r/cv	nerve	**neurolysis** (noo RALL ih sis)	separating a nerve by removing adhesions
-lysis	s	break apart		

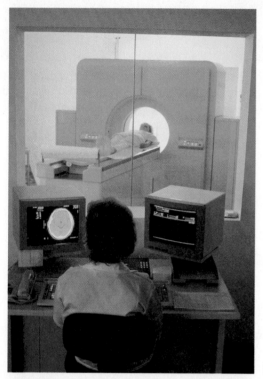
(a)

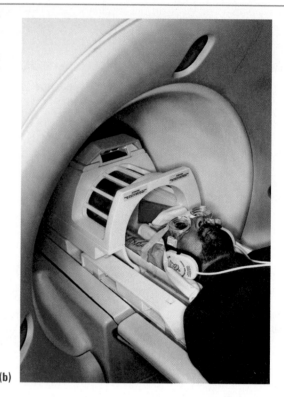
(b)

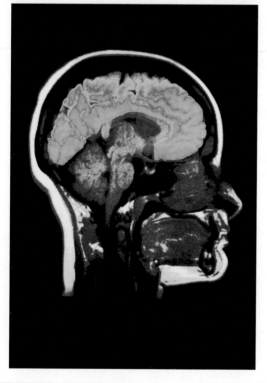
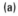
(c)

Figure 6.19 ::::

Magnetic resonance imaging (MRI).
(a) The MRI lab includes the scanning instrument and a computer station.
(b) An open chamber MRI, into which the patient is transported. The "cave" is surrounded by a series of magnets and detectors that rotate around the immobilized patient.
(c) Enhanced color MRI of the head at a lateral view.

WORD PARTS (WHEN APPLICABLE)			TERM	DEFINITION
Part	Type	Meaning		
neur/o -plasty	r/cv s	nerve surgical repair	**neuroplasty** (NOO roh plas tee)	surgical repair of a nerve
neur/o -rrhaphy	r/cv s	nerve suture	**neurorrhaphy** (noo ROR ah fee)	suture of a nerve
neur/o scien -ist	r/cv r s	nerve understanding one who practices	**neuroscientist** (noo roh SIGH en tist)	one who studies in the field of neuroscience
neur/o -tomy	r/cv s	nerve incision	**neurotomy** (noo ROT oh mee)	incision into a nerve
neur/o logist	r/cv s	nerve one who studies	**neurologist** (noo RAL oh jist)	a physician specializing in general disorders of the nervous system
tom/o -graphy	r/cv s	to cut recording	**positron emission tomography** (PAHZ ih tron ee MISH un toh MOG rah fee)	brain scan providing a map of blood flow within the brain that can be correlated to brain activity; abbreviated **PET scan**
psych -iatry	r s	mind treatment, specialty	**psychiatry** (sigh KIGH ah tree)	the branch of medicine that addresses disorders of the brain
psych/o -logy	r/cv s	mind study of	**psychology** (sigh KALL oh jee)	the field of study of human behavior
radic -otomy	r s	nerve root incision	**radicotomy** (ray dih KOT oh mee)	incision into a nerve root; also called rhizotomy (rye ZOT oh mee)
			reflex testing	diagnostic tests performed to observe the body's response to a touch stimulus, which are useful when assessing stroke, head trauma, and other neurological challenges; this includes deep tendon reflexes (DTR) involving percussion at the patellar (Achilles) tendon or elsewhere, and Babinski reflex involving stimulation of the plantar surface of the foot
			sedative (SED ah tiv)	an agent that quiets tension and anxiety
sub- dur -al	p r s	below hard pertaining to	**subdural** (sub DOO ral)	pertaining to below the dura mater

SELF QUIZ 6.5

SAY IT—SPELL IT!

Review the terms of the nervous system by speaking the phonetic pronunciations out loud, then writing the correct spelling of the term.

1. KRAY nee EK toh mee

2. GANG lee on EK toh mee

3. noo REK toh mee

4. noo ROL i siss

5. noo ROR ah fee

6. noo ROT oh mee

6.16 7. ray dih KOT oh mee

8. ek oh en SEFF ah LOG rah fee

MATCH IT!

Match the term on the left with the correct definition on the right.

_____1. PET   a. agent that relieves pain

_____2. MRI   b. agent with a calming effect

_____3. reflex testing   c. magnetic resonance imaging

_____4. sedative   d. deep tendon reflex and Babinski reflex

_____5. analgesic   e. diagnostic imaging of brain function

BREAK IT DOWN!

Analyze and separate each term into its word parts by labeling each word part using p = prefix, r = root, cv = combining vowel, and s = suffix.

1. craniectomy

2. craniotomy

3. ganglionectomy

4. neurolysis

5. neuroplasty

6. radicotomy

WORD BUILDING

Construct or recall medical terms from the following meanings.

1. excision of part of the skull

2. incision into the skull

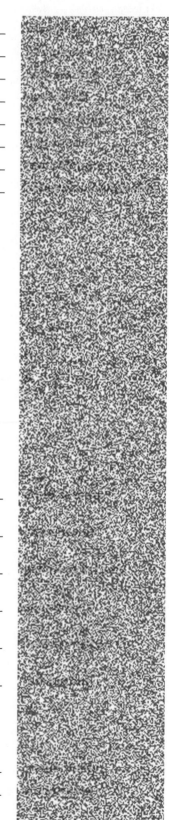

3. separating a nerve by removing adhesions

_____

4. suture of a nerve

_____

6.17 5. numbness or tingling without a known cause

_____

6. excision of a ganglion

_____

7. incision into a nerve root

_____

8. without feeling or sensation

_____

9. recording brain structures with sound waves

_____

10. measuring changes in brain wave activity

_____

11. x-ray of blood vessels in the brain

_____

12. abbreviated as CT or CAT scan

_____

13. an agent that quiets tension and anxiety

_____

6.18 14. a physician specializing in general disorders of the nervous system

_____

FILL IT IN!

Fill in the blanks with the correct terms.

1. To diagnose the extent of a brain injury, a computed _____ (CT) scan is often used initially. For additional structural details, often magnetic resonance imaging or _____ is provided. To test functional damage, _____ potential (EP) testing and positron emission tomography, also called a _____ scan may be used.

2. If a patient has slipped into a coma or "deep sleep," the level of consciousness can be determined with the use of an electroencephalogram or _____.

3. In some patients with reduced blood flow to the brain, a cerebral _____ can be used to determine the location of a blockage. Often, surgical intervention is necessary to prevent a stroke or CVA.

4. A patient with the brain disorder narcolepsy should not be given _____, which quiet tension and anxiety.

5. A computed tomography scan, or _____ scan, is one method of viewing brain structures without the need for invasive surgery.

6. _____ is administered during surgery to free the patient of pain.

abbreviations of the nervous system

The abbreviations that are associated with the nervous system are summarized here.
Study these abbreviations, and review them in the exercise that follows.

ABBREVIATION	DEFINITION	ABBREVIATION	DEFINITION
AD	Alzheimer's disease	EEG	electroencephalogram
ALS	amyotrophic lateral sclerosis	EP	evoked potential
CT (CAT) scan	computed (axial) tomography scan	MRI	magnetic resonance imaging
CP	cerebral palsy	MS	multiple sclerosis
CVA	cerebrovascular accident (stroke)	PD	Parkinson's disease
DTR	deep tendon reflexes	PET	positron emission tomography
EchoEG	echoencephalography	TIA	transient ischemic attack

SELF QUIZ 6.6

Fill in the blanks with the abbreviation or the complete medical term.

Abbreviation

Medical Term

1. _____   evoked potential

2. PET   _____

3. _____   transient ischemic attack

4. EEG   _____

6.19 5. _____   computed axial tomography scan

6. MRI   _____

7. _____   Parkinson's disease

8. CP   _____

9. _____   echoencephalography

10. DTR   _____

11. _____   multiple sclerosis

12. CVA   _____

13. _____   Alzheimer's disease

14. ALS   _____

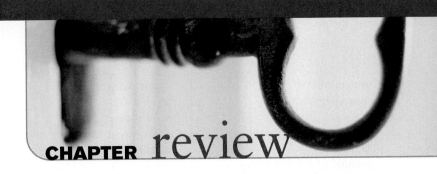

In this section, we will review all the word parts and medical terms from this chapter. As in earlier tables, the word roots are shown in **bold.**

Check each word part and medical term to be sure you understand the meaning. If any are not clear, please go back into the chapter and review that term. Then, complete the review exercises that follow.

[word parts **checklist**]

Prefixes

- ❑ a-
- ❑ di-
- ❑ dys-
- ❑ hemi-
- ❑ hydro-
- ❑ hyper-
- ❑ mono-
- ❑ pan-
- ❑ para-
- ❑ poly-
- ❑ pre-
- ❑ tetra-

Word Roots/Combining Vowels

- ❑ **alges**/o
- ❑ **astheni**/o
- ❑ **cephal**/o
- ❑ **cerebell**/o

- ❑ **cerebr**/o
- ❑ **cran**/o
- ❑ **crani**/o
- ❑ **dur**/o
- ❑ **embol**/o
- ❑ **encephal**/o
- ❑ **esthes**/o
- ❑ **gangli**/o
- ❑ **ganglion**
- ❑ **gli**/o
- ❑ **gnos**/o
- ❑ **lys**/o
- ❑ **mening**/o
- ❑ **ment**/o
- ❑ **myel**/o
- ❑ **neur**/o
- ❑ **phas**/o
- ❑ **plegi**/o
- ❑ **psych**/o

- ❑ **quadr**/i
- ❑ **radic**/o
- ❑ **radicul**/o
- ❑ **somat**/o
- ❑ **thalam**/o

Suffixes

- ❑ -algia
- ❑ -asthenia
- ❑ -cele
- ❑ -gram
- ❑ -iatry
- ❑ -itis
- ❑ -lepsy
- ❑ -oid
- ❑ -paresis
- ❑ -phagia
- ❑ -phasia
- ❑ -plegia

[medical terminology **checklist**]

- ❑ afferent
- ❑ a**gnos**ia
- ❑ Alzheimer's disease (AD)
- ❑ **amy**otrophic **late**ral **scler**osis (ALS)
- ❑ an**alges**ic
- ❑ an**esthes**ia
- ❑ a**phas**ia
- ❑ **arachn**oid
- ❑ axon
- ❑ **cephal**algia
- ❑ **cerebell**itis
- ❑ **cerebell**um
- ❑ **cerebr**al aneurism
- ❑ **cerebr**al **angi**ography

- ❑ **cerebr**al **arterio**scler**osis
- ❑ **cerebr**al **athero**scler**osis
- ❑ **cerebr**al cortex
- ❑ **cerebr**al **embol**ism
- ❑ **cerebr**al hemispheres
- ❑ **cerebr**al palsy (CP)
- ❑ **cerebr**al **thromb**osis
- ❑ **cerebr**ospinal fluid
- ❑ **cerebr**ovascular accident (CVA)
- ❑ **cerebr**ovascular disease
- ❑ **cerebr**um
- ❑ coma
- ❑ computed (axial) **tom**ography (CT or CAT scan)

- ❑ corpus callosum
- ❑ **crani**ectomy
- ❑ **crani**otomy
- ❑ dementia
- ❑ dendrites
- ❑ deep tendon reflexes (DTR)
- ❑ dia**gnos**tic imaging
- ❑ di**encephal**on
- ❑ **dur**a mater
- ❑ **dur**itis
- ❑ dys**phas**ia
- ❑ **echo**encephalography (EchoEG)
- ❑ efferent
- ❑ **electro**encephalogram (EEG)

❏ **encephal**itis
❏ **encephal**omalacia
❏ epilepsy
❏ evoked potential studies (EP studies)
❏ **gangli**a
❏ **gangli**itis
❏ **ganglion**ectomy
❏ **gli**oma
❏ hemi**pleg**ia
❏ hydro**cephal**y
❏ hyper**esthes**ia
❏ hypo**thalam**us
❏ **lumb**ar puncture
❏ magnetic resonance imaging (MRI)
❏ medulla
❏ **mening**ioma
❏ **mening**itis
❏ **mening**ocele
❏ **meningomyel**ocele
❏ mono**pleg**ia

❏ multiple **scler**osis (MS)
❏ **myel**itis
❏ **myel**ogram
❏ **narc**olepsy
❏ **neur**algia
❏ **neur**asthenia
❏ **neur**ectomy
❏ **neur**itis
❏ **neuroarthr**opathy
❏ **neur**olysis
❏ **neur**oma
❏ **neur**oplasty
❏ **neur**orrhaphy
❏ **neur**osis
❏ **neur**otomy
❏ **neur**otransmitter
❏ palsy
❏ para**pleg**ia
❏ par**esthes**ia
❏ Parkinson's disease (PD)
❏ pia mater
❏ **pleg**ia

❏ polio**myel**itis
❏ poly**neur**itis
❏ pons
❏ positron emission **tom**ography (PET)
❏ **psych**opathy
❏ **psych**osis
❏ **psychosom**atic
❏ **quadri**plegia
❏ **radic**otomy
❏ **radicul**itis
❏ reflex testing
❏ Schwann cells
❏ sciatica
❏ sedative
❏ shingles
❏ sub**dur**al
❏ synapse
❏ syncope
❏ **thalam**us
❏ transient ischemic attack (TIA)
❏ **ventr**icle

[show what **you know!**]

BREAK IT DOWN!

Analyze and separate each term into its word parts by labeling each word part using p = prefix, r = root, cv = combining vowel, and s = suffix.

		r s
Example:	1. psychiatry	psych/iatry
	2. dysphasia	_____
	3. hypothalamus	_____
	4. cerebellitis	_____
	5. cerebrovascular	_____
	6. encephalitis	_____
	7. hydrocephaly	_____
	8. meningomyelocele	_____
	9. hyperesthesia	_____
	10. myelitis	_____
	11. neurasthenia	_____
	12. neuroma	_____
	13. paraplegia	_____

14. polyneuritis _____

15. psychosomatic _____

16. craniectomy _____

17. craniotomy _____

18. neurolysis _____

19. radicotomy _____

20. psychopathy _____

21. neurorraphy _____

WORD BUILDING

Construct or recall medical terms from the following meanings.

Example:

1. inability to speak _____ aphasia _____

2. a pain in the head (headache) _____

3. inflammation of the cerebellum _____

4. a disease of blood vessels in the cerebrum _____

5. a tumor of neuroglial cells _____

6. softening of brain tissue _____

7. inflammation of the dura mater _____

8. increased sensitivity to a stimulus _____

9. inflammation of the brain _____

10. protrusion of the meninges _____

11. literally a *condition of many hardened areas* _____

12. inflammation of the spinal cord _____

13. literally *nerve weakness* _____

14. a tumor arising from nervous tissue _____

15. pain in a nerve _____

16. abnormal sensation of numbness _____

17. paralysis on one side of the body _____

18. inflammation of many nerves _____

19. a disease of the mind _____

20. paralysis of all four limbs _____

21. inflammation of the nerve roots _____

22. excision of part of the skull _____

23. incision into the skull _____

24. suture of a nerve _____

25. separating a nerve by removing adhesions _____

26. incision into a nerve _____

CASE STUDIES

Fill in the blanks with the correct terms.

1. The patient was examined following an automobile collision. At the time of admittance she reported symptoms of headache, or (a) _____, generalized pain in the nerves, or (b) _____, of the right shoulder and upper arm, and difficulty with speech, or (c) _____. Physical examination that included (d) _____ _____ _____ (DTR) showed an inflammation of multiple nerves, or (e) _____, of the shoulder and upper arm. Anti-inflammatory medication and pain relievers, or (f) _____, were prescribed for treatment. Two weeks after the first exam, the patient returned with reported episodes of fainting, or (g) _____, with abnormal sensations along the left side of the body that were without an objective cause, or (h) _____. Following a preliminary CT, or (i) _____ _____, scan, an MRI, or (j) _____ _____ _____ was ordered for a more complete evaluation. The MRI revealed bleeding below the dura mater, or a (k) _____ hemorrhage, which was increasing the (l) _____ (within the cranium) pressure. An incision into the cranium, or (m) _____, was performed to correct the hemorrhage and reduce the intracranial pressure. The patient made a complete recovery.

2. A (n) _____ (old age) patient was admitted following an apparent attempted suicide, in which he walked in front of a city bus on a busy street. The trauma of the accident triggered seizures, suggesting a condition of (o) _____. Other symptoms included difficulty speaking, or (p) _____, mental confusion, loss of short term memory, and a loss of the ability to interpret sensory information, or (q) _____. It was determined that the patient suffered from AD, or (r) _____ _____, in addition to the trauma injuries. Due to the accident trauma, the patient was evaluated further with CT scans and MRI. The MRI suggested the presence of a blood clot within the brain, or a (s) _____ _____. A (t) _____ _____ was scheduled to confirm the finding, which would reveal the status of blood vessels supplying the brain. However, before the test could be made, a stroke, or (u) _____ _____, occurred. The stroke was initially believed to be relatively minor, affecting half of the face to produce the condition of (v) _____. However, psychological testing soon determined that the patient had suffered a severe impairment of mental function, or (w) _____. The condition was diagnosed as a (x) _____, due to the incapacitating nature of the mental state. MRIs later showed a softening of brain tissue, or (y) _____, had resulted.

[piece it all **together!**]

CROSSWORD

From the chapter material, fill in the crossword puzzle with answers to the following clues.

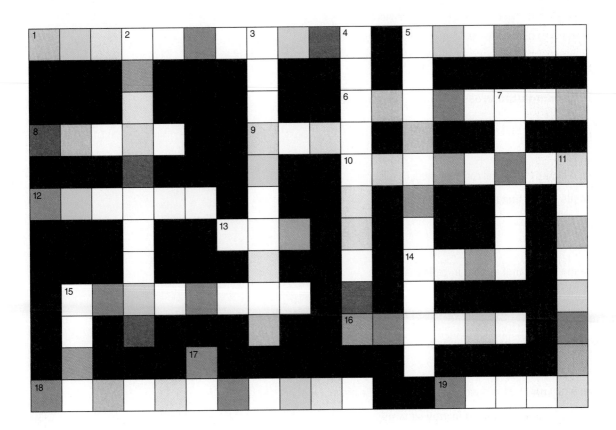

ACROSS

1. A physician specializing in neurology. (Find puzzle piece 6.18)
5. The fatty covering over some axons. (Find puzzle piece 6.2)
6. The membranes surrounding the brain and spinal cord. (Find puzzle piece 6.3)
8. Vaccines have nearly eliminated this disease. (Find puzzle piece 6.12)
9. A root word that means *glue*. (Find puzzle piece 6.9)
10. Where neuron cell bodies may congregate in the PNS. (Find puzzle piece 6.7)
12. The common term for cerebrovascular accident. (Find puzzle piece 6.15)
13. In Arabic, this word means *soft*. (Find puzzle piece 6.4)
14. A long, boring lecture might seem to put you in this state. (Find puzzle piece 6.13)
15. This term literally means *not in the mind*. (Find puzzle piece 6.14)
16. CSF bears a slight hue of this color. (Find puzzle piece 6.6)
18. Abnormal numbness or tingling without a known cause. (Find puzzle piece 6.17)
19. Transmit nerve impulses away from the cell body. (Find puzzle piece 6.1)

DOWN

2. A procedure also known as rhizotomy. (Find puzzle piece 6.16)
3. Inflammation of a ganglion. (Find puzzle piece 6.8)
4. What the "T" in CT scan stands for. (Find puzzle piece 6.19)
5. Protrusion of the meninges. (Find puzzle piece 6.10)
7. A tumor of supporting cells. (Find puzzle piece 6.9)
11. Inflammation of a nerve. (Find puzzle piece 6.11)
15. In Arabic, this term means *hard*. (Find puzzle piece 6.5)
17. An abbreviation for *computed tomography.* (Find puzzle piece 6.19)

WORD UNSCRAMBLE

From the completed crossword puzzle, unscramble:

1. All of the letters that appear in **green** squares

   __ __ ☐ __ __ __ __

   Clue: A blow to the spinal cord may produce this

2. All of the letters that appear in **red** squares

   ☐ __ __ __ __

   Clue: The mind

3. All of the letters that appear in **yellow** squares

   __ __ __ __ __ ☐ __

   Clue: Senseless

4. All of the letters in **orange** squares

   __ ☐ __ __ __ __

   Clue: A tumor that arises from supportive cells in the brain

5. All of the letters that appear in **gray** squares

   __ ☐ __ __ __ __ __

   Clue: Literally a *condition of a nerve,* it makes coping difficult

6. All of the letters in **purple** squares

   __ __ __ __ ☐ __ __ __ __ __ __ __

   Clue: Inflammation of the brain

7. All of the letters in **peach** squares

   __ __ __ __ __ __ ☐

   Clue: When *hard* becomes swollen

8. All of the letters in **pink** squares

   __ __ __ ☐

   Clue: The color of brain matter containing neuron cell bodies

Now write down each of the letters that are boxed and unscramble them to find the hidden medical term of the nervous system: __ __ __ __ __ __ __ __ .

MEDmedia wrap-up

www.prenhall.com/wingerd

Before you go on to the next chapter, take advantage of the free CD-ROM and study guide website that accompany this book. Simply load the CD-ROM for additional activities, games, animations, videos, and quizzes linked to this chapter. Then visit www.prenhall.com/wingerd for even more!

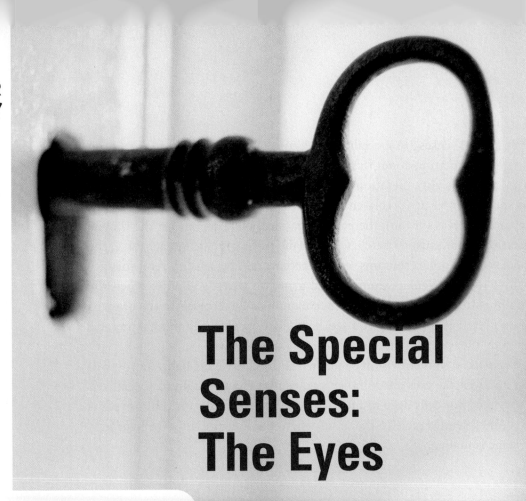

CHAPTER
7

The Special Senses: The Eyes

LEARNING OBJECTIVES

After completing this chapter, you will be able to:

- Define and spell the word parts used to create medical terms for the eyes

- Identify the parts of the eyes and describe their structure and function

- Define common medical terms used for the eyes

- Break down and define common medical terms used for symptoms, diseases, disorders, procedures, treatments, and devices for the eyes

MEDmedia

www.prenhall.com/wingerd

Enhance your study with the power of multimedia! Each chapter of this book links to activities, games, animations, videos, and quizzes that you'll find on your CD-ROM. Plus, you can click on www.prenhall.com/wingerd, to find a free chapter-specific companion website that's loaded with additional practice and resources.

 CD-ROM

- Audio Glossary
- Exercises & Activities
- Flashcard Generator
- Animations
- Videos

Companion Website

- Exercises & Activities
- Audio Glossary
- Drug Updates
- Current News Updates

A secure distance learning course is available at www.prenhall.com/onekey.

The special senses are specialized parts of the body that provide the brain with information about the outside environment. There are four special senses: vision (sight), audation (hearing), gustation (taste), and smell. The four special senses are perceived with the help of highly specialized organs. They are the eyes (vision), the ears (audation), taste organs on the tongue (gustation), and sensory patches within the nose (smell). In each case, the special sensory organ contains sensory receptors. The sensory receptors are sensitive to a particular stimulus, and generate a nerve impulse when the stimulus is sufficiently strong. The nerve impulse then travels to the brain to be interpreted as something you see, hear, taste, or smell. In this chapter, we will study the eyes and the special sense of vision.

The special sense of vision begins when the eyes detect light. As you will soon discover, the eyes are complex organs that channel light to specialized sensory receptor cells deep inside each eye. Once the receptor cells are stimulated, they send signals to the brain where the interpretation of light into an image is made.

word parts focus

Let's look at word parts. The following table contains a list of word parts that when combined build many of the terms of the eyes.

PREFIX	DEFINITION	PREFIX	DEFINITION
a-, an-	without	intra-	within
bi-, bin-	two	para-	near, alongside; departure from normal
e-	to remove		

WORD ROOT	DEFINITION	WORD ROOT	DEFINITION
blephar	eyelid	nyct, nyctal	night, nocturnal
conjunctiv	to bind together, conjunctiva	ocul	eye
cor, core	pupil	opt, ophthalm	eye
corne	horny, cornea	phac, phak	lens
dacry	tear	phot	light
dipl	double	presby	old age
fovea	small pit	retin	net, retina
humor	fluid	scler	thick, hard, sclera
ir, irid	rainbow, iris	stigmat	point
kerat	hard, cornea	ton	tone, tension, pressure
lacrim	tear	vitr, vitre	glassy

SUFFIX	DEFINITION	SUFFIX	DEFINITION
-algia	pain	-ptosis	condition of falling or drooping
-opia	vision	-rrhagia	bleeding, hemorrhage
-phobia	fear	-rrhea	excessive discharge (of fluid)
-plegia	paralysis		

SELF QUIZ 7.1

Review the word parts of terminology for the eyes by working carefully through the exercises that follow. Soon, we will apply this new information to build medical terms.

> **Success Hint:** Once you get to the crossword puzzle at the end of the chapter, remember to check back here for clues! Your clues are indicated by the puzzle icon.

A. Provide the definition of the following prefixes and suffixes.

1. bi-, bin- _____

2. intra- _____

3. -algia _____

4. -opia _____

5. -phobia _____

6. -plegia _____

7. -ptosis _____

8. para- _____

9. -rrhea _____

10. -rrhagia _____

B. Provide the word root for each of the following terms.

1. eyelid _____

2. conjunctiva _____

3. horny, cornea _____

4. tear _____

5. iris _____

7.1 6. hard or cornea _____

7. night or nocturnal _____

8. eye _____

9. lens _____

10. light _____

11. old age _____

12. hard or sclera _____

13. point _____

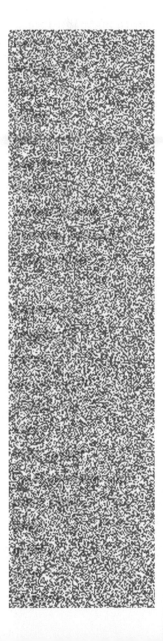

14. glassy   _____

15. fluid   _____

16. net, retina   _____

17. small pit   _____

18. pupil   _____

[anatomy and physiology overview]

The eyes are the organs of vision or sight. Each eye is set within a recession in the skull known as the **orbit**, and covered by the protective fold of the **eyelid** (Figure 7.1::::). The eye receives additional protection from a thin sheet of cells that cover the anterior surface of the eye and the inner surface of the eyelid. This layer is known as the **conjunctiva**, which means *to bind together*. The conjunctiva is kept moistened by watery secretions from the large **lacrimal glands**, which secrete tears, and the smaller **meibomian glands** located along the edges of the eyelids. When the eye is viewed internally (Figure 7.2::::), you can observe that its walls are made of three layers: a fibrous layer, a vascular layer, and a nervous layer.

The outermost layer of the eye is known as the **fibrous layer**. It contains the white part of the eye, called the **sclera**, and the transparent window of the eye, the **cornea**. The term *sclera* is derived from the Greek word *skleros*, which means *hard*. The term *cornea* is from the Latin word *corneus*, which means *made of horn*. Both parts of the fibrous layer are composed of tough fibrous connective tissue, giving the eye a tough, protective outer coat, as their names suggest. Behind the cornea is a narrow chamber known as the **anterior chamber**. It is filled with a watery fluid, the **aqueous humor**, which is continually produced and reabsorbed. The term *aqueous humor* literally means *watery fluid*.

The middle layer of the eye is called the **vascular layer**, due to the abundance of blood vessels it contains. The vascular layer includes the **iris**, **pupil**, **lens**, and **choroid**. The iris is the colored ring of the eye, and includes smooth muscle fibers. Muscles of the iris regulate the amount of light entering the eye through the pupil, the black opening in the center. The word pupil is from the Latin word *pupilla*, which means a *doll* or *little girl*. The lens is a transparent disk that is suspended behind the pupil by suspensory ligaments, which attach to ciliary muscles. The ciliary muscles pull on the lens when they contract, changing the lens shape to allow light to focus on the retina. Behind the lens is a large cavity, the **posterior cavity**, which is filled with a gelatinous material known as **vitreous humor**. The term *vitreous* means *glassy*,

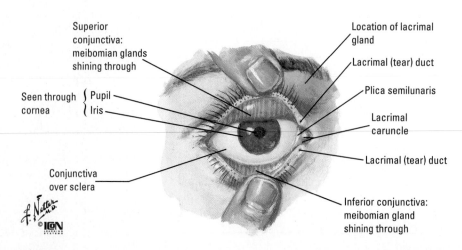

Superior conjunctiva: meibomian glands shining through

Seen through cornea { Pupil, Iris

Conjunctiva over sclera

Location of lacrimal gland

Lacrimal (tear) duct

Plica semilunaris

Lacrimal caruncle

Lacrimal (tear) duct

Inferior conjunctiva: meibomian gland shining through

Figure 7.1 ::::

Anterior surface of the eye.
Source: Icon Learning Systems.

enrichment module enrichment module enrichment module enrichment module enrichment module enrichment module enrichment module enrichm

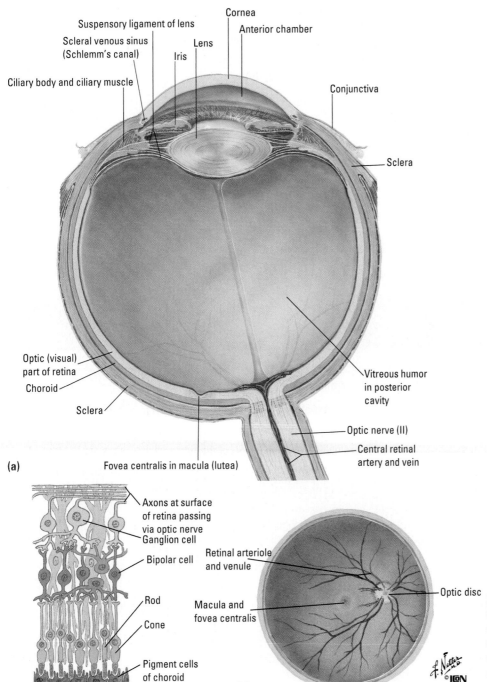

(a)

Suspensory ligament of lens
Scleral venous sinus
(Schlemm's canal)
Ciliary body and ciliary muscle
Iris
Lens
Cornea
Anterior chamber
Conjunctiva
Sclera
Optic (visual) part of retina
Choroid
Sclera
Fovea centralis in macula (lutea)
Vitreous humor in posterior cavity
Optic nerve (II)
Central retinal artery and vein

(b)

Axons at surface of retina passing via optic nerve
Ganglion cell
Bipolar cell
Rod
Cone
Pigment cells of choroid

(c)

Retinal arteriole and venule
Macula and fovea centralis
Optic disc

Figure 7.2 ::::

Eye structure.
(a) Structures of the eye in a sectioned, lateral view.
(b) The retina.
(c) Ophthalmic view of a normal retina.
Source: Icon Learning Systems.

and *humor* means *fluid.* The choroid is rich in blood vessels, whose blood supply nourishes the cells of the retina. The term *choroid* is derived from the Greek word meaning *resembling a membrane.*

The third, innermost layer of the eye is the **nervous layer.** It consists of a thin film at the back of the eye known as the **retina** (Figure 7.2). The term *retina* is derived from the Latin word for *net,* to describe its early appearance to scientists who noticed its thin structure. The retina is composed of neurons, including receptors sensitive to light. Known as **photoreceptors,** they include two types of cells that are descriptive of their shape: **rods** and **cones.** Rods are very sensitive to small amounts of light, but are limited to black and white shades. Cones require more light as a stimulus, but enable you to perceive color. The area of the retina that is the site for your sharpest vision is called the **fovea centralis,** which literally means *central pit.* Named

[thinking critically!]

What do you suppose would be the consequence of seeing with a retina that lacks cone cells?

from the slight depression it lies within, known as the **macula**, the fovea contains the highest concentration of cones in the retina. The neurons that form the retina send information out of the eye by way of the **optic nerve**, which travels to the brain. The exit point of the optic nerve is an area of the retina that lacks photoreceptors, which is why it is called the *blind spot*. Its technical name is the **optic disc**.

getting to the root of it | anatomy and physiology terms

Many of the anatomy and physiology terms are formed from roots that are used to construct the more complex medical terms of the eyes, including symptoms, diseases, and treatments. In this section, we will review the terms that describe the structure and function of the eyes *in relation to their word roots*, which are shown in **bold**.

Study the word roots and terms in this list and complete the review exercises that follow.

Word Root (Meaning)	Terms Formed from the Word Root (Pronunciation)	Definition
conjunctiv (to bind together)	**conjunctiv**a (kon junk TEE vah)	a layer of epithelium covering the inner surfaces of the eyelids and the anterior surface of the eye
corne (horny, cornea)	**corne**a (KOR nee ah)	the anterior part of the fibrous layer, it is a transparent covering over the iris and pupil
fovea (small pit)	**fovea** centralis (FOH vee ah sen TRAH lis)	a small depression in part of the retina where cones are in greatest abundance, making it the area of highest visual acuity
humor (fluid)	vitreous **humor** (VITT ree uss HYOO mer)	a gelatinous mass in the posterior cavity of the eye
	aqueous **humor** (AY kwee uss HYOO mer)	watery fluid in the anterior chamber of the eye
ir (rainbow, iris)	**ir**is (EYE riss)	a ring of smooth muscle that forms the colored part of the eye
lacrim (tear)	**lacrim**al glands (LAK rim al)	tear glands located near the dorsolateral surface of the eye; lacrimal ducts carry the tears from the glands to wash over the anterior surface of the eye
ocul (eye)	intra**ocul**ar (IN trah OK yoo lahr)	pertaining to within the eye
opt (eye)	**opt**ic nerve (OPP tik)	nerve pathway from the retina of both eyes to the brain
	optic disk (OPP tik)	the "blind spot," it is a small region of the retina where photoreceptors are absent due to the origin of the optic nerve
retin (net, retina)	**retin**a (RETT in ah)	a thin film of neurons at the back of the eye containing the photoreceptors
scler (thick, hard)	**scler**a (SKLAIR ah)	the tough, white outer covering of the eye

OTHER IMPORTANT TERMS
The terms in this table are related to the structure and function of the eyes, but are not built from word roots.

anterior chamber	a narrow cavity between the cornea and the iris
choroid (KOH royd)	a thin layer of connective tissue that is rich in blood vessels located behind the retina
cones	cone-shaped photoreceptors that enable color perception
fibrous layer	the outer layer of the eye, it is composed of fibrous connective tissue and includes the cornea and sclera
lens	the disc-shaped transparent structure located behind the pupil, which is suspended by ligaments that are attached to ciliary muscles (contraction of the ciliary muscles changes the shape of the lens)
meibomian glands (my BOH mee ahn)	named after Heinrich Meibom, who first described them in 1683, they are small oil glands in the edges of the eyelids that help lubricate the eyes
posterior cavity	the large cavity of the eye posterior to the lens
pupil (PYOO pill)	an opening at the center of the iris that allows light to pass through; the pupil size is regulated by nervous control of the iris
rods	rod-shaped photoreceptors that are very sensitive to light, but only perceive black and white
vascular layer (VAS kyoo lahr)	the middle layer of the eye, which includes the iris, pupil, lens, and choroid
visual acuity (VIZH oo al ah KYOO ih tee)	quality or sharpness of vision; abbreviated **VA**

SELF QUIZ 7.2

SAY IT—SPELL IT!

Review the terms of the eyes by speaking the phonetic pronunciation out loud, then writing the correct spelling of the term.

Success Hint: Use the audio glossary on the CD and CW for additional help with pronunciation of these terms.

1. AY kwee uss HYOO mer   _____
2. KOH royd   _____
3. EYE riss   _____
4. PYOO pill   _____
5. kon junk TEE vah   _____
6. KOR nee ah   _____
7. SKLAIR ah   _____
8. LAK rim al   _____
9. my BOH mee ahn   _____
10. RETT in ah   _____
11. VITT ree uss HYOO mer   _____

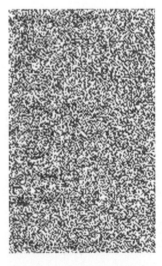

MATCH IT!

Match the term on the left with the correct definition on the right.

_____1. conjunctiva

a. the white outer covering of the eye

_____2. iris

b. carries information to the brain

_____3. cornea

c. literally, "resembling a membrane"

_____4. sclera

d. a transparent disc that changes form

_____5. optic nerve

e. the colored part of the vascular layer

_____6. orbit

f. a gelatinous mass in the posterior cavity

_____7. lens

g. a bony depression that houses the eye

_____8. choroid

h. a watery fluid

_____9. aqueous humor

i. the transparent part of the fibrous layer

_____10. retina

j. a protective epithelial covering

_____11. vitreous humor

k. the "blind spot"

_____12. fovea centralis

l. secretes tears

_____13. optic disc

m. a thin film containing the photoreceptors

_____14. lacrimal gland

n. located along the edge of the eyelids

_____15. meibomian glands

o. the area where vision is best

FILL IT IN!

Fill in the blanks with the correct terms.

1. The layer of epithelium covering the visible part of the eye and inner eyelid is the
   _____. It is lubricated with a watery secretion produced by the
   large _____ glands.

2. The fibrous layer of the eye includes the white _____ and the
   transparent _____.

7.2   3. The vascular layer of the eye includes a circular, colorful band of smooth muscle
   known as the _____, a transparent disc that can change shape

7.3   when ciliary muscles contract, known as the _____, and a thin
   layer of connective tissue behind the retina called the _____,
   which literally means *membrane-like*.

4. A round, black hole that allows light to pass into the eye is known as the

7.4   _____.

5. The _____ chamber is a space located between the cornea and
   iris that is filled with a clear fluid known as
   _____ _____. The cavity behind the lens is the
   _____ cavity and contains a gelatinous material called
   _____ _____.

6. The nervous layer consists of a thin film of nervous tissue known as the

_____. It contains the receptors sensitive to light, or

_____, known as the _____ and

_____. The area of the retina that provides the sharpest vision

is the _____ _____, whereas the area of the

retina where the optic nerve exits is the *blind spot,* or

_____ _____.

[medical terms of the

eyes]

The treatment of diseases associated with the eyes requires medical specialization. **Ophthalmology** is the medical discipline that treats conditions associated with the eyes and vision. This is a constructed term that can be written as

ophthalm/o/logy

where *ophthalm* is a word root that means eye, and -logy is a suffix that means study of, as we have seen before. A physician specializing in this field is called an **ophthalmologist.**

Another word root for eye is opt, which is used to form the term **optometry.** Note that the suffix in optometry is -metry, which means measurement. One who practices optometry is known as an optometrist. An optometrist is not a physician, but is professionally trained to examine eyes to correct vision problems and eye disorders.

As a complex organ that is partially exposed to the outside environment, the eye is subject to many diseases that can affect vision. Some diseases of the eye are inherited, while others may be acquired by injury, infection, or old age. In addition to the eye, diseases that affect other parts of the nervous system can also influence vision. For example, the optic nerve, the thalamus, and part of the occipital lobe of the cerebral cortex (called the visual cortex) all play critical roles in the transmission and interpretation of impulses sent from the retina. Consequently, a developmental defect, a lesion, or an injury that affects any one of these parts can wreak havoc on the sense of sight.

[thinking critically!]

If you were punched in the eye and experienced pain, swelling, and loss of vision to that eye as a result, from what type of eye specialist would you seek medical assistance?

let's construct terms!

In this section, we will assemble all of the word parts to construct medical terminology related to the eyes. Abbreviations are used to indicate each word part: **p** = prefix, **r** = root, **cv** = combining vowel, and **s** = suffix. Note that some terms are not constructed from word parts, but they are included here to expand your vocabulary.

The medical terms of the eyes are listed in the following three sections:

- Symptoms and Signs
- Diseases and Disorders
- Treatments, Procedures, and Devices

Each section is followed by review exercises. Study the lists in these tables and complete the review exercises that follow.

Symptoms and Signs

WORD PARTS (WHEN APPLICABLE)			TERM	DEFINITION
Part	Type	Meaning		
asthen	r	weakness	**asthenopia**	eyestrain
-opia	s	vision	(ass theh NOH pee ah)	
blephar/o	r/cv	eyelid	**blepharoptosis**	drooping of an eyelid (Figure 7.3::::)
-ptosis	s	condition of falling or drooping	(BLEF ah ropp TOH siss)	

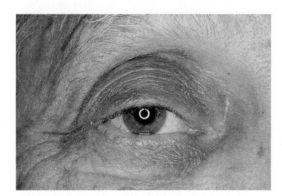

Figure 7.3 ::::

Blepharoptosis. Drooping of an eyelid.
Source: Leonard Lessen/Peter Arnold, Inc.

emmetr	r	according to measure	**emmetropia**	normal condition of the eye; abbreviated **Em**
-opia	s	vision	(em eh TROH pee ah)	(Figure 7.4::::)
leuk/o	r/cv	white	**leukocoria**	condition of white in the pupil
cor	r	pupil	(loo koh KOH ree ah)	
-ia	s	condition of		
ophthalm	r	eye	**ophthalmalgia**	pain associated with the eye
-algia	s	pain	(OFF thal MAHL jee ah)	
oph-thalm/o	r/cv	eye	**ophthalmorrhagia**	hemorrhage (bleeding) of the eye
-rrhagia	s	bleeding	(off THAL moh RAH jee ah)	

SELF QUIZ 7.3

SAY IT—SPELL IT!

Review the terms of the eyes by speaking the phonetic pronunciation guides out loud, then writing in the correct spelling of the term.

7.5 1. ass theh NOH pee ah   _____

2. BLEF ah ropp TOH siss   _____

3. em eh TROH pee ah   _____

4. loo koh KOH ree ah   _____

5. OFF thal MAHL jee ah   _____

6. off THAL moh RAH jee ah   _____

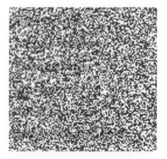

Emmetropia and Refractive Errors

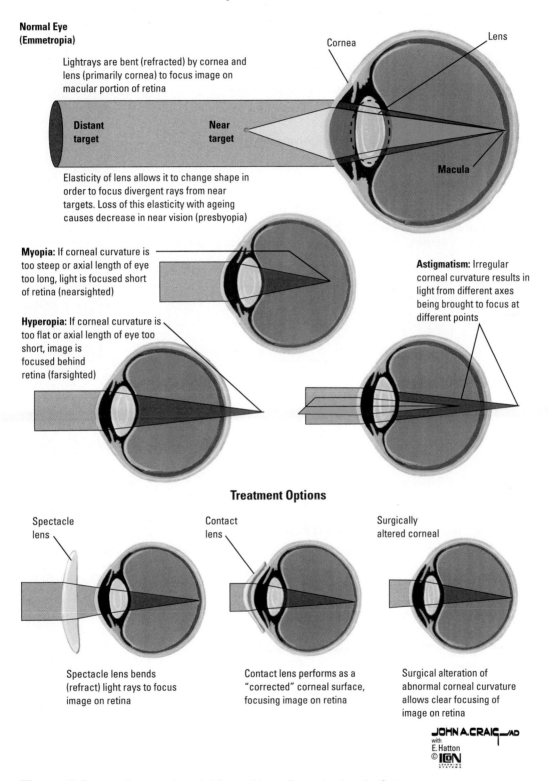

Normal Eye (Emmetropia)

Lightrays are bent (refracted) by cornea and lens (primarily cornea) to focus image on macular portion of retina

Distant target

Near target

Cornea

Lens

Macula

Elasticity of lens allows it to change shape in order to focus divergent rays from near targets. Loss of this elasticity with ageing causes decrease in near vision (presbyopia)

Myopia: If corneal curvature is too steep or axial length of eye too long, light is focused short of retina (nearsighted)

Hyperopia: If corneal curvature is too flat or axial length of eye too short, image is focused behind retina (farsighted)

Astigmatism: Irregular corneal curvature results in light from different axes being brought to focus at different points

Treatment Options

Spectacle lens

Contact lens

Surgically altered corneal

Spectacle lens bends (refract) light rays to focus image on retina

Contact lens performs as a "corrected" corneal surface, focusing image on retina

Surgical alteration of abnormal corneal curvature allows clear focusing of image on retina

JOHN A. CRAIG AD
with
E. Hatton
© ICON
LEARNING
SYSTEMS

Figure 7.4 :::: **Emmetropia and vision problems.** *Source: Icon Learning Systems.*

MATCH IT!

Match the term on the left with the correct definition on the right.

_____1. asthenopia

_____2. blepharoptosis

_____3. emmetropia

_____4. leukocoria

_____5. ophthalmalgia

_____6. ophthalmorrhagia

a. normal condition of the eye

b. hemorrhage of the eye

c. pain associated with the eye

d. eyestrain

e. condition of white in the pupil

f. drooping of an eyelid

BREAK IT DOWN!

Analyze and separate each term into its word parts by labeling each word part using p = prefix, r = root, cv = combining vowel, and s = suffix.

1. asthenopia _____

2. blepharoptosis _____

3. emmetropia _____

4. leukocoria _____

5. ophthalmalgia _____

6. ophthalmorrhagia _____

WORD BUILDING

Construct or recall medical terms from the following meanings.

1. normal condition of the eye _____

2. hemorrhage of the eye _____

3. pain associated with the eye _____

4. eyestrain _____

5. condition of white in the pupil _____

6. drooping of an eyelid _____

Diseases and Disorders

WORD PARTS (WHEN APPLICABLE)			TERM	DEFINITION
Part	Type	Meaning		
a- stigmat -ism	p r s	without point condition of	**astigmatism** (ah STIG mah tizm)	defective curvature of the refractive surface of the eye; abbreviated **Ast** (Figure 7.4)
blephar -itis	r s	eyelid inflammation	**blepharitis** (BLEF ah RYE tiss)	inflammation of the eyelid
			cataract (KAT ah rakt)	a reduction of transparency of the lens (Figure 7.5▦)
			chalazion (kah LAY zee on)	a localized swelling at the edge of an eyelid caused by obstruction of a meibomian gland (Figure 7.6▦)

[FYI]

Cataract

There are more than 30 types of cataracts, most of which arise from time (old age) as the intricate protein structure of the lens gradually breaks down. The term *cataract* is from the Latin word for *waterfall*. It was an ancient belief that the gradual loss of vision was due to a veil that fell between the lens and the cornea, spilling over vision *like a waterfall*.

Chalazion

The Greek word for hailstone, *chalaza*, was used to describe a small skin swelling like a pimple in ancient times. Adding the diminutive ending -ion forms our term, which literally means "a small pimple." Although small, a chalazion is usually a chronic condition of a meibomian gland that can cause local pain to the affected eye and surrounding tissues.

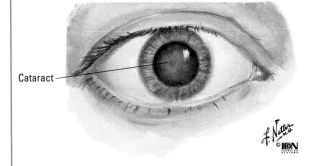

Cataract

Figure 7.5 ▦ **Cataract.** *Source: Icon Learning Systems.*

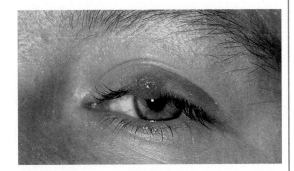

Figure 7.6 ▦ **Chalazion.** *Source: Custom Medical Stock Photo, Inc.*

WORD PARTS (WHEN APPLICABLE)			TERM	DEFINITION
Part	Type	Meaning		
conjuntiv	r	to bind together, conjunctiva	**conjunctivitis** (kon JUNK tih VYE tiss)	inflammation of the conjunctiva; also called pinkeye (Figure 7.7)
-itis	s	inflammation		

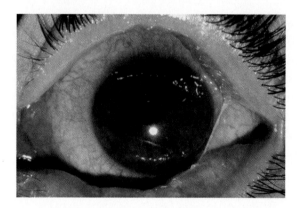

Figure 7.7
Conjunctivitis, with the characteristic "pink eye" appearance. *Source: Buddy Crofton/Medical Images, Inc.*

Part	Type	Meaning	TERM	DEFINITION
corne/o	r/cv	horny, cornea	**corneoiritis** (KOR nee oh eye RYE tiss)	inflammation of the cornea and iris
ir	r	rainbow, iris		
-itis	s	inflammation		
dacry/o	r/cv	tear	**dacryocystitis** (DAK ree oh sist EYE tiss)	inflammation of the lacrimal sac
cyst	r	bladder, sac		
-itis	s	inflammation		
			detached retina (RETT in ah)	separation of the retina from the choroid at the back of the eye
dipl	r	double	**diplopia** (dih PLOH pee ah)	double vision
-opia	s	vision		
endo-	p	within	**endophthalmitis** (ehn doff thal MYE tiss)	inflammation of internal tissues of the eye
ophthalm	r	eye		
-itis	s	inflammation		
			glaucoma (glaw KOH mah)	a loss of vision resulting from increased intraocular pressure, which damages the optic nerve (Figure 7.8)
			hordeolum (hor DEE oh lum)	an infection of a meibomian gland causing a local swelling of the eyelid; also called **sty** (Figure 7.9)
hyper-	p	excessive	**hyperopia** (HIGH per OH pee ah)	reduced vision with nearby objects; also called farsightedness (Figure 7.4)
-opia	s	vision		
irid/o	r/cv	rainbow, iris	**iridoplegia** (ir ih doh PLEE jee ah)	paralysis of the eye
-plegia	s	paralysis		
ir	r	rainbow, iris	**iritis** (eye RYE tiss)	inflammation of the iris
-itis	s	inflammation		
kerat	r	hard, cornea	**keratitis** (kair aht EYE tiss)	inflammation of the cornea
-itis	s	inflammation		
			macular degeneration (MAK yoo lahr de jenn er AY shun)	progressive deterioration of an area of the retina known as the macula lutea, leading to a loss of central vision; the most common cause is age—this is called age-related macular degeneration, and abbreviated **ARMD**

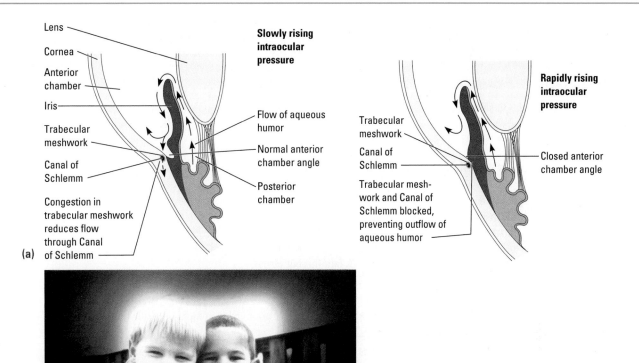

Lens

Cornea

Anterior chamber

Iris

Trabecular meshwork

Canal of Schlemm

Congestion in trabecular meshwork reduces flow through Canal of Schlemm

(a)

Slowly rising intraocular pressure

Flow of aqueous humor

Normal anterior chamber angle

Posterior chamber

Rapidly rising intraocular pressure

Trabecular meshwork

Canal of Schlemm

Trabecular mesh-work and Canal of Schlemm blocked, preventing outflow of aqueous humor

Closed anterior chamber angle

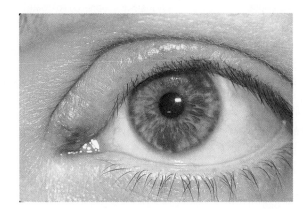

(b)

Figure 7.8 :::: **Glaucoma.**

(a) Two alternate forms of glaucoma, both of which result in the accumulation of aqueous humor in the anterior chamber.
(b) Narrowing of the optical fields is a typical symptom of untreated glaucoma.
Source: Pearson Education.

Figure 7.9 ::::
Hordeolum (or sty).

Source: Science Photo Library/Photo Researchers, Inc.

WORD PARTS (WHEN APPLICABLE)			TERM	DEFINITION
Part	Type	Meaning		
myo -opia	r s	to shut vision	**myopia** (my OH pee ah)	reduced vision with distant objects; also called nearsightedness (Figure 7.4)

> **[FYI]**
>
> **Myopia**
> You may recall from Chapter 5 that my/o is the word root and combining form for muscle. It is derived from the Greek word for muscle, *myos*. However, in the word myopia, the root word myo is derived from the similar Greek word *myo*, which means to shut. When followed by the suffix -opia, the term myopia translates into "to shut vision."

WORD PARTS			TERM	DEFINITION
nyctal -opia	r s	night vision	**nyctalopia** (NIK tah LOH pee ah)	poor vision at night or in dim light
			nystagmus (niss TAG muss)	involuntary, rhythmic movements of the eye
ocul/o myc -osis	r/cv r s	eye fungus condition of	**oculomycosis** (ok yoo loh my KOH siss)	fungal infection of the eye
ophthalm/o -pathy	r/cv s	eye disease	**ophthalmopathy** (OFF thal MOPP ah thee)	a general term for a disease of the eye
ophthalm/o -plegia	r/cv s	eye paralysis	**ophthalmoplegia** (off thal moh PLEE jee ah)	paralysis of the eye affecting the muscles that move the eyeball
phot/o -phobia	r/cv s	light fear	**photophobia** (FOH toh FOH bee ah)	abnormal fear of light
phot/o retin -itis	r/cv r s	light net, retina inflammation	**photoretinitis** (FOH toh RETT in EYE tiss)	inflammation of the retina caused by extreme light intensity
presby -opia	r s	old age vision	**presbyopia** (PRESS bee OH pee ah)	impaired vision due to aging
			pterygium (teh RIJ ee um)	abnormal fold of fibrous tissue extending between the conjunctiva and cornea
retin -itis	r s	net, retina inflammation	**retinitis pigmentosa** (rett in EYE tiss pig men TOH sah)	an inherited disease characterized by night blindness, progressive atrophy, and retinal pigment changes
retin/o blast -oma	r/cv r s	net, retina germ, bud tumor	**retinoblastoma** (RETT in noh blast OH mah)	a malignant tumor that originates from a developing retinal cell
retin/o -pathy	r/cv s	net, retina disease	**retinopathy** (RETT in OPP ah thee)	a general term for any disease of the retina (Figure 7.10::::)
scler/o kerat -itis	r/cv r s	thick, hard, sclera hard, cornea inflammation	**sclerokeratitis** (sklair oh kair aht EYE tiss)	inflammation of the sclera and cornea

WORD PARTS (WHEN APPLICABLE)			TERM	DEFINITION
Part	Type	Meaning		
scler/o -malacia	r/cv s	thick, hard, sclera softening	**scleromalacia** (sklair oh mah LAY she ah)	softening of the sclera
			scotoma (skoh TOH mah)	an abnormal blind spot in vision
			strabismus (strah BIZ muss)	a condition of crossed eyes that is caused by the visual axes failing to meet at the same point; the condition causes a noticeable squint: heterotropia if both eyes deviate inward or outward, esotropia if one eye deviates inward, and exotropia if one eye deviates outward (Figure 7.11)

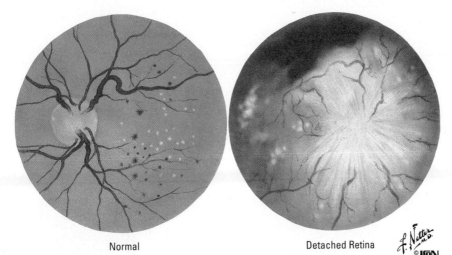

Normal   Detached Retina

Figure 7.10
Retinopathy. Illustration of a normal retina (left) and a diseased retina (right). *Source: Icon Learning Systems.*

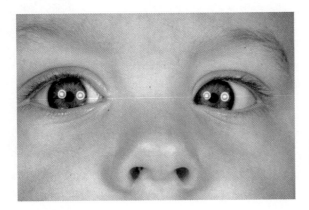

Figure 7.11
Strabismus in an infant.

Source: Barts Medical Library/ Phototake NYC.

disease focus | Glaucoma and Intraocular Pressure

Glaucoma is a group of diseases in which the optic nerve is damaged, resulting in vision loss. A common cause of glaucoma is an increase in intraocular pressure, which refers to the fluid pressure inside the eye.

In healthy eyes, a watery secretion called aqueous humor is continually produced when plasma leaks across capillary walls. The fluid first enters the posterior chamber of the eye (between the iris and the lens), then flows into the anterior chamber (between the cornea and the iris). Normally, aqueous humor drains through the trabecular meshwork located at the corner where the iris and the cornea meet, into an expanded vein called the canal of Schlemm, where it reenters the bloodstream (see Figure 7.8).

If problems develop that slow or block fluid drainage, fluid inside the eye builds up and intraocular pressure increases, which can damage the optic nerve if the pressure is not relieved. Damage to the optic nerve results in gradual vision loss until blindness occurs.

While there is no cure for glaucoma and no way to restore vision lost because of it, treatment is available to prevent further damage to the optic nerve. Treatments for most types of glaucoma include eye drops, laser surgery, and conventional surgery. These treatments are aimed at reducing intraocular pressure by either reducing the production rate of aqueous humor or by increasing its drainage rate.

SELF QUIZ 7.4

SAY IT—SPELL IT!

Review the terms of the eyes by speaking the phonetic pronunciation guides out loud, then writing in the correct spelling of the term.

1. ah STIG mah tizm _____
2. kah LAY zee on _____
3. kon JUNK tih VYE tiss _____
4. KOR nee oh eye RYE tiss _____
5. DAK ree oh sist EYE tiss _____
6. dih PLOH pee ah _____
7. ehn doff thal MYE tiss _____
8. glaw KOH mah _____
9. HIGH per OH pee ah _____
10. ir ih doh PLEE jee ah _____
7.6 11. my OH pee ah _____
12. NIK tah LOH pee ah _____
13. niss TAG muss _____
14. FOH toh RETT in EYE tiss _____
7.7 15. PRESS bee OH pee ah _____
16. teh RIJ ee um _____
17. RETT in noh blast OH mah _____
18. RETT in OPP ah thee _____
19. sklair oh kair aht EYE tiss _____
7.8 20. sklair oh mah LAY she ah _____
21. strah BIZ muss _____

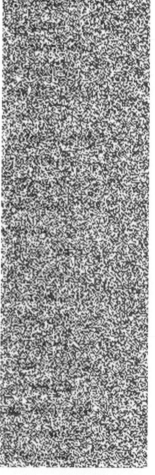

MATCH IT!

Match the term on the left with the correct definition on the right.

_____ 1. blepharitis

_____ 2. corneoiritis

_____ 3. endophthalmitis

_____ 4. hordeolum

_____ 5. iritis

_____ 6. macular degeneration

_____ 7. nystagmus

_____ 8. ophthalmopathy

_____ 9. presbyopia

_____10. scleromalacia

a. an infection of a meibomian gland

b. deterioration of the macula lutea leading to a loss of central vision

c. a general term for a disease of the eye

d. inflammation of the eyelid

e. involuntary, rhythmic movements of the eye

f. inflammation of the cornea and iris

g. impaired vision due to aging

h. inflammation of the iris

i. softening of the sclera

j. inflammation of internal tissues of the eye

BREAK IT DOWN!

Analyze and separate each term into its word parts by labeling each word part using p = prefix, r = root, cv = combining vowel, and s = suffix.

1. astigmatism   _____

2. corneoiritis   _____

3. dacryocystitis   _____

4. hyperopia   _____

5. iridoplegia   _____

6. oculomycosis   _____

7. ophthalmoplegia   _____

8. photoretinitis   _____

9. retinopathy   _____

10. sclerokeratitis   _____

11. scleromalacia   _____

WORD BUILDING

Construct or recall medical terms from the following meanings.

1. a reduction of transparency of the lens _____

2. a localized swelling at the edge of an eyelid caused by obstruction of a meibomian gland _____

3. separation of the retina from the choroid _____

4. abnormal fear of light _____

5. abnormal fold of fibrous tissue extending between the conjunctiva and cornea _____

6. inherited disease characterized by night blindness, progressive atrophy, and retinal pigment changes _____

7. an abnormal blind spot in vision _____

FILL IT IN!

Fill in the blanks with the correct terms.

1. The temporary condition you may suffer from after studying all night for an exam is clinically called _____. This condition can lead to double vision, _____, if the eyes don't receive the rest they need.

2. An eyelid that droops, or _____, is often caused by a local inflammation, or _____.

3. A condition that is common among children is inflammation of the conjunctiva, or _____. If it is not treated with antibiotics, the infection and inflammation that follows can spread to a lacrimal sac producing the condition _____, the cornea resulting in _____, the iris causing _____, or to both the cornea and iris to form the condition of _____.

4. Failure to arrest infection in the eye can lead to the more serious condition _____, in which the muscles of the iris become paralyzed.

7.9   5. An increase in intraocular pressure is often the cause of _____, which is one of the most common forms of eye disease, or _____.

6. A somewhat common crossing of the eyes, or _____, occurs among children, in which one eye deviates inward, called _____.

7.10   The condition often causes double vision, or _____, which leads to learning disabilities.

7. Impaired vision due to old age is known as _____. In many seniors, this condition is coupled with disease of the retina, or _____, where the retina separates from the choroid, called a _____ _____. Another common affliction of

7.11   old age is a clouding of the lens, or _____.

Treatments, Procedures, and Devices

WORD PARTS (WHEN APPLICABLE)			TERM	DEFINITION
Part	Type	Meaning		
blephar/o -plasty	r/cv s	eyelid surgical repair	**blepharoplasty** (BLEF ah roh plass tee)	surgical repair of an eyelid
			cataract extraction (KAT ah rakt)	excision of a lens that has lost its clarity (Figure 7.12::::)

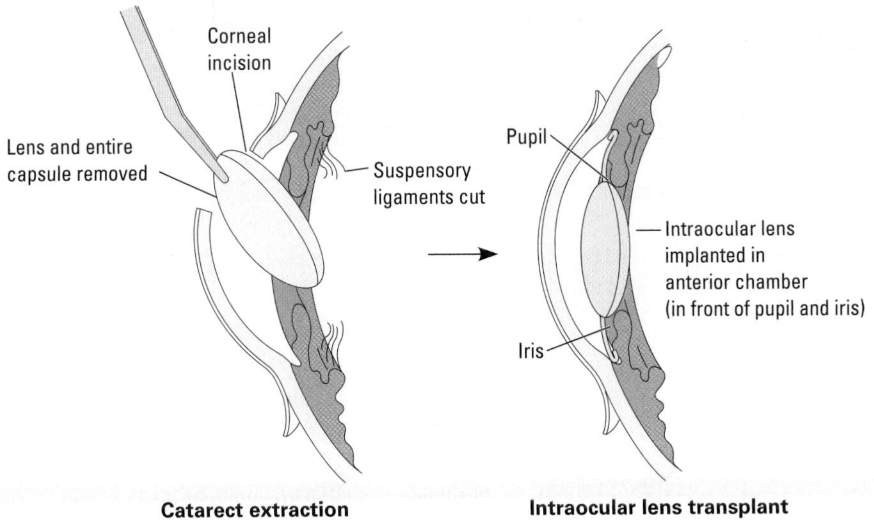

Corneal incision

Lens and entire capsule removed

Suspensory ligaments cut

Pupil

Intraocular lens implanted in anterior chamber (in front of pupil and iris)

Iris

Catarect extraction

Intraocular lens transplant

Figure 7.12 ::::

Cataract extraction. The procedure involves surgical removal of a cataract lens and its replacement with an artificial lens. The artifical lens is usually an acrylic (Plexiglass) material.
Source: Pearson Education

WORD PARTS (WHEN APPLICABLE)			TERM	DEFINITION
			distance visual acuity (VIZH oo al ah KYOO ih tee)	a test of the ability to see the details and shape of objects from recorded distances
e- nucle -ation	p r s	to remove kernel process	**enucleation** (ee noo klee AY shun)	excision of an eyeball from the socket
fluorescein angi/o -graphy	r/cv s	a dye blood vessel recording process	**fluorescein angiography** (floo oh RESS ee in an jee OH grah fee)	visual recording of blood vessels in the retina and choroid using fluorescein dye, which is injected into a vein and circulates through the eye
intra- ocul -ar	p r s	within eye pertaining to	**intraocular lens transplant** (in trah AHK yoo lahr)	surgical implantation of an artificial lens to replace a defective natural lens (Figure 7.12)
irid -ectomy	r s	rainbow, iris surgical removal	**iridectomy** (ir id EK toh mee)	excision of a portion of the iris
irid/o -tomy	r/cv s	rainbow, iris cutting into, incision	**iridotomy** (ir id AHT oh mee)	incision into the iris to allow the aqueous humor to drain from the anterior chamber; usually performed with a laser to treat glaucoma
kerat/o -metry	r/cv s	hard, cornea measurement	**keratometry** (kair ah TOM eh tree)	a procedure using a hand-held device called a keratometer (kair ah TOM eh ter), which measures the curvature of the cornea, usually for fitting contact lenses
kerat/o -plasty	r/cv s	hard, cornea surgical repair	**keratoplasty** (KAIR ah toh plass tee)	corneal transplant (Figure 7.13::::)

WORD PARTS (WHEN APPLICABLE)			TERM	DEFINITION
Part	**Type**	**Meaning**		

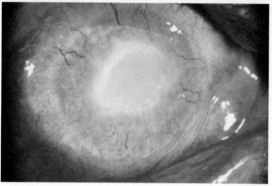 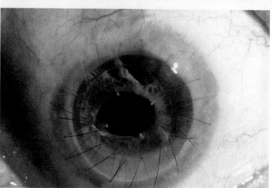

Figure 7.13 ⠿ **Keratoplasty, or corneal transplant.**
(a) The diseased, nontransparent cornea prior to the procedure.
(b) During the keratoplasty, the cornea is removed and replaced with one obtained from a cadaver of an uninfected adult under the age of 65 years. The sutures used to attach the replacement are finer than a human hair.
Source: Custom Medical Stock Photo, Inc.

Part	Type	Meaning	TERM	DEFINITION
			LASIK (LAY sik)	acronym for laser-assisted in situ keratomileusis; it is the use of a laser to reshape the corneal tissue beneath the surface of the cornea to correct vision abnormalities, such as myopia, hyperopia, and astigmatism
			mydriatic (MID ree ATT ik)	a chemical agent that dilates the pupils
ophthalm -ic	r s	eye pertaining to	**ophthalmic evaluation** (off THAL mik)	a variety of procedures using specialized instruments to assist in the diagnosis of eye disorders
ophthalm/o -logist	r/cv s	eye one who studies	**ophthalmologist** (off thal MALL oh jist)	a physician specializing in the treatment of eyes
ophthalm/o -logy	r/cv s	eye study of	**ophthalmology** (off thal MALL oh jee)	the field of medicine focusing on the study of disease related to the eyes
ophthalm/o -scopy	r/cv s	eye viewing, process	**ophthalmoscopy** (off thal MOSS koh pee)	use of a hand-held instrument with a light, called an **ophthalmoscope** (off THAL moh skope) to view the eye's interior (Figure 7.14⠿)
opt -ic -ian	r s s	eye pertaining to pertaining to	**optician** (opp TISH ahn)	a technician trained in filling prescriptions for corrective lenses
opt/o -metry	r/cv s	eye measurement	**optometry** (opp TOM eh tree)	measurement of vision, usually to test acuity for prescribing corrective lenses; the process includes the use of an **optometer** (opp TOM eh ter), which measures the range and sharpness of vision (Figure 7.15⠿)
opt/o -metrist	r/cv s	eye one who measures	**optometrist**	a professional—not a physician—trained to examine eyes to correct vision problems and eye disorders

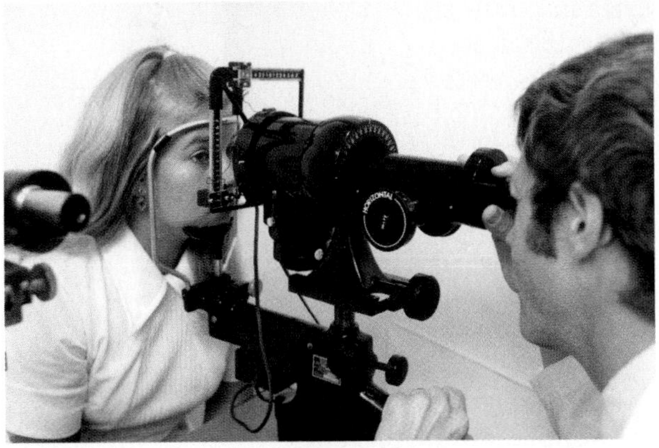

WORD PARTS (WHEN APPLICABLE)			TERM	DEFINITION
Part	**Type**	**Meaning**		

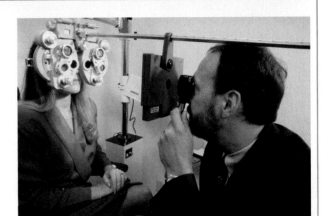

Figure 7.14 :::: Ophthalmoscopy.
Source: Pearson Education.

Figure 7.15 :::: Optometry, which measures visual acuity for corrective lenses.
Source: David Weintraub/Photo Researchers, Inc.

Part	Type	Meaning	TERM	DEFINITION
phac/o	r/cv	lens	**phacoemulsification**	use of ultrasound frequencies to break up a cataract, which is then aspirated and removed
emulsif	r	a process of combining two liquids	(FAK oh ee mull sih fih KAY shun)	
-ic	s	pertaining to		
-ation	s	process of		
phot/o	r/cv	light	**photorefractive keratectomy**	use of a laser to flatten the corneal surface in an effort to correct myopia, abbreviated **PRK**
refract	r	to bend light		
-ive	s	pertaining to	(foh toh ree FRAK tiv	
kerat	r	hard, cornea	kair ah TEK toh mee)	
-ectomy	s	excision		
rad/i	r/cv	spoke of a wheel	**radial keratotomy**	incisions into the cornea to produce a spoke-like effect, which serves to flatten the cornea and correct for myopia; abbreviated **RK**
-al	s	pertaining to	(RAY dee all	
kerat/o	r/cv	hard, cornea	kair ah TOTT oh mee)	
-tomy	s	incision		
scler	r	thick, hard, sclera	**scleral buckling**	repair of a detached retina, in which a portion of the sclera is resected and an implant inserted; the suturing of the implant causes the sclera to buckle slightly
-al	s	pertaining to	(SKLAIR al)	
son/o	r/cv	sound	**sonography**	high-frequency sound waves used to detect problems associated with the eye, like foreign objects, detached retina, etc.
-graphy	s	recording, process	(son OG rah fee)	
			strabotomy	incision into the tendon of an eye's extrinsic muscle to correct strabismus (crossed eyes)
			(strah BOTT oh mee)	
ton/o	r/cv	tone, tension, pressure	**tonometry**	measurement of intraocular pressure, primarily used to test for glaucoma; an instrument called a **tonometer** (toh NOM eh ter) is used for this test
-metry	s	measurement	(tohn OM eh tree)	
vitr	r	glassy	**vitrectomy**	surgical removal of the vitreous humor
-ectomy	s	excision	(vih TREK toh mee)	

> **[FYI]**
>
> **Keratotomy**
> Radial keratotomy is a conventional procedure for reshaping the cornea to correct for near-sightedness (myopia). First used in 1965, it is now outdated and is being replaced by PRK, or photorefractive keratotomy, which removes tissue from the corneal surface using a special laser, and LASIK, or laser-assisted in situ keratomileusis, which reshapes the cornea, also using a special laser. Both procedures integrate the use of a computer and laser to reduce the risk of accidental injury.

SELF QUIZ 7.5

SAY IT—SPELL IT!

Review the terms of the eyes by speaking the phonetic pronunciation out loud, then writing the correct spelling of the term.

1. off thal MALL oh jee _____

2. BLEF ah roh plass tee _____

3. kair ah TOM eh tree _____

4. off thal MOSS koh pee _____

7.12 5. off thal MALL oh jist _____

BREAK IT DOWN!

Analyze and separate each term into its word parts by labeling each word part using p = prefix, r = root, cv = combining vowel, and s = suffix.

1. optometry _____

2. blepharoplasty _____

3. keratoplasty _____

4. keratectomy _____

5. iridectomy _____

6. tonometry _____

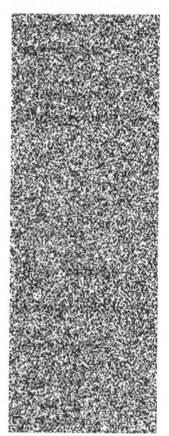

MATCH IT!

Match the term on the left with the correct definition on the right.

_____ 1. enucleation

_____ 2. ophthalmologist

_____ 3. optician

_____ 4. blepharoplasty

_____ 5. intraocular lens transplant

_____ 6. iridectomy

_____ 7. LASIK

_____ 8. tonometry

_____ 9. phacoemulsification

_____10. scleral buckling

_____11. strabotomy

_____12. vitrectomy

a. surgical repair of an eyelid

b. excision of a portion of the iris

c. laser-assisted in situ keratomileusis

d. measurement of intraocular pressure

e. physician specializing in the treatment of eyes

f. incision into the tendon of an eye's extrinsic muscle

g. repair of a detached retina

h. excision of an eyeball from the socket

i. surgical implantation of an artificial lens

j. surgical removal of the vitreous humor

k. a technician trained in filling prescriptions for corrective lenses

l. use of ultrasound frequencies to break up a cataract

FILL IT IN!

Fill in the blanks with the correct terms.

1. To correct the damage from iridoplegia an _____ to remove a part of the iris can be performed.

2. Myopia can often be corrected by a relatively outdated technique that includes incisions into the cornea, called a _____ _____.
   Alternatively, a laser can be used to flatten the corneal surface in a procedure called _____ _____. A more radical procedure involves

   the surgical replacement of the cornea, called a _____.

3. Glaucoma is usually diagnosed with a device called a _____.
   In extreme cases, a procedure that removes the vitreous humor, called a _____, can be performed.

4. Strabismus can be corrected in a surgical procedure called a _____.

abbreviations of the eyes

The abbreviations that are associated with the eyes are summarized here. Study these abbreviations, and review them in the exercise that follows.

ABBREVIATION	DEFINITION	ABBREVIATION	DEFINITION
Ast	astigmatism	OS	oculus sinister, or left eye
Em	emmetropia	OU	oculus uterque, or each eye
EENT	eye, ear, nose, and throat	PRK	photorefractive keratotomy
LASIK	laser-assisted in situ keratomileusis	RK	radial keratotomy
ARMD	age-related macular degeneration	VA	visual acuity
OD	oculus dexter, or right eye		

SELF QUIZ 7.6

Fill in the blanks with the abbreviation or the complete medical term.

Abbreviation	Medical Term
1. _____	left eye
2. Em	_____
3. _____	each eye
4. OD	_____
5. _____	eye, ear, nose, and throat
6. VA	_____
7. _____	photorefractive keratotomy
8. RK	_____
9. _____	astigmatism

7.13

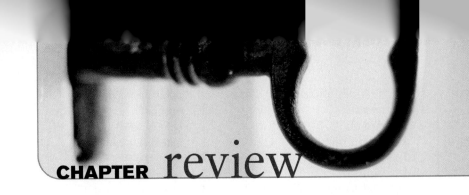
In this section, we will review all the word parts and medical terms from this chapter. As in earlier tables, the word roots are shown in **bold**.

Check each word part and medical term to be sure you understand the meaning. If any are not clear, please go back into the chapter and review that term. Then, complete the review exercises that follow.

[word parts **checklist**]

Prefixes

- ❏ a-, an-
- ❏ bi-, bin-,
- ❏ e-
- ❏ intra-
- ❏ para-

Word Roots/Combining Vowels

- ❏ **blephar**/o
- ❏ **conjunctiv**/o
- ❏ **cor**/o, **core**/o
- ❏ **corne**/o
- ❏ **dacry**/o

- ❏ **dipl**/o
- ❏ **fovea**
- ❏ **humor**/o
- ❏ **ir**/i, **irid**/o
- ❏ **kerat**/o
- ❏ **lacrim**/o
- ❏ **nyct**/o, **nyctal**/o
- ❏ **ocul**/o
- ❏ **opt**/o, **opthalm**/o
- ❏ **phac**/o, **phak**/o
- ❏ **phot**/o
- ❏ **presby**/o
- ❏ **retin**/o

- ❏ **scler**/o
- ❏ **stigmat**/o
- ❏ **ton**/o
- ❏ **vitre**/o

Suffixes

- ❏ -algia
- ❏ -opia
- ❏ -phobia
- ❏ -plegia
- ❏ -ptosis
- ❏ -rrhagia
- ❏ -rrhea

[medical terminology **checklist** WWW]

- ❏ age-related macular degeneration (ARMD)
- ❏ **anter**ior chamber
- ❏ **aque**ous **humor**
- ❏ **asthen**opia
- ❏ a**stigmat**ism (Ast)
- ❏ **blephar**itis
- ❏ **blephar**oplasty
- ❏ **blephar**optosis
- ❏ cataract
- ❏ cataract extraction
- ❏ chalazion
- ❏ **choroid**
- ❏ **cili**ary muscles
- ❏ cones
- ❏ **conjunctiv**a
- ❏ **conjunctiv**itis
- ❏ **corne**a

- ❏ **corne**o**ir**itis
- ❏ **dacry**o**cyst**itis
- ❏ detached **retin**a
- ❏ **dipl**opia
- ❏ distance visual acuity
- ❏ emmetropia (Em)
- ❏ end**ophthalm**itis
- ❏ e**nucle**ation
- ❏ esotropia
- ❏ exotropia
- ❏ eyes, ears, nose, and throat (EENT)
- ❏ **fibr**ous layer
- ❏ fluorescein **angi**ography
- ❏ **fovea** centralis
- ❏ glaucoma
- ❏ heterotropia
- ❏ hordeolum

- ❏ hyperopia
- ❏ intra**ocul**ar
- ❏ intra**ocul**ar lens transplant
- ❏ **irid**ectomy
- ❏ **irid**oplegia
- ❏ **irid**otomy
- ❏ **ir**is
- ❏ **ir**itis
- ❏ **kerat**itis
- ❏ **kerat**ometer
- ❏ **kerat**ometry
- ❏ **kerat**oplasty
- ❏ **lacrim**al glands
- ❏ laser-assisted in situ **kerat**omileusis (LASIK)
- ❏ lens
- ❏ **leuk**o**cor**ia
- ❏ macular degeneration

- ❏ meibomian glands
- ❏ mydriatic
- ❏ **myo**pia
- ❏ nervous layer
- ❏ **nyctal**opia
- ❏ nystagmus
- ❏ **oculomyc**osis
- ❏ **ocul**us dexter, or right, eye (OD)
- ❏ **ocul**us sinister, or left, eye (OS)
- ❏ **ocul**us uterque, or each, eye (OU)
- ❏ **ophthalm**algia
- ❏ **ophthalm**ic evaluation
- ❏ **ophthalm**opathy
- ❏ **ophthalm**oplegia
- ❏ **ophthalm**orrhagia
- ❏ **ophthalm**oscope

- ❏ **ophthalm**oscopy
- ❏ **opt**ic disk
- ❏ **opt**ic nerve
- ❏ **opt**ician
- ❏ **opt**ometer
- ❏ **opt**ometry
- ❏ **phac**oemulsification
- ❏ **phot**ophobia
- ❏ **phot**orefractive **kerat**ectomy (PRK)
- ❏ **phot**oretinitis
- ❏ **presby**opia
- ❏ pterygium
- ❏ **radial kerat**otomy (RK)
- ❏ **retin**a
- ❏ **retin**itis pigmentosa
- ❏ **retin**oblastoma

- ❏ **retin**opathy
- ❏ rods
- ❏ **scler**a
- ❏ **scler**al buckling
- ❏ **sclerokerat**itis
- ❏ **scler**omalacia
- ❏ scotoma
- ❏ **son**ography
- ❏ **strab**ismus
- ❏ **strab**otomy
- ❏ **ton**ometer
- ❏ **ton**ometry
- ❏ **vasc**ular layer
- ❏ visual acuity (VA)
- ❏ **vitr**ectomy
- ❏ **vitr**eous **humor**

[show what **you know!**]

BREAK IT DOWN!

Analyze and separate each term into its word parts by labeling each word part using p = prefix, r = root, cv = combining vowel, and s = suffix.

		r cv s
Example:	1. ophthalmology	ophthalm/o/logy
	2. presbyopia	
	3. sclerokeratinitis	
	4. retinoblastoma	
	5. blepharoptosis	
	6. hyperopia	
	7. iridoplegia	
	8. conjunctivitis	
	9. ophthalmalgia	
	10. photoretinitis	
	11. oculomycosis	
	12. diplopia	
	13. dacryocystitis	
	14. corneoiritis	
	15. keratitis	
	16. iridectomy	

WORD BUILDING

Construct or recall medical terms from the following meanings.

Example: 1.   defective curvature of the eye _____astigmatism_____

2.   localized swelling of the eyelid _____

3.   abnormal increase in intraocular pressure _____

4.   an infection of a meibomian gland _____

5.   involuntary, rhythmic eye movements _____

6.   eyestrain _____

7.   drooping of an eyelid _____

8.   normal condition of the eye _____

9.   double vision _____

10.   paralysis of the eye _____

11.   nearsightedness _____

12.   bleeding of the eye _____

13.   fungal infection of the eye _____

14.   fibrous tissue between cornea and conjunctiva _____

15.   condition of crossed eyes _____

16.   surgical repair of an eyelid _____

17.   removal of the vitreous humor _____

CASE STUDY

Fill in the blanks with the correct terms.

1.   A female patient was admitted to the emergency room complaining of pain associated with the eye, a condition called

(a) _____, that followed a minor head trauma during a fall. An initial exam revealed a mild

inflammation of the conjunctiva, or (b) _____, with a slight deviation of the left eye inward, or

(c) _____. Some paralysis of the right eye's iris, or (d) _____, was possible.

The patient was referred for examination by a physician specializing in eye disorders, or an (e) _____,

who used an (f) _____ to view the eye's interior. Vision was also measured using an

(g) _____, and intraocular pressure was determined using a (h) _____. The

specialist found that the trauma caused the retina to separate from the choroid, called a (i) _____

_____, but determined that all other conditions were temporary and a state of normality, or

(j) _____, would return after minimal treatment. However, the detached retina would require more

careful analysis using a fluorescein dye, in a procedure known as (k) _____

_____. Treatment would probably include resection of the sclera and insertion of an implant in a

procedure known as (l) _____ _____.

[piece it all **together!** 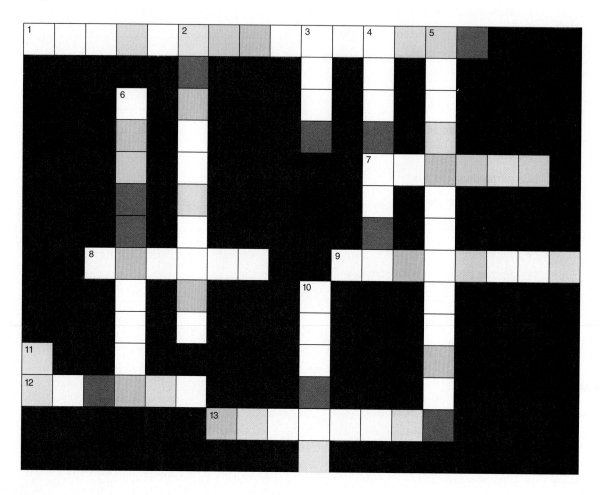]

CROSSWORD

From the chapter material, fill in the crossword puzzle with answers to the following clues.

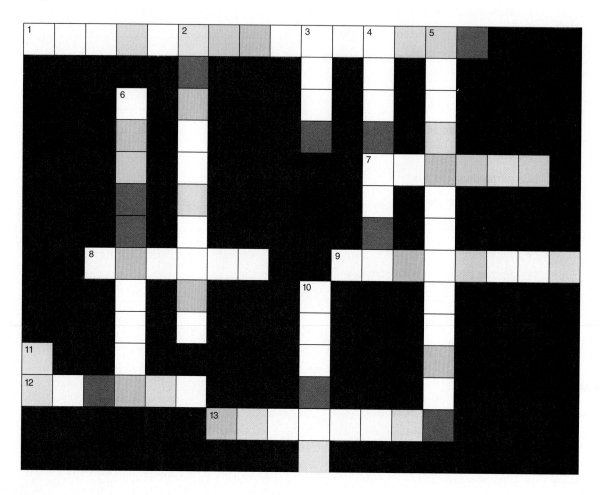

ACROSS

1. A physician specializing in eye disorders. (Find puzzle piece 7.12)
7. The transparent portion of the fibrous eye layer. (Find puzzle piece 7.2)
8. Reduced vision with distant objects, or nearsightedness. (Find puzzle piece 7.6)
9. A loss of transparency of the lens. (Find puzzle piece 7.11)
12. Combining form that means "hard." (Find puzzle piece 7.1)
13. A condition of double vision. (Find puzzle piece 7.10)

DOWN

2. A medical term for eyestrain. (Find puzzle piece 7.5)
3. This part of the eye is normally transparent, although it loses transparency with a cataract condition. (Find puzzle piece 7.3)
4. A condition that can often be treated with an iridotomy. (Find puzzle piece 7.9)
5. Abnormal softening of the white outer covering of the eye. (Find puzzle piece 7.8)
6. A common eye condition of old age. (Find puzzle piece 7.7)
10. Openings in the center of the colorful, circular muscles in both eyes. (Find puzzle piece 7.4)
11. Incisions into the cornea in order to flatten it to correct for myopia (abbreviation). (Find puzzle piece 7.13)

WORD UNSCRAMBLE

From the completed crossword puzzle, unscramble:

1. All of the letters that appear in **green** squares

   ☐ __ __ __

   Clue: Normally transparent, it loses its transparency when a cataract develops

2. All of the letters that appear in **gray** squares

   __ __ __ __ __ ☐ __ __ __

   Clue: A chemical agent that dilates the pupils

3. All of the letters that appear in **red** squares

   ☐ __ __ __ __ __ __ __ __

   Clue: A condition of crossed eyes that literally means *to squint*

4. All of the letters that appear in **yellow** squares

   __ ☐ __ __ __

   Clue: The "net" within the eye that contains rod cells and cone cells

5. All of the letters that appear in **peach** squares

   ☐ __

   Clue: A procedure that flattens the cornea as a treatment for myopia (abbreviation)

   Now write down each of the letters that are boxed and unscramble them to find the hidden medical term of the eyes:

   __ __ __ __ __

   Clue: The hidden word is an acronym.

MEDmedia **wrap-up**

www.prenhall.com/wingerd
Before you go on to the next chapter, take advantage of the free CD-ROM and study guide website that accompany this book. Simply load the CD-ROM for additional activities, games, animations, videos, and quizzes linked to this chapter. Then visit www.prenhall.com/wingerd for even more!

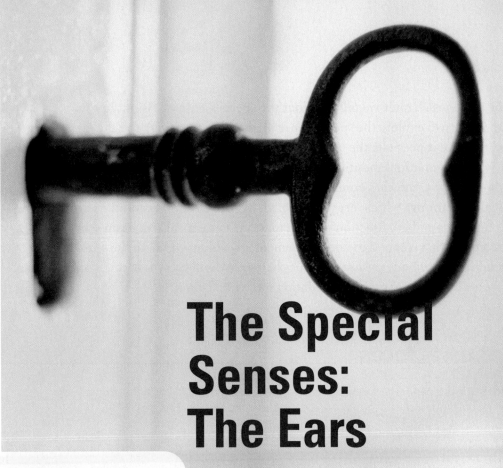

CHAPTER
8

The Special Senses: The Ears

LEARNING OBJECTIVES

After completing this chapter, you will be able to:

- Define and spell the word parts used to create medical terms for the ears

- Identify the parts of the ears and describe their structure and function

- Define common medical terms used for the ears

- Break down and define common medical terms used for symptoms, diseases, disorders, procedures, treatments, and devices for the ears

MEDmedia

www.prenhall.com/wingerd
Enhance your study with the power of multimedia! Each chapter of this book links to activities, games, animations, videos, and quizzes that you'll find on your CD-ROM. Plus, you can click on www.prenhall.com/wingerd, to find a free chapter-specific companion website that's loaded with additional practice and resources.

CD-ROM
- Audio Glossary
- Exercises & Activities
- Flashcard Generator
- Animations
- Videos

 Companion Website
- Exercises & Activities
- Audio Glossary
- Drug Updates
- Current News Updates

A secure distance learning course is available at www.prenhall.com/onekey.

In the previous chapter we talked about the special sense of vision. In this chapter we will explore the special sense of audation (hearing) and the organs that make it possible: the ears. Similar to the eyes, the ears provide the brain with information about the outside environment, but instead of responding to light, the ears contain sensory receptors that respond to mechanical vibrations, which are interpreted by the brain as sound. The perception of sound is a function called audation. The ears also contain sensory receptors that respond to body movement, providing you with the sense of equilibrium and body position. In this chapter, we will focus our study on the ears and the special senses of audation and equilibrium.

word parts focus

Let's look at word parts. The following table contains a list of word parts that when combined build many of the terms of the ears, audation, and equilibrium.

PREFIX	DEFINITION	PREFIX	DEFINITION
a-, an-	without	para-	near, alongside; departure from normal

WORD ROOT	DEFINITION	WORD ROOT	DEFINITION
acou, acoust	hearing	ot	ear
aud, audi	hearing	salping	tube (usually the Eustachian
aur	ear		or fallopian tubes)
labyrinth	maze or inner ear	staped	stirrup, or stapes
mast	breast	tympan	eardrum
myring	membrane or eardrum		

SUFFIX	DEFINITION	SUFFIX	DEFINITION
-acusis, -cusis	hearing condition	-rrhagia	bleeding or hemorrhage
-algia	pain	-rrhea	excessive discharge (of fluid)
-itis	inflammation		

SELF QUIZ 8.1

Review the word parts of terminology for the ears by working carefully through the exercises that follow. Soon, we will apply this new information to build medical terms.

A. Provide the definition of the following prefixes and suffixes.

1. -algia _____

2. an- _____

3. para- _____

4. -acusis, -cusis _____

5. -rrhea _____

6. -rrhagia _____

7. a- _____

8. -itis _____

B. Provide the word root for each of the following terms.

1. ear _____

2. breast _____

3. membrane, eardrum _____

4. tube _____

5. stirrup _____

6. eardrum _____

7. maze, internal ear _____

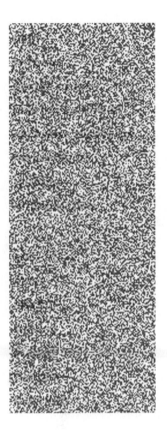

[anatomy and physiology overview]

The ears are the organs of hearing, or **audation**. Each ear contains sensory receptors that respond to sound waves, or mechanical vibrations, by generating a nerve impulse. Once generated, the impulse is carried to the brain. The temporal lobes of the cerebral cortex receive this information and interpret it into sound. In addition to mechanical vibrations, the ears also contain sensory receptors that are sensitive to body position and equilibrium.

The structures of the ears include a series of channels and chambers that direct mechanical vibrations to the sensory receptors (Figure 8.1) There are three portions of each ear: outer, middle, and inner. In general, the outer ear is partially external, the middle ear is located within a cavity that is surrounded by the **mastoid process** of the temporal bone, and the inner ear is embedded within the mastoid process.

The **outer ear** consists of the flap-like appendages on the sides of your head that are commonly referred to as the ears, and a skin-lined canal. The appendages are called **auricles,** a term which literally means *pertaining to the ear*. The canal extends from its external opening to the eardrum and is called the **external auditory canal.** Along its way are specialized glands that secrete earwax, or **cerumen.** The auricles collect sound waves and direct them to the external auditory canal. The canal channels the sound waves to the eardrum, which is the entrance to the middle ear.

[FYI]

Mast

Mast is derived from the Greek word, *mastos,* which means breast. Although there is no female breast associated with the ears, the word part is used with the suffix -oid as the term for a part of the skull surrounding the ears, called the mastoid. The mastoid points downward to form a projection (called the mastoid process), which reminded its namers of the shape of a female breast.

enrichment module enrichment modul

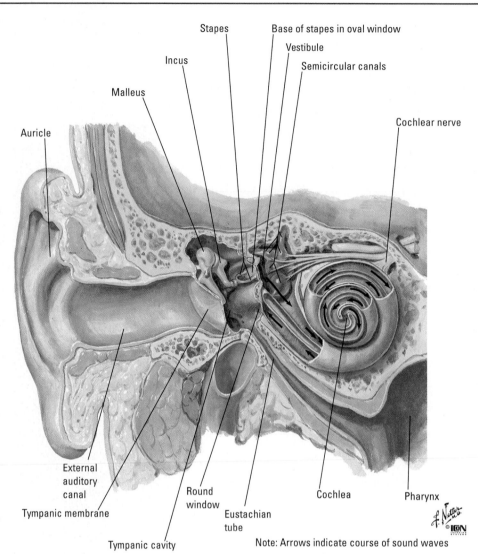

Stapes   Base of stapes in oval window

Vestibule

Incus   Semicircular canals

Malleus

Cochlear nerve

Auricle

External auditory canal

Tympanic membrane

Round window

Tympanic cavity

Eustachian tube

Cochlea   Pharynx

Note: Arrows indicate course of sound waves

Figure 8.1 ::::

Anatomy of the ear. The cochlea is shown partially sectioned to reveal its internal structure. *Source: Icon Learning Systems.*

    The **middle ear** consists of the eardrum, or **tympanic membrane** (Figure 8.2::::) and a series of small bones called **ossicles.** The term *tympanic* is derived from the Greek word *tympanon,* which means *drum,* and the term *ossicles* means *little bones.* The ossicles lie in a small, air-filled cavity between the inside wall of the eardrum and the inner ear. The cavity, which is known as the **tympanic cavity,** receives the distal opening of the **Eustachian tube,** which begins at the throat. For this reason, the middle ear is subject to infections that can travel from the mouth and throat. The three ossicles are the **malleus** or *hammer,* the **incus** or *anvil,* and the **stapes** or *stirrup.* These three Latin terms are very descriptive of the shapes of these tiny bones, as you can see in Figure 8.1. The eardrum converts sound waves to mechanical vibrations, which are transmitted to the inner ear by the ossicles. The stapes passes the vibrations to the inner ear by contacting a thin membrane that separates them, called the oval window.

    The **labyrinth** or inner ear consists of a series of winding, twisting channels within the temporal bone. The channels are lined with a membrane, and form three structures: the **cochlea,** the **vestibule,** and the **semicircular canals.**

[FYI]

Tympanic

The word *tympanic* is derived from *tympanon,* the Greek word for a percussion instrument like a drum or tambourine. The term was first used in 1255 by the medieval anatomist Gabrielle Fallopius when he noticed the similarity between the tight skin covering the eardrum and the percussion instrument.

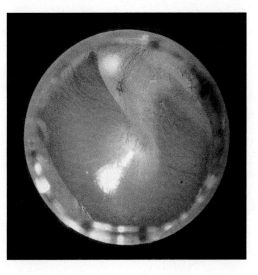

Figure 8.2 ::::

Tympanic membrane. A normal tympanic membrane is shown in this photograph through an otoscope.
Source: Pearson Education.

[FYI]

Labyrinth

The term labyrinth is believed to have originated from the ancient Lydian language that preceded the Golden Age of Greece, where it was used as the label for "house of the double-axe." This house was a maze designed to protect the inner sanctum from invaders, which served as the throne room for Minos, the King of Crete. Over the years, the labyrinth became synonymous with the word "maze." When early scientists first observed the twisting chambers of the inner ear, they were struck by its resemblance to a twisting maze, leading to the use of the term labyrinth.

[**thinking critically!**]

How are sound waves converted to mechanical vibrations within the middle ear?

[**thinking critically!**]

What is triggered when the hair cells within the organ of Corti move in response to vibrations?

The term cochlea means *snail shell* in Latin. As you can see in Figure 8.1, the cochlea closely resembles a snail's spiral shell. Internally, it is divided into two channels that run parallel and are filled with fluid. Vibrations are passed from the stapes of the middle ear to the cochlear channels, which are then carried by the fluid through the cochlea like small waves on a tiny ocean (Figure 8.3::::). Deep within the cochlea is an area containing sensory neurons, whose dendrites (neuron extensions) appear like small hairs poking into the fluid. The area is known as the **organ of Corti.** When the vibrations reach the organ of Corti, they cause the dendrites to change position, which triggers a nerve impulse that travels to the brain. The temporal lobe of the brain translates the impulse into sound.

The semicircular canals are the three loops of the inner ear, which you can see in Figure 8.1. At their base is the vestibule, which is a chamber that joins the semicircular canals with the cochlea. Like the cochlea, the canals are filled with fluid. This fluid moves through the tubular canals when you change body position. When the fluid contacts sensory receptors embedded within the vestibule, it triggers a nerve impulse. The impulse travels to the cerebellum, where it is interpreted as body position to help you to maintain muscle coordination and equilibrium.

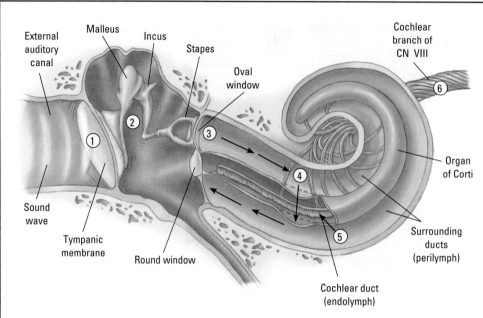

Figure 8.3 ::::

Transmission of sound waves to the cochlea and the organ of Corti. *Step 1:* sound waves contact the tympanic membrane, causing it to vibrate. *Step 2:* The vibration is transmitted to the three middle ear ossicles. *Step 3:* The vibration is passed from the stapes to the oval window, generating waves in the fluid (perilymph). *Step 4:* The perilymph waves push against the cochlear duct, causing the fluid (endolymph) to move. *Step 5:* Movement of the endolymph causes movement of the sensory receptor cells within the organ of Corti. *Step 6:* A nerve impulse travels to the CNS for interpretation as sound. *Source: Icon Learning Systems.*

getting to the root of it | anatomy and physiology terms

Many of the anatomy and physiology terms are formed from roots that are used to construct the more complex medical terms of the ears, including symptoms, diseases, and treatments. In this section, we will review the terms that describe the structure and function of the ears *in relation to their word roots,* which are shown in blue.

Study the word roots and terms in this list and complete the review exercises that follow.

Word Root (Meaning)	Terms Formed from the Word Root (Pronunciation)	Definition
aur (ear)	**aur**icle (AW rih kl)	the external appendages on the sides of the head that are commonly referred to as the ears; also called pinna (PINN ah)
aud, audi (hearing)	**aud**ation (aw DAY shun)	the process of hearing
	external **audi**tory canal (AW dih tor ee)	the skin-lined tube extending from the auricle to the eardrum
labyrinth (maze, inner ear)	**labyrinth** (LAB ih rinth)	a series of fluid-filled channels within the mastoid process of the temporal bone; also called the inner ear
mast (breast)	**mast**oid process (MASS toyd)	a breast-shaped projection near the base of the temporal bone that houses the middle and inner ears
tympan (eardrum)	**tympan**ic membrane (tihm PAHN ik)	a membrane-covered disk that receives sound waves, amplifies them, and transmits them to the first ossicle, the malleus; also called the eardrum; abbreviated TM
	tympanic cavity (tihm PAHN ik)	a small, air-filled cavity between the inside wall of the eardrum and the inner ear

OTHER IMPORTANT TERMS
The terms in this table are related to the structure and function of the ears, but are not built from word roots.

cerumen (seh ROO men)	the waxy substance produced by glands lining the external auditory canal; the term is the Latin word for *wax*
cochlea (KOHK lee ah)	a spiral snail shell-shaped series of fluid-filled channels of the inner ear that contains the organ of Corti
Eustachian tube (yoo STAY she ehn)	first described by Bartolommeo Eustachio in 1565, this tube connects the throat with the tympanic cavity of the middle ear
outer ear	the part of the ear that includes the auricle and the external auditory canal
incus (ING kuss)	the middle of the three auditory ossicles and is shaped like a blacksmith's anvil
malleus (MALL ee us)	is the first of the three auditory ossicles of the middle ear, and is shaped like a hammer
middle ear	the midsection of the ear that lies within the tympanic cavity of the temporal bone; it includes the tympanic membrane and the ossicles
organ of Corti (KOR tee)	an area within the cochlea that contains the sensory receptors for audation, which is connected to sensory nerves that send impulses to the brain
semicircular canals (seh mee SER kyoo ler)	three loop-shaped, fluid-filled canals that detect changes in body position
stapes (STAY peez)	the third of the three auditory ossicles and is shaped like the stirrup of a horse's saddle
vestibule (VESS tih byool)	a chamber joining the semicircular canals with the cochlea and containing sensory receptors that respond to changes in body position for the sense of equilibrium

SELF QUIZ 8.2

SAY IT—SPELL IT!

Review the terms of the ears by speaking the phonetic pronunciation guides out loud, then writing in the correct spelling of the term.

Success Hint: Once you get to the crossword puzzle at the end of the chapter, remember to check back here for clues! Your clues are indicated by the puzzle icon.

1. STAY peez   _____
2. yoo STAY she ehn   _____
3. VESS tih byool   _____
4. ING kuss   _____
5. KOHK lee ah   _____
6. MALL ee us   _____
7. tihm PAHN ik   _____
8. AW rih kl   _____
9. LAB ih rinth   _____

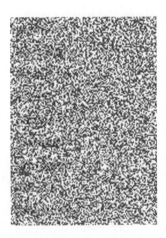

MATCH IT!

Match the term on the left with the correct definition on the right.

_____1. three loop-shaped, fluid-filled canals that detect   a. middle ear
           changes in body position

_____2. an area within the cochlea that contains the sensory   b. Eustachian tube
           receptors for audation

_____3. the midsection of the ear that lies within the tympanic   c. mastoid process
           cavity of the temporal bone; it includes the tympanic
           membrane and the ossicles

_____4. Latin for _hammer_, the first of the three auditory ossicles   d. semicircular canals
           of the middle ear, and is shaped like a hammer

_____5. the part of the ear that includes the auricle and the   e. audation
           external auditory canal

_____6. first described by Bartolommeo Eustachio in 1565,   f. organ of Corti
           this tube connects the throat with the tympanic cavity
           of the middle ear

_____7. the external appendages on the sides of the head that   g. outer ear
           are commonly referred to as the ear

_____8. the process of hearing   h. malleus

_____9. a breast-shaped projection near the base of the   i. auricle
           temporal bone that houses the middle and inner ears

WORD BUILDING

Construct or recall medical terms from the following meanings.

1. the skin-lined tube extending from
   the auricle to the eardrum   _____

2. houses the middle and inner ears   _____

3. the eardrum   _____

4. a small, air-filled cavity between
   the inside wall of the eardrum
   and the inner ear   _____

5. the Latin word for _wax_   _____

FILL IT IN!

Fill in the blanks with the correct terms.

1. The ear is the organ of _____, commonly called hearing, and
   equilibrium. The outer ear is exposed to the external environment, the middle
   ear is located within the _____ cavity, and the inner ear is
   embedded within a projection of the temporal bone known as the
   _____ process.

2. The external appendage of the outer ear is known as the _____.
   It channels sound waves into the external _____ canal, which
   carries the waves to the eardrum. Glands lining the canal deposit a waxy secretion,
   known as _____.

8.13. The middle ear includes the eardrum, which is called the _____ membrane, a tube connecting the middle ear to the throat called the _____ tube, and three tiny bones called _____. The first bone is in the shape of a hammer and is called the _____. The second or middle bone is shaped like an anvil and is known as the _____. The third bone is shaped like a stirrup for a horse's saddle and is called the _____.

4. The _____ or inner ear gets its name from its winding channels,

8.2 which resemble a maze. It includes the snail-shaped _____, three fluid-filled loops called the _____ canals, and the central chamber known as the _____. The cochlea contains sensory receptors within an area called the _____ _____ _____ which detect mechanical vibrations that are interpreted as sound by the brain.

[medical terms of the]
ears

Diseases of the ear may affect the functions of hearing or equilibrium, or in some cases both. They include inherited defects, damage caused by infection and inflammation, and damage from injury. Hearing and equilibrium may also be challenged by tumors affecting nerve impulse transmission to the brain, and by diseases of the brain that affect the interpretation of sound or equilibrium.

The treatment of diseases of the ear is usually performed by a physician specializing in ear conditions. The medical field of study that focuses on diseases of the ear is called **otology,** which can be written as:

ot/o/logy

where *ot* is the word root for ear. A physician specializing in otology is an **otologist.**

Ear disorders may also be treated by a physician specializing in disorders of the ear, nose, and throat. This field of study is called **otorhinolaryngology,** which can be written as:

ot/o/rhin/o/laring/o/logy

which includes the word root *ot* for ear, *rhin* for nose, and *laryng* for larynx or throat. As you might guess, a physician in this field is called an **otorhinolaryngologist** or an **ENT,** which is an abbreviation for ears, nose, and throat.

The general study of hearing disorders is known as **audiology.** This term uses the word root *aud,* which means *hearing*. Audiology can be written as:

audi/o/logy

A specialist in this field is an **audiologist.** An audiologist is professionally trained but is not a physician.

[**thinking critically!**]

Which type of ear specialist would you seek medical advice from if you suddenly experienced a loss of hearing in one ear that was associated with sharp local pain, a sore throat, bleeding from the nose, and nausea?

let's construct terms!

In this section, we will assemble all of the word parts to construct medical terminology related to the ears. Abbreviations are used to indicate each word part: **p** = prefix, **r** = root, **cv** = combining vowel, and **s** = suffix. Note that some terms are not constructed from word parts, but they are included here to expand your vocabulary.

The medical terms of the ears are listed in the following three sections:

- Symptoms and Signs
- Diseases and Disorders
- Treatments, Procedures, and Devices

Each section is followed by review exercises. Study the lists in these tables and complete the review exercises that follow.

Symptoms and Signs

WORD PARTS (WHEN APPLICABLE)			TERM	DEFINITION
Part	Type	Meaning		
an- -acusis	p s	without hearing	**anacusis** (AN ah KOO siss)	total hearing loss
hyper- -acusis	p s	excessive hearing	**hyperacusis** (HIGH per ah KOO siss)	overly sensitive hearing
ot -algia	r s	ear pain	**otalgia** (oh TALL jee ah)	pain in the ear, or earache
ot/o -rrhagia	r/cv s	ear bleeding or hemorrhage	**otorrhagia** (oh toh RAY jee ah)	bleeding, or hemorrhage, from the ear
ot/o -rrhea	r/cv s	ear excessive discharge	**otorrhea** (oh toh REE ah)	abnormal drainage from the ear
para- -cusis	p s	departure from normal hearing condition	**paracusis** (PAIR ah KOO siss)	partial loss or impaired hearing
			tinnitus (tinn EYE tuss)	a ringing or buzzing sensation in the ears
			vertigo (VER tih goh)	a sensation of dizziness

SELF QUIZ 8.3

SAY IT—SPELL IT!

Review the terms of the ears by speaking the phonetic pronunciation guides out loud, then writing in the correct spelling of the term.

> **Success Hint:** Use the audio glossary on the CD and CW for additional help with pronunciation of these terms.

1. tinn EYE tuss _____

2. VER tih goh _____

3. oh TALL jee ah _____

4. AN ah KOO siss _____

5. HIGH per ah KOO siss _____

6. PAIR ah KOO siss _____

7. oh toh RAY jee ah _____

8. oh toh REE ah _____

MATCH IT!

Match the term on the left with the correct definition on the right.

_____1. tinnitus   a. a sensation of dizziness

_____2. vertigo   b. pain in the ear, or earache

_____3. otalgia   c. a ringing or buzzing sensation in the ears

_____4. anacusis   d. partial loss or impaired hearing

_____5. hyperacusis   e. total hearing loss

_____6. paracusis   f. overly sensitive hearing

_____7. otorrhea   g. bleeding from the ear

_____8. otorrhagia   h. fluid discharge from the ear

BREAK IT DOWN!

Analyze and separate each term into its word parts by labeling each word part using p = prefix, r = root, cv = combining vowel, and s = suffix.

1. paracusis _____

2. otalgia _____

3. anacusis _____

4. hypercusis _____

5. otorrhea _____

WORD BUILDING

Construct or recall medical terms from the following meanings.

1. total hearing loss _____

2. overly sensitive hearing _____

3. pain in the ear, or earache _____

4. partial loss or impaired hearing _____

5. a ringing or buzzing sensation in the ears _____

6. a sensation of dizziness _____

7. fluid discharge from the ear _____

8. bleeding from the ear _____

FILL IT IN!

Fill in the blanks with the correct terms.

1. A common symptom of an inner ear infection is the loss of equilibrium (dizziness), which is called _____. If the condition persists and is associated with ringing in the ear it is called _____,

2. A symptom of total hearing loss is known as _____, and a symptom of partial or impaired hearing is called _____.

3. With the symptom _____, hearing is excessively sensitive, often causing pain in the ear, or _____.

4. The symptom of a fluid discharge from the ear is called _____. When the fluid is blood, the symptom is known as _____

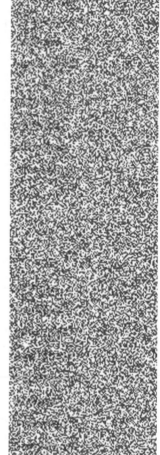

Diseases and Disorders

WORD PARTS (WHEN APPLICABLE)			TERM	DEFINITION
Part	Type	Meaning		
acoust	r	hearing	**acoustic neuroma**	a benign tumor that arises from the auditory nerve,
-ic	s	pertaining to	(ah KOOS tik	which may cause hearing impairment
neur	r	nerve	noo ROH mah)	
-oma	s	tumor		
cerumen	r	ear wax	**cerumen impaction**	excessive buildup of ear wax in the external auditory
impact	r	to fasten	(seh ROO men	canal
-ion	s	condition of	ihm PAK shun)	
labyrinth	r	maze, inner ear	**labyrinthitis**	inflammation of the labyrinth (inner ear)
-itis	s	inflammation	(LAB ih rinn THYE tiss)	
mast	r	breast	**mastoiditis**	inflammation of the mastoid process and associated
-oid	s	resemble	(mass toy DYE tiss)	tissues
-itis	s	inflammation		
			Menière's disease	a chronic disease of the inner ear that includes
			(men YERZ)	symptoms of dizziness and ringing in the ear

8.3

8.4

WORD PARTS (WHEN APPLICABLE)			TERM	DEFINITION
Part	Type	Meaning		
myring	r	membrane, eardrum	**myringitis** (mihr in JYE tiss)	inflammation of the eardrum; also called tympanitis (tihm pah NYE tiss) (Figure 8.4::::)
-itis	s	inflammation		

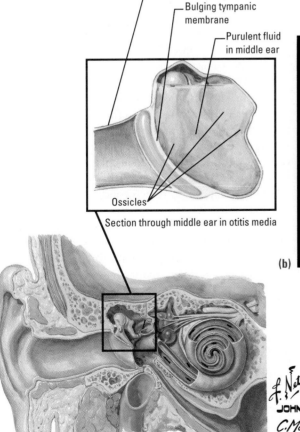

Figure 8.4 ::::

Myringitis. Scarring of the tympanic membrane can be seen through the otoscope.
Source: Professor Tony Wright, Institute of Laryncology and Otology/SPL/Photo Researchers, Inc.

WORD PARTS			TERM	DEFINITION
ot	r	ear	**otitis externa** (oh TYE tiss eks TER nah)	inflammation of the external auditory canal
-itis	s	inflammation		
extern	r	exterior		
-a	s	singular		
ot	r	ear	**otitis media** (oh TYE tiss MEH dee ah)	inflammation of the middle ear; abbreviated **OM** (Figure 8.5::::)
-itis	s	inflammation		
med	r	middle		
-ia	s	condition of		

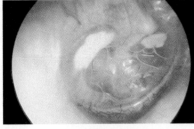

External auditory canal
Bulging tympanic membrane
Purulent fluid in middle ear
Ossicles
Section through middle ear in otitis media

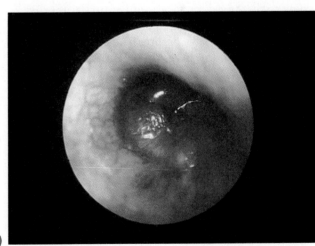

(b)

Figure 8.5 ::::

Otitis media.
(a) This illustration shows an inflamed tympanic membrane, which is the most common source of ear pain in this infection. The TM may also become inflamed due to a perforation.
Source: Icon Learning Systems.
(b) A photograph of the tympanic membrane from a patient with otitis media.
Source: Janet Hayes/Medical Images, Inc.

(a)

WORD PARTS (WHEN APPLICABLE)			TERM	DEFINITION
Part	Type	Meaning		
ot/o -pathy	r/cv s	ear disease	**otopathy** (oh TOPP ah thee)	any disease of the ear
ot/o scler -osis	r/cv r s	ear thick, hard condition of	**otosclerosis** (OH to skleh ROH siss)	abnormal formation of bone between the stapes and the oval window, causing a progressive loss of hearing
presby -acusis	r s	old age hearing	**presbyacusis** (PREZ bee ah KOO siss)	hearing impairment that is associated with old age

disease focus | Otitis Media in Children

Otitis media (OM) is the most common type of ear inflammation among children. Usually caused by a bacterial infection, it often begins as a sore throat or cold. Once the bacteria become established in the throat, they are capable of spreading along the Eustachian tube to the middle ear. The condition is extremely common: according to the American Society of Pediatrics, approximately 75 percent of children experience at least one episode of OM by the age of three years. When left untreated, the condition can result in permanent damage and hearing loss.

The symptoms of OM in young children are often difficult to identify, since most victims are too young to communicate their discomfort. They include irritability, fever, and tugging or pulling of the ear. In more advanced conditions, fluid may drain from the ear, and the ear may become sensitive to touch. Loss of balance may also be present, and in severe cases, the child may exhibit a lack of responsiveness to sounds resulting from hearing loss.

Children are more susceptible to OM than adults for several reasons. Children tend to be more susceptible to infections. Their developing immune systems leave them less capable of fending off bacteria and viruses than adults. In children, the Eustachian tube is shorter in length than in adults, making the journey between the throat and the middle ear easier for bacteria. The Eustachian tube swells as an early, normal response to infection, but when this happens, fluids become trapped in the middle ear where they do not belong.

Unfortunately, this creates a comfortable environment for the growth of bacteria. Also, the palatine tonsils are relatively larger in young children than in adults. They also swell as a normal response to an infection, and when they do there is increased pressure pinching the Eustachian tube, making drainage from the middle ear even more difficult.

As fluid accumulates within the middle ear, bacteria are able to proliferate into surrounding tissues. As a result, white blood cells migrate to the infection site to battle the bacteria, producing additional swelling, pus, and pain. The pressure within the middle ear increases, pushing against the tympanic membrane and round window. Too much pressure can damage both structures, eventually tearing them and producing hearing loss. Although the anacusis resulting from OM is usually temporary, an untreated condition can lead to permanent anacusis.

Fortunately, treatment for OM in children can defeat the infection and, in most cases, any damage. Treatments include ear drops to numb the pain, over the counter medications to reduce fever and inflammation, and antibiotics to challenge the infection. In cases in which the tympanic membrane has been damaged, surgery may be required to provide repairs in a procedure called a **tympanoplasty** or **myringoplasty**. Surgery is often accompanied with the temporary placement of a drainage tube to reduce the fluid pressure within the middle ear.

SELF QUIZ 8.4

SAY IT—SPELL IT!

Review the terms of the ears by speaking the phonetic pronunciation guides out loud, then writing in the correct spelling of the term.

1. mass toy DYE tiss   _____
2. mihr in JYE tiss   _____
3. oh TYE tiss MEH dee ah   _____
4. OH to skleh ROH siss   _____
5. PREZ bee ah KOO siss   _____
6. men YERZ   _____

MATCH IT!

Match the term on the left with the correct definition on the right.

_____1. acoustic neuroma

_____2. cerumen impaction

_____3. otitis externa

_____4. myringitis

_____5. otopathy

_____6. otosclerosis

_____7. presbyacusis

_____8. otitis media

_____9. Menière's disease

a. chronic disease of the inner ear that includes symptoms of dizziness and ringing in the ear

b. inflammation of the middle ear

c. excessive buildup of ear wax

d. abnormal formation of bone between the stapes and the oval window

e. hearing impairment due to old age

f. benign tumor of the auditory nerve

g. any disease of the ear

h. inflammation of the external auditory canal

i. also known as tympanitis

BREAK IT DOWN!

Analyze and separate each term into its word parts by labeling each word part using p = prefix, r = root, cv = combining vowel, and s = suffix.

1. acoustic neuroma   _____

2. labyrinthitis   _____

3. mastoiditis   _____

4. otalgia   _____

5. myringitis   _____

6. presbycusis   _____

WORD BUILDING

Construct or recall medical terms from the following meanings.

8.5   1. a benign tumor that arises from the
          auditory nerve, which may cause
          hearing impairment   _____

      2. inflammation of the eardrum   _____

      3. inflammation of the external
          auditory canal   _____

8.6   4. any disease of the ear   _____

      5. a chronic disease of the inner ear
          that includes symptoms of dizziness
          and ringing in the ear   _____

      6. inflammation of the labyrinth
          (inner ear)   _____

      7. inflammation of the mastoid process
          and associated tissues   _____

      8. inflammation of the middle ear   _____

      9. excessive buildup of ear wax in the
          external auditory canal   _____

     10. hearing impairment that is
          associated with old age   _____

8.7 11. abnormal formation of bone between
          the stapes and the oval window,
          causing a progressive loss of hearing   _____

FILL IT IN!

Fill in the blanks with the correct terms.

1. An infection of the throat sometimes spreads to the middle ear to produce the

    condition of _____ _____, which is caused

    when bacteria migrate along the _____ tube. If not treated, the

    infection may spread to the cells of the mastoid process to produce

    _____, which can result in impaired hearing loss or

    _____. In severe cases, surgical removal of infected air cells

    called a mastoidectomy may become necessary.

2. An inflammation of the eardrum is called _____, and an

    inflammation of the middle ear is _____ _____.

3. Any disease of the ear, or _____, can result in hearing

    impairment, or _____, or in more severe cases, a complete

    loss of hearing, or _____. The gradual hearing loss that is

    common with old age is known as _____.

Treatments, Procedures, and Devices

WORD PARTS (WHEN APPLICABLE)			TERM	DEFINITION
Part	Type	Meaning		
acou	r	hearing	**acoumetry**	a procedure that measures hearing using an
-metry	s	measurement	(ah KOO meh tree)	instrument called an acoumeter (ah KOOM eh ter)
audi/o	r/cv	hearing	**audiologist**	one who specializes in hearing disorders and
-logist	s	one who studies	(aw dee ALL oh jist)	treatment
audi/o	r/cv	hearing	**audiology**	the study of hearing disorders
-logy	s	study of	(aw dee ALL oh jee)	
audi/o	r/cv	hearing	**audiometry**	a procedure that measures hearing using an
-metry	s	measurement	(aw dee AH meh tree)	audiometer (aw dee AH meh ter); a recording of the measurement is called an audiogram (AW dee oh gram) (Figure 8.6::::)
labyrinth	r	maze, inner ear	**labyrinthectomy**	excision of the labyrinth from the temporal bone
-ectomy	s	surgical removal	(LAB ih rinn THEK toh mee)	(Figure 8.7::::)

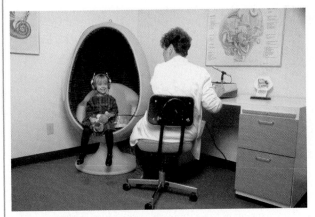

Figure 8.6 :::: **Audiometry.**
Source: Merrill Education.

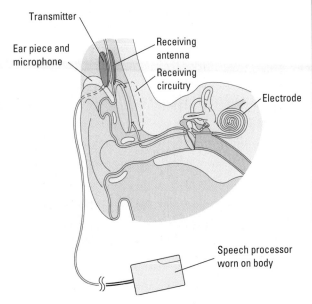

Figure 8.7 :::: **Labyrinthectomy.** The surgical removal of the cochlea of the inner ear is often followed by its replacement with an implant.

mast	r	breast	**mastoidectomy**	excision of the mastoid process, which involves
-oid	s	resemble	(MASS toy DEK toh mee)	removing the air cells from within the mastoid
-ectomy	s	surgical removal		process by cutting or drilling away the bony interconnections
mast	r	breast	**mastoidotomy**	incision into the mastoid process
-oid	s	resemble	(MASS toy DOTT oh mee)	
-otomy	s	cut into, incision		

WORD PARTS (WHEN APPLICABLE)			TERM	DEFINITION
Part	**Type**	**Meaning**		
myring/o	r/cv	membrane, eardrum	**myringoplasty** (mih RING goh plass tee)	surgical repair of the tympanic membrane
-plasty	s	surgical repair		
myring/o	r/cv	membrane, eardrum	**myringotomy** (mih ring OTT oh mee)	incision into the tympanic membrane, usually to release pus and relieve pressure in the middle ear; sometimes temporary tubes are inserted during this procedure to reduce middle ear pressure
-tomy	s	incision		
ot/o	r/cv	ear	**otology** (oh TALL oh jee)	the medical field of ear disorders and treatment
-logy	s	study of		
ot/o	r/cv	ear	**otorhinolaryngologist** (OH toh RYE noh LAIR in GALL oh jist)	a physician specializing in the treatment of ear, nose, and throat disorders; abbreviated ENT
rhin/o	r/cv	nose		
laryng/o	r/cv	voicebox, larynx		
-logist	s	one who studies		
ot/o	r/cv	ear	**otorhinolaryngology** (OH toh RYE noh LAIR in GALL oh jee)	the field of medicine that manages disorders of the ear, nose, and throat
rhin/o	r/cv	nose		
laryng/o	r/cv	voicebox, larynx		
-logy	s	study of		
ot/o	r/cv	ear	**otoscopy** (oh TOSS koh pee)	a visual examination of the ear using a hand-held device called an otoscope (OH toh skope) (Figure 8.8 ::::)
-scopy	s	process of viewing		

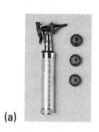 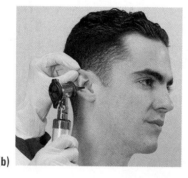

(a)   **(b)**

Figure 8.8 ::::
Otoscopy.
(a) An otoscope.
(b) Use of the otoscope.
Source: Pearson Education.

staped	r	stirrup, stapes	**stapedectomy** (stay pee DEK toh mee)	excision of the stapes; this procedure is often performed to restore hearing and may involve replacement of the stapes with a prosthesis
-ectomy	s	surgical removal		
tympan/o	r/cv	eardrum	**tympanometry** (tihm pahn AH meh tree)	a procedure that evaluates tympanic membrane elasticity by measuring its movement, using an instrument called a tympanometer (tihm pah NAH meh ter)
-metry	s	measurement		
tympan/o	r/cv	eardrum	**tympanoplasty** (tihm pahn oh PLASS tee)	surgical repair of the tympanic membrane
-plasty	s	surgical repair		

SELF QUIZ 8.5

SAY IT—SPELL IT!

Review the terms of the ears by speaking the phonetic pronunciation guides out loud, then writing in the correct spelling of the term.

1. OH toh RYE noh LAIR in GALL oh jee   _____

2. ah KOO meh tree   _____

3. LAB ih rinn THEK toh mee   _____

4. MASS toy DOTT oh mee   _____

5. mih RING goh plass tee   _____

6. oh TOSS koh pee   _____

7. tihm pahn AH meh tree   _____

MATCH IT!

Match the term on the left with the correct definition on the right.

_____1. otoscopy   a. ear, nose, and throat

_____2. myringotomy   b. incision into the mastoid process

_____3. tympanoplasty   c. excision of the mastoid process

_____4. ENT   d. surgical repair of the eardrum

_____5. mastoidectomy   e. incision into the eardrum

_____6. mastoidotomy   f. visual examination of the ear

BREAK IT DOWN!

Analyze and separate each term into its word parts by labeling each word part using p = prefix, r = root, cv = combining vowel, and s = suffix.

1. acoumetry   _____

2. audiometry   _____

3. mastoidectomy   _____

4. myringotomy   _____

5. otoscopy   _____

6. tympanoplasty   _____

WORD BUILDING

Construct or recall medical terms from the following meanings.

1. a procedure that measures hearing using an instrument called an acoumeter   _____

2. a procedure that measures hearing using an audiometer; a recording of the measurement is called an audiogram _____

3. excision of the labyrinth from the temporal bone _____

4. excision of the mastoid process, which involves removing the air cells from within the mastoid process by cutting or drilling away the bony interconnections _____

5. incision into the mastoid process _____

6. surgical repair of the tympanic membrane _____

7. incision into the tympanic membrane _____

8.8 8. a visual examination of the ear _____

9. excision of the stapes _____

10. a procedure that evaluates tympanic membrane elasticity by measuring its movement _____

11. surgical repair of the tympanic membrane _____

FILL IT IN!

Fill in the blanks with the correct terms.

1. Many of the diseases and disorders associated with the ears can be diagnosed with the help of _____, which uses an acoumeter, or the help of _____, in which a recording is made that is called an _____.

8.9 2. Surgical removal of the stapes, called a _____, is sometimes necessary to correct a birth defect.

3. Surgical removal of the mastoid air cells may become necessary to treat a chronic condition of mastoiditis, in the procedure called a _____. The first step in this procedure is an incision, known as a _____.

4. Listening to extremely loud music with headphones on can damage the eardrum, in some cases requiring a _____ to correct it.

5. To relieve pressure within the tympanic cavity, an incision through the eardrum in the procedure _____ is sometimes needed, followed by insertion of a temporary drainage tube.

6. A visual examination of the ear, or _____, is often used by a physician specializing in ear disorders, or an _____, as a first step in a physical examination.

abbreviations of the ear

The abbreviations that are associated with the ear are summarized here. Study these abbreviations, and review them in the exercise that follows.

ABBREVIATION	DEFINITION	ABBREVIATION	DEFINITION
AD	right ear (in Latin, *auris dexter*)	ENT	ear, nose, and throat
AS	left ear (in Latin, *auris sinister*)	EENT	eye, ear, nose, and throat
AU	both ears (in Latin, *aures unitas*)	OM	otitis media
TM	tympanic membrane	Oto	otology

SELF QUIZ 8.6

Fill in the blanks with the abbreviation or the complete medical term.

Abbreviation   **Medical Term**

1. AD   _____

2. _____   left ear

3. Oto   _____

4. TM   _____

8.10 5. _____   both ears

6. ENT   _____

8.11 7. _____   otitis media

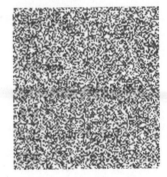

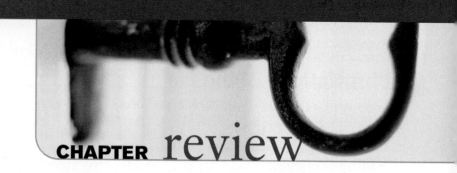

CHAPTER review

In this section, we will review all the word parts and medical terms from this chapter. As in earlier tables, the word roots are shown in **bold.**

Check each word part and medical term to be sure you understand the meaning. If any are not clear, please go back into the chapter and review that term. Then, complete the review exercises that follow.

[word parts **checklist**]

Prefixes

- ❏ a-, an-
- ❏ para-

Word Roots/Combining Vowels

- ❏ **acou**/o, **acoust**/o
- ❏ **aud**/o, **audi**/o
- ❏ **aur**/i

- ❏ **labyrinth**/o
- ❏ **mast**/o
- ❏ **myring**/o
- ❏ **ot**/o
- ❏ **salping**/o
- ❏ **staped**/o
- ❏ **tympan**/o

Suffixes

- ❏ -acusis
- ❏ -algia
- ❏ -rrhagia
- ❏ -rrhea

[medical terminology **checklist**]

- ❏ **acou**metry
- ❏ **acou**stic neuroma
- ❏ anacusis
- ❏ **aud**ation
- ❏ **audi**ometry
- ❏ **aur**icle
- ❏ both ears, **aur**es unitas (AU)
- ❏ cerumen
- ❏ cerumen impaction
- ❏ cochlea
- ❏ ears, nose, and throat (ENT)
- ❏ Eustachian tube
- ❏ **extern**al **audit**ory canal
- ❏ incus
- ❏ **labyrinth**
- ❏ **labyrinth**ectomy
- ❏ **labyrinth**itis
- ❏ left ear, **aur**is sinister (AS)

- ❏ malleus
- ❏ **mast**oid process
- ❏ **mast**oidectomy
- ❏ **mast**oiditis
- ❏ **mast**oidotomy
- ❏ Menière's disease
- ❏ middle ear
- ❏ **myring**itis
- ❏ **myring**oplasty
- ❏ **myring**otomy
- ❏ organ of Corti
- ❏ **ot**algia
- ❏ **ot**itis externa
- ❏ **ot**itis media (OM)
- ❏ **ot**ology (Oto)
- ❏ **ot**opathy
- ❏ **ot**orrhagia
- ❏ **ot**orrhea

- ❏ **ot**osclerosis
- ❏ **ot**oscopy
- ❏ outer ear
- ❏ paracusis
- ❏ presbyacusis
- ❏ right ear, **aur**is dexter (AD)
- ❏ semicircular canals
- ❏ **staped**ectomy
- ❏ stapes
- ❏ tinnitus
- ❏ **tympan**ic cavity
- ❏ **tympan**ic membrane (TM)
- ❏ **tympan**ometry
- ❏ **tympan**oplasty
- ❏ vertigo
- ❏ vestibule

[show what **you know!**]

BREAK IT DOWN!

Analyze and separate each term into its word parts by labeling each word
part using p = prefix, r = root, cv = combining vowel, and s = suffix.

		r s
Example:	1. otalgia	ot/algia
	2. mastoidotomy	_____
	3. anacusis	_____
	4. labyrinthitis	_____
	5. otosclerosis	_____
	6. otopathy	_____

WORD BUILDING

Construct or recall medical terms from the following meanings.

Example:	1. surgical repair of the tympanic membrane	tympanoplasty
	2. total hearing loss	_____
	3. inflammation of the inner ear	_____
	4. pain in the ear	_____
	5. inflammation of the middle ear	_____
	6. abnormal drainage from the ear	_____
	7. any disease of the ear	_____
	8. partial loss of hearing	_____
	9. excessive buildup of earwax	_____
	10. excision of the stapes	_____

CASE STUDIES

Fill in the blanks with the correct terms.

1. An elderly patient was admitted to a clinic following complaints of impaired hearing, called

   (a) _____, ear pain, or (b) _____, and abnormal fluid drainage from the ears,

   or (c) _____, that included an occasional blood loss, or (d) _____. During an

   examination, the patient indicated that she had fallen recently when she became very dizzy from a ringing in the ears. After

   identifying the condition of (e) _____ by the ringing sensation and (f) _____

   from symptoms of dizziness, further exams were made. Following exams that involved the use of an audiometer to produce

   an (g) _____ reading and an acoumeter, it was determined that the patient was suffering from a middle ear infection, or (h) _____ _____, that had spread to the inner ear to

produce (i) _____. The infection had been initiated from a streptococcus throat infection, traveling

to the middle ear by way of the (j) _____ tube. The infection had become advanced, and the removal

of the mastoid process, or (k) _____, had become necessary. During the surgery, it was found that

the labyrinth was severely infected and its removal in a (l) _____ proceeded immediately. Although

the infection and all decaying tissue was successfully eliminated, the patient was left with total hearing loss, or

(m) _____.

[piece it all **together!**]

CROSSWORD

From the chapter material, fill in the crossword puzzle with answers to the following clues.

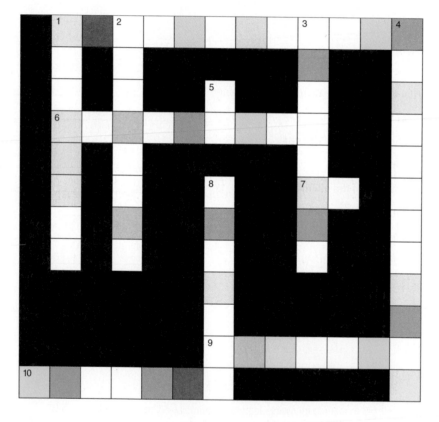

ACROSS

1. Abnormal formation of bone in the ear. (Find puzzle piece 8.7)
6. Partially impaired hearing. (Find puzzle piece 8.3)
7. Abbreviation for a middle ear infection. (Find puzzle piece 8.11)
9. Common name for the tympanic membrane. (Find puzzle piece 8.1)
10. A cancer that can cause anacusis. (Find puzzle piece 8.5)

DOWN

1. Any disease of the ear. (Find puzzle piece 8.6)

2. Excessive discharge from the ear. (Find puzzle piece 8.4)

3. A physical exam performed with an otoscope. (Find puzzle piece 8.8)

4. Surgical removal of the stapes. (Find puzzle piece 8.9)

5. Abbreviation meaning both ears. (Find puzzle piece 8.10)

8. The part of the inner ear that houses the organ of Corti. (Find puzzle piece 8.2)

WORD UNSCRAMBLE

From the completed crossword puzzle, unscramble:

1. All of the letters that appear in **green** squares

   _ _ _ _ ☐

   Clue: The anvil of the middle ear

2. All of the letters that appear in **red** squares

   ☐ _

   Clue: Abbreviation for the eardrum

3. All of the letters that appear in **gray** squares

   _ ☐ _

   Clue: The special sensory organ for hearing and equilibrium

4. All of the letters that appear in **peach** squares

   _ _ _ ☐ _ _ _

   Clue: Any disease of the ear

5. All of the letters that appear in **yellow** squares

   ☐ _ _

   Clue: Includes outer, middle, and inner parts

6. All of the letters that appear in **pink** squares

   _ _ _ ☐ _ _ _

   Clue: An instrument used during otoscopy

Now write down each of the letters that are boxed to find the hidden medical term of the ears:

_ _ _ _ _ _

MEDmedia wrap-up

www.prenhall.com/wingerd

Before you go on to the next chapter, take advantage of the free CD-ROM and study guide website that accompany this book. Simply load the CD-ROM for additional activities, games, animations, videos, and quizzes linked to this chapter. Then visit www.prenhall.com/wingerd for even more!

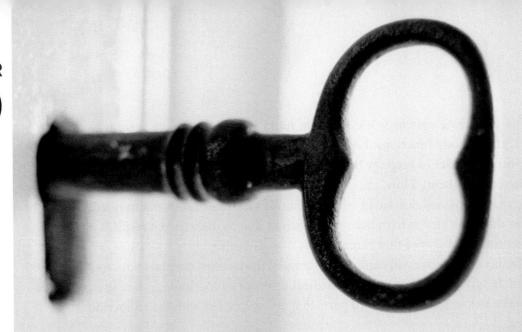

The Endocrine System

LEARNING OBJECTIVES

After completing this chapter, you will be able to:

- Define and spell the word parts used to create terms for the endocrine system

- Identify the major organs of the endocrine system and describe their structure and function

- Break down and define common medical terms used for symptoms, diseases, disorders, procedures, treatments, and devices associated with the endocrine system

- Build medical terms from the word parts associated with the endocrine system

- Pronounce and spell common medical terms associated with the endocrine system

MEDmedia

www.prenhall.com/wingerd

Enhance your study with the power of multimedia! Each chapter of this book links to activities, games, animations, videos, and quizzes that you'll find on your CD-ROM. Plus, you can click on www.prenhall.com/wingerd, to find a free chapter-specific companion website that's loaded with additional practice and resources.

CD-ROM

- Audio Glossary
- Exercises & Activities
- Flashcard Generator
- Animations
- Videos

 Companion Website

- Exercises & Activities
- Audio Glossary
- Drug Updates
- Current News Updates

A secure distance learning course is available at www.prenhall.com/onekey.

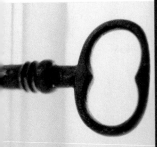

The endocrine system works hand in hand with the nervous system to regulate body functions. Like the nervous system, it provides a method of control in order to keep the body functioning despite changing conditions in the environment. Thus, the primary role of the endocrine system is to achieve homeostasis, a state in which the body's equilibrium is maintained. When the endocrine system becomes deficient due to disease, the result is a homeostatic imbalance that often affects overall health.

In this chapter, we will explore the terms of the healthy, normal endocrine system before proceeding with the medical terms of endocrinology. But first, let's take a close look at the word parts that are associated with the endocrine system.

word parts focus

PREFIX	DEFINITION	PREFIX	DEFINITION
ad-	toward	hyper-	excessive, above normal
anti-	against, opposing	hypo-	under, below normal
endo-	within, absorbing	para-	near, alongside; departure from normal
ex-, exo-	outside, away from	syn-	together

[FYI]

para-
The prefix para- may become a root word when placed in the center of a constructed word.

WORD ROOTS	DEFINITION	WORD ROOTS	DEFINITION
acr	extremity, or extreme	kal	potassium
aden	gland	ket	ketone bodies (a byproduct of protein metabolism)
andr	male		
calc	calcium	lob	lobe
cortic	tree bark, outer covering, cortex	megal	abnormally large
crin	to secrete	myx	mucus
dips	thirst	natr	sodium
gluc	glucose, or sugar	pancreat	sweetbread, pancreas
glyc, glycos	glycogen (a storage form of sugar), glucose or sugar	ren	kidney
		thyr	shield, thyroid
hormon	to set in motion	tox	poison

SUFFIX	DEFINITION	SUFFIX	DEFINITION
-drome	run, running	-oid	resemblance to
-emia	blood	-osis	condition of
-ism	condition or disease	-plasia	shape, formation

SELF QUIZ 9.1

Review the word parts of endocrine system terminology by working carefully through the exercises that follow. Soon, we will apply this new information to build medical terms.

A. Provide the definition of the following prefixes and suffixes.

1. anti-   _____

2. endo-   _____

3. ex-   _____

4. syn-   _____

5. -drome   _____

6. -emia   _____

7. -oid   _____

8. -plasia   _____

B. Provide the word root for each of the following terms.

1. extremity   _____

2. gland   _____

3. kidney   _____

4. male   _____

5. calcium   _____

6. cortex   _____

7. to secrete   _____

8. thirst   _____

9. glucose   _____

10. potassium   _____

11. abnormally large _____

12. sodium   _____

13. thyroid gland   _____

14. poison   _____

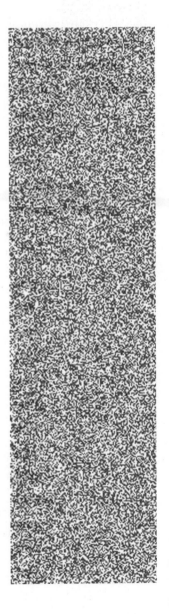

[anatomy and physiology *overview*]

The endocrine system communicates to the body by secreting chemicals into the bloodstream. The chemicals are called **hormones,** which are produced by special organs known as endocrine glands.

Endocrine glands secrete hormones directly into the watery environment surrounding each cell. From there, the hormones enter the bloodstream, which carries them throughout the body's circulation until they reach the part of the body they are to affect (Figure 9.1::::). Because blood flows much more slowly than the conduction of a nerve impulse, a hormone takes longer to reach its destination. As a result, the control provided by the endocrine system occurs more slowly, and also lasts longer, when compared to the nervous system.

Endocrine control is initiated when a hormone contacts a cell, known as a **target cell,** and begins a chemical chain reaction within the cell that results in a change in the cell's metabolism or protein synthesis. **Metabolism** means *a condition of change,* and refers to the exchange of energy within a cell. Protein synthesis is the process of new protein construction within a cell.

Hormones are extremely potent chemicals. In many cases, a single hormone molecule can change the function of a cell, which can affect many other cells. That potency is like changing the color of Lake Michigan from blue to red by dropping a few drops of red food coloring into the lake! Once millions of cells are stimulated by a hormone to change their metabolism or protein synthesis, an organ, a system, or even the entire body may respond, resulting in the hormonal control of body function.

Endocrine Glands

Structurally, the endocrine system consists of the organs of the body that secrete hormones (Figure 9.2::::). The organs are also called glands, since their primary function is the secretion of a product. As you are about to discover, the endocrine glands are scattered throughout the body.

The pea-sized **pituitary gland** is located within the cranial cavity immediately below the brain and is connected to the hypothalamus. Due to its location beneath the brain, it is also called the hypophysis, which is a Greek word that means *undergrowth.* Although it is the size of a small pea, it is often called the *master gland* due

[FYI]

Hormone
The term *hormone* is derived from the Greek word *hormon,* which means *to set in motion.* The term's meaning refers to the profound impact hormones can have on body function: A single hormone molecule can set off a chain reaction of events that can alter body function.

[thinking critically!]

What two cellular functions may undergo change due to the influence of a hormone?

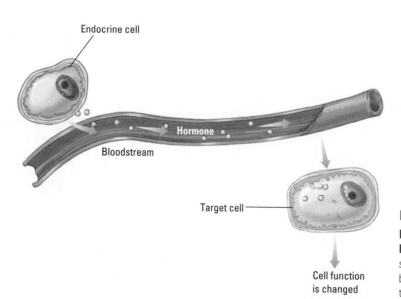

Endocrine cell

Hormone

Bloodstream

Target cell

Cell function is changed

Figure 9.1 ::::

Endocrine glands secrete hormones. The hormones are secreted and diffuse into the bloodstream. Once they contact a target cell, a change may begin.

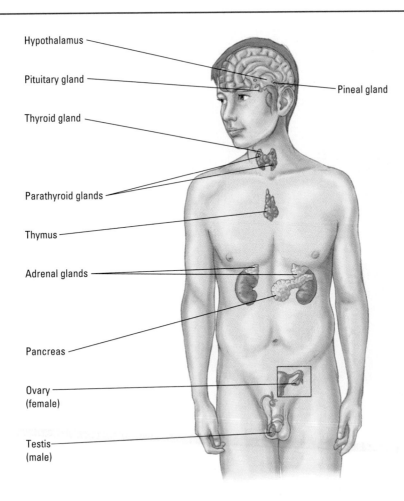

Hypothalamus

Pituitary gland

Pineal gland

Thyroid gland

Parathyroid glands

Thymus

Adrenal glands

Pancreas

Ovary
(female)

Testis
(male)

Figure 9.2 :::::

The endocrine glands are distributed throughout the body.

to the control it maintains over other glands. The pituitary gland consists of two lobes, the anterior lobe and the posterior lobe. The anterior lobe is also called the adenohypophysis, and is made up of soft glandular tissue that produces the following hormones (Figure 9.3:::::):

- growth hormone (GH), which regulates metabolism and body growth
- adrenocorticotrophic (add DREE noh kor tih koh TROH fik) hormone (ACTH), which activates the adrenal gland
- melanocyte-stimulating (mell AN oh sight) hormone (MSH),which stimulates skin pigment production
- thyroid-stimulating hormone (TSH), which stimulates the thyroid gland
- prolactin (proh LAK tinn) (PRL), which stimulates milk secretion by the mammary glands
- follicle-stimulating (FALL ih kl) hormone (FSH), which stimulates development of ova and sperm
- luteinizing (LOO teh NIGH zing) hormone (LH), which stimulates secretion of sex hormones by the gonads

The posterior lobe of the pituitary gland is called the neurohypophysis and consists of nervous tissue. It secretes two hormones:

- oxytocin (AHK see TOH sin) (OT), which stimulates contractions of the uterus and milk secretion by the mammary glands
- antidiuretic (AN tye dye yoo RET ik) hormone (ADH), which stimulates water reabsorption in the kidneys and reduces urine volume

[**thinking critically!**]

Which endocrine glands are regulated by the anterior pituitary gland?

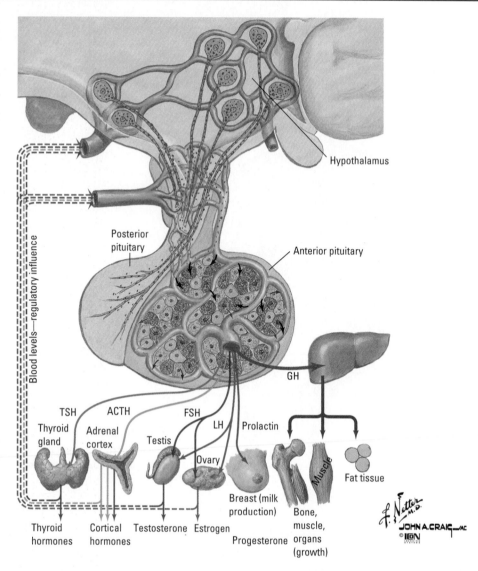

Figure 9.3 ::::

The pituitary gland, which hangs below the hypothalamus at the base of the brain. The hormones secreted by the anterior pituitary gland and their targets are illustrated.
Source: Icon Learning Systems.

Like the pituitary gland, the small **pineal gland** is also located within the cranial cavity, but it is located within the center of the brain. The pineal gland secretes one hormone, melatonin (MELL ah TOH ninn), which regulates body rhythms, including sleep cycles.

Located in the anterior part of the neck are the **thyroid gland** and **parathyroid glands.** The thyroid gland is a butterfly-shaped endocrine organ that wraps around the larynx (Figure 9.4::::). It consists of a right and left lobe connected by a narrow band called the isthmus. The thyroid gland secretes three primary hormones:

- thyroxine (thigh ROK seen) (T_4) regulates the breakdown of glucose and the synthesis of most cells of the body

- triiodothyronine (try eye oh doh THIGH roh neen) (T_3) works in conjunction with thyroxine to produce the same effects (note: T_4 and T_3 are together referred to as thyroid hormone)

- calcitonin (KAL sih TOH ninn) (CT) stimulates the production of new bone material to reduce calcium levels in the blood

The parathyroid glands consist of three or four pea-sized organs embedded within the posterior side of the larger thyroid gland. The parathyroid glands secrete parathyroid hormone (PAIR ah THIGH royd) (PTH), which increases calcium levels in the blood (the opposite effect of calcitonin).

[FYI]

Thyroid
The shape of the thyroid gland must have reminded Hippocrates of a shield, since the term is derived from the Greek word for this defensive warrior gear, *thyreos.*

[thinking critically!]

Which two hormones help control calcium levels in the blood?

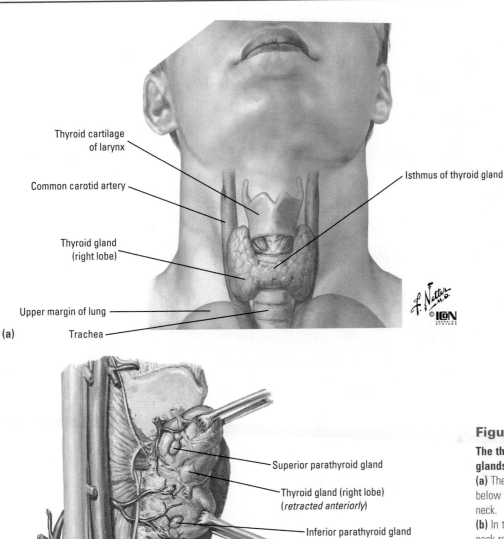

Thyroid cartilage of larynx

Common carotid artery

Thyroid gland (right lobe)

Upper margin of lung

(a) Trachea

Isthmus of thyroid gland

Superior parathyroid gland

Thyroid gland (right lobe) (*retracted anteriorly*)

Inferior parathyroid gland

Trachea

(b)

Figure 9.4 ::::

The thyroid and parathyroid glands.
(a) The thyroid gland is located just below the thyroid cartilage in the neck.
(b) In this right lateral view of the neck region, the thyroid gland is shown pulled aside to reveal two parathyroid glands.
Source: Icon Learning Systems.

Located within the abdominal cavity are the paired **adrenal glands,** also called the suprarenals. The adrenal glands are located on top of each kidney. Each includes a **cortex,** or outer part and a **medulla,** or inner part. The adrenal cortex secretes:

- aldosterone (al DOSS ter ohn), which regulates body fluid balance and blood pressure
- glucocorticoids (GLOO koh KOR tih koydz), which reduce inflammation
- androgens (AN droh jennz) and estrogens (ESS troh jennz), which stimulate the development of sex characteristics

The adrenal medulla secretes two hormones, epinephrine (EP ih NEFF rinn), also called adrenaline (ah DREHN ah linn), and norepinephrine (NOR ep ih NEFF rinn). Both hormones prolong the conditions for a "fight or flight" response, which includes an increase in metabolism, heart rate, blood pressure, etc.

Like the adrenals, the **pancreas** is also located in the abdominal cavity, but immediately behind the stomach (Figure 9.5::::). It is a soft, oblong organ that performs two functions: the secretion of hormones and the secretion of digestive enzymes. (We will consider its digestive function later in the chapter on the digestive system.)

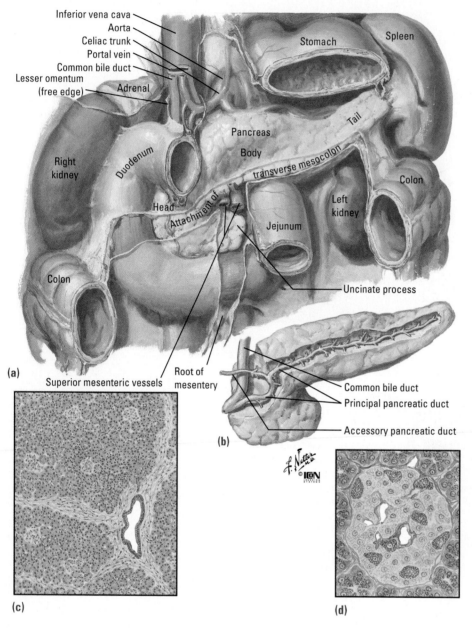

(a)

(b)

(c)

(d)

Figure 9.5 ::::

The pancreas and islets of Langerhans.
(a) Location of the pancreas, with the stomach and small intestine cut away.
(b) The pancreas, with its central duct exposed.
(c) Microscopic section of the pancreas, low power.
(d) Microscopic section of a single islet of Langerhans, high power.
Source: Icon Learning Systems.

The part of the pancreas that secretes hormones consists of clusters of cells, which produce hormones that regulate sugar levels in the blood. These clusters are distributed throughout the organ. Each cluster is called an **islet of Langerhans,** named after the scientist who first identified them. Each islet secretes two primary hormones:

- insulin (IN soo linn), which reduces blood sugar levels by stimulating the conversion of glucose to glycogen (a storage form) and facilitating the uptake of glucose into body cells

- glucagon (GLOO kah gahn), which increases blood sugar levels by stimulating the conversion of glycogen into glucose in the liver, releasing glucose into the bloodstream

The **thymus gland** is a soft gland that shrinks in size after puberty; it is located anterior to and above the heart in the thoracic cavity. The thymus gland secretes the hormone thymosin (THIGH moh sin), which helps to establish the immune response during early childhood.

[thinking critically!]

What do you suppose would result from a failure of the pancreas to secrete insulin?

enrichment module enrichment

The **gonads** are the endocrine glands that produce sex hormones and the reproductive cells, or gametes. The gonads of the male are the **testes,** which secrete testosterone (tess TOSS ter ohn). The female gonads are the **ovaries,** which secrete estrogen (ESS troh jenn) and progesterone (proh JESS ter ohn).

In addition to the primary endocrine organs, other organs of the body contain endocrine cells that secrete hormones. These organs include the heart, stomach, and kidneys, which are covered in other chapters. We will study the gonads in the chapter on the reproductive system. In this chapter, we will confine our study of the endocrine system to the pituitary gland, pineal gland, thyroid gland, parathyroid glands, adrenal glands, pancreas, and thymus gland.

[FYI]

Pancreas
The term pancreas comes from Greek for *sweetbread* due to the characteristically sweet taste of the pancreas of certain animals.

getting to the root of it | anatomy and physiology terms

Many of the anatomy and physiology terms are formed from roots that are used to construct the more complex medical terms of the endocrine system, including symptoms, diseases, and treatments. In this section, we will review the terms that describe the structure and function of the endocrine system *in relation to their word roots,* which are shown in **bold.**

Study the word roots and terms in this list and complete the review exercises that follow.

Word Root (Meaning)	Terms Formed from the Word Root (Pronunciation)	Definition
crin (to secrete)	endo**crin**e system (EHN doh krinn)	the system of the body that functions in homeostasis by releasing hormones from endocrine glands
hormon (to set in motion)	**hormon**e (HOR mohn)	a chemical substance secreted by certain cells that travel through the bloodstream to eventually trigger changes in target cells
ren (kidney)	ad**ren**al glands (add REE nal)	a pair of glands, each located on top of a kidney, which consist of the adrenal cortex and the adrenal medulla; they are also called the suprarenals
	ad**ren**al cortex (ad REE nal KOR teks)	the outer region of the adrenal gland, which secretes hormones that regulate fluid balance and blood pressure, reduce inflammation, and stimulate the development of sex characteristics
	ad**ren**al medulla (ad REE nal meh DULL lah)	the inner part of the adrenal gland, which secretes hormones that prolong the conditions for a "fight or flight" response, including an increase in metabolism, heart rate, blood pressure, etc.
thyr (shield, thyroid)	para**thyr**oid (PAIR ah THIGH royd) glands	the four or five pea-sized glands embedded within the posterior side of the larger thyroid gland, which secrete parathyroid hormone to increase calcium levels in the blood
	thyroid (THIGH royd) gland	a large, butterfly-shaped soft gland on the anterior side of the neck, which consists of a right and left lobe connected by a narrow band called the isthmus; it secretes three primary hormones that regulate the breakdown and synthesis of glucose in most cells of the body, and stimulate the production of new bone material to reduce calcium levels in the blood

OTHER IMPORTANT TERMS

The terms in this table are related to the structure and function of the endocrine system, but are not built from word roots.

gonads	organs that secrete sex hormones and produce sex cells; male gonads are called testes and female gonads are called ovaries
islets of Langerhans (EYE letts ov LAHNG er hahnz)	named after the scientist who first identified them, these clusters of cells are distributed throughout the pancreas and are responsible for the secretion of the pancreatic hormones, insulin and glucagon
metabolism (meh TAB oh lizm)	the sum of all energy-activities in the body; the term literally means *a condition of change*
pancreas (PAN kree ass)	a soft, oblong organ located behind the stomach in the abdominal cavity, which secretes hormones that regulate blood sugar levels
pineal gland (pih NEE al)	a small, pea-sized gland within the center of the brain that secretes one hormone, melatonin, which regulates body rhythms
pituitary gland (pih TOO ih tair ee)	located at the base of the brain and connected to the hypothalamus, this *master gland* consists of the anterior lobe and the posterior lobe and maintains control over other glands; also called the hypophysis
target cell	any cell of the body that is affected by a particular hormone; the effects of a hormone upon a target cell are a change in metabolism or protein synthesis
thymus gland (THIGH muss)	a soft gland located anterior and above the heart, it shrinks in size after puberty and secretes the hormone thymosin, which initiates the immune response

SELF QUIZ 9.2

Success Hint: Once you get to the crossword puzzle at the end of the chapter, remember to check back here for clues! Your clues are indicated by the puzzle icon.

SAY IT—SPELL IT!

Review the terms of the endocrine system by speaking the phonetic pronunciation guides out loud, then writing in the correct spelling of the term.

1. pih TOO ih tair ee _____

2. pih NEE al _____

3. THIGH royd _____

4. PAIR ah THIGH royd _____

5. add REE nal _____

6. PAN kree ass _____

7. EYE letts ov LAHNG er hahnz _____

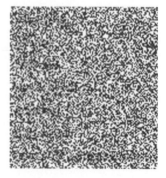

MATCH IT!

Match the term on the left with the correct definition on the right.

_____1. islets of Langerhans   a. reduces sugar levels in the blood

_____2. target cell   b. the adenohypophysis

_____3. pituitary gland   c. located on the anterior side of the neck

_____4. neurohypophysis   d. secretes insulin and glucagon

_____5. anterior lobe   e. embedded within the thyroid gland

_____6. insulin   f. a powerful gland attached to the brain

_____7. adrenal medulla   g. a general site of hormone action

_____8. thyroid gland   h. secretes epinephrine

_____9. parathyroid gland   i. secretes antidiuretic hormone

FILL IT IN!

Fill in the blanks with the correct terms.

9.1 1. The endocrine gland that regulates the release of _____ by several other endocrine glands is the _____ gland. It includes an anterior lobe, or the _____, which secretes seven hormones and a posterior lobe, which secretes two hormones. One of them is

9.2 _____, which stimulates contractions of the uterus and milk secretion by the mammary glands.

9.3 2. The _____ gland secretes the hormone melatonin, which regulates rhythms that include sleep patterns.

3. The large butterfly-shaped organ in the neck is the _____ gland. It secretes two hormones that regulate the breakdown of _____ and synthesis of proteins in cells.

4. The four or five small organs embedded within the thyroid gland are the _____ glands. These small glands secrete parathyroid hormone, which increases _____ levels in the blood.

5. The _____ glands are located above each kidney. They include two portions, an outer _____ and an inner medulla.

6. The _____ includes clusters of cells that secrete two primary

9.4 hormones. The islets of Langerhans produce _____, which reduces blood sugar levels, and _____, which raises blood sugar levels.

[medical terms of the

endocrine system]

An array of disorders can occur when an endocrine gland fails to deliver the quantity of hormones needed to regulate body functions. In general, endocrine disease results in either an abnormal increase in hormone production, called **hypersecretion,** or an abnormal decrease, called **hyposecretion.** Either condition upsets the homeostatic balance of the body. Hypersecretion may arise due to an inherited disease or a tumor. Often, hyposecretion occurs if an endocrine gland suffers trauma due to an injury or infection, although it also may be caused by an inherited disorder or a tumor.

Sometimes, an endocrine disorder includes an array of symptoms and involves multiple organs. This type of disease is generally known as a **syndrome.**

The treatment of endocrine diseases is a focused discipline within medicine. The field of study is known as **endocrinology.** This is a constructed word that can be written as

endo/crin/o/logy

in which endo- is a prefix meaning *within or absorbing, crin* is a word root that means *to secrete,* and -logy is a suffix that means *study of.* Thus, endocrinology is the science concerned with internal secretions and their pathologic and physiologic relationships. A physician who practices the *study of secreting within,* or endocrinology, is called an **endocrinologist. Endocrinopathy** is a term used to describe a disease or disorder in the function of an endocrine gland and the related consequences.

> [**thinking critically!**]
>
> Can you think of a syndrome that is *not* an endocrine disorder?

let's construct terms!

In this section, we will assemble all of the word parts to construct medical terminology related to the endocrine system. Abbreviations are used to indicate each word part: **p** = prefix, **r** = root, **cv** = combining vowel, and **s** = suffix. Note that some terms are not constructed from word parts, but they are included here to expand your vocabulary.

The medical terms of the endocrine system are listed in the following three sections:

- Symptoms and Signs
- Diseases and Disorders
- Treatments, Procedures, and Devices

Each section is followed by review exercises. Study the lists in these tables and complete the review exercises that follow.

Symptoms and Signs

WORD PARTS (WHEN APPLICABLE)			TERM	DEFINITION
Part	Type	Meaning		
acid	r	acid	**acidosis**	an abnormal accumulation of waste materials that are acidic, often a symptom of diabetes mellitus; acidosis may also be caused by respiratory or kidney disorders
-osis	s	condition of	(ass ih DOH siss)	

WORD PARTS (WHEN APPLICABLE)			TERM	DEFINITION
Part	Type	Meaning		
ex	p	outside, away from	**exophthalmos** (eks off THAL mohs)	abnormal protrusion of the eyes (Figure 9.6::::)
ophthalm/o	r/cv	eye		
-s	s	plural		
			goiter (GOY ter)	an abnormal enlargement of the thyroid gland caused by a tumor, lack of iodine in the diet, or infection (Figure 9.7::::)

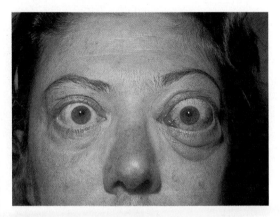

Figure 9.6 :::: **Exophthalmos, in which the eyes protrude.** It is a symptom of hyperthyroidism (Graves' disease).
Source: University of Ilinois, Custom Medical Stock Photo, Inc.

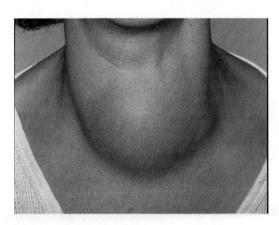

Figure 9.7 :::: **Goiter.** The formation of numerous nodules in the thyroid gland cause the characteristic enlargement of the neck, which is a symptom of iodine deficiency or tumors.
Source: Custom Medical Stock Photo, Inc.

			TERM	DEFINITION
			hypersecretion (HIGH per seh KREE shun)	abnormal increase in hormone production, often the result of an inherited disease or a tumor
			hyposecretion (HIGH poh seh KREE shun)	abnormal decrease in hormone production, which often occurs when an endocrine gland suffers trauma due to an injury or infection; may also be caused by an inherited disorder or a tumor
ket	r	ketone bodies	**ketosis** (kee TOH siss)	excessive amount of ketone bodies in the blood and urine, which is a symptom of an abnormal metabolism of carbohydrates as seen in uncontrolled diabetes and starvation; also known as ketoacidosis (KEE toh ass ih DOH siss)
-osis	s	condition of		
poly-	p	many	**polydipsia** (PALL ee DIP see ah)	abnormal state of excessive thirst
dips	r	thirst		
-ia	s	condition		
poly-	p	many	**polyuria** (PALL ee YOO ree ah)	excretion of abnormally large volumes of urine
ur	r	urine		
-ia	s	condition		

SELF QUIZ 9.3

Success Hint: Use the audio glossary on the CD and CW for additional help with pronunciation of these terms.

SAY IT—SPELL IT!

Review the terms of the endocrine system by speaking the phonetic pronunciation guides out loud, then writing in the correct spelling of the term.

1. ass ih DOH siss   _____

2. kee TOH siss   _____

9.5 3. PALL ee DIP see ah   _____

4. PALL ee YOO ree ah   _____

9.6 5. eks off THAL mohs   _____

6. GOY ter   _____

7. HIGH per seh KREE shun   _____

8. HIGH po seh KREE shun   _____

MATCH IT!

Match the term on the left with the correct definition on the right.

_____1. *acidosis*   a. abnormal state of excessive thirst

_____2. *ketosis*   b. excretion of large quantities of urine

_____3. *polydipsia*   c. enlargement at the throat

_____4. *polyuria*   d. abnormal accumulation of waste materials
                                     that are acidic

_____5. *exophthalmos*   e. excessive amount of ketone bodies in
                                     the blood and urine

_____6. *goiter*   f. protrusion of the eyes

BREAK IT DOWN!

Analyze and separate each term into its word parts by labeling each word part using p = prefix, r = root, cv = combining vowel, and s = suffix.

1. acidosis   _____

2. ketosis   _____

3. polydipsia   _____

4. polyuria   _____

5. exophthalmos   _____

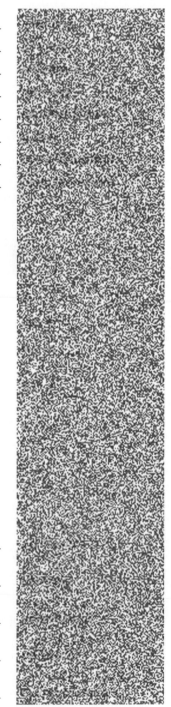

WORD BUILDING

Construct or recall medical terms from the following meanings.

1. abnormal state of excessive thirst _____

2. excretion of large quantities of urine _____

3. excessive amount of ketone bodies
   in the blood and urine _____

4. abnormal accumulation of waste
   materials that are acidic _____

5. protrusion of the eyes _____

6. abnormal enlargement of the
   thyroid gland _____

FILL IT IN!

Fill in the blanks with the correct terms.

1. A medical term that literally means a *condition of acid* is known as

   _____, in which body fluids drop dangerously in pH. A related

   condition is known as _____, and includes the accumulation of

   ketone bodies in body fluids.

2. Urinating more frequently than normal is a symptom known as

   _____, while the symptom of being thirsty more than normal

   is called _____.

3. The eyes protruding from the face is a symptom of an endocrine disorder, and is

   known as _____.

4. A lack of iodine in the diet is a common cause of _____, which

   looks like an enlarged throat.

Diseases and Disorders

WORD PARTS (WHEN APPLICABLE)			TERM	DEFINITION
Part	Type	Meaning		
acr/o	r/cv	extreme	**acromegaly**	an enlargement of bone structure most prominent in
megal	r	large	(ak roh MEG ah lee)	the face and hands, resulting in disfigurement, and
-y	s	process of		caused by the hypersecretion of growth hormone
				from the pituitary gland after puberty (Figure 9.8⬚⬚⬚⬚)
			Addison's disease	a chronic syndrome caused by hyposecretion of the
				adrenal cortex, characterized by darkening of the
				skin, loss of appetite, mental depression, and
				muscle weakness (Figure 9.9⬚⬚⬚⬚)

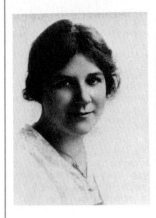
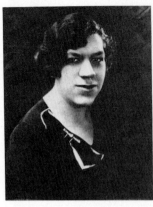
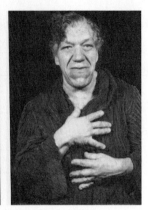

Figure 9.8 ::::

Acromegaly. Acromegaly is a metabolic disorder in which excessive amounts of growth hormone are secreted during adulthood, resulting in enlarged bones, mostly apparent in the face and hands.
Courtesy of Clinical Pathological Conference, American Journal of Medicine.

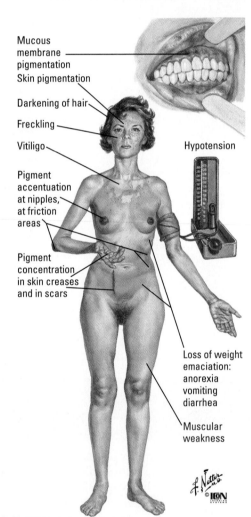

Mucous membrane pigmentation
Skin pigmentation
Darkening of hair
Freckling
Vitiligo
Pigment accentuation at nipples, at friction areas
Pigment concentration in skin creases and in scars

Hypotension

Loss of weight emaciation: anorexia vomiting diarrhea

Muscular weakness

Figure 9.9 ::::

Addison's disease. Caused by chronic hyposecretion of the adrenal cortex, it produces the illustrated symptoms.
Source: Icon Learning Systems.

[FYI]

Addison's Disease

In 1855, a series of signs and symptoms were connected for the first time into a common cause. They included "feeble heart action, anemia, irritability of the stomach, and a peculiar change in the color of the skin." The syndrome was named to recognize its discoverer, the English physician Thomas Addison, who correlated the symptoms and signs to a failure of the adrenal cortex.

WORD PARTS (WHEN APPLICABLE)			TERM	DEFINITION
Part	**Type**	**Meaning**		
aden	r	gland	**adenitis**	inflammation of a gland
-itis	s	inflammation	(add eh NYE tiss)	
aden	r	gland	**adenosis**	abnormal condition of a gland
-osis	s	condition of	(add eh NOH siss)	
ad-	p	toward	**adrenal virilism**	excessive production of androgen (male sex hormone) by the adrenal cortex, usually caused by adrenal hyperplasia or a tumor in adult women; symptoms include masculinization
ren	r	kidney	(add REE nal	
-al	s	pertaining to	VIHR ill izm)	
viril	r	masculine		
-ism	s	condition		
ad-	p	toward	**adrenalitis**	inflammation of the adrenal gland
ren	r	kidney	(add REE nah LYE tiss)	
-al	s	pertaining to		
-itis	s	inflammation		
ad-	p	toward	**adrenocortico-hyperplasia**	abnormal development of the adrenal cortex resulting in its excessive size and hypersecretion of its hormones
ren/o	r/cv	kidney		
cortic/o	r/cv	outer covering, cortex	(ah DREE noh KOR tih koh high per PLAY zee ah)	
hyper-	p	excessive		
-plasia	s	shape, formation		
ad-	p	toward	**adrenomegaly**	abnormal enlargement of the adrenal glands
ren/o	r/cv	kidney	(add ree noh MEG ah lee)	
megal	r	large		
-y	s	process of		
ad-	p	toward	**adrenopathy**	general disease of the adrenal gland
ren/o	r/cv	kidney	(ADD ren OPP ah thee)	
-pathy	s	disease		
calc/i	r/cv	calcium	**calcipenia**	deficiency of calcium; also called **hypocalcemia** (HIGH poh kal SEE mee ah)
-penia	s	deficiency	(kal sih PEE nee ah)	
			cretinism	congenital hypothyroidism in children, which results in reduced mental development and dwarfed physical stature
			(KREE tin izm)	
			Cushing's syndrome	a syndrome resulting from hypersecretion of the adrenal cortex, characterized by obesity, moon face, hyperglycemia, and muscle weakness (Figure 9.10▦)
			(KUSH ingz SIN drohm)	
			diabetes insipidus	caused by hyposecretion of ADH by the posterior lobe of the pituitary gland, its symptoms include polydipsia and polyuria; abbreviated **DI**
			(DYE ah BEE teez in SIP ih duss)	
			diabetes mellitus	a chronic disorder of carbohydrate metabolism, it includes type I, which requires hormone replacement therapy with insulin, and type II, which can usually be managed with diet and exercise programs; abbreviated **DM** (Figure 9.11▦)
			(DYE ah BEE teez MELL ih tuss)	

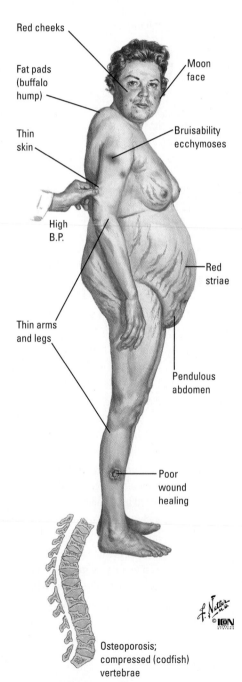

Red cheeks

Fat pads (buffalo hump)

Thin skin

High B.P.

Thin arms and legs

Moon face

Bruisability ecchymoses

Red striae

Pendulous abdomen

Poor wound healing

Osteoporosis; compressed (codfish) vertebrae

Figure 9.10 ::::

Cushing's syndrome. Caused by hypersecretion of the adrenal cortex, it produces the illustrated symptoms.
Source: Icon Learning Systems.

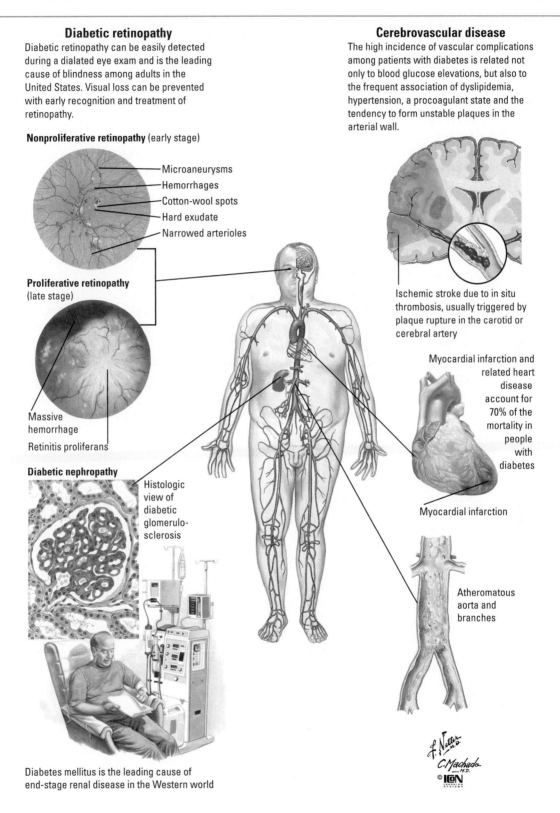

Diabetic retinopathy

Diabetic retinopathy can be easily detected during a dialated eye exam and is the leading cause of blindness among adults in the United States. Visual loss can be prevented with early recognition and treatment of retinopathy.

Nonproliferative retinopathy (early stage)

- Microaneurysms
- Hemorrhages
- Cotton-wool spots
- Hard exudate
- Narrowed arterioles

Proliferative retinopathy (late stage)

Massive hemorrhage

Retinitis proliferans

Diabetic nephropathy

Histologic view of diabetic glomerulo-sclerosis

Diabetes mellitus is the leading cause of end-stage renal disease in the Western world

Cerebrovascular disease

The high incidence of vascular complications among patients with diabetes is related not only to blood glucose elevations, but also to the frequent association of dyslipidemia, hypertension, a procoagulant state and the tendency to form unstable plaques in the arterial wall.

Ischemic stroke due to in situ thrombosis, usually triggered by plaque rupture in the carotid or cerebral artery

Myocardial infarction and related heart disease account for 70% of the mortality in people with diabetes

Myocardial infarction

Atheromatous aorta and branches

Figure 9.11 ::::

Diabetes mellitus. The abnormally high blood sugar levels that result in this disease produce many complications, some of which are illustrated here.
Source: Icon Learning Systems.

WORD PARTS (WHEN APPLICABLE)			TERM	DEFINITION
Part	**Type**	**Meaning**		
endo- crin/o -pathy	p r/cv s	within to secrete disease	**endocrinopathy** (ehn doh krin OPP ah thee)	general disease of the endocrine system
hirsut[e] -ism	r s	hairy condition	**hirsutism** (HER soot izm)	the presence of excessive body hair; in women it is caused by the hypersecretion of androgens by the adrenal cortex
hyper- calc -emia	p r s	excessive calcium blood	**hypercalcemia** (HIGH per kal SEE mee ah)	abnormally high calcium levels in the blood
hyper- glyc -emia	p r s	excessive glycogen, sugar blood	**hyperglycemia** (HIGH per glye SEE mee ah)	abnormally high glucose (sugar) levels in the blood
hyper- insulin -ism	p r s	excessive insulin condition	**hyperinsulinism** (HIGH per IN soo linn izm)	excessive amounts of insulin in the blood, resulting in low levels of sugar in the blood, fainting, and convulsions
hyper- kal -emia	p r s	excessive potassium blood	**hyperkalemia** (HIGH per kal EE mee ah)	abnormally high potassium levels in the blood
hyper- para- thyr -oid -ism	p p r s s	excessive near, alongside shield resemblance to condition	**hyperparathyroidism** (HIGH per pair ah THIGH royd izm)	hypersecretion of the parathyroid glands, usually due to a tumor
hyper- thyr -oid -ism	p r s s	excessive shield resemblance to condition	**hyperthyroidism** (HIGH per THIGH royd izm)	hypersecretion of the thyroid gland, which is characterized by exophthalmos, goiter, rapid heart rate, and weight loss (Figure 9.12::::); also called Graves' disease or thyrotoxicosis (THIGH roh tahk sih KOH siss)
hypo- calc -emia	p r s	under, below normal calcium blood	**hypocalcemia** (HIGH poh kal SEE mee ah)	abnormally low calcium levels in the blood
hypo- glyc -emia	p r s	under, below normal glycogen, sugar blood	**hypoglycemia** (HIGH poh glye SEE mee ah)	abnormally low blood sugar levels
hypo- kal -emia	p r s	under, below normal potassium blood	**hypokalemia** (HIGH poh kal EE mee ah)	abnormally low potassium levels in the blood
hypo- natr -emia	p r s	under, below normal sodium blood	**hyponatremia** (HIGH poh nah TREE mee ah)	abnormally low sodium levels in the blood

WORD PARTS (WHEN APPLICABLE)			TERM	DEFINITION
Part	**Type**	**Meaning**		

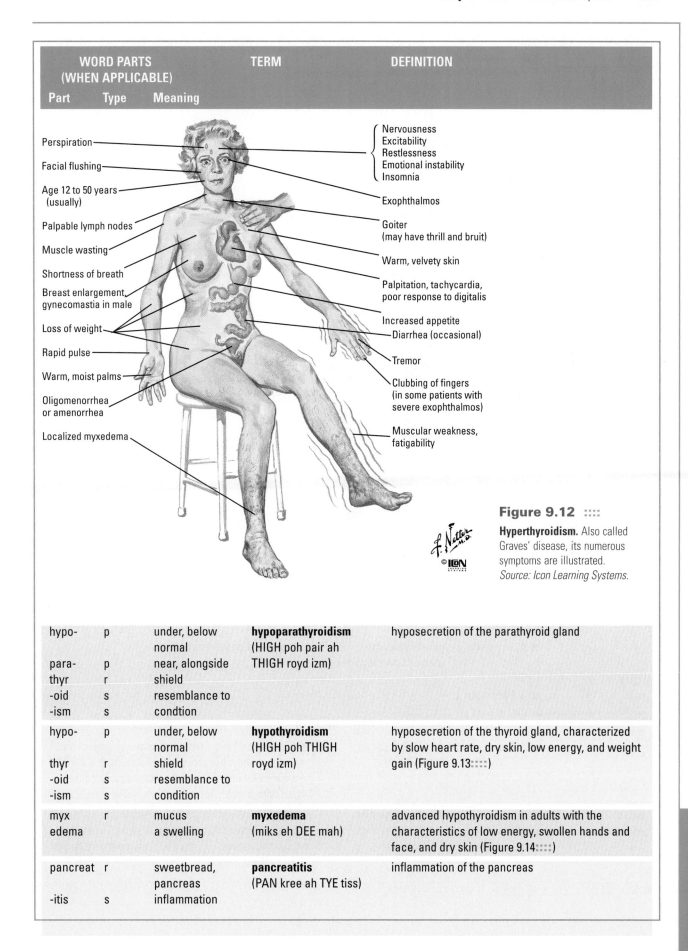

Perspiration

Facial flushing

Age 12 to 50 years (usually)

Palpable lymph nodes

Muscle wasting

Shortness of breath

Breast enlargement, gynecomastia in male

Loss of weight

Rapid pulse

Warm, moist palms

Oligomenorrhea or amenorrhea

Localized myxedema

Nervousness
Excitability
Restlessness
Emotional instability
Insomnia

Exophthalmos

Goiter
(may have thrill and bruit)

Warm, velvety skin

Palpitation, tachycardia, poor response to digitalis

Increased appetite
Diarrhea (occasional)

Tremor

Clubbing of fingers
(in some patients with severe exophthalmos)

Muscular weakness, fatigability

Figure 9.12 ::::

Hyperthyroidism. Also called Graves' disease, its numerous symptoms are illustrated. *Source: Icon Learning Systems.*

Part	Type	Meaning	Term	Definition
hypo-	p	under, below normal	**hypoparathyroidism** (HIGH poh pair ah THIGH royd izm)	hyposecretion of the parathyroid gland
para-	p	near, alongside		
thyr	r	shield		
-oid	s	resemblance to		
-ism	s	condtion		
hypo-	p	under, below normal	**hypothyroidism** (HIGH poh THIGH royd izm)	hyposecretion of the thyroid gland, characterized by slow heart rate, dry skin, low energy, and weight gain (Figure 9.13::::)
thyr	r	shield		
-oid	s	resemblance to		
-ism	s	condition		
myx	r	mucus	**myxedema** (miks eh DEE mah)	advanced hypothyroidism in adults with the characteristics of low energy, swollen hands and face, and dry skin (Figure 9.14::::)
edema		a swelling		
pancreat	r	sweetbread, pancreas	**pancreatitis** (PAN kree ah TYE tiss)	inflammation of the pancreas
-itis	s	inflammation		

WORD PARTS (WHEN APPLICABLE)			TERM	DEFINITION
Part	Type	Meaning		

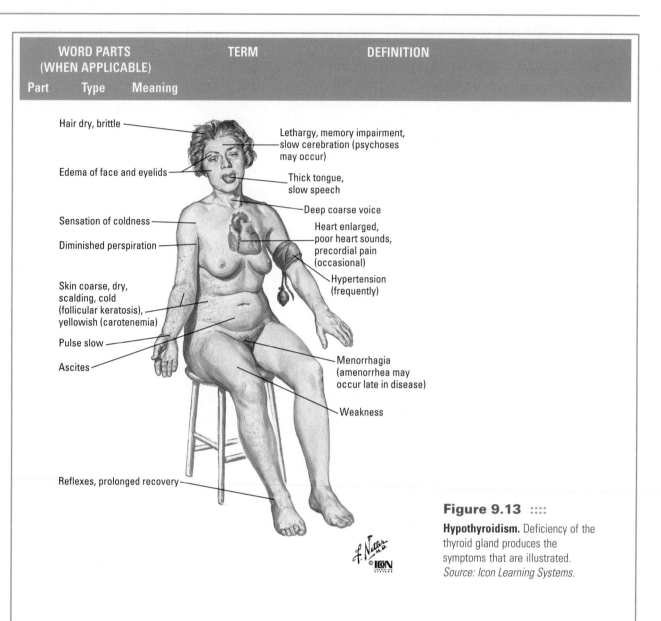

Hair dry, brittle

Edema of face and eyelids

Sensation of coldness

Diminished perspiration

Skin coarse, dry, scalding, cold (follicular keratosis), yellowish (carotenemia)

Pulse slow

Ascites

Reflexes, prolonged recovery

Lethargy, memory impairment, slow cerebration (psychoses may occur)

Thick tongue, slow speech

Deep coarse voice

Heart enlarged, poor heart sounds, precordial pain (occasional)

Hypertension (frequently)

Menorrhagia (amenorrhea may occur late in disease)

Weakness

Figure 9.13 ::::

Hypothyroidism. Deficiency of the thyroid gland produces the symptoms that are illustrated. *Source: Icon Learning Systems.*

para-	p	near, alongside	**parathyroidoma** (pair ah thigh royd OH mah)	tumor of the parathyroid gland
thyr	r	shield		
-oid	s	resemblance to		
-oma	s	tumor		
dwarf	r	small	**pituitary dwarfism** (pih TOO ih tair ee DWARF izm)	caused by hyposecretion of growth hormone by the pituitary gland at an early age, slowing growth and causing a short but proportional stature; it is a congenital condition that can be treated during childhood with growth hormone therapy (Figure 9.15::::)
-ism	s	condition		
gigant	r	giant	**pituitary gigantism** (pih TOO ih tair ee JYE gahnt izm)	caused by hypersecretion of growth hormone that begins before puberty, leading to an abnormally increased growth of bones to produce a very large stature (Figure 9.15)
-ism	s	condition		

WORD PARTS (WHEN APPLICABLE)			TERM	DEFINITION
Part	**Type**	**Meaning**		

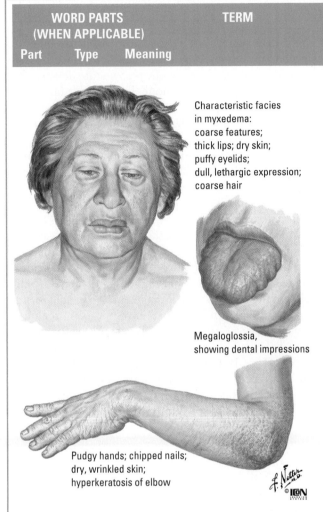

Characteristic facies in myxedema: coarse features; thick lips; dry skin; puffy eyelids; dull, lethargic expression; coarse hair

Megaloglossia, showing dental impressions

Pudgy hands; chipped nails; dry, wrinkled skin; hyperkeratosis of elbow

Figure 9.14 :::: **Myxedema, which is characterized by swollen hands and face and dry skin.**
Source: Icon Learning Systems.

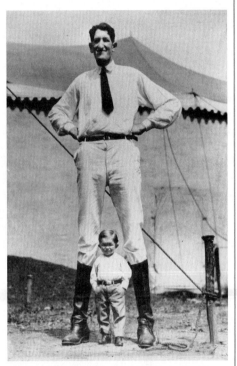

Figure 9.15 :::: **Growth hormone disorders.** Photograph of a pituitary giant and a pituitary dwarf, both adults of about the same age.
Source: Ewing Galloway, Inc.

Part	Type	Meaning	Term	Definition
tetan	r	convulsive muscle tension	**tetany** (TETT ah nee)	caused by a deficiency of parathyroid hormone, the low calcium levels in the blood lead to excitation of nerves and muscle spasms
-y	s	process of		
thyr/o	r/cv	shield	**thyrotoxicosis** (THIGH roh toks ih KOH siss)	a condition resulting from excessive thyroid hormone levels
tox	r	poison		
-ic	s	pertaining to		
-osis	s	condition of		
syn-	p	together	**syndrome** (SIN drohm)	a disorder with an array of symptoms and involving multiple organs
drome	r	a running		

disease focus | Diabetes Mellitus

Diabetes mellitus is the most common disease of the pancreatic **islets of Langerhans.** In fact, about 10 million people in the United States suffer from this disorder, and it is a major contributor to other conditions including heart disease, kidney disease, blindness, and hypertension. If it is not carefully controlled, its long-term complications can reduce life expectancy by as much as one-third. Almost 50,000 people die each year as a result of diabetes mellitus and its complications, making it the fourth most common cause of death in the United States.

Two distinct clinical varieties of diabetes mellitus are recognized. They are **type I diabetes** (insulin-dependent diabetes) and **type II diabetes** (noninsulin-dependent diabetes or maturity-onset diabetes). Type I diabetes usually develops before 40 years of age, most frequently during adolescence. It usually is marked by a dramatic decrease in the number of beta cells, which are one of several types of secretory cells in the islets of Langerhans. The decline in beta cells results in a deficiency of insulin (hyposecretion). Recent investigations clearly indicate the beta cells are destroyed by antibodies produced by the body's own white blood cells. Exactly how this autoimmune condition arises has not yet been determined, but it is probably due to an inherited genetic mutation. Type I diabetes is managed by daily injections of insulin in an effort to restore deficient levels of this important hormone. Insulin must be injected because it is a protein molecule; it cannot be taken orally, as it would be digested by enzymes in the digestive tract.

Type II diabetes makes up about 90 percent of all diabetic cases. In contrast to type I diabetes, it develops gradually throughout adulthood and is most common in overweight persons over 40 years of age. It is characterized by the inability of target cells to take up insulin and utilize it, even though sufficient insulin levels may be released. This causes **hyperglycemia,** (unusually high levels of glucose in the blood) and **acidosis** (excessively low blood pH). Investigators have recently shown the cause of type II diabetes to be related to a decrease in the number of insulin receptors on the target cells. The decrease of insulin receptors reduces the ability of the cells to take up insulin from the blood and use it. Type II diabetes is usually milder than Type I, and often can be treated by careful diet management and maintaining an appropriate body weight. Daily injections of insulin are required in more severe cases.

SELF QUIZ 9.4

SAY IT—SPELL IT!

Review the terms of the endocrine system by speaking the phonetic pronunciation guides out loud, then writing in the correct spelling of the term.

1. SIN drohm _____
2. ak roh MEG ah lee _____
3. add REE nal EYE tiss _____
4. add ree noh MEG ah lee _____
5. kal sih PEE nee ah _____
6. HIGH per kal SEE mee ah _____
7. HIGH per IN soo linn izm _____
8. HIGH per kal EE mee ah _____
9. HIGH per THIGH royd izm _____
10. HIGH poh glye SEE mee ah _____
11. HIGH poh nah TREE mee ah _____
12. HIGH poh pair ah THIGH royd izm _____
13. pair ah thigh royd OH mah _____
14. miks eh DEE mah _____

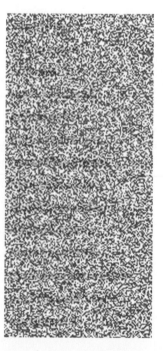

MATCH IT!

Match the term on the left with the correct definition on the right.

_____ 1. adrenalitis

_____ 2. hyperthyroidism

_____ 3. exophthalmos

_____ 4. endocrinology

_____ 5. acromegaly

_____ 6. adrenomegaly

_____ 7. adrenocorticohyperplasia

_____ 8. parathyroidoma

_____ 9. hypothyroidism

_____ 10. hyperparathyroidism

_____ 11. hypoglycemia

_____ 12. hypercalcemia

_____ 13. hypokalemia

9.7 _____ 14. Addison's disease

_____ 15. Cushing's syndrome

_____ 16. cretinism

_____ 17. acidosis

_____ 18. hirsutism

_____ 19. goiter

_____ 20. pituitary gigantism

_____ 21. pituitary dwarfism

_____ 22. diabetes insipidus

_____ 23. diabetes mellitus

a. caused by too much GH in adulthood

b. excessive development of adrenal cortex

c. tumor of the parathyroid gland

d. abnormally low blood sugar

e. too much calcium in the blood

f. protrusion of the eyes

g. a medical specialization

h. hyperactive thyroid gland

i. inflammation of the adrenals

j. abnormally low potassium levels

k. enlargement of an adrenal gland

l. advanced state causes myxedema

n. too much calcitonin production

m. abnormal enlargement of the thyroid gland

o. excessive body hair growth in a female

p. caused by hypothyroidism during childhood

q. produces the symptom of polydipsia

r. symptoms include obesity, hyperglycemia

s. caused by high levels of GH during childhood

t. includes type I and type II

u. when blood levels become too acidic

v. caused by low levels of GH early in life

w. caused by hyposecretion of adrenal cortex

BREAK IT DOWN!

Analyze and separate each term into its word parts by labeling each word part using p = prefix, r = root, cv = combining vowel, and s = suffix.

9.8   1. endocrinology   _____

2. acromegaly   _____

3. adrenocorticohyperplasia   _____

4. adrenopathy   _____

5. endocrinopathy   _____

6. hyperglycemia   _____

7. hyperinsulinism   _____

8. hyperkalemia   _____

9. hyperparathyroidism _____

10. hypoglycemia   _____

11. hypothyroidism   _____

12. parathyroidoma   _____

FILL IT IN!

Fill in the blanks with the correct terms.

1. An adult with hypersecretion of growth hormone from the pituitary gland that strikes after puberty has a condition known as _____. If growth hormone is hypersecreted during childhood, it causes pituitary _____. When GH is secreted in abnormally low amounts during early childhood, the result is pituitary _____. The generalized term that includes each of these conditions and other endocrine disorders is _____.

9.9

2. Inflammation of the adrenal gland, or _____, is one of several possible conditions. It causes increased size or _____ of the adrenals and is a form of general disease of the adrenals called an

9.10

_____.

3. A tumor of the parathyroid gland, called a _____, may lead to hypersecretion, known as _____, which causes abnormally high levels of calcium in the blood, or _____. In some cases, a tumor may produce the opposite effect, or _____, which causes abnormally low calcium levels in the blood, or _____.

9.11 4. Acute inflammation of the pancreas, or _____, can be a life-threatening disease. It can lead to the excessive release of insulin into the bloodstream, or _____, which can elevate blood pressure to dangerous levels. A symptom of pancreatic failure is abnormally high glucose

9.12 levels in the bloodstream, or _____.

9.13 5. One symptom of _____ _____, abbreviated DM, is the accumulation of acid byproducts in the blood, a condition known as acidosis. This condition may coincide with the accumulation of ketone bodies, known

9.14 as _____. Both conditions can be life-threatening to the patient, and are more common in patients with type _____ diabetes.

The injection of the hormone _____ can return blood levels to homeostasis, but only temporarily.

6. Hyposecretion of the adrenal cortex can produce symptoms characteristic of the syndrome _____ disease, which include darkening of the skin, mental depression, and loss of appetite. In contrast, hypersecretion of the adrenal cortex can produce excessive body hair growth in women, or _____, which is a symptom of the syndrome known as adrenal _____. If cortical hormones other than androgens are excessively produced, the result is a syndrome known as _____ syndrome, which produces a moon face appearance.

⟡ **9.15** 7. A _____ is a symptom of deficient levels of iodine in the diet, or a tumor of the _____ gland. If hypothyroidism strikes early in life, it can produce the permanent symptoms of the syndrome known as

_____.

8. Hypersecretion of the pituitary growth hormone during childhood can result in the condition known as pituitary _____, whereas hyposecretion of growth hormone during childhood years causes pituitary _____.

9. A drop in PTH causes a reduction of calcium in the blood, which leads to muscle spasms in the condition known as _____.

Treatments, Procedures, and Devices

WORD PARTS (WHEN APPLICABLE)			TERM	DEFINITION
Part	Type	Meaning		
ad- ren -al -ectomy	p r s s	toward kidney pertaining to surgical removal	**adrenalectomy** (add REE nal EK toh mee)	excision of the adrenal gland
			fasting blood sugar	a diagnostic test to determine blood sugar levels following a 12-hour fast; extreme variations in blood sugar is an indication of diabetes mellitus; abbreviated **FBS**
endo- crin/o -logist	p r/cv s	within to secrete one who studies	**endocrinologist** (ehn doh krin ALL oh jist)	a physician specializing in the treatment of endocrine disorders
endo- crin/o -logy	p r/cv s	within to secrete study of	**endocrinology** (ehn doh krin ALL oh jee)	a field of medicine focusing on the study and treatment of endocrine disorders
endo- crin/o -pathy	p r/cv s	within to secrete disease	**endocrinopathy** (ehn doh krin OPP ah thee)	a disease or disorder in the function of an endocrine gland and the related consequences

WORD PARTS (WHEN APPLICABLE)			TERM	DEFINITION
Part	Type	Meaning		
			glucose tolerance test (GLOO kohs)	a diagnostic test to confirm a diagnosis of diabetes mellitus and to determine other abnormalities in glucose metabolism; usually following an FBS, the patient is given glucose either orally or intravenously, then at timed intervals, blood samples are taken and glucose levels determined and charted; abbreviated **GTT**
post- prand/i -al	p r/cv s	after, behind midday meal pertaining to	**postprandial blood sugar** (post PRAN dee al)	a measurement of blood sugar levels after a meal, usually over two hours; abbreviated **PPBS** (Figure 9.16 ::::)
			radioactive iodine uptake (RAY dee oh AK tihv EYE oh dyne)	a diagnostic procedure measuring thyroid function, in which radioactive iodine uptake into the thyroid gland is measured; abbreviated **RAIU**
			thyroid scan (THIGH royd)	a diagnostic procedure that records an image of the thyroid gland following the oral administration of a labeled substance, usually iodine; used to detect thyroid tumors (Figure 9.17 ::::)

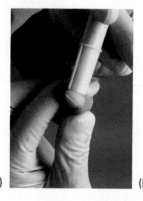
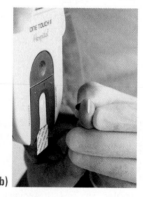
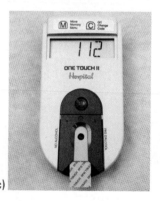

(a) (b) (c)

Figure 9.16 :::: **Blood glucose measurement.** A postprandial test may be self-administered.
(a) A lance pierces the skin of a finger.
(b) A small blood sample is gently squeezed onto a reagent strip.
(c) The glucose meter will display the glucose concentration in the blood sample. A reading of 80 to 130 mg/dL is a normal range.

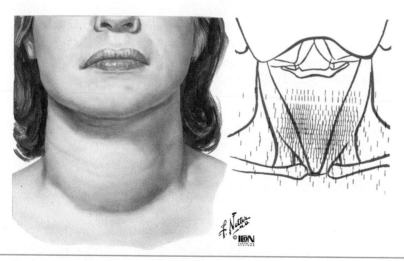

Figure 9.17 ::::

Thyroid scan. The right image is the data from a thyroid scan, printed on a superimposed map of the thyroid gland from the subject patient, shown on the left with a goiter.
Source: Icon Learning Systems.

WORD PARTS (WHEN APPLICABLE)			TERM	DEFINITION
Part	**Type**	**Meaning**		
			thyroxine test (thigh ROK sihn)	a direct measurement of the amount of thyroxine in the blood to determine hyperthyroidism (high levels) or hypothyroidism (low levels)
			hormone replacement therapy (HOR mohn)	the use of a drug that replaces a hormone to correct a hormone deficiency; abbreviated **HRT**
para- thyr -oid -ectomy	p r s s	near, alongside shield resemblance to surgical removal	**parathyroidectomy** (PAIR ah THIGH royd EK toh mee)	excision of one or more parathyroid glands
			radioiodine therapy (RAY dee oh EYE oh dyne THAIR ah pee)	the use of radioactive iodine to treat a disease of the thyroid gland, such as a thyroid tumor
thyr -oid -ectomy	r s s	shield resemblance to surgical removal	**thyroidectomy** (THIGH royd EK toh mee)	excision of the thyroid gland (Figure 9.18::::)

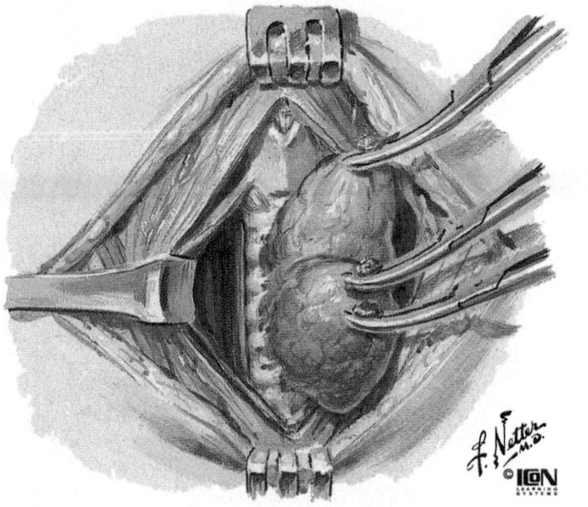

Figure 9.18 ::::

Thyroidectomy. In this procedure, the thyroid gland is accessed by a vertical incision through the neck and removed.
Source: Icon Learning Systems.

WORD PARTS			TERM	DEFINITION
thyr -oid -otomy	r s s	shield resemblance to cutting into	**thyroidotomy** (THIGH royd OTT oh mee)	incision into the thyroid gland
thyr/o para- thyr -oid -ectomy	r/cv p r s s	shield near, alongside shield resemblance to surgical removal	**thyroparathyroidectomy** (THIGH roh pair ah THIGH royd EK toh mee)	excision of the thyroid and parathyroid glands

SELF QUIZ 9.5

SAY IT—SPELL IT!

Review the terms of the endocrine system by speaking the phonetic pronunciation guides out loud, then writing in the correct spelling of the term.

1. add REE nal EK toh mee _____

2. HIGH poff ih SEK toh mee _____

3. PAIR ah THIGH royd EK toh mee _____

4. THIGH royd OTT oh mee _____

5. RAY dee oh EYE oh dyne _____

6. THIGH royd EK toh mee _____

MATCH IT!

Match the term on the left with the correct definition on the right.

_____ 1. adrenalectomy   a. records an image of the thyroid gland

_____ 2. fasting blood sugar   b. measurement of blood glucose after a meal

_____ 3. glucose tolerance test   c. use of a drug to correct deficient hormone levels

_____ 4. postprandial blood sugar   d. excision of an adrenal gland

_____ 5. radioactive iodine uptake e. measures blood sugar levels after a 12 hour fast

_____ 6. thyroid scan   f. removal of the pituitary gland

_____ 7. thyroxine test   g. often used to confirm diabetes mellitus

_____ 8. hormone replacement
     therapy   h. excision of the thyroid gland

_____ 9. thyroparathyroidectomy   i. measurement of thyroxine levels in the blood

_____ 10. hypophysectomy   j. removal of the thyroid and parathyroid glands

_____ 11. thyroidectomy   k. measures thyroid function using labeled iodine

BREAK IT DOWN!

Analyze and separate each term into its word parts by labeling each word part using p = prefix, r = root, cv = combining vowel, and s = suffix.

1. endocrinologist   _____

2. thyroidotomy   _____

3. thyroparathyroidectomy   _____

4. endocrinopathy   _____

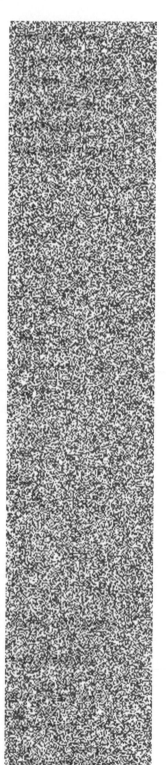

WORD BUILDING

Construct or recall medical terms from the following meanings.

9.16 1. a blood test taken 12 hours after eating _____

9.17 2. evaluates sugar metabolism by its administration _____

3. a diagnostic procedure measuring radioactive iodine uptake into the thyroid gland _____

4. measurement of blood sugar levels after a meal _____

5. measurement of the amount of thyroxine in the blood to determine hyperthyroidism or hypothyroidism _____

6. use of a drug that replaces a hormone to correct a hormone deficiency _____

7. procedure that records an image of the thyroid gland following the oral administration of a labeled substance, usually iodine; used to detect thyroid tumors _____

8. excision of one or more parathyroid glands _____

9. use of radioactive iodine to treat a disease of the thyroid gland, such as a thyroid tumor _____

10. incision into the thyroid gland _____

FILL IT IN!

Fill in the blanks with the correct terms.

1. Surgical removal of the endocrine glands becomes necessary in severe cases, often resulting from the development of a tumor that cannot be removed without excising the organ itself. Removal of the adrenal glands is a procedure known as _____. Excision of the thyroid gland is a more common procedure, and is known as _____, while excision of one or more parathyroid glands is called a _____. The excision of the thyroid gland and the embedded parathyroids is a _____.

9.18 2. Grave's disease is also called _____. One of its symptoms is protrusion of the eyes, or _____. The disease can be confirmed in a radiation lab using a _____ procedure, such as the radioactive _____ uptake procedure, and scanning the organ to produce an image, a procedure known as a _____ _____. If the thyroid is excised, hormone replacement therapy is often prescribed, abbreviated _____.

3. A diagnostic test that evaluates blood sugar levels after a 12-hour fast is called a

_____ _____ _____ test. The

results may be confirmed by a _____ _____ test,

in which blood samples are taken at timed intervals. A third test for diabetes

mellitus is called a _____ _____ sugar test, in

which blood sugar is measured following a meal.

abbreviations of the endocrine system

The abbreviations that are associated with the endocrine system are summarized here. Study these abbreviations, and review them in the exercise that follows.

ABBREVIATION	DEFINITION	ABBREVIATION	DEFINITION
DI	diabetes insipidus	HRT	hormone replacement therapy
DM	diabetes mellitus	PPBS	postprandial blood sugar
FBS	fasting blood sugar	RAIU	radioactive iodine uptake
GTT	glucose tolerance test		

SELF QUIZ 9.6

Fill in the blanks with the abbreviation or the complete medical term.

Abbreviation	Medical Term
1. GTT	_____
2. _____	radioactive iodine uptake
3. PPBS	_____
4. _____	diabetes insipidus
5. FBS	_____
6. _____	hormone replacement therapy
7. DM	_____

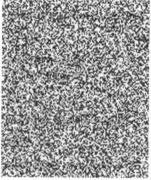

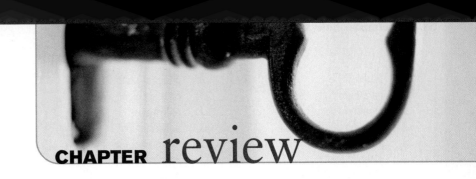

CHAPTER review

In this section, we will review all the word parts and medical terms from this chapter. As in earlier tables, the word roots are shown in **bold.**

Check each word part and medical term to be sure you understand the meaning. If any are not clear, please go back into the chapter and review that term. Then, complete the review exercises that follow.

[word parts **checklist**]

Prefixes

- ❑ ad-
- ❑ anti-
- ❑ endo-
- ❑ ex-, exo-
- ❑ hyper-
- ❑ hypo-
- ❑ para-
- ❑ syn-

Word Roots/Combining Vowels

- ❑ **acr**/o
- ❑ **aden**/o

- ❑ **andr**/o
- ❑ **calc**/i
- ❑ **cortic**/o
- ❑ **crin**/o
- ❑ **dips**/o
- ❑ **gluc**/o
- ❑ **glyc**/o, **glycos**/o
- ❑ **hormon**/o
- ❑ **kal**/i
- ❑ **ket**/o
- ❑ **lob**/o
- ❑ **megal**/o
- ❑ **myx**/o

- ❑ **natr**/o
- ❑ **pancreat**/o
- ❑ **ren**/o
- ❑ **thyr**/o
- ❑ **tox**/o

Suffixes

- ❑ -drome
- ❑ -emia
- ❑ -ism
- ❑ -oid
- ❑ -osis
- ❑ -plasia

[medical terminology **checklist**]

- ❑ acidosis
- ❑ **acr**omegaly
- ❑ Addison's disease
- ❑ **aden**ohypo**phys**is
- ❑ ad**ren**al gland
- ❑ ad**ren**al virilism
- ❑ ad**ren**alectomy
- ❑ ad**ren**aline
- ❑ ad**ren**alitis
- ❑ ad**ren**o**cortic**ohyperplasia
- ❑ ad**ren**o**cortic**o**troph**ic hormone
- ❑ ad**ren**omegaly
- ❑ ad**ren**opathy
- ❑ aldosterone
- ❑ androgen
- ❑ **anteri**or lobe
- ❑ antidiuretic hormone
- ❑ **calc**ipenia
- ❑ **calc**itonin
- ❑ cortex

- ❑ cortisol
- ❑ cortisone
- ❑ cretinism
- ❑ Cushing's syndrome
- ❑ diabetes insipidus
- ❑ diabetes mellitus
- ❑ endo**crin**opathy
- ❑ epinephrine
- ❑ estrogen
- ❑ ex**ophthalm**os
- ❑ follicle-stimulating hormone
- ❑ glucagon
- ❑ **gluc**o**cortic**oids
- ❑ **gluc**ose
- ❑ goiter
- ❑ growth hormone
- ❑ **hirsut**ism
- ❑ **hormon**e
- ❑ hyper**calc**emia
- ❑ hyper**glyc**emia

- ❑ hyperinsulinism
- ❑ hyperpara**thyr**oidism
- ❑ hypersecretion
- ❑ hyper**thyr**oidism
- ❑ hypo**calc**emia
- ❑ hypo**glyc**emia
- ❑ hypo**glyc**emia
- ❑ hypo**natr**emia
- ❑ hypopara**thyr**oidism
- ❑ hyposecretion
- ❑ insulin
- ❑ islets of Langerhans
- ❑ **ket**osis
- ❑ luteinizing hormone
- ❑ melanocyte-stimulating hormone
- ❑ melatonin
- ❑ **myx**edema
- ❑ **neur**ohypo**phys**is
- ❑ oxytocin

❑ pancreas	❑ pituitary gigantism	❑ **thyr**oid gland
❑ para**thyr**oid glands	❑ pituitary gland	❑ **thyr**oidectomy
❑ para**thyr**oidectomy	❑ poly**dips**ia	❑ **thyr**oidotomy
❑ para**thyr**oiditis	❑ **posteri**or lobe	❑ **thyr**onine
❑ para**thyr**oidoma	❑ radioiodine therapy	❑ **thyr**opara**thyr**oidectomy
❑ pineal gland	❑ thymosin	
❑ pituitary dwarfism	❑ thymus gland	

[show what **you know!**]

BREAK IT DOWN!

Analyze and separate each term into its word parts by labeling each word part using p = prefix, r = root, cv = combining vowel, and s = suffix.

```
                                        p      r  cv  s
```

Example: 1. endocrinology   endo/crin/o/logy

2. adrenalitis   _____

3. hyperthyroidism   _____

4. pancreatic   _____

5. hypoglycemia   _____

6. adrenocorticohyperplasia _____

7. adrenomegaly   _____

8. endocrinopathy   _____

9. exophthalmos   _____

10. hyperinsulinism   _____

11. hyperparathyroidism _____

12. hypocalcemia   _____

13. hyponatremia   _____

14. parathyroidoma   _____

15. hypophysectomy   _____

16. parathyroidectomy   _____

17. thyroidotomy   _____

18. thyroparathyroidectomy _____

WORD BUILDING

Construct or recall medical terms from the following meanings.

Example: 1. generalized disease of the endocrine system   endocrinopathy

2. excessive production of thyroid hormones   _____

3. surgical removal of the pituitary gland   _____

4. inflammation of the adrenal gland   _____

5. reduced sodium levels in the blood   _____

6. increased calcium levels in the blood   _____

7. a tumor of the parathyroid gland   _____

8. caused by too much GH in adulthood   _____

9. generalized disease of the adrenal gland   _____

10. excessive body hair   _____

11. reduced production of PTH   _____

12. excessive insulin levels in the blood   _____

13. inflammation of the pancreas   _____

14. abnormally high glucose levels in the blood   _____

CASE STUDIES

Fill in the blanks with the correct terms.

1. A 12-year-old patient was referred by her personal physician for an endocrinological evaluation in the

    (a) _____ department, following a four-week history of symptoms of energy loss between meals,

    excessive thirst, or (b) _____, headache, polyuria (excessive urination), and sleeplessness. A routine

    blood test had also been recorded by the physician, and had shown ketone bodies in the blood, or

    (c) _____, combined with a lowered blood pH, or (d) _____. Endocrinological

    evaluation included a FBS, or (e) _____ _____ _____,

    followed by a (f) _____ tolerance test, and a urinalysis. The tests indicated the patient suffered from

    excessive sugar levels in the blood, or (g) _____, that was due to a failure of islet beta cells to

    produce proper levels of the hormone (h) _____. A diagnosis of (i) _____

    _____ _____ was recorded. The patient was treated with regular insulin and

    trained in self-glucose testing and insulin administration, and referred to a local educational program in diabetes manage-

    ment to include her parent's participation.

2. A 30-year-old patient was admitted for hospitalization following reports of symptoms that included frequent headaches, loss

    of energy, unexplained weight gain, and tenderness in the upper left back region. More recently, increased body hair, or

    (j) _____, was an additional cause for concern. An early diagnosis was made of

    (k) _____, or a generalized disease of the adrenals, and possible (l) _____,

    since the attending physician believed the series of symptoms could be traced to a developmental defect of the adrenals. The

    physician also believed the back tenderness could be explained by the increased size of the adrenal, or

    (m) _____. However, the weight gain had produced a redistribution of body fat, establishing a _moon

    face_ that characterizes (n) _____ syndrome. On this basis, a third diagnosis was made. This diagnosis

    also explained the excessive blood sugar levels, or (o) _____, combined with energy loss and muscle

    weakness. However, the cause remained a mystery until the patient's tender area was examined with MRI. This diagnostic tool revealed a tumor of the left adrenal gland, or (p) _____. Apparently, the tumor had caused the

adrenal gland to hypersecrete male sex hormones, known as (q) _____, which had caused the body

hair; a condition known as adrenal (r) _____. It had also caused the hypersecretion of other adrenal

(s) _____ hormones, which lead to the metabolic disturbance.

[piece it all **together!**]

CROSSWORD

From the chapter material, fill in the crossword puzzle with answers to the following clues.

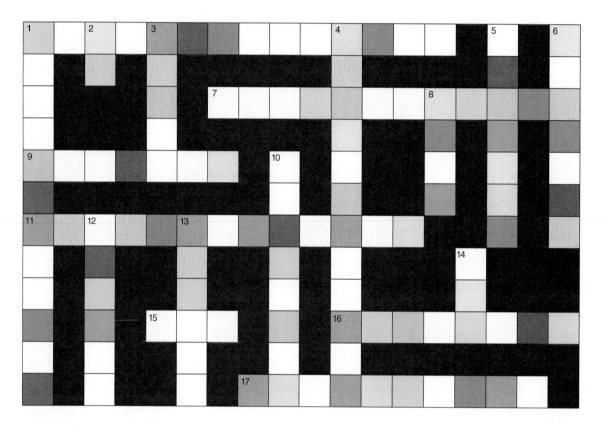

ACROSS

1. In general, any disease of the endocrine system. (Find puzzle piece 9.9)
7. Inflammation of the organ whose word root means *sweetbread*. (Find puzzle piece 9.11)
9. A potent chemical that is *set in motion*. (Find puzzle piece 9.1)
11. Abnormally high glucose levels in the blood. (Find puzzle piece 9.12)
15. An abbreviation for a test for carbohydrate metabolism that may follow an FBS. (Find puzzle piece 9.17)
16. A chronic syndrome caused by hyposecretion of the adrenal cortex. (Find puzzle piece 9.7)
17. A symptom of diabetes insipidus. (Find puzzle piece 9.5)

DOWN

1. When he stared at the camera, the wide-eyed actor Peter Lorre appeared to have this symptom of thyroid disease. (Find puzzle piece 9.18)

2. Abbreviation for a disease of carbohydrate metabolism. (Find puzzle piece 9.13)

3. A word root with combining vowel that means *to secrete.* (Find puzzle piece 9.8)

4. Abnormal enlargement of the adrenal glands. (Find puzzle piece 9.10)

5. Often a symptom of uncontrolled diabetes mellitus. (Find puzzle piece 9.14)

6. A hormone that decreases glucose levels in the blood; it must be injected in type I diabetes. (Find puzzle piece 9.4)

8. The emphasized syllable in exophthalmos. (Find puzzle piece 9.6)

10. A pituitary hormone that stimulates uterine contractions, spelled backwards. (Find puzzle piece 9.2)

12. A small gland in the brain that regulates sleep rhythms. (Find puzzle piece 9.3)

13. A disease of the thyroid gland that can be caused by a diet deficient in iodized salt. (Find puzzle piece 9.15)

14. Abbreviation for a common test of diabetes mellitus. (Find puzzle piece 9.16)

WORD UNSCRAMBLE

From the completed crossword puzzle, unscramble

1. All of the letters that appear in **red** squares ☐ __ __ __ __ __ __ __ __

   Clue: Severe hypothyroidism in children causes this syndrome

2. All of the letters that appear in **purple** squares __ __ __ __ ☐ __ __ __ __

   Clue: The bearded lady of circuses probably had this symptom

3. All of the letters that appear in **peach** squares __ __ __ __ __ __ ☐

   Clue: Although two diseases share this word, they are unrelated

4. All of the letters that appear in **blue** squares __ ☐ __ __ __ __ __

   Clue: Literally, a Greek warrior's shield

5. All of the letters that appear in **yellow** squares __ __ ☐ __ __ __ __ __

   Clue: When the blood becomes dangerously acidic

6. All of the letters that appear in **green** squares __ __ __ __ ☐ __

   Clue: A chemical, that when deficient, can cause a goiter

7. All of the letters that appear in **pink** squares __ __ __ __ ☐ __ __ __ __ __ __ __

   Clue: Eating hard candy can temporarily cure this condition

8. All of the letters that appear in **gray** squares ☐ __ __ __ __ __ __ __

   Clue: A cluster of signs and symptoms related to a single condition

Now write down each of the letters that are boxed and unscramble them to find the hidden medical term of the endocrine system: __ __ __ __ __ __ __ __.

MEDmedia wrap-up

www.prenhall.com/wingerd

Before you go on to the next chapter, take advantage of the free CD-ROM and study guide website that accompany this book. Simply load the CD-ROM for additional activities, games, animations, videos, and quizzes linked to this chapter. Then visit www.prenhall.com/wingerd for even more!

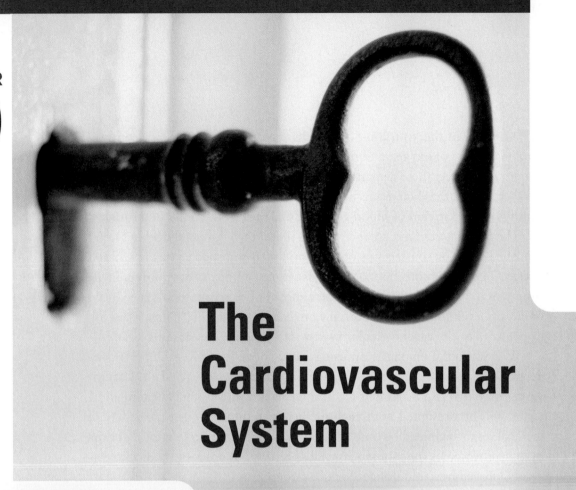

The Cardiovascular System

LEARNING OBJECTIVES

After completing this chapter, you will be able to:

- Define and spell the word parts used to create medical terms for the cardio-vascular system

- Identify the organs of the cardio-vascular system and describe their structure and function

- Define common medical terms used for the cardiovascular system

- Break down and define common medical terms used for symptoms, diseases, disorders, procedures, treatments, and devices for the cardiovascular system

MEDmedia

www.prenhall.com/wingerd

Enhance your study with the power of multimedia! Each chapter of this book links to activities, games, animations, videos, and quizzes that you'll find on your CD-ROM. Plus, you can click on www.prenhall.com/wingerd, to find a free chapter-specific companion website that's loaded with additional practice and resources.

CD-ROM

- Audio Glossary
- Exercises & Activities
- Flashcard Generator
- Animations
- Videos

 Companion Website

- Exercises & Activities
- Audio Glossary
- Drug Updates
- Current News Updates

A secure distance learning course is available at www.prenhall.com/onekey.

Every one of the 30 trillion or so cells in your body requires a continuous supply of oxygen and nutrients, and an unending removal of waste materials. To meet these demands, the blood, which we will study in the next chapter, carries these materials in the body's circulation. How does the constantly flowing stream of blood get from one part of the body to another?

The *cardiovascular system* circulates blood throughout the body. Blood is pushed along by contractions of the heart and is transported through blood vessels. The continuous flow of blood is vital to a body's functioning. If the supply of oxygen and nutrients or the removal of waste materials is reduced or cut off, even for a few minutes, the affected cells may die. Thus, a disease or disorder of the cardiovascular system can pose life-threatening risks.

With an initial emphasis on using word roots, we will establish a connection between the terms for the anatomy and physiology of the cardiovascular system and its related medical terms in this chapter. Then, medical terms will be presented with each of their component word parts. These medical terms include the symptoms, diseases, and disorders that afflict normal cardiovascular functioning, as well as terms that describe medical treatments, procedures, and devices for these conditions.

word parts focus

Let's look at word parts. The following table contains a list of word parts that when combined build the terms of the cardiovascular system.

PREFIX	DEFINITION	PREFIX	DEFINITION
brady-	slow	inter-	between
endo-	within, inner	peri-	around, about
epi-	upon	tachy-	rapid, fast

WORD ROOT	DEFINITION	WORD ROOT	DEFINITION
angi, angin	blood vessel	coron	crown or circle
aort	aorta	cyan	blue
arter, arteri	windpipe, artery	ech	to bounce
ather	fat	electr	electricity
atri	atrium	isch	to hold back
card, cardi	heart	my, myos	muscle

WORD ROOT	DEFINITION	WORD ROOT	DEFINITION
occlus	to close up	thromb	clot of blood
pector	chest	valvul	little valve
phleb	vein	varic	dilated vein
pulmon	lung	vas	blood vessel
sphygm	pulse	vascul	little blood vessel
sten	narrowness, constriction	ven	vein
steth	chest	ventricul	little belly or cavity

[FYI]

Artery

It may seem strange that the term **artery** is derived from the Greek word *arteria*, which means *windpipe*. In the days of Aristotle when it was named, it was thought that arteries carried air because after death these vessels were bloodless, air-filled tubes. Veins, on the other hand, retain blood after death due to their lower blood pressure. The early Greeks wrongly concluded that veins were the only carriers of blood in the living body.

SUFFIX	DEFINITION	SUFFIX	DEFINITION
-ac	pertaining to	-is	pertaining to
-apheresis	removal	-lytic	pertaining to dissolution
-dynia	pain	-rrhexis	rupture
-gram	recording	-sclerosis	hardening
-graph	instrument used to record		

SELF QUIZ 10.1

Review the word parts of cardiovascular system terminology by working carefully through the exercises that follow. Soon, we will apply this new information to build medical terms.

A. Provide the definition of the following prefixes and suffixes.

1. brady- _____

2. endo- _____

3. inter- _____

4. peri- _____

5. tachy- _____

6. -ac _____

7. -apheresis _____

8. -dynia _____

9. -sclerosis _____

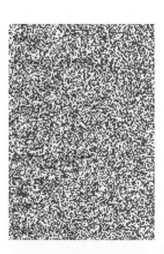

B.   Provide the word root for each of the following terms.

1. blood vessel   _____

2. aorta   _____

3. artery   _____

4. fat   _____

5. atrium   _____

6. heart   _____

7. crown or circle   _____

8. blockage   _____

9. chest   _____

10. vein   _____

11. pulse   _____

12. narrowness   _____

13. clot   _____

14. dilated vein   _____

15. blood vessel   _____

16. vein   _____

17. to bounce   _____

18. electricity   _____

[anatomy and physiology overview]

The cardiovascular system is composed of the heart and blood vessels, which circulate blood throughout the body to bring it into close proximity to every living cell. The term *cardiovascular* is made up of two word roots: **cardi** meaning *heart* and **vascul** meaning *little blood vessels*. The heart pumps blood through the blood vessels, which include the arteries, veins, and capillaries.

Blood circulation is a complete loop. **Arteries** carry blood from the heart to body parts, and **veins** carry blood back to the heart. **Capillaries** are microscopic blood vessels located between arteries and veins. Their walls are composed of only a single layer of thin cells allowing the passage of nutrients, oxygen, and carbon dioxide between the blood and body cells (Figure 10.1▪▪▪).

The Heart

The heart is a fist-sized, hollow muscular pump located in the thoracic cavity (Figure 10.2▪▪▪). It is covered externally by a thick, parchment-like membrane known as the **pericardial sac** or **parietal pericardium.** The term *parietal* is from the Latin word for *wall of a house,* and refers to an outer anatomical wall or layer. The pericardial sac encloses a potential space known as the **pericardial cavity,** which is nearly filled by the presence of the heart. A small amount of fluid is also present, which reduces friction between the heart wall and the pericardial sac during heart contractions. A thinner membrane forms the outer surface of the heart, and is called the **epicardium** or **visceral pericardium.** Many of the blood vessels that provide the heart with nutritious blood course through the epicardium.

[FYI]

Pericardium

Notice that the term *pericardium* is a constructed term that literally means *pertaining to surrounding the heart.* Be aware that pericardium is also the anatomical term for the heart membranes.

enrichment module enrichment module enrich

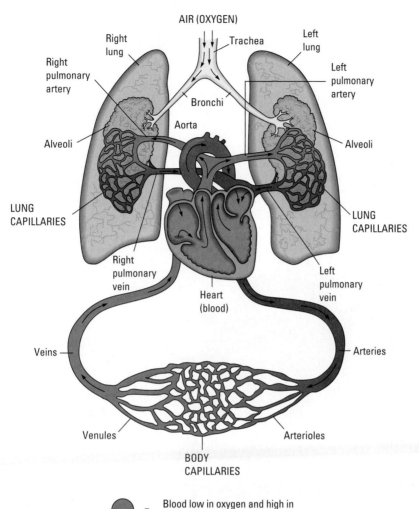

AIR (OXYGEN)

Right lung

Trachea

Left lung

Right pulmonary artery

Left pulmonary artery

Bronchi

Aorta

Alveoli

Alveoli

LUNG CAPILLARIES

LUNG CAPILLARIES

Right pulmonary vein

Left pulmonary vein

Heart (blood)

Veins

Arteries

Venules

Arterioles

BODY CAPILLARIES

⬤ = Blood low in oxygen and high in carbon dioxide (deoxygenated).

⬤ = Blood high in oxygen and low in carbon dioxide (oxygenated).

Figure 10.1 ⁞⁞⁞⁞

The cardiovascular system.
A schematic view of the closed circulation of blood. The heart is sectioned, and the capillaries are enlarged to enable you to see them.
Source: Pearson Education.

When the heart is sectioned, its wall structure and internal chambers can be studied (Figure 10.3⁞⁞⁞⁞). The heart wall consists of the outermost epicardium, a thick **myocardium** composed of cardiac muscle, and a thin inner lining called the **endocardium.** The endocardium lines each of the four heart chambers. The chambers include two thin-walled **atria** that receive incoming blood, and two thick-walled **ventricles** that push blood out of the heart. The right atrium receives blood from two large veins known as the **vena cavae,** and also from the **coronary sinus** that drains the heart. The right ventricle receives this blood and pumps it to the lungs where the blood is oxygenated. The left atrium receives blood from the lungs, by way of four pulmonary veins (two from each lung). The left ventricle then pumps blood to the entire body, except the lungs.

When blood flows through the heart, it moves from the atria to the ventricles. This one-way flow is maintained by the **atrioventricular (AV) valves:** the **mitral valve** or **bicuspid valve** on the left side, and the **tricuspid valve** on the right side. Blood that is pumped from the ventricles passes through the **semilunar (SL) valves,** which mark the junction between the two ventricles and the two major arteries. The two arteries are the **pulmonary trunk** on the right side and the **aorta** on the left side.

The pulmonary trunk divides into the right and left pulmonary arteries, which carry blood to the lungs. Once within the lungs, the arteries branch extensively to

[FYI]

Atrium
The term *atrium* is derived from the Latin word that means *entrance hall*, the room where guests would enter and be received by their host. In the heart there are two atria, which receive the blood coming into the heart.

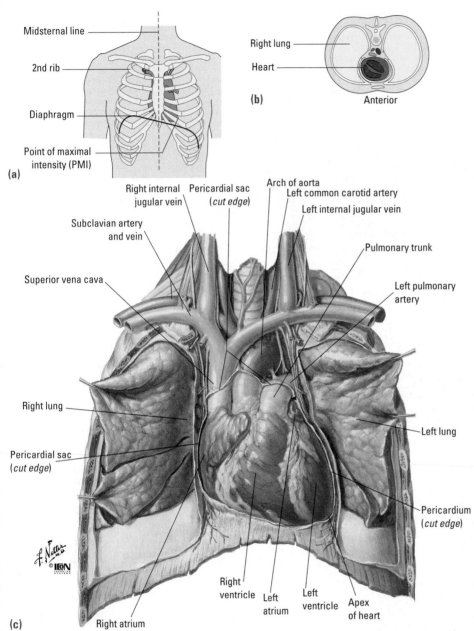

Midsternal line

2nd rib

Diaphragm

Point of maximal
intensity (PMI)

(a)

Right lung

Heart

(b)

Anterior

Right internal
jugular vein

Pericardial sac
(*cut edge*)

Arch of aorta
Left common carotid artery

Left internal jugular vein

Subclavian artery
and vein

Pulmonary trunk

Superior vena cava

Left pulmonary
artery

Right lung

Left lung

Pericardial sac
(*cut edge*)

Pericardium
(*cut edge*)

Right
ventricle

Left
atrium

Left
ventricle

Apex
of heart

(c)

Right atrium

Figure 10.2 :::::

External anatomy of the heart.
(a) Location of the heart in the
thoracic cavity in relation to the
sternum, ribs, and diaphragm.
Source: Pearson Education.
(b) Cross-sectional view of the
chest showing the position of the
heart.
Source: Pearson Education.
(c) Relationship of the heart and its
great vessels, with the lungs pulled
slightly away. The pericardial sac
surrounds the heart and forms the
pericardial cavity.
Source: Icon Learning Systems.

form a vast capillary network. Here the blood gases, oxygen and carbon dioxide, are exchanged between the capillaries and the air sacs of the lungs. As a result, the blood is refreshed with oxygen. Blood circulation associated with the lungs is known as the **pulmonary circulation.**

The aorta is the largest vessel of the body, since it carries blood from the left ventricle to every part of the body (except the lungs) by way of its many branches. The distribution network of the aorta serves to transport oxygen, nutrients, and other substances to the cells of the body other than the lungs. The distribution of the aortic branches and the return of blood to the heart by way of veins is called the **systemic circulation.** A small branch of the aorta near its base carries blood to the heart, beginning a local circulatory loop supplying the heart that is known as the **coronary circulation.** The volume of blood that enters the systemic circulation by way of the aorta with each heart beat is a measurable amount, and is known as the **cardiac output (CO).**

[**thinking critically!**]

What are the two main
types of circulation,
and how do the levels
of oxygen and carbon
dioxide vary between
them?

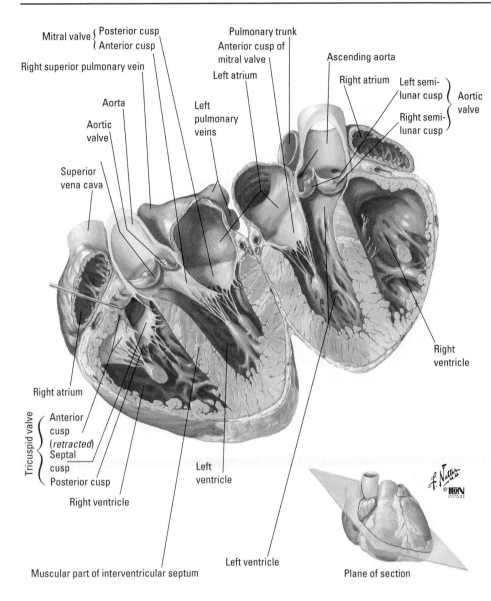

Mitral valve { Posterior cusp / Anterior cusp

Right superior pulmonary vein

Aorta

Aortic valve

Superior vena cava

Pulmonary trunk

Anterior cusp of mitral valve

Left atrium

Left pulmonary veins

Ascending aorta

Right atrium

Left semi-lunar cusp

Right semi-lunar cusp

} Aortic valve

Right ventricle

Right atrium

Tricuspid valve { Anterior cusp (*retracted*) / Septal cusp / Posterior cusp

Right ventricle

Muscular part of interventricular septum

Left ventricle

Left ventricle

Plane of section

Figure 10.3 ⠿

Internal anatomy of the heart.
The heart is sectioned to reveal its internal features.
Source: Icon Learning Systems.

The heart includes specialized cells that generate or carry impulses, which stimulate the heart to contract. The cells are collectively known as the **heart conduction system,** which consists of:

- a cluster of cells in the right atrium that serve as the pacemaker of the heart—known as the **sinoatrial (SA) node**

- a second cluster of cells that relay the signal to the ventricles, called the **atrioventricular (AV) node**

- cells that form a conduction pathway through the walls of the ventricles known as the **atrioventricular (AV) bundle,** also called **bundle of His**

The heart conduction system maintains the rhythmic cardiac cycle of atrial filling, atrial contraction, ventricular filling, and ventricular contraction by coordinating the sequence of these events.

The Blood Vessels

The blood vessels transport blood throughout the body. They include three main types: arteries, veins, and capillaries. In general, arteries carry blood away from the heart while veins carry blood toward the heart. The walls of arteries and veins have a similar composition, both with several layers that include an inner **endothelium,** a middle layer of smooth muscle, and an outer layer of connective tissue (Figure 10.4 :::). Capillaries are located between arteries and veins, and their walls are composed of only a single layer of thin cells.

The walls of arteries are thick with smooth muscle and elastic fibers, enabling them to change in diameter to accommodate changing volumes of blood. The changing blood volumes are due to large pressure differences that occur as the heart proceeds through its rhythmic cycle of contraction and relaxation. Ventricular contraction, or **systole,** causes the pressure to rise, while ventricular relaxation, or **diastole,** causes pressure to drop. The term *systole* means *contracting,* whereas the term *diastole* means *drawing apart.* The pressure differences that are produced by alternating states of systole and diastole are referred to as **blood pressure,** which is measured routinely to aid in the diagnosis of heart or vascular disease. Arteries may actively participate in blood pressure by either **vasoconstriction** (contracting their walls to reduce their diameter) or **vasodilation** (relaxing their walls to increase diameter). As arteries extend farther and farther from the heart, they branch into smaller vessels called **arterioles,** which means *little arteries.*

The walls of veins are much thinner than artery walls, since they contain less smooth muscle. Also, veins are larger than arteries in diameter. They carry blood sluggishly, often against gravity. As a result, blood tends to pool in veins. Contractions of your skeletal muscles and breathing activity help to push blood toward the heart. Some veins also contain valves, which help prevent the back flow of blood. Veins form as smaller vessels converge as they extend closer to the heart. These smaller vessels are called **venules,** or *little veins.*

The exchange of substances between the blood and body cells occurs exclusively across the walls of capillaries. Capillaries are located between arteries and veins, and their walls are composed of only a single layer of thin cells. Since capillaries have only a thin cell layer, substances such as oxygen, carbon dioxide, and nutrients can pass between the blood and the fluid that surrounds body cells. This fluid is called **interstitial** (*between tissues*) **fluid.** Capillaries often form densely branching beds within organs, which maximizes the amount of material exchange.

Capillary
The term *capillary* means *minute, resembling a hair,* which is very descriptive of the microscopic size of these blood vessels.

[thinking critically!]

Why don't substances, such as oxygen and nutrients, diffuse across the walls of arteries and veins?

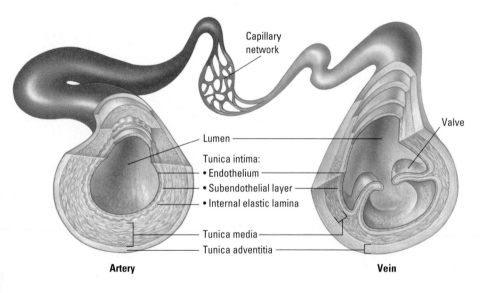

Capillary network

Valve

Lumen

Tunica intima:
• Endothelium
• Subendothelial layer
• Internal elastic lamina

Tunica media
Tunica adventitia

Artery

Vein

Figure 10.4 ::::

The structure of blood vessels: arteries, veins, and capillaries.
Source: Pearson Education.

getting to the root of it | anatomy and physiology terms

Many of the anatomy and physiology terms are formed from roots that are used to construct the more complex medical terms of the cardiovascular system, including symptoms, diseases, and treatments. In this section, we will review the terms that describe the structure and function of the cardiovascular system *in relation to their word roots,* which are shown in **bold.**

Study the word roots and terms in this list and complete the review exercises that follow.

Word Root (Meaning)	Terms Formed from the Word Root (Pronunciation)	Definition
aort (aorta)	**aort**a (ay OR tah)	the large artery that emerges from the left ventricle
	aortic valve (ay OR tik)	the left semilunar (semi LOO nahr) valve
arter (artery)	**arter**iole (ahr TEE ree ohl)	a vessel that is transitional between arteries and capillaries
	artery (AHR ter ee)	blood vessels that carry blood away from the heart
atri (atrium)	**atri**um (AY tree um)	the two superior chambers of the heart that receive incoming blood from veins; the plural form is *atria*
	atrioventricular bundle (ay tree oh vehn TRIK yoo lahr)	arising from modified heart cells, a bundle of cell extensions that serve as conducting pathways for impulses in the heart conduction system; also called *AV bundle* and *bundle of His*
	atrioventricular node (ay tree oh vehn TRIK yoo lahr)	a cluster of modified heart cells that slow the impulse to the ventricles; also called *AV node*
	atrioventricular valve (ay tree oh vehn TRIK yoo lahr)	two heart valves, right and left, that channel blood to flow in one direction from an atrium to a ventricle
	left **atri**oventricular valve (ay tree oh vehn TRIK yoo lahr)	the left heart valve that channels blood to flow in one direction from the left atrium to the left ventricle; also called *bicuspid valve* or *mitral valve*
	right **atri**oventricular valve (ay tree oh ven TRIK yoo lahr)	the right heart valve that channels blood to flow in one direction from the right atrium to the right ventricle; also called the *tricuspid valve*
	sino**atri**al node (sigh noh AY tree al)	a cluster of modified heart cells in the right atrial wall that originates each cardiac cycle; also called *SA node*

Word Root (Meaning)	Terms Formed from the Word Root (Pronunciation)	Definition
card, cardi (heart)	**cardi**ac cells (KAR dee ak)	cells of the heart's myocardium
	endo**cardi**um (ehn doh KAR dee um)	a thin layer of connective tissue that lines the heart chambers
	epi**cardi**um (ep ih KAR dee um)	the membrane forming the outer layer of the heart wall, which is also known as the visceral pericardium
	myo**cardi**um (my oh KAR dee um)	the bulk of the heart wall, it is composed of cardiac muscle tissue and is the functional part of the heart that produces contractions
	peri**cardi**al cavity (pair ih KAR dee al CAV ih tee)	a space enclosed by the pericardial sac that contains the heart and fluid
	peri**cardi**al sac (pair ih KAR dee al)	the outer membrane surrounding the heart, which is also known as the parietal pericardium
coron (crown or circle)	**coron**ary circulation (KOR ah nair ee)	the circulatory pathway that supplies the cells of the heart
cusp (point)	bi**cusp**id valve (bye CUSS pid)	the left atrioventricular valve of the heart, also known as the mitral valve, which consists of two flaps that point downward into the left ventricle
	tri**cusp**id valve (try CUSS pid)	the right atrioventricular valve of the heart, which consists of three flaps that point downward into the right ventricle
diast (to expand)	**diast**ole (dye ASS toe lee)	dilation of the heart chambers during which their walls relax and they fill with blood
pulmon (lung)	**pulmon**ary circulation (PULL mon air ee ser kew LAY shun)	the circulatory route associated with the lungs, in which blood releases its CO_2 load and becomes oxygenated
	pulmonary trunk (PULL mon air ee)	the major artery arising from the right ventricle
	pulmonary valve (PULL mon air ee)	the right semilunar valve
syst (contraction)	**syst**ole (SISS toh lee)	contraction of the heart resulting in expulsion of blood from the heart chambers
	systemic circulation (siss TEM ik ser kyoo LAY shun)	the circulatory route that begins from the left ventricle at the aorta, extends throughout the body except the lungs, and returns to the right atrium
thel (nipple)	endo**thel**ium (ehn doh THEE lee um)	the lining of the heart chambers and blood vessels, it is composed of flattened epithelial cells and a thin layer of connective tissue
vas (blood vessel)	**vas**oconstriction (vaz oh kon STRIK shun)	narrowing of a blood vessel that is produced when the vessel wall contracts
	vasodilation (vaz oh DYE lay shun)	dilation of a blood vessel that is produced when the vessel wall relaxes

Word Root (Meaning)	Terms Formed from the Word Root (Pronunciation)	Definition
vascul (little blood vessel)	cardio**vascul**ar system (kar dee oh VAS kyoo lahr)	body system comprised of the heart and blood vessels
ven (vein)	**ven**in (VAYN)	a blood vessel that carries blood toward the heart
	venule (VEHN yool)	a small, transitional blood vessel between a capillary and a vein
ventricul (little belly or cavity)	**ventricl**e (VEHN trih kull)	a general term that means a chamber, in the heart it refers to the two thick-walled chambers (right and left) that contract to push blood through arteries

OTHER IMPORTANT TERMS
The terms in this table are related to the structure and function of the cardiovascular system, but are not built from word roots.

blood	watery fluid consisting of plasma, blood cells, and platelets, which suspends materials in its fluid medium as it is carried throughout the body by way of the cardiovascular system
blood pressure	pressure within a blood vessel caused by blood volume within the confined space
blood vessels	tube-shaped organs that carry blood
bundle of His (HISS)	arising from modified heart cells, a bundle of cell extensions that serve as conducting pathways for impulses in the heart conduction system; also called atrioventricular bundle
capillaries (KAP ih lair eez)	microscopic blood vessels located between arteries and veins
heart	the fist-sized, hollow muscular pump located in the thoracic cavity responsible for circulating blood throughout the body
heart conduction system (kon DUK shun)	specialized cells that generate or carry impulses stimulating the heart to contract, which include the sinoatrial node, atrioventricular node, and the atrioventricular bundle
mitral valve (MY tral)	the heart valve that directs blood flow in one direction from the left atrium to the left ventricle, which is also called left atrioventricular valve or bicuspid valve

[FYI]

Mitral
The term *mitral* is derived from the Latin word *miter,* which refers to a two-leafed hat worn by Catholic bishops. The two-leafed valve resembles the shape of the bishop's miter.

SELF QUIZ 10.2

SAY IT—SPELL IT!

Review the terms of the cardiovascular system by speaking the phonetic pronunciation guides out loud, then writing in the correct spelling of the term.

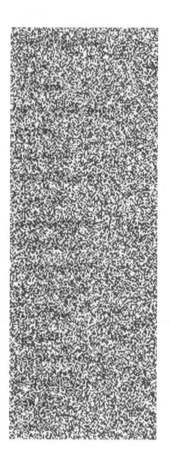

> **Success Hint:**   Use the audio glossary on the CD and CW for additional help with pronunciation of these terms.

1. kar dee oh VAS kyoo lar   _____

2. ay OR tah   _____

3. ahr TEE ree ohl   _____

4. ay tree oh vehn TRIK yoo lahr   _____

5. AY tree um   _____

6. bye CUSS pid   _____

7. KAP ih lair eez   _____

8. dye ASS toe lee   _____

9. ehn doh KAR dee um   _____

10. ehn doh THEE lee um   _____

11. my oh KAR dee um   _____

12. semi LOO nahr   _____

13. sigh noh AY tree al   _____

14. SIS toe lee   _____

15. vaz oh kon STRIK shun   _____

16. vaz oh dye LAY shun   _____

17. VEHN trih kull   _____

18. VEHN yool   _____

MATCH IT!

Match the term on the left with the correct definition on the right.

_____ 1. artery   a. sinoatrial node

_____ 2. capillary   b. increases diameter of an artery

_____ 3. venule   c. receives blood from vena cavae

_____ 4. left ventricle   d. composed of cardiac muscle tissue

_____ 5. right atrium   e. outer membrane of the heart

_____ 6. aortic valve   f. epicardium

_____ 7. SA node   g. is increased by vasoconstriction

_____ 8. endocardium   h. transitional between capillary and vein

_____ 9. myocardium   i. heart valve at the origin of the aorta

_____10. vasodilation   j. lines the heart chambers

_____11. pericardial sac   k. form the myocardium

_____12. visceral pericardium   l. a potential space containing the heart

_____13. pericardial cavity   m. pushes blood through the aorta

_____14. cardiac cells   n. its wall is one cell layer thick

_____15. blood pressure   o. carries blood away from the heart

FILL IT IN!

Fill in the blanks with the correct anatomy and physiology terms.

Success Hint: Once you get to the crossword puzzle at the end of the chapter, remember to check back here for clues! Your clues are indicated by the puzzle icon.

1. The cardiovascular system is a constructed term that literally means

   _____ and blood vessels, which are its two major types of

   organs. It functions in the transport of _____.

2. The heart is pocketed within a space contained by the thoracic cavity, which is

   called the _____ cavity. It is surrounded by an outer, thick

   membrane, which is known as the _____ _____

   or the parietal _____. Forming the outermost wall of the heart

   is a thinner membrane called the _____, or visceral pericardium.

3. The wall of the heart is dominated by a thick layer of cardiac muscle tissue,

   known as the _____. The thin lining of the heart chambers is

   called the _____. The heart chambers include the two

   thin-walled _____, which receive blood entering the heart, and

   the two thick-walled _____, which expel blood from the heart.

4. During the heart cycle, blood passes from the right atrium through the

   _____ valve into the right ventricle. The right ventricle contracts

   to push blood through the _____ valve into the pulmonary trunk,

   which carries blood to the lungs. The circulation of blood through the lungs is

   called the _____ circulation.

5. Blood entering the _____ _____ arrives from

   the lungs in an oxygenated state. Blood then passes through the

   _____ valve to enter the left ventricle. Contraction of the left

   ventricle pushes blood through the _____ valve to enter the

   largest artery of the body, the _____.

6. The coordination of the heart cycle is provided by the heart

   _____ system. The cycle is initiated by the

   _____ node, and the spread of impulses to the ventricles is

   slowed by the _____ node. The bundle of

   _____ carries electrical impulses to the myocardium of the

   ventricles.

10.1

7. Blood vessels that carry blood away from the heart are called

10.2   _____, while those that carry blood toward the heart are called

10.3   _____. The microscopic vessels that serve as the only site of

   material exchange between the blood and _____ fluid are the

   _____. Arteries carry blood under pressure, and their smooth

   _____ and elastic fibers enable them to become smaller in

   diameter, or perform _____, or to dilate during vasodilation,

   which helps to regulate blood pressure. The farther arteries branch, the smaller

   they become; these blood vessels are called _____. On the

   other hand, veins are formed when smaller vessels, called

10.4   _____, converge on the way to the heart.

LABEL IT!

Label the figures below by filling in the blanks.

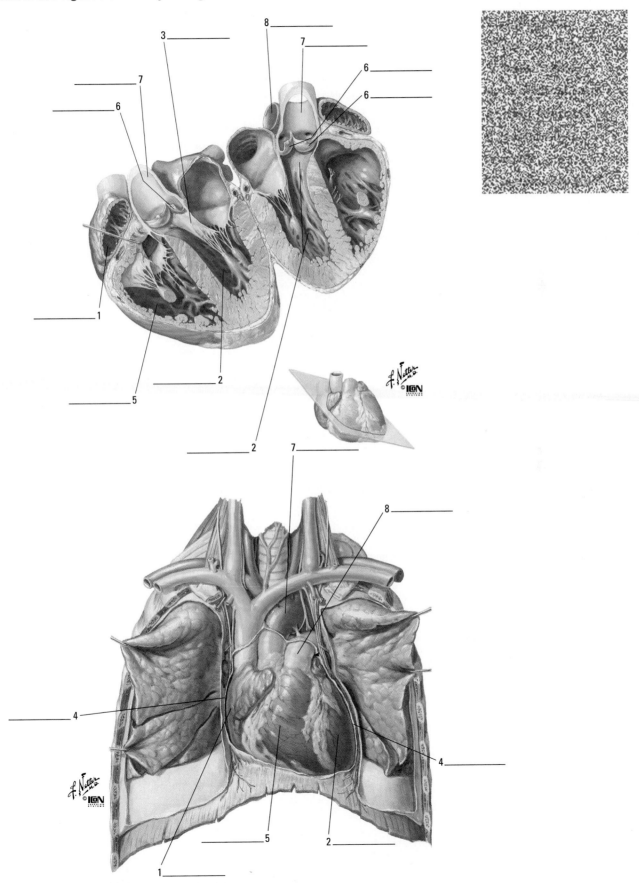

[medical terms of the

[cardiovascular system]

Many diseases and disorders of the cardiovascular system have a profound effect on the body's overall health. The result of cardiovascular disease is often the reduction or stoppage of blood flow to one or more body parts. As you learned earlier in this chapter, the loss of blood flow to a part of the body results in the death of cells. If blood flow reduction affects a large area or a critical organ like the brain, kidneys, or the heart itself, the resulting cell death can produce a condition that is life-threatening.

A division of medicine known as **cardiology** provides clinical treatment for heart disease. Cardiology is a constructed term, which can be written as:

cardi/o/logy

where the word root *cardi* means *heart,* and the suffix -logy means *study of.* A physician specializing in this field is called a **cardiologist.** Generally, a cardiologist also treats conditions associated with blood vessels, due to the close functional relationship between blood vessels and the heart.

In "Getting to the Root of It" in the previous section, you saw how learning just one word root helps you to understand some of the anatomy and physiology terms. Now, we will take you a step further, and show you that, by adding a combining vowel to those word roots to make a combining form, then using a prefix and suffix, you can form many of the medical terms related to the cardiovascular system. You are on your way to mastery of the medical terms related to the cardiovascular system!

let's construct terms!

In this section, we will assemble all of the word parts to construct medical terminology related to the cardiovascular system. Abbreviations are used to indicate each word part: **p** = prefix, **r** = root, **cv** = combining vowel, and **s** = suffix. Note that some terms are not constructed from word parts, but they are included here to expand your vocabulary.

The medical terms of the cardiovascular system are listed in the following three sections:

- Symptoms and Signs
- Diseases and Disorders
- Treatments, Procedures, and Devices

Each section is followed by review exercises. Study the lists in these tables and complete the review exercises that follow.

Symptoms and Signs

WORD PARTS (WHEN APPLICABLE)			TERM	DEFINITION
Part	Type	Meaning		
angin -a pector -is	r s r s	blood vessel singular chest pertaining to	**angina pectoris** (an JYE nah PECK tor iss)	chest pain usually caused by an insufficient supply of blood to the heart
angi/o -spasm	r/cv s	blood vessel contraction	**angiospasm** (AN jee oh spazm)	abnormal contractions (spasms) of a blood vessel wall
angi/o sten/o -sis	r/cv r/cv s	blood vessel narrowness state of	**angiostenosis** (an jee oh sten OH siss)	narrowing of a blood vessel
a- rrhythm -ia	p r s	absence rhythm condition of	**arrhythmia** (ah RITH mee ah)	any loss of rhythm in the heart beat
brady- card -ia	p r s	slow heart condition of	**bradycardia** (brad ee KAR dee ah)	an abnormally slow heart rate, usually under 50 beats per minute
cardi/o -dynia	r/cv s	heart pain	**cardiodynia** (kar dee oh DIN ee ah)	a sensation of pain in the heart
cardi/o -genic	r/cv s	heart pertaining to formation	**cardiogenic** (kar dee oh JENN ik)	a condition originating in the heart
cardi/o -megaly	r/cv s	heart large	**cardiomegaly** (kar dee oh MEG ah lee)	abnormal hypertrophy (enlargement) of the heart
cyan -osis	r s	blue condition of	**cyanosis** (sigh ah NOH siss)	a symptom in which a blue tinge is seen in the skin and mucous membranes, which is caused by oxygen deficiency
dys- rhythm -ia	p r s	abnormal rhythm condition of	**dysrhythmia** (diss RITH mee ah)	a disturbance or abnormality of the heart's normal rhythmic cycle
			palpitation (pal pih TAY shun)	an experience of pounding, racing, or skipping of the heart beat
			perfusion deficit (per FYOO zhun DEFF ih sitt)	a reduction of blood flow through a vessel, which may be caused by an occlusion or narrowing
tachy- card -ia	p r s	rapid, fast heart condition of	**tachycardia** (tak ee KAR dee ah)	a fast heartbeat

SELF QUIZ 10.3

SAY IT—SPELL IT!

Review the terms of the cardiovascular system by speaking the phonetic pronunciation guides out loud, then writing in the correct spelling of the term.

1. AN jee oh spazm _____

2. ah RITH mee ah _____

3. an jee oh sten OH siss _____

4. brad ee KAR dee ah _____

5. kar dee oh DIN ee ah _____

6. kar dee oh JENN ik _____

7. diss RITH mee ah _____

8. tak ee KAR dee ah _____

BREAK IT DOWN!

Analyze and separate each term into its word parts by labeling each word part using p = prefix, r = root, cv = combining vowel, and s = suffix.

1. angiostenosis _____

2. arrhythmia _____

3. bradycardia _____

4. cardiodynia _____

5. dysrhythmia _____

FILL IT IN!

Fill in the blanks with the correct terms.

10.5 1. _____ is a loss of heart rhythm that can lead to stoppage of the heart.

2. Atherosclerosis is characterized by a plaque formation on the inside of a vessel, causing a narrowing of the artery, or _____, which reduces blood flow. When this condition affects an artery supplying the brain, it leads to a stroke, or cerebrovascular accident (CVA).

3. A factor that originates from the heart is known as _____. It may refer to chest pain originating from the heart. A generalized pain in the heart is a _____.

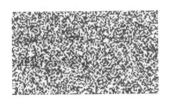

4. If a pain in the chest is accompanied by a rapid heart rate, or

    _____, it could result in severe heart disease. If pain is

    accompanied by a slow heart rate, or _____, it may be a sign

    that critical organs are not receiving an adequate blood supply.

Diseases and Disorders

WORD PARTS (WHEN APPLICABLE)			TERM	DEFINITION
Part	Type	Meaning		
aneurysm	r	bulging of a vessel wall	**aneurysm** (AN yoo rizm)	bulging of an arterial wall caused by a congenital defect or an acquired weakness of the arterial wall produced as blood is pushed against it (Figure 10.5 ::::)
angi/o card -itis	r/cv r s	blood vessel heart inflammation	**angiocarditis** (AN jee oh kar DYE tiss)	inflammation of the heart and blood vessels
angi -oma	r s	blood vessel tumor	**angioma** (an jee OH mah)	tumor arising from a blood vessel
arteri/o -rrhexis	r/cv s	artery rupture	**arteriorrhexis** (ahr TEE ree oh REK siss)	rupture of an artery

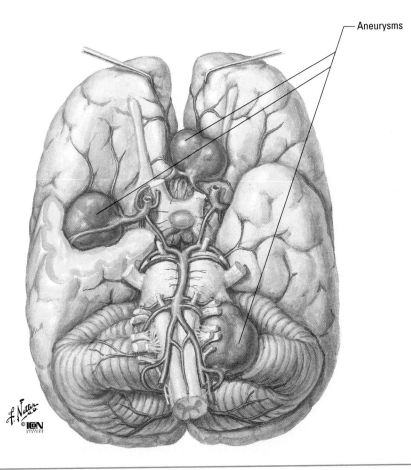

— Aneurysms

Figure 10.5 ::::

Aneurysm. In this illustration of the ventral side of the brain, three large aneurysms are clearly present. *Source: Icon Learning Systems.*

WORD PARTS (WHEN APPLICABLE)			TERM	DEFINITION
Part	**Type**	**Meaning**		
arteri/o	r/cv	artery	**arteriosclerosis**	hardening of the arteries, in which the artery walls
scler	r	hardening	(ahr tee ree oh skleh	lose their elasticity and become brittle
-osis	s	condition of	ROH siss)	
ather/o	r/cv	fatty	**atherosclerosis**	narrowing of an artery due to the deposition of a
scler	r	hardening	(ath er oh skleh ROH siss)	fatty plaque along the internal wall (Figure 10.6 ::::)
-osis	s	condition of		

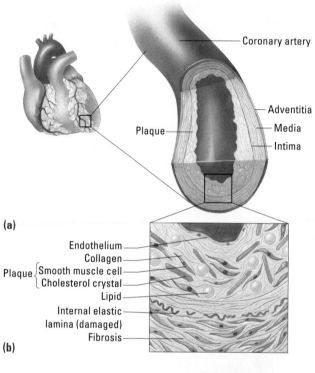

Coronary artery

Adventitia

Media

Intima

Plaque

(a)

Endothelium
Collagen
Plaque { Smooth muscle cell
Cholesterol crystal
Lipid
Internal elastic lamina (damaged)
Fibrosis

(b)

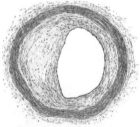

Moderate atherosclerotic narrowing of lumen

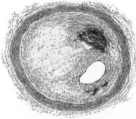

Almost complete occlusion by intimal atherosclerosis with calcium deposition

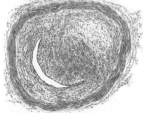

(c) Hemorrhage into atheroma, leaving only a slitlike lumen

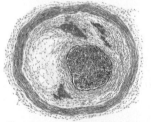

Complete occlusion by thrombus in lumen greatly narrowed by atheroma

Figure 10.6 ::::

Atherosclerosis.
(a) A sectioned coronary artery that exhibits an accumulation of fatty plaque, which reduces the internal diameter of the vessel.
Source: Pearson Education.
(b) In this close-up, you can see that the plaque consists of cholesterol, triglycerides, phospholipids, collagen, and smooth muscle cells.
Source: Pearson Education.
(c) Four types and degrees of atherosclerotic narrowing.
Source: Icon Learning Systems.

WORD PARTS (WHEN APPLICABLE)			TERM	DEFINITION
Part	Type	Meaning		
atri	r	atrium	**atrial septal defect** (AY tree al)	congenital condition characterized by an opening in the septum that separates the right and left atria, allowing blood to pass between them; abbreviated **ASD**
-al	s	pertaining to		
sept	r	wall		
-al	s	pertaining to		
atri/o	r/cv	atrium	**atrioventricular defect** (ay tree oh vehn TRIK yoo lahr)	a defect, usually congenital, that alters the structure of both an atrium and a ventricle
ventricul	r	little belly		
-ar	s	pertaining to		
cardi	r	heart	**cardiac arrest** (KAR dee ak)	cessation of heart activity
-ac	s	pertaining to		
cardi	r	heart	**cardiac tamponade** (KAR dee ak tam poh NAHD)	acute compression of the heart due to the accumulation of fluid within the pericardial cavity
-ac	s	pertaining to		
tampon	r	plug		
-ade	s	process		
cardi/o	r/cv	heart	**cardiomyopathy** (kar dee oh my OPP ah thee)	a general disease of the heart muscle
my/o	r/cv	muscle		
-pathy	s	disease		
cardi/o	r/cv	heart	**cardiovalvulitis** (kar dee oh val vyoo LYE tiss)	inflammation of the heart valves
valvul	r	little valve		
-itis	s	inflammation		
			claudication (klah dih KAY shun)	a pain in a limb, usually the lower leg, caused by poor circulation
			coarctation of the aorta (koh ark TAY shun)	congenital disease in which the aorta is narrowed, causing reduced systemic circulation and fluid accumulation in the lungs
			congestive heart failure	a chronic condition characterized by the inability of the left ventricle to pump enough blood through the body to adequately supply systemic tissues; abbreviated **CHF**; also called left ventricular failure
			cor pulmonale (KOR pull moh NAY lee)	literally "heart lung" in French, this chronic enlargement of the right ventricle results from congestion within the pulmonary circulation; also called right ventricular failure
coron	r	crown, circle	**coronary artery disease** (KOR ah nair ee AHR ter ee)	a generalized condition of the arteries of the heart characterized by a reduction of blood flow to the heart wall for which the most common cause is atherosclerosis; abbreviated **CAD**
-ary	s	pertaining to		
coron	r	crown, circle	**coronary occlusion** (KOR ah nair ee oh KLOO zhun)	blockage of an artery supplying the heart, often due to atherosclerosis (Figure 10.6)
-ary	s	pertaining to		
occlus	r	to close up		
-ion	s	process		
thromb	r	clot of blood	**deep vein thrombosis** (throm BOH siss)	the abnormal presence of stationary blood clots within the deep veins of the leg; abbreviated **DVT**
-osis	s	condition of		
embol	r	a throwing in	**embolism** (EM boh lizm)	a blood clot or foreign particle (including air or fat) that moves through the circulation, which can produce a severe circulatory restriction when it becomes lodged in an artery (plural = emboli)
-ism	s	condition of		

WORD PARTS (WHEN APPLICABLE)			TERM	DEFINITION
Part	Type	Meaning		
endo- card -itis	p r s	within heart inflammation	**endocarditis** (EHN doh kar DYE tiss)	inflammation of the endocardium; a common cause is a bacterial infection, in which case it is called bacterial endocarditis (Figure 10.7)

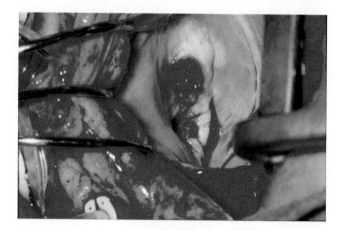

Figure 10.7

Endocarditis. Photograph of a surgical procedure repairing a heart valve that has been scarred by bacterial endocarditis. The valve is the white tissue; the red and black areas on the valve are lesions. *Source: M. English/Custom Medical Stock Photo, Inc.*

WORD PARTS (WHEN APPLICABLE)			TERM	DEFINITION
Part	Type	Meaning		
			fibrillation (fih brill AY shun)	uncoordinated, rapid contractions of the ventricles or atria, resulting in circulatory collapse
			heart flutter	extremely rapid, but regular, contractions of the heart; either atrial or ventricular
			heart attack	an acute episode during which the heart fails to pump blood effectively, usually caused by a myocardial infarction (MI)
			heart block	an interference with the normal electrical conduction of the heart, often the result of an MI affecting the SA or AV node
			heart murmur	an abnormal soft, blowing or rasping sound heard through auscultation of the heart
			hemorrhoid (HEM oh royd)	varicose vein in the anal region, which produces symptoms of local pain and itching
hyper- tens -ion	p r s	excessive, above pressure process of	**hypertension** (HIGH per TEN shun)	persistently high blood pressure which includes essential hypertension where the condition is not traceable to a single cause, and secondary hypertension where the high blood pressure is caused by the effects of another disease, such as atherosclerosis
hypo- tens -ion	p r s	deficient, below pressure process of	**hypotension** (HIGH poh TEN shun)	a chronic condition of low blood pressure
isch -emia	r s	to hold back blood condition	**ischemia** (iss KEE mee ah)	an abnormally low flow of blood to tissues
my/o cardi -al	r/cv r s	muscle heart pertaining to	**myocardial infarction** (my oh KAR dee al in FARK shun)	death of a portion of the myocardium usually caused by an occluded vessel interrupting blood flow, it often results in a heart attack; abbreviated **MI** (Figure 10.8)

WORD PARTS (WHEN APPLICABLE)			TERM	DEFINITION
Part	**Type**	**Meaning**		

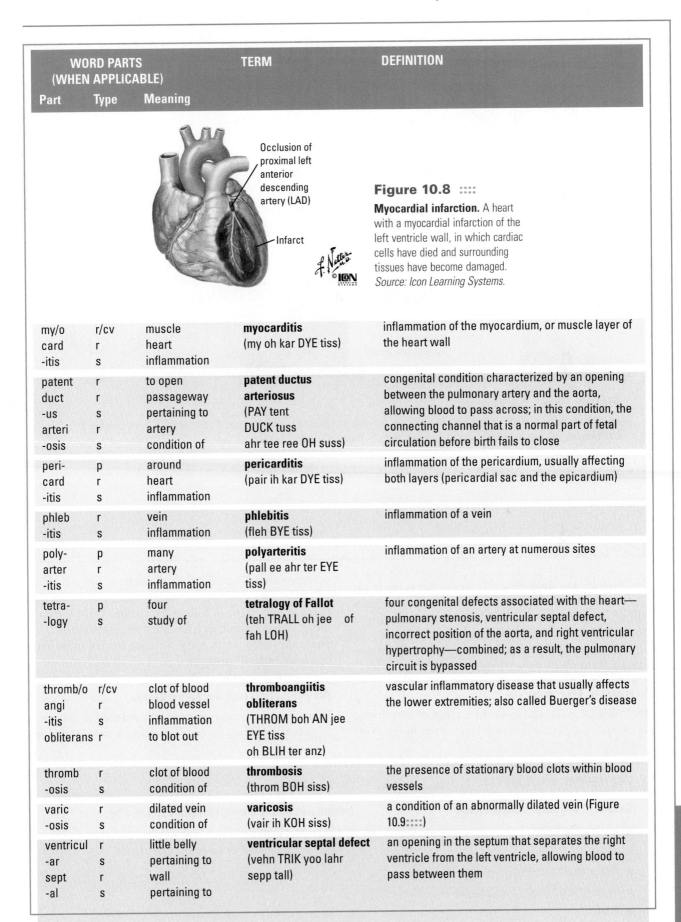

Occlusion of proximal left anterior descending artery (LAD)

Infarct

Figure 10.8 ⸬

Myocardial infarction. A heart with a myocardial infarction of the left ventricle wall, in which cardiac cells have died and surrounding tissues have become damaged. *Source: Icon Learning Systems.*

Part	Type	Meaning	TERM	DEFINITION
my/o card -itis	r/cv r s	muscle heart inflammation	**myocarditis** (my oh kar DYE tiss)	inflammation of the myocardium, or muscle layer of the heart wall
patent duct -us arteri -osis	r r s r s	to open passageway pertaining to artery condition of	**patent ductus arteriosus** (PAY tent DUCK tuss ahr tee ree OH suss)	congenital condition characterized by an opening between the pulmonary artery and the aorta, allowing blood to pass across; in this condition, the connecting channel that is a normal part of fetal circulation before birth fails to close
peri- card -itis	p r s	around heart inflammation	**pericarditis** (pair ih kar DYE tiss)	inflammation of the pericardium, usually affecting both layers (pericardial sac and the epicardium)
phleb -itis	r s	vein inflammation	**phlebitis** (fleh BYE tiss)	inflammation of a vein
poly- arter -itis	p r s	many artery inflammation	**polyarteritis** (pall ee ahr ter EYE tiss)	inflammation of an artery at numerous sites
tetra- -logy	p s	four study of	**tetralogy of Fallot** (teh TRALL oh jee of fah LOH)	four congenital defects associated with the heart—pulmonary stenosis, ventricular septal defect, incorrect position of the aorta, and right ventricular hypertrophy—combined; as a result, the pulmonary circuit is bypassed
thromb/o angi -itis obliterans	r/cv r s r	clot of blood blood vessel inflammation to blot out	**thromboangiitis obliterans** (THROM boh AN jee EYE tiss oh BLIH ter anz)	vascular inflammatory disease that usually affects the lower extremities; also called Buerger's disease
thromb -osis	r s	clot of blood condition of	**thrombosis** (throm BOH siss)	the presence of stationary blood clots within blood vessels
varic -osis	r s	dilated vein condition of	**varicosis** (vair ih KOH siss)	a condition of an abnormally dilated vein (Figure 10.9⸬)
ventricul -ar sept -al	r s r s	little belly pertaining to wall pertaining to	**ventricular septal defect** (vehn TRIK yoo lahr sepp tall)	an opening in the septum that separates the right ventricle from the left ventricle, allowing blood to pass between them

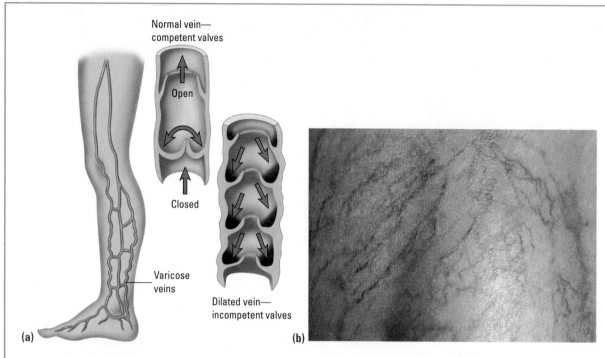

Figure 10.9 :::: **Varicosis.**

(a) Varicose veins, one type of varicosis, develops due to the failure of valves in the superficial veins of the leg, which leads to blood accumulation in response to gravity and vein dilation. *Source: Pearson Education.*
(b) Photograph of spider veins of the leg. *Courtesy of Jason L. Smith, MD.*

disease focus | Heart Disease

The statistics are staggering. Heart disease is the leading cause of death in the United States for men and women. According to the American Heart Association, someone in the U.S. suffers from a heart disease-related event about every 29 seconds, and someone dies from such an event about every minute.

Angina Pectoris

Heart disease is the end result of a series of conditions that stem from circulation problems in the heart. Poor coronary circulation deprives the heart of oxygen, damaging cardiac cells, and causing acute pain. When this damage falls short of killing the cardiac cells, the condition is experienced as pain called angina pectoris. This pain may often be an early warning sign of more serious heart-related problems.

Myocardial Infarction

When the heart's oxygen supply is reduced to the point of actually killing myocardial cells, a myocardial in-

Angina Pectoris

Causes of angina pectoris include:

- atherosclerosis
- stress
- heavy exercise following a meal
- hypertension (high blood pressure)
- anemia
- thyroid disease

Angina pectoris is a symptom characterized by:

- chest pain with tightness in the chest, which is often accompanied by dizziness and nausea

farction (MI) occurs. About 90 percent of the time, an MI is caused by a thrombus (a stationary blood clot) in one of the coronary arteries, an embolus (a drifting blood clot), or a spasm in one of the coronary arteries. Also, conditions such as atherosclerosis dramatically increase the chances of having a MI because it narrows the opening of one or more coronary vessels and encourages the formation of clots that break off to form emboli.

Heart Attack

The cardiac cells that die during an MI are not replaced by new functional cells, but by scar tissue that cannot contract. As a result, the heart muscle loses at least some of its strength. The degree of effect is dependent on the size and location of the infarcted, or dead, area. Often an MI leads to an episode where the heart's inability to supply its own circulation results in an acute loss of heart function. This episode is called a heart attack. In extreme cases, an MI can cause complete heart stoppage, called **cardiac arrest.**

Treatment of Heart Disease

Improvements in the areas of the treatment and prevention of heart disease have dramatically reduced the number of people who experience a heart attack and also the number of related fatalities. Surgical treatments such as **coronary artery bypass grafts** and **balloon angioplasty** have become routine procedures, and in even severe cases **heart transplants** can extend lives. Drug treatments are also important in reducing and managing the effects of heart disease. New classes of drugs are being used to dissolve clots in thrombolytic therapy procedures, and the oral administration of heart stimulants combined with blood thinners is reducing the frequency and severity of heart attacks. Perhaps most significantly, patients suffering from heart disease or conditions that may lead to it can lessen the chance of a heart attack by reducing their risk factors.

Lowering Risk through Patient Education

Education can be critical in helping patients implement measures that will lower their risks of heart disease and, ultimately, heart attack. These measures involve reducing the risk factors that can lead to heart disease, including high blood cholesterol, high blood pressure, cigarette smoking, and obesity. Preventive measures include losing weight if obese, maintaining a healthy, low-cholesterol diet, not smoking, and exercising regularly. Results can be dramatic. For example:

- every 1 percent decline in serum cholesterol level is accompanied by a 2 to 3 percent decline in the risk for a heart attack
- quitting smoking provides a 50 to 70 percent lowered risk within five years of cessation
- regular exercise has been shown to reduce the chance of a heart attack by 35 to 55 percent

---

Avoiding Heart Disease

Risk Factors	Preventive Measures
■ high blood cholesterol	■ implementing a diet low in cholesterol
■ high blood pressure	■ regular exercise
■ cigarette smoking	■ maintaining a healthy weight; losing weight if obese
■ obesity	

SELF QUIZ 10.4

SAY IT—SPELL IT!

Review the terms of the cardiovascular system by speaking the phonetic pronunciation guides out loud, then writing in the correct spelling of the term.

1. AN jee oh kar DYE tiss _____

2. an jee OH mah _____

3. ahr TEE ree oh REK siss _____

4. ahr tee ree oh skleh ROH siss _____

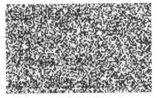

5. ath er oh skleh ROH siss _____

6. kar dee oh my OPP ah thee _____

7. kar dee oh val vyoo LYE tiss _____

8. EHN doh kar DYE tiss _____

9. high per TEN shun _____

10. my oh KAR dee al in FARK shun _____

11. my oh kar DYE tiss _____

12. pair ih kar DYE tiss _____

13. fleh BYE tiss _____

14. pall ee ahr ter EYE tiss _____

15. THROM boh AN jee EYE tiss
    oh BLIH ter anz _____

BREAK IT DOWN!

Analyze and separate each term into its word parts by labeling each word part using p = prefix, r = root, cv = combining vowel, and s = suffix.

1. angiocarditis _____

2. cardiovascular _____

10.6 3. angioma _____

4. arteriosclerosis _____

5. cardiomyopathy _____

6. cardiovalvulitis _____

7. endocarditis _____

8. pericarditis _____

9. polyarteritis _____

10. thromboangiitis _____

MATCH IT!

Match the term on the left with the correct definition on the right.

_____1. aneurysm

_____2. cardiac tamponade

_____3. cor pulmonale

_____4. angina pectoris

_____5. cardiac arrest

_____6. coronary artery disease

_____7. coronary occlusion

_____8. atrial septal defect

_____9. congestive heart failure

_____10. embolus

_____11. fibrillation

_____12. heart attack

_____13. heart block

_____14. hemorrhoid

_____15. perfusion deficit

_____16. varicosis

a. a disease afflicting coronary vessels

b. a congenital heart disease

c. interference of heart conduction system

d. reduction of blood flow through a vessel

e. literally, "a dilation"

f. a mobile blood clot

g. cessation of heart beat

h. uncoordinated, rapid heart beat

i. varicose vein in the anal region

j. an abnormally dilated vein condition

k. caused by fluid within pericardial cavity

l. literally, "heart lung"

m. left ventricular failure

n. a blockage in a coronary vessel

o. an acute episode often caused by an MI

p. chest pain due to blood flow reduction

FILL IT IN!

Fill in the blanks with the correct terms.

1. The area of a hospital that treats patients with heart disease is called

10.7 _____.

2. Inflammation of the heart and blood vessels is a condition known as

_____.

3. An inflammatory condition that affects an artery, but not the heart, and at multiple

sites is called _____. On the other hand, inflammation of the

heart muscle only is _____, and inflammation of the lining of

the heart chambers is _____. Inflammation of one or more

heart valves is known as _____. Another inflammatory

condition associated with the heart is _____, in which the

membrane surrounding the heart becomes affected. In each of these

inflammatory conditions, bacterial infection is the most common cause. If not

treated with antibiotics effectively, each condition can become life threatening.

4. Inflammation of a vein is known as _____. This condition can be very painful. When the condition is localized to the lower extremities, it is called _____ obliterans. Inflammation of a blood vessel can be

10.8   caused by a tumor, called an _____, or by a generalized deterioration of blood vessels that causes a progressive weakening of the walls, leaving them inelastic and brittle. This condition is known as _____.

5. The gradual development of fatty plaques on the inner wall of arteries is known

10.9   as _____. It is the leading cause of cardiac cell death, or

10.10 _____ _____, which is abbreviated MI. In most

10.11 cases, an _____ leads to a heart attack, which is a loss of normal heart rhythm.

10.12 6. A disease affecting the heart, in general, is called a _____.

7. _____ is a relatively common condition in older age, and is characterized by a persistent high blood pressure. The opposite condition, that of chronic low blood pressure, is called _____.

10.13 8. An _____ occurs when an arterial wall bulges outward at a particular site, due to congenital defect or acquired weakness of the wall.

9. Often an early warning of serious heart disease, _____ _____ is chest pain caused by the lack of blood supply to the

10.14 heart, or _____. If left untreated, it will often result in a myocardial infarction (MI). If the MI is severe, the heart may stop, called cardiac _____. An acute episode during which the heart fails to pump blood effectively, usually due to an MI, is a _____ _____.

10. The disease atherosclerosis often produces a blockage in a coronary vessel, called a coronary _____. The generalized condition that results is known as _____ _____ _____, or CAD. The narrowed opening can become completely blocked by a blood clot that

10.15 moves through the circulation, causing an _____. A fixed blood

10.16 clot, called a _____, causes a condition called _____.

11. In the disease _____ _____, the right ventricle becomes enlarged due to congestion within the pulmonary circulation. In _____ heart failure, the left ventricle fails to pump blood adequately, resulting in poor blood supply to many tissues. An uncoordinated, rapid heartbeat also reduces blood supply to tissues, and is called _____. However, a heart experiencing _____ does not reduce blood supply to tissues, since the heart beat is coordinated.

12. A disease of the heart that is present at birth is called a _____

heart disease. It may include an opening in the septum that separates the two

atria, known as _____ _____ defect; a

narrowed aorta, which is known as _____ of the aorta; patent

ductus arteriosus, in which an opening is present between the pulmonary artery

and the _____; or ventricular _____ defect, in

which a hole is present in the septum that separates the two ventricles. In

tetralogy of _____, four conditions are combined that result

in a bypass of the pulmonary circulation.

WORD BUILDING

Construct or recall medical terms from the following meanings.

1. A blood clot condition that circulates
   with blood flow   _____

2. A sound that may be a sign of heart
   valve problems   _____

3. Extremely rapid, but regular, heart
   contractions   _____

4. A result of damage to the SA node   _____

5. Obstruction of an artery supplying
   the heart   _____

10.17 6. Cessation of heart activity   _____

10.18 7. Pressure within a blood vessel _____

8. Pounding, racing, or skipping of the
   heart beat   _____

9. Literally "to hold back blood"   _____

10. Chronic failure of the left ventricle   _____

11. A congenital opening in the interatrial
    septum   _____

12. Pain in the lower limb due to poor
    circulation   _____

13. Congenital narrowing of the aorta   _____

Treatments, Procedures, and Devices

WORD PARTS (WHEN APPLICABLE)			TERM	DEFINITION
Part	**Type**	**Meaning**		
aneurysm	r	bulging of a vessel wall	**aneurysmectomy** (AN yoo riz MEK toh mee)	surgical removal (excision) of an aneurysm (a bulging of an arterial wall)
-ectomy	s	excision		
angi/o	r/cv	blood vessel	**angiogram** (AN jee oh gram)	recording obtained from an angiography (an jee OG rah fee) procedure, it is an x-ray of a blood vessel after injection of a contrast medium (Figure 10.10 ::::)
-gram	s	record		
angi/o	r/cv	blood vessel	**angioplasty** (AN jee oh plas tee)	general surgical repair of a blood vessel (Figure 10.11 ::::); it includes procedures to reopen blocked vessels (for example, balloon angioplasty is the insertion of an inflatable balloon into a vessel that is expanded to open the vessel, and laser angioplasty is the use of a laser beam to open blocked arteries)
-plasty	s	surgical repair		

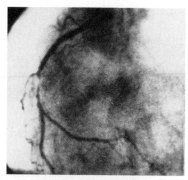

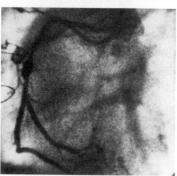

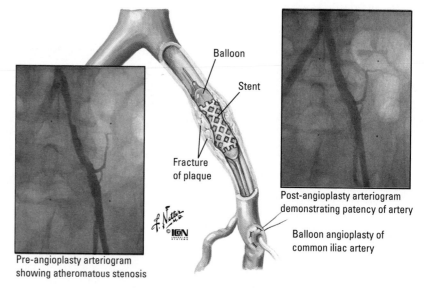

Pre-angioplasty arteriogram showing atheromatous stenosis

Balloon

Stent

Fracture of plaque

Post-angioplasty arteriogram demonstrating patency of artery

Balloon angioplasty of common iliac artery

Figure 10.11 :::: **Balloon angioplasty.** Balloon angioplasty is the insertion of a balloon-tipped catheter through a vein in the leg until it reaches an occluded vessel, and once in place, the balloon is inflated to compress the plaque against the vessel wall.
Source: Icon Learning Systems.

Figure 10.10 :::: **Angiogram, which reveals details of blood vessels supplying the heart.**

The upper image shows a blockage, which was opened by angioplasty as confirmed in the lower image.
Source: Icon Learning Systems.

WORD PARTS (WHEN APPLICABLE)			TERM	DEFINITION
Part	**Type**	**Meaning**		
angi/o	r/cv	blood vessel	**angiorrhaphy**	suturing a blood vessel to close an incision
-rrhaphy	s	to suture	(an jee OR rah fee)	
angi/o	r/cv	blood vessel	**angioscopy**	use of a flexible fiberoptic instrument, or
-scopy	s	examination	(AN jee OS koh pee)	endoscope, to observe a diseased blood vessel in order to assess the lesion and decide upon a mode of treatment; the procedure also includes use of a camera, video recorder, and monitor (Figure 10.12⋮⋮⋮⋮)

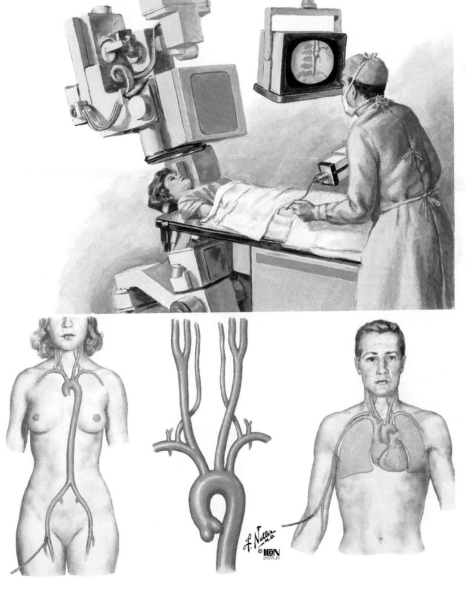

Figure 10.12 ⋮⋮⋮⋮ **Angioscopy.** The fiber optic end of the endoscope is located at the end of a catheter, which may be inserted either through a vessel in the arm or in the leg and guided by thin cables to its destination. The camera may then photograph the interior of the vessel, which is displayed on a monitor. *Source: Icon Learning Systems.*

WORD PARTS (WHEN APPLICABLE)			TERM	DEFINITION
Part	Type	Meaning		
aort/o -gram	r/cv s	aorta recording	**aortogram** (ay OR toh gram)	a recording of an x-ray of the aorta
arteri/o -gram	r/cv s	artery recording	**arteriogram** (ahr TEE ree oh gram)	a recording of an x-ray of a particular artery
arteri/o -tomy	r/cv s	artery incision	**arteriotomy** (ahr TEE ree OTT oh mee)	an incision into an artery
ather -ectomy	r s	fat excision	**atherectomy** (ath er EK toh mee)	surgical removal of a fatty plaque within a blood vessel using a specialized rotary knife and a catheter (a flexible tube) (Figure 10.13::::)
			auscultation (oss kull TAY shun)	physical examination consisting of listening to internal sounds using a stethoscope (STETH oh skope); sounds that suggest abnormalities are often caused by dysrhythmias (Figure 10.14::::)

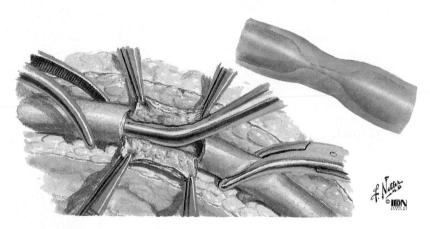

Figure 10.13 :::: **Atherectomy.** The surgical procedure includes the removal of fatty plaque from within an artery to correct an occlusion.
Source: Icon Learning Systems.

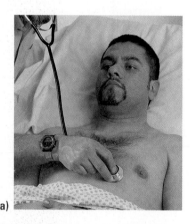

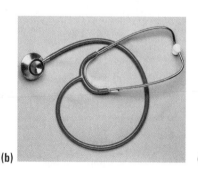

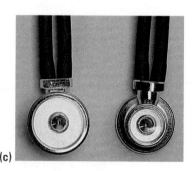

(a) (b) (c)

Figure 10.14 :::: **Auscultation.**

(a) Ausculation is an important part of a complete physical examination.
(b) The procedure involves the use of a stethoscope, shown here.
(c) The metal disc amplifies sound, and may consist of a flat disc (left) or a bell (right).
Source: Elena Dorfman

WORD PARTS (WHEN APPLICABLE)			TERM	DEFINITION
Part	**Type**	**Meaning**		

[FYI]

Auscultation

Auscultation is derived from the Latin word *ausculto,* which means *to listen.* During the ancient times of Aristotle, early physicians practiced this form of evaluation by pressing an ear against the patient's chest. The stethoscope, which literally means *to view the chest,* is a device that made this procedure much more efficient after its first use around 1725.

cardi	r	heart	**cardiac catheterization**	insertion of a narrow flexible tube, or catheter,
-ac	s	pertaining to	(KAR dee ak cath eh ter ih ZAY shun)	through a coronary blood vessel to withdraw blood samples, measure pressures, and inject contrast medium for imaging purposes (Figure 10.15:::::)

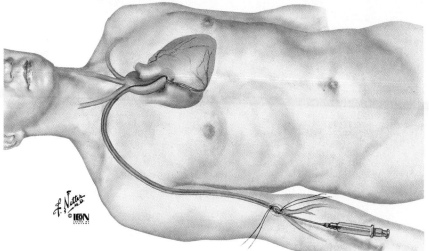

Figure 10.15 :::::

Cardiac catheterization.
The procedure consists of the insertion of a catheter into a blood vessel, such as the brachial artery in the arm, and its passage to the heart.
Source: Icon Learning Systems.

cardi	r	heart	**cardiac pacemaker**	a battery-powered device that is implanted under
-ac	s	pertaining to	(KAR dee ak)	the skin and wired to the SA node; it produces timed electric pulses that replace the pacemaking function of the SA node (Figure 10.16:::::)
cardi/o	r/cv	hear	**cardiopulmonary**	an emergency response procedure that includes
pulmon	r	lung	**resuscitation**	artificial ventilation and external heart massage;
-ary	s	pertaining to	(KAR dee oh PULL	abbreviated **CPR**
resuscitat	r	to revive	mon air ee	
-ion	s	process	ree suss ih TAY shun)	
coron	r	crown, circle	**coronary angiogram**	a recording of an x-ray of the heart's circulation
-ary	s	pertaining to	(KOR ah nair ee	
angi/o	r/cv	blood vessel	AN jee oh gram)	
-gram	s	recording		
coron	r	crown, circle	**coronary artery bypass**	surgical procedure in which a blood vessel is
-ary	s	pertaining to	**graft**	removed from another part of the body and inserted in the coronary circulation to bypass blood flow around an occluded (blocked) coronary artery; abbreviated **CABG** (Figure 10.17:::::)

WORD PARTS (WHEN APPLICABLE)			TERM	DEFINITION
Part	Type	Meaning		

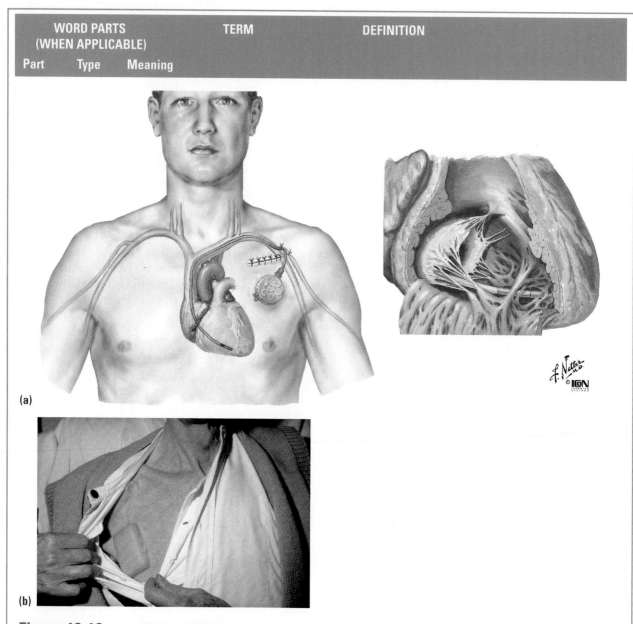

Figure 10.16 :::: **Cardiac pacemaker.**
(a) The pacemaker device is implanted beneath the skin near the heart, and the electrode is surgically connected to the heart wall. In this illustration, the electrode is inserted through the right ventricle, as shown in the opened heart. *Source: Icon Learning Systems.*
(b) Photograph of a pacemaker in a patient's chest. *Source: Photo Researchers Inc./Science Photo Library.*

Part	Type	Meaning	TERM	DEFINITION
coron	r	crown, circle	**coronary stent**	a plastic scaffold that is used to anchor a surgical implantation (graft); in this case it is implanted in a coronary artery to prevent closure of the artery after angioplasty or atherectomy (Figure 10.18::::)
-ary	s	pertaining to		
			defibrillation (dee fib rih LAY shun)	electrical charge to the heart in an effort to defibrillate, or to stop fibrillation, of the heart delivered by paddles onto the skin of the chest, or to the heart muscle directly if the chest has been opened (Figure 10.19::::)

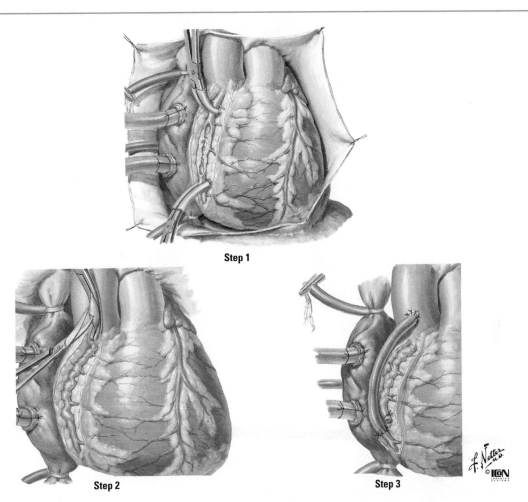

Step 1

Step 2

Step 3

Figure 10.17 :::: **Coronary bypass artery graft.** The procedure involves isolation of the occluded coronary artery (step 1) and the grafting of a vessel to bypass it (steps 2, 3). The graft vessel is usually a portion of the saphenous vein of the leg or the internal mammary artery, and it is grafted with extremely fine sutures.
Source: Icon Learning Systems.

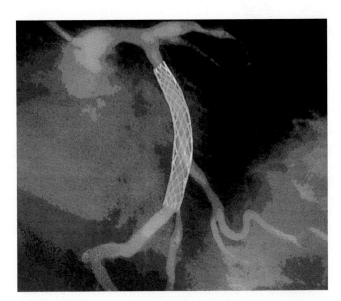

Figure 10.18 ::::

Coronary stent. An angiogram revealing a stent, which helps prevent closure of the vessel following procedures to correct a stenosis.

WORD PARTS (WHEN APPLICABLE)			TERM	DEFINITION
Part	Type	Meaning		

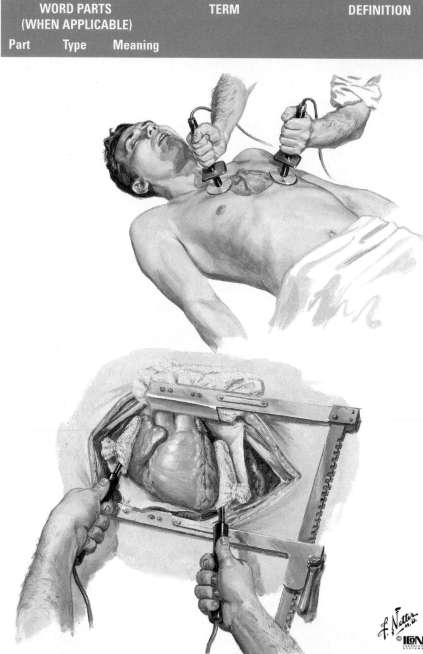

Figure 10.19 :::

Defibrillation. An emergency procedure in which paddles may be used on the outside of the chest wall (upper figure) or electrodes inserted into the heart wall (lower figure). The purpose of the procedure is to abruptly stop the heart from fibrillating. Once the heart restarts, the cardiac cycle is often more regular.
Source: Icon Learning Systems.

Part	Type	Meaning	TERM	DEFINITION
son/o -graphy	r/cv s	sound recording procedure	**Doppler sonography** (DOP ler son OG rah fee)	an ultrasound procedure that evaluates blood flow in an effort to determine the cause of a localized reduction in blood flow (Figure 10.20 :::)
ech/o cardi/o -graphy	r/cv r/cv s	to bounce heart recording procedure	**echocardiography** (EK oh kar dee OG rah fee)	an ultrasound procedure where sound waves are directed through the heart to evaluate heart anomalies—the recorded data is called an echocardiogram (ek oh kar dee OH gram); if performed during exercise to identify heart conditions, it is called a stress echocardiogram, or stress ECHO

WORD PARTS (WHEN APPLICABLE)			TERM	DEFINITION
Part	Type	Meaning		

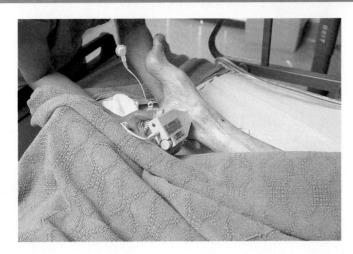

Figure 10.20 ::::
Doppler sonography.
The photograph demonstrates the use of a Doppler ultrasound device to assess pulse rate (in this case, the tibial pulse).
Source: Pearson Education.

Part	Type	Meaning	TERM	DEFINITION
electr/o	r/cv	electricity	**electrocardiography** (ee lek troh kar dee OG rah fee)	procedure in which the electrical events associated with the beating of the heart are evaluated, represented by deflections of a pen on a graph known as an electrocardiogram (ee lek troh kar dee OH gram); abbreviated ECG or EKG (the "K" is from the German term); when it is measured during physical activity using a treadmill or ergometer, it is called a stress electrocardiogram, and is useful in detecting heart conditions (Figure 10.21::::)
cardi/o	r/cv	heart		
-graphy	s	recording procedure		
embol	r	a throwing in	**embolectomy** (EM boh LEK toh mee)	surgical removal of a floating blood clot, or embolus (EM boh luss)
-ectomy	s	excision		
end-	p	within	**endarterectomy** (END ahr teh REK toh mee)	incision into an artery usually to remove fatty plaque or a blood clot
arter	r	artery		
-ectomy	s	excision		
			hemorrhoidectomy (hem oh royd EK toh mee)	surgical removal of hemorrhoids
			Holter ambulatory monitor (AM byoo lah tor ee)	a portable electrocardiograph worn by the patient, which monitors electrical activity of the heart over 24-hour periods, proving useful in detecting periodic or transient abnormalities
angi/o	r/cv	blood vessel	**magnetic resonance angiography**	magnetic resonance imaging of the heart and coronary blood vessels; abbreviated **MRA**
-graphy	s	recording procedure		
my/o	r/cv	muscle	**myocardial radionuclide perfusion scan**	following injection of an isotope, blood flow (perfusion) to cardiac cells is monitored; the test may be performed while the patient is under stress or at rest
cardi	r	heart		
-al	s	pertaining to		
			nuclear medicine imaging of the heart	visualization of the heart following administration of radioactive isotopes to aid in diagnosis

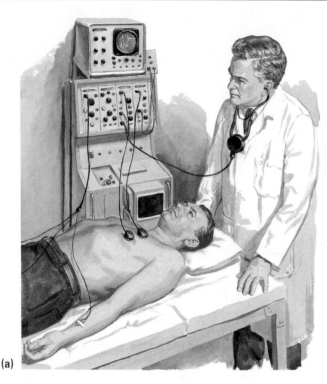

(a)

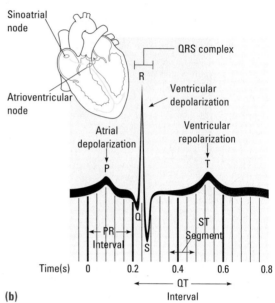

Sinoatrial node

Atrioventricular node

QRS complex

R

Ventricular depolarization

Atrial depolarization

Ventricular repolarization

P

T

Q

S

PR Interval

ST Segment

Time(s)   0   0.2   0.4   0.6   0.8

QT Interval

(b)

Normal sinus rhythm (NSR)

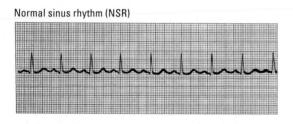

Sinus tachycardia

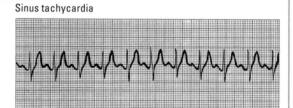

Sinus arrhythmia

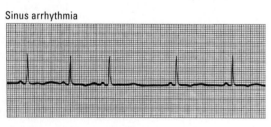

Sinus bradycardia

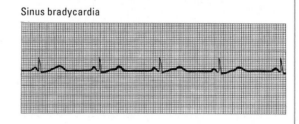

(c)

Figure 10.21 :::: **Electrocardiography.**
(a) The electrocardiogram is obtained by applying skin electrodes to the chest wall, which send electrical signals to a computer that interprets them into a graph form. *Source: Icon Learning Systems.*
(b) Illustration of the electrical events of the heart and a normal EKG. *Source: Pearson Education.*
(c) The EKG is useful in identifying arrhythmias, which are shown. *Source: Pearson Education.*

WORD PARTS (WHEN APPLICABLE)			TERM	DEFINITION
Part	**Type**	**Meaning**		
peri- cardi/o -stomy	p r/cv s	around heart surgical creation of an opening	**pericardiostomy** (pair ih KAR dee OS toh mee)	surgical creation of an opening in the pericardial sac, usually to relieve pressure resulting from pericarditis
phleb -ectomy	r s	vein excision	**phlebectomy** (fleh BEK oh mee)	excision (surgical removal) of a vein
phleb/o -tomy	r/cv s	vein incision	**phlebotomy** (fleh BOT oh mee)	incision into a vein, usually to remove blood for sampling or to donate blood; a technician who performs this procedure is called a phlebotomist (fleh BOT oh mist)
tom/o -graphy	r/cv s	to cut recording procedure	**positron emission tomography (PET) scan**	procedure that provides blood flow images using PET scan techniques with radioactive isotope labeling
sphygm/o man/o -metry	r/cv r/cv s	pulse thin measurement	**sphygmomanometry** (SFIG moh mah NOM eh tree)	procedure that measures arterial blood pressure using a device called a sphygmomanometer (sfig moh mah NOM eh ter), which consists of an arm cuff and air pressure pump with a mercury pressure gauge (Figure 10.22::::)

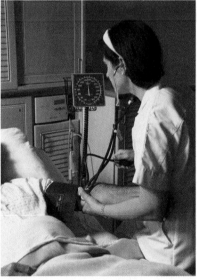

Figure 10.22 ::::

Sphygmomanometry. Taking blood pressure readings with the use of a sphygmomanometer, which includes an arm cuff and pressure gauge. A stethoscope is used to listen for sounds within the brachial artery. *Source: Pearson Education.*

WORD PARTS			TERM	DEFINITION
thromb/o -lytic	r/cv s	clot of blood pertaining to dissolution	**thrombolytic therapy** (throm boh LITT ik)	treatments dissolving blood clots, or thrombi, using drugs such as streptokinase or tissue plasminogen activator (TPA); this treatment is often applied within 6 hours of an MI—if possible—and has been credited with saving many lives
valvul/o -plasty	r/cv s	little valve surgical repair	**valvuloplasty** (VAL vyoo loh plass tee)	surgical repair of a heart valve; if repair is not possible, a valve replacement may be required using an artificial valve or a porcine (pig) valve (Figure 10.23::::)
ven/o -gram	r/cv s	vein recording	**venogram** (VEE noh gram)	a recording of an x-ray of a vein

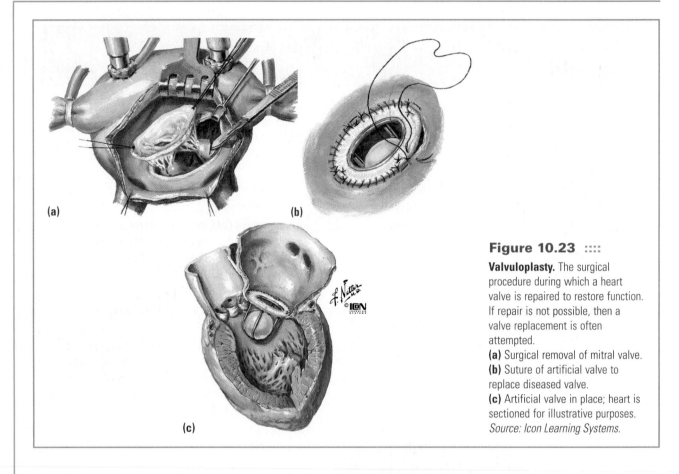

(a)

(b)

(c)

Figure 10.23 ::::

Valvuloplasty. The surgical procedure during which a heart valve is repaired to restore function. If repair is not possible, then a valve replacement is often attempted.
(a) Surgical removal of mitral valve.
(b) Suture of artificial valve to replace diseased valve.
(c) Artificial valve in place; heart is sectioned for illustrative purposes.
Source: Icon Learning Systems.

SELF QUIZ 10.5

SAY IT—SPELL IT!

Review the terms of the cardiovascular system by speaking the phonetic pronunciation guides out loud, then writing in the correct spelling of the term.

1. AN yoo riz MEK toh mee _____

2. AN jee oh gram _____

3. ahr TEE ree oh gram _____

4. ay OR toh gram _____

10.19 5. VEE noh gram _____

6. AN jee oh plas tee _____

7. an jee OR rah fee _____

8. AN jee OS koh pee _____

9. ahr TEE ree OTT oh mee _____

10. ath er EK toh mee _____

11. oss kull TAY shun _____

12. cath eh ter ih ZAY shun _____

13. dee fib rih LAY shun _____

14. EK oh kar dee OG rah fee _____

15. ee lek troh KAR dee *oh* gram _____

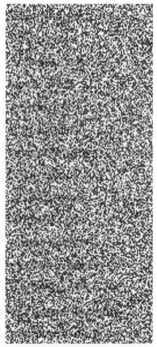

16. EM boh LEK toh mee _____

17. END ahr teh REK toh mee _____

18. hem oh royd EK toh mee _____

19. pair ih KAR dee OS toh mee _____

20. fleh BEK toh mee _____

21. fleh BOT oh mee _____

22. VAL vyoo loh plass tee _____

BREAK IT DOWN!

Analyze and separate each term into its word parts by labeling each word part using p = prefix, r = root, cv = combining vowel, and s = suffix.

1. angiostenosis _____

2. aneurysmectomy _____

3. angiogram _____

4. arteriogram _____

5. angioplasty _____

6. angiorrhaphy _____

7. arteriotomy _____

8. atherectomy _____

9. echocardiography _____

10. electrocardiogram _____

11. embolectomy _____

12. endarterectomy _____

13. pericardiostomy _____

14. valvuloplasty _____

MATCH IT!

Match the term on the left with the correct definition on the right.

_____1. phlebectomy

a. abbreviated MRA

_____2. atherectomy

b. suturing an artery

_____3. angiogram

c. stops the heart from fibrillating

_____4. electrocardiogram

d. removal of anal varicosities

_____5. thrombolytic therapy

e. a type of nuclear medicine imaging

_____6. Holter ambulatory monitor

f. using sound waves to monitor blood flow

_____7. magnetic resonance angiography

g. incision into an artery

_____8. endarterectomy

h. excision of a vein

_____9. hemorrhoidectomy

i. repair or replacement of heart valves

_____10. angiorrhaphy

j. excision of fatty plaque

_____11. myocardial radionuclide perfusion scan

k. abbreviated ECG or EKG

_____12. stress ECHO

l. x-ray of a blood vessel

_____13. defibrillation

m. an echocardiogram while exercising

_____14. Doppler sonography

n. a portable electrocardiograph

_____15. valvuloplasty

o. treatments to dissolve blood clots

FILL IT IN!

Fill in the blanks with the correct terms.

1. Surgical removal of a weakened blood vessel that threatens to blow open with blood pressure is called an _____. This condition is often identified in the procedure known as _____. An x-ray with contrasting medium of the aorta is an _____, and an x-ray that addresses the heart's own circulation is a _____ _____.

2. In the condition atherosclerosis, a fatty plaque causes a reduction of blood flow. This condition is often evaluated using an endoscopic camera in a procedure known as an _____. If warranted, the surgical removal of the plaque may be recommended, called an _____. If the procedure involves scraping of the inside of an artery, it is known as an _____. A nonsurgical technique to reopen clogged arteries is known as balloon _____. This procedure often includes placement of a plastic scaffold to stabilize the vessel, known as a coronary _____. In extreme cases, a surgical technique that involves bypassing blocked coronary arteries may become necessary. This procedure is a coronary artery _____ _____.

3. Often the first diagnostic evaluation performed on the heart is an

   _____, during which a _____ is used.

4. Following an auscultation, a cardiologist will often evaluate the electrical activity

   10.21   of the heart with the use of _____, which will obtain a reading

   known as an _____ (abbreviation). Another diagnostic tool

   utilizes sound waves to observe the heart, called _____. If a

   condition appears, this procedure will be performed during physical duress, and

   is called a _____ _____. If a problem appears

   with coronary circulation, a second type of ultrasound technique can be used to

   evaluate blood flow, known as a _____ sonography.

5. To correct a dysrhythmia, a battery-powered device can be implanted beneath

   the skin to replace the SA node. This device is a cardiac _____.

   Implantation of the device often follows a preliminary period during which a

   portable electrocardiograph is used to monitor the condition, known as a

   _____ ambulatory monitor.

abbreviations of the cardiovascular system

The abbreviations that are associated with the cardiovascular system are summarized
here. Study these abbreviations, and review them in the exercise that follows.

ABBREVIATION	DEFINITION	ABBREVIATION	DEFINITION
ASD	atrial septal defect	ECG, EKG	electrocardiogram
AV	atrioventricular	HHD	hypertensive heart disease
BP	blood pressure	MI	myocardial infarction
CABG	coronary artery bypass graft	MRA	magnetic resonance
CAD	coronary artery disease		angiography
CHF	congestive heart failure	SA	sinoatrial
CPR	cardiopulmonary resuscitation	SL	semilunar (pertaining to
DVT	deep vein thrombosis		the heart valve)

SELF QUIZ 10.6

Fill in the blanks with the abbreviation or the complete medical term.

Abbreviation	Medical Term
1. ASD	_____
2. _____	hypertensive heart disease
3. MI	_____
4. _____	magnetic resonance angiography
5. ECG	_____
6. _____	congestive heart failure

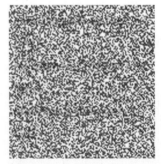

7. CAD   _____

8. _____   cardiopulmonary resuscitation

9. CABG   _____

10. _____   atrioventricular

11. BP   _____

12. _____   sinoatrial

13. DVT   _____

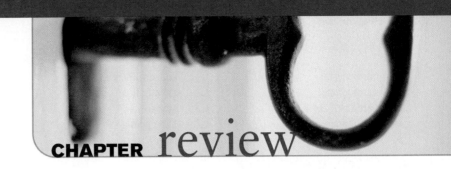

In this section, we will review all the word parts and medical terms from this chapter. As in earlier tables, the word roots are shown in **bold.**

Check each word part and medical term to be sure you understand the meaning. If any are not clear, please go back into the chapter and review that term. Then, complete the review exercises that follow.

[word parts **checklist**]

Prefixes

- ❑ brady-
- ❑ endo-
- ❑ epi-
- ❑ inter-
- ❑ peri-
- ❑ tachy-

Word Roots/Combining Vowels

- ❑ **angi**/o
- ❑ **angin**/o
- ❑ **aort**/o
- ❑ **arter**/o
- ❑ **arteri**/o
- ❑ **ather**/o
- ❑ **atri**/o

- ❑ **card**/o
- ❑ **cardi**/o
- ❑ **coron**/o
- ❑ **cyan**/o
- ❑ **ech**/o
- ❑ **electr**/o
- ❑ **isch**/o
- ❑ **my**/o
- ❑ **myos**/o
- ❑ **occlus**/o
- ❑ **pector**/o
- ❑ **phleb**/o
- ❑ **sphygm**/o
- ❑ **sten**/o
- ❑ **steth**/o
- ❑ **thromb**/o
- ❑ **valvul**/o

- ❑ **varic**/o
- ❑ **vas**/o
- ❑ **vascul**/o
- ❑ **ven**/o
- ❑ **ventricul**/o

Suffixes

- ❑ -ac
- ❑ -apheresis
- ❑ -dynia
- ❑ -gram
- ❑ -graph
- ❑ -is
- ❑ -lytic
- ❑ -rrhexis
- ❑ -sclerosis

[medical terminology **checklist**]

- ❑ aneurysm
- ❑ aneurysmectomy
- ❑ **angi**na **pector**is
- ❑ **angi**o**cardi**tis
- ❑ **angi**ogram
- ❑ **angi**ography
- ❑ **angi**oma
- ❑ **angi**oplasty
- ❑ **angi**orrhaphy
- ❑ **angi**oscopy
- ❑ **angi**ospasm
- ❑ **angi**o**sten**osis
- ❑ **aort**a
- ❑ **aort**ogram

- ❑ arrhythmia
- ❑ **arteri**ogram
- ❑ **arteri**oles
- ❑ **arteri**orrhexis
- ❑ **arteri**otomy
- ❑ **arter**y
- ❑ **arteri**osclerosis
- ❑ **ather**ectomy
- ❑ **ather**osclerosis
- ❑ **atri**al **sept**al defect (ASD)
- ❑ **atri**o**ventricul**ar (AV)
- ❑ **atri**o**ventricul**ar defect
- ❑ **atri**o**ventricul**ar node
- ❑ **atri**o**ventricul**ar valve

- ❑ **atri**um
- ❑ auscultation
- ❑ bi**cusp**id valve
- ❑ blood pressure (BP)
- ❑ blood vessel
- ❑ bone marrow transplant
- ❑ brady**cardi**a
- ❑ bundle of His
- ❑ capillary
- ❑ **cardi**ac arrest
- ❑ **cardi**ac catheterization
- ❑ **cardi**ac cells
- ❑ **cardi**ac pacemaker
- ❑ **cardi**ac **tampon**ade

- ☐ **cardi**odynia
- ☐ **cardi**ogenic
- ☐ **cardi**omegaly
- ☐ **cardi**o**my**opathy
- ☐ **cardi**o**pulmon**ary resuscitation (CPR)
- ☐ **cardi**o**valvul**itis
- ☐ claudication
- ☐ coarctation of the aorta
- ☐ con**gen**ital heart disease
- ☐ congestive heart failure (CHF)
- ☐ cor pulmonale
- ☐ **coron**ary **angi**ogram
- ☐ **coron**ary artery bypass graft (CABG)
- ☐ **coron**ary artery disease (CAD)
- ☐ **coron**ary circulation
- ☐ **coron**ary **occlus**ion
- ☐ **coron**ary stent
- ☐ deep vein **thromb**osis (DVT)
- ☐ defibrillation
- ☐ diastole
- ☐ Doppler **son**ography
- ☐ dys**rhythm**ia
- ☐ echo**cardi**ogram
- ☐ echo**cardi**ography
- ☐ electro**cardi**ogram (ECG, EKG)
- ☐ electro**cardi**ography
- ☐ **embol**ectomy
- ☐ **embol**us
- ☐ end**arter**ectomy
- ☐ endo**cardi**tis

- ☐ endo**cardi**um
- ☐ endo**theli**um
- ☐ epi**cardi**um
- ☐ fibrillation
- ☐ flutter
- ☐ heart attack
- ☐ heart block
- ☐ heart murmur
- ☐ hemorrhoid
- ☐ hemorrhoidectomy
- ☐ Holter ambulatory monitor
- ☐ hyper**tens**ion
- ☐ hyper**tens**ive heart disease (HHD)
- ☐ hypo**tens**ion
- ☐ interstitial fluid
- ☐ ischemia
- ☐ magnetic resonance **angi**ography (MRA)
- ☐ mitral valve
- ☐ **myocardi**al infarction (MI)
- ☐ **myocardi**al radionuclide perfusion scan
- ☐ **myocardi**tis
- ☐ **myocardi**um
- ☐ nuclear medicine imaging
- ☐ palpitation
- ☐ parietal peri**cardi**um
- ☐ patent ductus **arteri**osus
- ☐ perfusion defect
- ☐ peri**cardi**al sac
- ☐ peri**cardi**ostomy

- ☐ peri**cardi**tis
- ☐ **phleb**ectomy
- ☐ **phleb**itis
- ☐ **phleb**otomy
- ☐ poly**arter**itis
- ☐ positron emission **tom**ography scan
- ☐ **pulmon**ary circulation
- ☐ **pulmon**ary trunk
- ☐ semilunar (SL)
- ☐ semilunar valve
- ☐ sino**atri**al (SA)
- ☐ sino**atri**al node
- ☐ stress ECHO
- ☐ **system**ic circulation
- ☐ systole
- ☐ tachy**cardi**a
- ☐ **tetra**logy of Fallot
- ☐ **thromb**o**angii**tis obliterans
- ☐ **thromb**olytic therapy
- ☐ **thromb**us
- ☐ tri**cusp**id valve
- ☐ **valvul**oplasty
- ☐ **varic**osis
- ☐ **vas**oconstriction
- ☐ **vas**odilation
- ☐ vein
- ☐ **ven**ogram
- ☐ ventricle
- ☐ **ventricul**ar septal defect
- ☐ **ven**ule
- ☐ visceral peri**cardi**um

[show what **you know!**]

BREAK IT DOWN!

Analyze and separate each term into word parts by labeling each word part using p = prefix, r = root, cv = combining vowel, and s = suffix.

Example:

		r cv r s
1.	cardiovascular	cardi/o/vascul/ar
2.	atrioventricular	_____
3.	pericardium	_____
4.	angiocarditis	_____
5.	angioma	_____
6.	arteriosclerosis	_____
7.	angiostenosis	_____
8.	arrhythmia	_____

9. bradycardia   _____

10. cardiodynia   _____

11. cardiomyopathy   _____

12. cardiovalvulitis   _____

13. endocarditis   _____

14. hypertension   _____

15. hypophysectomy   _____

16. myocarditis   _____

17. polyarteritis   _____

18. aneurysmectomy   _____

19. angiogram   _____

20. angiorrhaphy   _____

21. electrocardiography   _____

WORD BUILDING

Construct or recall medical terms from the following meanings.

Example: 1. generalized disease of the heart muscle   _____cardiomyopathy_____

2. inflammation of the heart and blood vessels   _____

3. narrowing of a blood vessel   _____

4. tumor arising from a blood vessel   _____

5. hardening of the arteries   _____

6. abnormally slow heart rate   _____

7. a sensation of pain in the heart   _____

8. originating from the heart   _____

9. abnormal hypertrophy of the heart   _____

10. inflammation of the inner heart membrane   _____

11. an abnormal heart rhythm   _____

12. high blood pressure that is persistent   _____

13. death of a portion of the myocardium   _____

14. inflammation of the myocardium   _____

15. inflammation of the outer heart membrane   _____

16. inflammation of a vein   _____

17. a recording of an x-ray of an artery   _____

18. general surgical repair of a blood vessel   _____

19. use of an endoscope to evaluate a blood vessel   _____

20. an incision into an artery   _____

21. listening to heart sounds with a stethoscope   _____

22. use of sound waves to diagnose a heart condition

_____

23. a measurement of heart electrical activity

_____

24. incision into an artery to remove plaque

_____

25. surgical opening into the pericardial sac

_____

CASE STUDIES

Fill in the blanks with the correct terms.

1. A patient complained of pain in the heart area of the chest, or (a) _____

_____, and was subsequently referred to (b) _____ for immediate diagnosis

and treatment. The specialist, a (c) _____, diagnosed the pain as having a cause from insufficient

blood supply to the heart, known as (d) _____ _____. The patient was given

medication and educated about heart disease management. Several weeks later, the patient was readmitted due to

continued complaints of chest pain. After evaluating heart electrical events with (e) _____, the

physician performed a technique using sound waves to evaluate heart activity during physical exercise, known as a

(f) _____ _____. The EKG showed a normal conduction system, thereby ruling

out damage to the conduction system, or a heart (g) _____. The stress ECHO also showed normal

results, ruling out damage to the heart muscle, or a (h) _____ _____, since the

heart muscle was receiving sufficient levels of oxygen. Since blood flow was normal, the narrowing of a coronary artery,

generally called an (i) _____, was eliminated as a cause, which also eliminated the common plaque-

forming disease that causes a stenosis, known as (j) _____. However, the stress ECHO did reveal an

abnormal contact with the pericardial sac with each heartbeat, suggesting inflammation of the membrane or

(k) _____. Inflammation of the inner heart membrane, a condition known as

(l) _____, was also suspected. A blood analysis was ordered, and found to be positive for bacterial

infection. A course of treatment was ordered that began with a surgical technique to create an opening in the pericardial sac,

called a (m) _____, and followed with antibiotic therapy to destroy the infectious microorganisms and

counter the inflammation.

2. A patient with a history of persistently high blood pressure, or (n) _____, complained of intermittent

pain sensations in the upper abdomen. Upon evaluation in which an x-ray was taken of the local arteries, called an

(o) _____, it became apparent that the source of the pain was from abnormal spasms of the aorta

wall, which is generally called (p) _____, due to an abnormal dilation of the vessel wall, called an

(q) _____. To avoid a possible rupture of the artery, an event known as an

(r) _____, surgery was required. The procedure is known as an (s) _____. After

repair, the vessel is closed with sutures in a procedure called an (t) _____.

3. The most common cause of acute events associated with heart disease is a (u) _____

_____, or MI. In most cases, a MI is the result of narrowed coronary arteries, a condition known as

(v) _____ _____ _____, or CAD, that leads to a reduction

of oxygen to the heart muscle, or (w)_____. The stenosis usually leads to complete blockage, or

(x) _____ _____, and is often caused by the accumulation of a fatty plaque

along the inner wall of arteries, called (y) _____. In some cases, the artery wall may also become

brittle and weak, resulting in the condition of (z) _____. In most cases, the narrowing can be corrected

using a balloon device in a noninvasive procedure called (aa) _____ _____. In

more serious cases, one or more grafts must be surgically inserted that bypass the occlusion in a procedure called a

(bb) _____ _____ _____ _____,

or CABG. In certain instances, a heart transplant may be necessary to extend the life of the patient.

[piece it all **together!** 🧩]

CROSSWORD

From the chapter material, fill in the crossword puzzle with answers to the following clues.

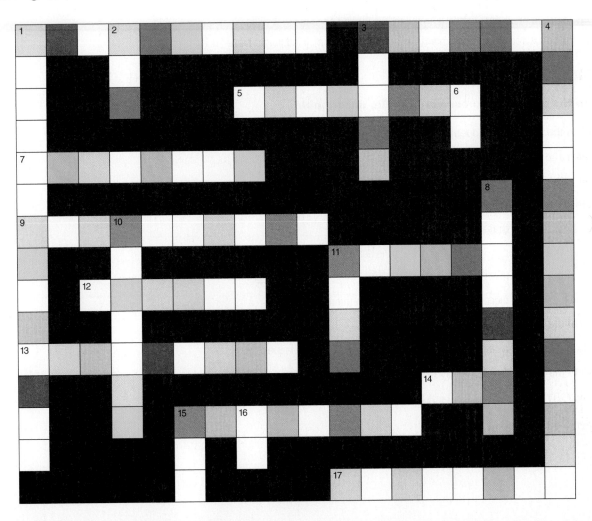

ACROSS

1. Where heart patients receive special attention. (Find puzzle piece 10.7)

3. A tumor arising from a blood vessel. (Find puzzle piece 10.8)

5. A recording of an x-ray of a vein. (Find puzzle piece 10.19)

7. Abnormally low supply of blood. (Find puzzle piece 10.14)

9. Pertaining to the muscle of the heart. (Find puzzle piece 10.10)

11. A connecting tube between capillaries and a vein. (Find puzzle piece 10.4)

12. A blood vessel capable of vasoconstriction. (Find puzzle piece 10.2)

13. An x-ray that helps diagnose problems with arteries. (Find puzzle piece 10.20)

14. A bundle that conducts electricity in the heart wall. (Find puzzle piece 10.1)

15. A "floater" that can cause an occlusion. (Find puzzle piece 10.15)

17. A blood clot that is stationary. (Find puzzle piece 10.16)

DOWN

1. A disease of the heart muscle. (Find puzzle piece 10.12)

2. The prefix to the term describing an uncoordinated heartbeat. (Find puzzle piece 10.5)

3. A word root and combining vowel that mean *blood vessel*. (Find puzzle piece 10.6)

4. A disease that causes an angiostenosis. (Find puzzle piece 10.9)

6. Abbreviation for the death of heart tissue. (Find puzzle piece 10.11)

8. A bulging of an arterial wall. (Find puzzle piece 10.13)

10. A heart stoppage is known as a _____ arrest. (Find puzzle piece 10.17)

11. Any blood vessel that carries blood toward the heart. (Find puzzle piece 10.3)

15. An abbreviation of the German term for an important diagnostic tool. (Find puzzle piece 10.21)

16. Can be measured with a sphygmomanometer (abbreviation). (Find puzzle piece 10.18)

WORD UNSCRAMBLE

From the completed crossword puzzle, unscramble:

1. All of the letters that appear in **red** squares ☐ _ _ _ _

   Clue: The largest artery in the body

2. All of the letters that appear in **purple** squares _ _ ☐ _ _ _ _ _ _ _

   Clue: The node that begins every heartbeat

3. All of the letters that appear in **peach** squares ☐ _ _ _ _ _ _ _ _ _ _ _ _

   Clue: Often caused by bacteria, it inflames the heart's inner lining

4. All of the letters that appear in **blue** squares _ _ _ _ _ ☐ _

   Clue: Literally, a "piece" or "patch" that flows with the bloodstream

5. All of the letters that appear in **yellow** squares _ _ _ _ ☐ _ _ _ _ _ _

   Clue: Often using a catheter, a procedure that removes arterial plaque

6. All of the letters that appear in **green** squares _ _ _ _ _ _ _ ☐

   Clue: The "c" word in CAD

7. All of the letters that appear in **pink** squares __ __ __ __ __ __ ☐ __

   Clue: A condition of unwanted "visible" veins

8. All of the letters that appear in **gray** squares __ __ __ __ __ __ __ __ __ ☐

   Clue: Abnormal smooth muscle activity in a blood vessel

Now write down each of the letters that are boxed to find the hidden medical term of the cardiovascular system:

__ __ __ __ __ __ __ __.

MEDmedia wrap-up

www.prenhall.com/wingerd

Before you go on to the next chapter, take advantage of the free CD-ROM and study guide website that accompany this book. Simply load the CD-ROM for additional activities, games, animations, videos, and quizzes linked to this chapter. Then visit www.prenhall.com/wingerd for even more!

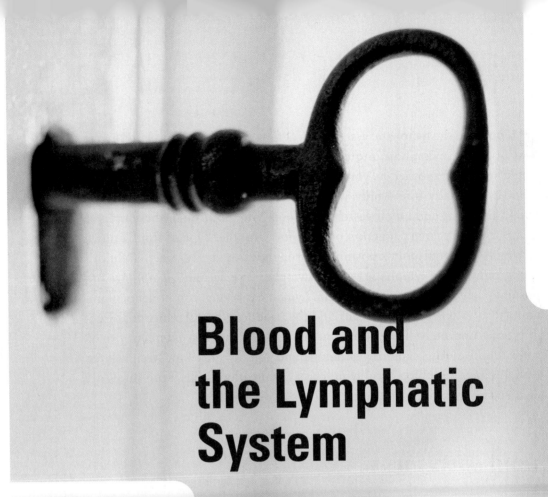

CHAPTER 11

Blood and the Lymphatic System

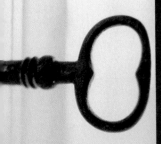

LEARNING OBJECTIVES

After completing this chapter, you will be able to:

- Define and spell the word parts used to create medical terms for blood and the lymphatic system

- Identify the organs of blood and the lymphatic system and describe their structure and function

- Define common medical terms used for blood and the lymphatic system

- Break down and define common medical terms used for symptoms, diseases, disorders, procedures, treatments, and devices for blood and the lymphatic system

Blood and the lymphatic system may at first seem like an unrelated group of topics to combine into one chapter. However, they are closely associated with one another, as you are about to discover. In the human body, blood is normally found only within the cardiovascular system—that is, within the heart and blood vessels. As blood courses through these organs, it performs its primary function of transport. Another type of fluid, known as lymph, also transports substances throughout the body, but this fluid is found only within lymphatic vessels. Lymphatic vessels and lymph are important parts of the lymphatic system. Lymph carries the components of immunity, such as white blood cells and the products they produce that fight infection. Amazingly, the two fluids are intertwined, because lymph is formed from blood during capillary exchange and rejoins the bloodstream later. And, because both blood and lymph carry white blood cells, both fluids are involved in the immune response.

word parts focus

Let's look at word parts. The following table contains a list of word parts that when combined build many of the terms of blood and the lymphatic system.

PREFIX	DEFINITION	PREFIX	DEFINITION
ana-	up, toward	macro-	large
homo-	same	micro-	small
iso-	equal	pro-	forward, preceding

WORD ROOT	DEFINITION	WORD ROOT	DEFINITION
aden	gland	path	disease
aut	self	poikil	irregular
bacter	bacteria	splen	spleen
blast	germ or bud (may also be used as a suffix)	staphyl	grape-like clusters; *Staphylococcus* (a bacterium)
erythr	red	strept	twisted or gnarled; *Streptococcus* (a bacterium)
hem, hemat	blood		
immun	exempt; immunity	therm	heat
leuk	white	thromb	clot
lymph	clear water or fluid	thym	wart-like; thymus gland
mon	one	tox	poison

SUFFIX	DEFINITION	SUFFIX	DEFINITION
-crit	to separate	-penia	abnormal reduction in number
-cyte	cell	-pexy	surgical fixation, suspension
-emia, -hemia	condition of blood	-phil, -philia	loving, affinity for
-lysis	to dissolve	-phylaxis	protection
-osis	condition of	-poiesis	formation

SELF QUIZ 11.1

Review the word parts of blood and the lymphatic system terminology by working carefully through the exercises that follow. Soon, we will apply this new information to build medical terms.

A. Provide the definition of the following prefixes and suffixes.

1. macro- _____
2. micro- _____
3. -crit _____
4. -emia _____
5. -penia _____
6. -phil _____
7. -poiesis _____
8. ana- _____
9. pro- _____
10. -phylaxis _____
11. -lysis _____
12. iso- _____
13. homo- _____
14. -cyte _____
15. -osis _____
16. -pexy _____

B. Provide the word root for each of the following terms.

1. germ or bud _____
2. red _____
3. blood _____
4. white _____
5. irregular _____
6. heat _____
7. clot _____

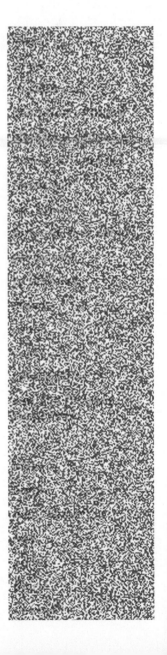

8. gland _____

9. exempt, immunity _____

10. clear water _____

11. grape-like clusters, *Staphylococcus* _____

12. disease _____

13. twisted or gnarled, *Streptococcus* _____

14. spleen _____

15. wart-like, thymus gland _____

16. bacter _____

17. mon _____

[anatomy and physiology overview]

You may recognize blood as the vital body fluid that transports substances necessary for survival, including oxygen, nutrients, enzymes, hormones, and waste materials. Recall from Chapter 10 that blood is transported within blood vessels of the cardiovascular system, and is propelled by the heart. As blood circulates, some of the fluid that passes through capillaries does not return to the bloodstream. Instead, this fluid finds its way into another series of vessels: the lymphatic vessels. They serve to channel the fluid, known as lymph, back into the cardiovascular system—a sort of "recycling system" of body fluid. Before reaching the cardiovascular system on its way toward the heart, the lymph passes through numerous lymphatic organs. The organs contain millions of white blood cells, which filter the lymph by removing bacteria and other unwanted materials. The white blood cells are the functional components of the immune response, which serves to defend us against viruses, bacteria, protozoa, fungi, and nonliving substances that can cause disease.

Blood

As you know, the blood transports materials throughout the body by way of the cardiovascular system. The blood is ideally suited to perform its transport function. It consists of a watery fluid and a combination of several types of formed elements that are suspended in the fluid (Figure 11.1::::).

The fluid part of blood is known as **plasma,** which is a Greek word that means *a shape or form.* Plasma is slightly more viscous (thicker) than water. It is thickened by the presence of dissolved proteins. The dissolved proteins also give plasma a slightly yellowish color. One of these proteins begins the blood clotting process, and is called **fibrinogen.** The removal of fibrinogen from a blood sample produces **serum,** which means *watery fluid or whey.* Serum is easier to store than whole blood since it does not clot, and is therefore a convenient blood replacement.

The formed elements that are carried along in the plasma current include three types: red blood cells, white blood cells, and platelets. **Red blood cells (RBCs),** or **erythrocytes,** are the most abundant cells, numbering about 4,200,000 to 6,200,000 per cc in adults. The cells are the shape of dinner plates, with a depression in the center (Figure 11.2::::). Each cell is filled to the brim with a specialized protein called **hemoglobin.** This abundant protein contains iron molecules, which enable the protein to bind to oxygen and carbon dioxide, providing an efficient vehicle for

[FYI]

Serum
The discovery of serum was made during World War I by a Red Cross team. It saved many lives on the battlefield because its availability as a blood substitute made storage and use under those conditions much more feasible.

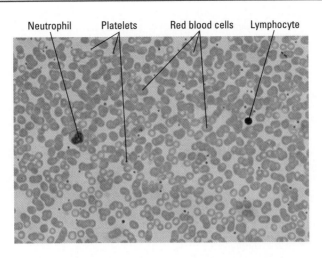

Neutrophil Platelets Red blood cells Lymphocyte

Figure 11.1 ⸬

A blood smear. The smear reveals representative cells from each formed element group: red blood cells, a platelet, and two white blood cells (shown is a lymphocyte and a neutrophil).

capturing and conveying these important gases. Along with other blood cell types, red blood cells are produced from precursor cells, called **stem cells,** in the red bone marrow during the process known as **hematopoiesis** (HEE mah toh poy EE siss). As a result, millions of small, disc-shaped red blood cells are released into the bloodstream each second (Figure 11.3⸬).

Red blood cells are usually a reddish mud-brick color when they are deprived of oxygen, and turn crimson red when their hemoglobin is saturated with oxygen. Because of the abundance of red blood cells in the blood, blood is red. Contrary to some beliefs, human blood is never blue or green in color.

Red blood cells contain specific proteins on their cell membranes that provide a unique "fingerprint" in each person. The combination of these proteins serves as the basis for blood typing. The most common blood type systems are the ABO system and the Rh system.

The second most abundant formed elements in blood are the **platelets,** or **thrombocytes.** Actually fragments from huge cells that break apart during development in the bone marrow, platelets are considerably smaller than red blood cells. They are also fewer in number, ranging between 150,000 and 360,000 cells per cc of blood. Platelets perform the role of preventing fluid loss that would otherwise follow an injury. They do this by releasing proteins in a process known as **coagulation,** which results in the formation of **blood clots** (Figure 11.4⸬).

The fewest cells in a normal sample of blood are the **white blood cells (WBCs),** or **leukocytes.** White blood cells perform an important role in protecting your body from infectious microorganisms and other foreign, unwanted materials. They are the

[**FYI**]

Hematopoiesis
Since red blood cells live only about 120 days and your body contains about 3 trillion of them, the red bone marrow must churn out about 10 billion cells every hour through the process of hematopoiesis just to keep pace.

[**thinking critically!**]

What would be the immediate result of a reduction in the rate of hematopoiesis?

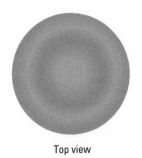

Top view

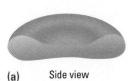

(a) Side view

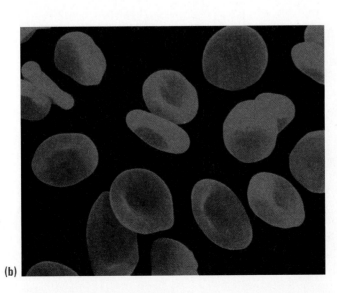

(b)

Figure 11.2 ⸬

Red blood cells.
(a) An illustration of red blood cell shape. Note the depression in the center. Red blood cells lack a nucleus; its loss during development produces the depression.
(b) Color-enhanced scanning electron mircograph of red blood cells.
Source: Custom Medical Stock Photo, Inc.

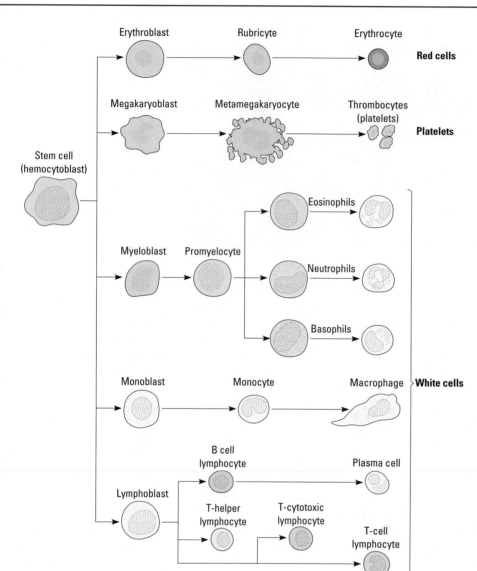

Figure 11.3 ::::

Hematopoiesis. All adult blood cells, shown at the right, arise from stem cells within the red bone marrow.

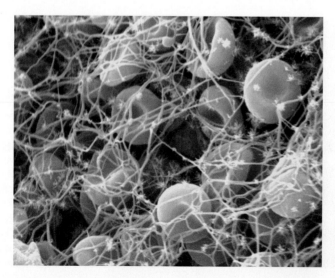

Figure 11.4 ::::

A blood clot. This photograph taken with an electron microscope shows the fibrin protein threads that have trapped red blood cells, forming the clot.

key players in the body's immune response. Several types of white blood cells exist in the blood, with names that are mostly based on their histological features. One group of white blood cells contain tiny, pebble-like objects in their cytoplasm, known as granules. They are called granulocytes, and include **eosinophils** (with granules that stain red), **basophils** (with granules that stain blue), and **neutrophils** (with granules that stain pink in a neutral stain). Of these, the neutrophils are the most abundant. They actively attack and "eat" bacteria and other unwanted cells. The cellular process of "eating" substances is known as **phagocytosis**. Eosinophils are also phagocytic, while basophils release substances that trigger an allergic reaction.

Another major group of white blood cells do not contain granules in their cytoplasm, and so are called agranulocytes. They include large cells called **monocytes,** and smaller cells called **lymphocytes.** The monocytes are aggressive "eaters" of bacteria and other unwanted cells, especially once they transform into macrophages, which literally means *large eater.* The lymphocytes provide you with the most powerful immune reactions of your body. Two types of lymphocytes exist: **T cells** and **B cells.** The T cells are capable of destroying unwanted substances by a variety of means, and are important in activating the B cells. The B cells produce the most effective weapon in the fight against infection: tiny molecules called **antibodies.** Antibodies attach to unwanted substances, called **antigens,** rendering them ineffective.

> **[thinking critically!]**
>
> What two cell types participate in the most powerful immune reactions of the body?

> **[FYI]**
>
> **Phagocytosis**
> Phagocytosis is a Latin word that literally means "condition of cell eating." Only certain cells are capable of this process, which involves the movement of the cell to the particle, surrounding the particle, ingesting the particle into a vacuole within the cytoplasm of the cell, and the secretion of acid and enzymes that digest the particle. Particles that are phagocytized include bacteria, dead or diseased cells, and other unwanted substances. A cell that performs this process is called a phagocyte.

The Lymphatic System

The lymphatic system is closely associated with the blood and its circulation, and includes components that play a key role in protecting the body against infection. Like the cardiovascular system, the lymphatic system also includes a series of vessels that carry a fluid through the body. However, there is no central pumping organ, and the fluid does not contain red blood cells or platelets. Also, the fluid, which is a yellowish liquid known as **lymph,** flows in a one-way direction toward the heart, rather than in a circulatory loop.

Lymph originates when interstitial fluid finds its way into microscopic **lymphatic capillaries.** The pressure that is generated by the incoming flow of lymph propels the fluid forward. From the capillaries, the lymph flows into larger **lymphatic vessels** (Figure 11.5▶), which are similar in structure to veins and often course alongside them. The lymphatic vessels deliver lymph into larger channels known as **lymphatic trunks,** which eventually merge with the subclavian veins near the heart. The largest lymphatic trunk is known as the **thoracic duct.** At the union with the veins, lymph flows into the blood circulation.

As lymph flows slowly through the lymphatic vessels, it is channeled through small, pea-sized organs called **lymph nodes** (Figure 11.6▶). The lymph nodes contain millions of white blood cells, which remove foreign materials from the lymph as it passes through them. Other organs of the lymphatic system include the **spleen,** located lateral to the stomach in the abdominal cavity; the **thymus gland** in the chest; three pairs of **tonsils** in the throat; and **lymphatic nodules** embedded within the wall of the large intestine. Each organ shares the characteristic of containing large quantities of white blood cells, which serve to protect against infection.

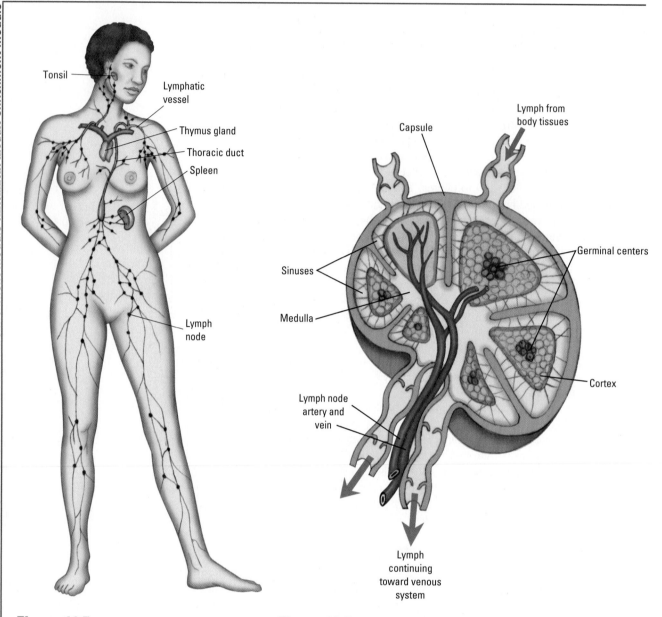

Figure 11.5 ::::

The lymphatic system. Lymphatic vessels, major lymph nodes, and lymphatic organs. The direction of lymph flow is toward the heart.

Figure 11.6 ::::

A lymph node. The interior of the node consists of white blood cells, which attack foreign substances as they pass through with the flow of lymph.

In summary, the two key functions of the lymphatic system are:

- recycling fluid back to the bloodstream
- fighting infection with the white blood cells it contains

We will discuss the latter role of the lymphatic system—the immune response—next.

Our bodies are continuously exposed to substances that can harm us, such as pathogenic (disease-causing) microorganisms, poisonous molecules, foreign particles, and even our own dying or diseased cells. Pathogenic microorganisms, or **pathogens,** are disease-causing agents that include viruses, bacteria, fungi, protozoans, and worm-like organisms (Figure 11.7::::). Pathogens may cause harm by physically destroying cells or by releasing poisonous substances that interfere with cell function. These substances are harmful molecules called **toxins.**

[thinking critically!]

Does lymph normally contain red blood cells?

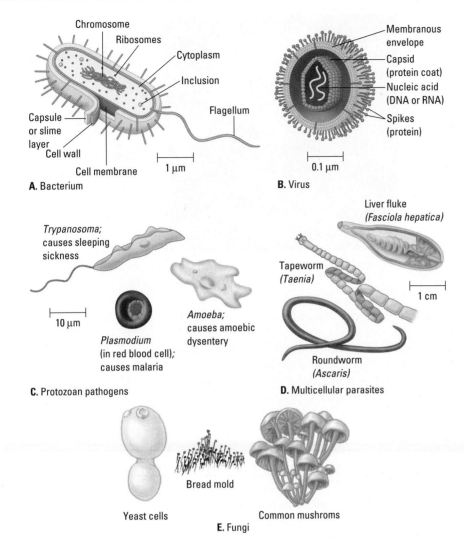

Figure 11.7 ::::

Pathogens.

(a) A bacterium is a single-celled organism that lacks a nucleus, and is much smaller than human cells.
(b) A virus consists of an outer protein coat that encloses RNA or DNA, and is smaller than bacteria.
(c) Protozoan pathogens are single-celled organisms that ingest other cells to survive.
(d) Multicellular parasites incude worm-like organisms, which ingest cells and the body's nutrients.
(e) Fungi are multicellular organisms that absorb nutrients and cells from the body for their survival.

Pathogens, toxins, and other harmful particles can severely disrupt your health if left unchecked by the body's defenses, leading to any one of a variety of immunological diseases. An immunological disease resulting from a pathogen is commonly called an **infection.** The mechanisms the body employs to battle infections are collectively called the **immune response.**

The immune response is a series of reactions against infections that are orchestrated by white blood cells. Initially, unwanted pathogens are attacked by white blood cells that are phagocytic, such as neutrophils, monocytes, and macrophages (Figure 11.8::::). The process occurs mainly within lymphatic organs, like the lymph nodes and spleen. It often results in inflammation, which produces local redness, swelling, heat, and pain at the site of the infection. However, in aggressive infections, phagocytosis cannot control the invaders alone. In these cases, lymphocytes are brought into the battle by chemical signals. During this process, the phagocytes produce chemical signals that result in the rapid growth of lymphocyte populations.

Two different mechanisms of lymphocyte activation take place during an infection. In the innate immune response, T cells become activated. Their activation results in the rapid growth of T cell populations within lymphatic tissue, resulting in the formation of specialized T cells that can destroy the pathogens effectively. One population group is called helper T cells, which are required for the activation of B cells during the second mechanism, known as the acquired immune response. During this reaction, B cells are transformed into larger cells, called plasma cells, which secrete enormous amounts of antibodies. Within days, the blood and lymph

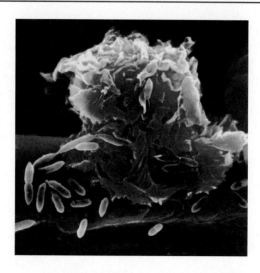

Figure 11.8 ::::

Macrophage. Enhanced color photograph from a scanning electron microscope of a phagocyte, in this case a macrophage, attacking and ingesting rod-shaped bacteria.

fill with these powerful molecules, which render the antigens ineffective and halt the infection.

Following an infection, certain lymphocytes remain in the lymph and bloodstream that can "remember" the pathogen's molecular signals. These "memory cells" provide you with immunity, which gives you additional protection because it enables your immune response to activate much more rapidly during subsequent exposures to the same antigen.

getting to the root of it | anatomy and physiology terms

Many of the anatomy and physiology terms are formed from roots that are used to construct the more complex medical terms of blood and the lymphatic system, including symptoms, diseases, and treatments. In this section, we will review the terms that describe the structure and function of blood and the lymphatic system *in relation to their word roots,* which are shown in **bold.**

Study the word roots and terms in this list and complete the review exercises that follow.

Word Root (Meaning)	Terms Formed from the Word Root (Pronunciation)	Definition
erythr (red)	**erythr**ocytes (ee RITH roh sights)	blood cells that specialize in transporting oxygen and carbon dioxide; also called **red blood cells (RBCs)**
hem, hemat (blood)	**hemat**opoiesis (HEE mah toh poy EE siss)	the process of blood cell formation within the red bone marrow
	hemoglobin (HEE moh GLOH binn)	an abundant protein in red blood cells that has a high bonding affinity for oxygen and carbon dioxide

Word Root (Meaning)	Terms Formed from the Word Root (Pronunciation)	Definition
immun (exempt; immunity)	**immun**ity (im YOO nih tee)	the status of being immune, or successfully resistant to infection
leuk (white)	**leuk**ocytes (LOO koh sights)	blood cells specializing in protecting the body from infection; also called **white blood cells (WBCs)**
lymph (clear water or fluid)	**lymph** (LIMF)	a yellowish fluid channeled through lymphatic capillaries, vessels, and trunks; similar in composition to plasma
	lymph nodes (LIMF nohdz)	pea-sized organs filled with white blood cells that filter out foreign materials from the lymph; nodes that are actively fighting an infection often swell, producing swollen glands that can be felt to aid in a diagnosis
	lymphatic capillaries (lim FAT ik)	microscopic, blind-ended vessels into which interstitial fluid diffuses; they are present in most tissues and often parallel blood capillaries
	lymphatic nodules (lim FAT ik NOD yoolz)	clusters of lymphatic tissue, composed of white blood cells that are embedded within the walls of the large intestine; also known as Peyer's patches
	lymphatic trunks (lim FAT ik)	large vessels that carry lymph to the subclavian veins near the heart
	lymphatic vessels (lim FAT ik)	vessels that carry lymph from lymphatic capillaries to lymphatic trunks; they are similar in structure to veins, and link lymph nodes to form a chain that leads toward the heart
	lymphocyte (LIMF oh sight)	a type of white blood cell that plays the primary role in conferring immunity and forms the bulk of lymphatic tissue; includes T cells and B cells
path (disease)	**path**ogen (PATH oh jenn)	any microorganism that causes disease, such as a virus, bacterium, protozoan, or fungus
thym (wart-like; thymus gland)	**thym**us gland (THIGH muss)	the soft organ located in the chest superior to the heart in which some white blood cells (known as "T" lymphocytes) become mature before entering the circulation; it is also part of the endocrine system (see Chapter 9)
tox (poison)	**tox**in (TAHKS inn)	a poisonous substance produced by a cell or tissue that affects various parts of the body

OTHER IMPORTANT TERMS
The terms in this table are related to the structure and function of the blood and the lymphatic system, but are not built from word roots.

antibody (AN tee bahd ee)	proteins released by activated B cells (known as **plasma cells**), which selectively bind to antigens during an immune response
antigen (AN tih jenn)	any foreign substance, usually a protein, against which an immune response is directed; abbreviation of "antibody-generating"
basophil (BAY soh fill)	a white blood cell that responds to antigens by releasing substances including histamine and serotonin, which cause inflammation
B cell	one of two types of lymphocytes, B cells respond to an infection by secreting antibodies which require activation by a helper T cell; B cell activity is called an **acquired immune response**
blood clot	a combination of protein fibers and trapped blood cells produced to slow or stop blood loss after an injury (see Figure 11.4)
coagulation (koh ahg yoo LAY shun)	the process of blood clot formation
fibrinogen (fye BRINN oh jenn)	a dissolved protein in blood that is the precursor for fibrin, which is the main protein component in a blood clot
neutrophil (NOO troh fill)	white blood cells that fight infection by phagocytizing unwanted foreign particles
phagocytosis (fag oh sigh TOH siss)	the process of "cell eating," during which a particle is ingested into the cell's cytoplasm and digested
plasma (PLAZ mah)	the liquid portion of blood
platelets (PLAYT lets)	cell fragments in the blood that facilitate the formation of blood clots; also called **thrombocytes** (THROM boh sights)
serum (SEE rum)	the fluid portion of plasma after fibrinogen has been removed
spleen	a soft, oblong organ located lateral and slightly posterior to the stomach in the abdominal cavity; it serves as a storage site for red blood cells and white blood cells
T cell	a type of lymphocyte that mounts an immune response that includes activation of other white blood cells, direct destruction of foreign cells, and establishment of a memory of the infection to create immunity; T cell activity is called an **innate immune response**
thoracic duct (thoh RASS ik)	the main lymphatic trunk, located alongside the aorta as it extends from the diaphragm behind the heart; it unites with the left subclavian vein, where it channels about three-quarters of the body's lymph drainage into the bloodstream
tonsils (TAHN sillz)	small, oval organs in the throat region that are filled with white blood cells that fight infection; they include one **pharyngeal tonsil** in the upper throat, which may be called **adenoids** when it swells with infection; two **palatine tonsils** near the union of the oral cavity (mouth) and throat; and two **lingual tonsils** at the back of the tongue

SELF QUIZ 11.2

SAY IT—SPELL IT!

Review the terms of blood and the lymphatic system by speaking the pronunciation out loud, then writing in the correct spelling of the term.

> **Success Hint:** Use the audio glossary on the CD and CW for additional help with pronunciation of these terms.

  1. HEE moh GLOH binn   _____

  2. LOO koh sights   _____

11.1 3. HEE mah toh poy EE siss   _____

  4. fye BRINN oh jenn   _____

  5. koh ahg yoo LAY shun   _____

  6. eh RITH roh sights   _____

  7. AN tih bahd ee   _____

  8. AN tih jenn   _____

  9. im YOO nih tee   _____

10. LIMF   _____

11. LIMF oh sight   _____

12. thoh RASS ik   _____

13. NOO troh fill   _____

MATCH IT!

Match the term on the left with the correct definition on the right.

_____ 1. erythrocytes	a. thrombocytes
_____ 2. leukocytes	b. occurs within the red bone marrow
_____ 3. platelets	c. the liquid portion of blood
_____ 4. plasma	d. oxygen-carrying protein in erythrocytes
_____ 5. serum	e. the process of blood clot formation
_____ 6. coagulation	f. the most abundant formed elements in blood
_____ 7. fibrinogen	g. protein fibers and trapped blood cells
_____ 8. hematopoiesis	h. form the basis of the immune response
_____ 9. blood clot	i. plasma without the clotting proteins
_____ 10. hemoglobin	j. precursor protein to fibrin
_____ 11. pharyngeal tonsils	k. a clear, yellowish fluid within lymphatic vessels
_____ 12. thoracic duct	l. pea-sized organs filled with leukocytes
_____ 13. spleen	m. called adenoids when they become inflamed
_____ 14. lymph	n. tubes that transport lymph
_____ 15. thymus gland	o. a soft organ lateral to the stomach
_____ 16. lymph nodes	p. the main collecting duct of lymphatic circulation
_____ 17. lymphatic vessels	q. located at the back of the throat
_____ 18. palatine tonsils	r. a soft gland located superior to the heart
_____ 19. phagocyte	s. any cell that ingests foreign particles

BREAK IT DOWN!

Analyze and separate each term into its word parts by labeling each word part using p = prefix, r = root, cv = combining vowel, and s = suffix.

1. erythrocyte   _____

2. leukocyte   _____

3. hematopoiesis   _____

4. lymphocyte   _____

FILL IT IN!

Fill in the blanks with the correct terms.

1. Red blood cells, or _____, form the major portion of blood. Other formed elements are white blood cells, or _____, and _____, or thrombocytes.

11.2   2. The liquid portion of blood is known as _____. When the clotting proteins, or _____, are removed from a sample of whole blood, the result is called _____.

3. The process of blood clot formation is known as _____.

11.3   4. The fluid within lymphatic vessels is known as _____. It originates from interstitial fluid that leaks into _____ _____, where its circulation toward the heart begins. The fluid passes through numerous pea-size organs called _____

11.4   _____ as it flows, where foreign material is filtered.

5. Most of the lymphatic circulation empties into the _____ _____ which is the main collecting trunk. This large vessel merges with the left subclavian vein, where lymph enters the blood circulation.

6. Organs of the lymphatic system include the _____, located lateral to the stomach, and the _____ _____, which is located above the heart. They also include _____ _____ in the intestinal walls, which are also called Peyer's

11.5   patches. The three pairs of _____ in the mouth and throat are also lymphatic organs.

7. An _____ occurs when a pathogen invades the body. It causes an initial response by cells that ingest foreign particles, called _____, which include _____ and neutrophils. If the infection persists, other white blood cells often housed within lymph nodes, known as

11.6   _____, will engage. This is a common _____ response.

8. Lymphocytes include two main types, _____

   and _____. Once the foreign substances, or

   _____, have been identified, the T cells destroy them directly,

   signal other white blood cells to the site, and activate B cells. Once activated,

   B cells produce special proteins called _____, which further

   deactivate the invaders.

9. Inflammation is a response to an infection that produces local swelling in an

   effort to increase the migration of white blood cells to the site. It occurs when

   11.7 _____ release substances including histamine and serotonin.

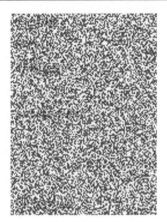

[medical terms of

blood and the lymphatic system]

Because blood is a vital body fluid, making sure it is healthy is an important part of health management. Like any other tissue, blood can experience disease from any one of several sources, including inherited abnormalities, infection, or tumor development. The loss of blood itself can become a life-threatening situation if intervention is not provided in time. Blood also serves as an important diagnostic tool. Because blood can be conveniently removed from a blood vessel and analyzed, it is an important avenue for testing body chemistry during a diagnostic evaluation.

The general field of medicine focusing on blood-related disease is known as **hematology.** You should recognize this term as a word constructed of the following parts:

hemat/o/logy

in which the word root *hemat* means *blood* from its Greek derivative *haima,* and the suffix -logy means study of. A physician specializing in the treatment of disease associated with the blood is called a **hematologist,** or alternatively, a **hematopathologist.**

You have already learned that the lymphatic system has dual functions: the recycling of fluid to the bloodstream, and the battle against infection. A disease of the lymphatic system may affect either function. Also, because the lymphatic system components are distributed throughout the body, a disease affecting this system can spread quickly to surrounding tissues, and often through the entire body. In fact, metastasizing cancer cells often use the low-pressure current of lymph to travel from one area of the body to another. In addition to tumors, lymphatic disease also includes infections that overwhelm the immune response, and inherited conditions that result in deficiencies.

The understanding of infectious diseases has been growing rapidly during the past 50 years, due mainly to new information coming from research labs. The field of medicine that focuses on these diseases is generally called **immunology** or, at some hospitals, **infectious diseases.**

The term immunology refers to the body's ability to defend against infection, and includes a variety of mechanisms. It is a constructed word, written as

immun/o/logy

where *immun* is a word root derived from the Latin word *immunis,* which means *exempt,* and -logy is the often-used suffix that means *a study of.* Its sub-disciplines include **virology** (study of viruses), **bacteriology** (study of bacteria), and **toxicology** (study of toxins).

The most important discovery in this field, and perhaps of any medical field, was made when Sir Alexander Fleming first reported the effects of the *Penicillium* mold on bacterial cultures. Fleming's work led to the discovery that bacterial infections could be treated with substances produced by their natural enemies, the fungi. When this was understood and **antibiotics** became available to patients suffering from bacterial infections of many types, millions of lives were saved. Although some bacteria have been able to develop resistance to antibiotics, this form of therapy remains our most effective weapon against bacterial infections.

[FYI]

Discovery of Antibiotics

The first antibiotic was discovered in 1926 by Sir Alexander Fleming, who found that a common bread mold (a fungus) could produce toxins capable of killing bacterial colonies. The *Penicillium* mold produces an antibacterial toxin that is now known as penicillin. In time, the fungal toxins were proven to be effective against many strains of bacteria, and their use as antibiotics have been hailed as the single most important treatment against bacterial infections ever.

Because many bacteria mutate and develop a resistance to antibiotics, the current challenge is to find new antibiotic varieties and techniques that can counter antibiotic resistance.

[thinking critically!]

If you are suffering from a virus, such as influenza, in combination with a secondary infection, and a physician writes you a prescription for antibiotics, what does that tell you about the secondary infection?

Unfortunately, bactericidal antibiotics have no effect upon viruses, another common source of infection. More recently, research on **HIV** (the virus that causes AIDS) has provided immunologists with a new battery of weapons to use against viral infections. The treatments for viral infections include a "cocktail," or mixture, of chemicals that interfere with the virus's ability to infect a cell or to reproduce once viruses have gained entry into a cell.

let's construct terms!

In this section, we will assemble all of the word parts to construct medical terminology related to blood and the lymphatic system. Abbreviations are used to indicate each word part: **p** = prefix, **r** = root, **cv** = combining vowel, and **s** = suffix. Note that some terms are not constructed from word parts, but they are included here to expand your vocabulary.

The medical terms of blood and the lymphatic system are listed in the following three sections:

- Symptoms and Signs
- Diseases and Disorders
- Treatments, Procedures, and Devices

Each section is followed by review exercises. Study the lists in these tables and complete the review exercises that follow.

Symptoms and Signs

WORD PARTS (WHEN APPLICABLE)			TERM	DEFINITION
Part	**Type**	**Meaning**		
an- iso- cyt -osis	p p r s	without equal cell condition of	**anisocytosis** (an EYE soh sigh TOH siss)	presence of red blood cells of unequal size
bacter -emia	r s	bacteria condition of blood	**bacteremia** (bak teer EE mee ah)	presence of bacteria in the bloodstream
erythr/o -penia	r/cv s	red abnormal reduction in number	**erythropenia** (ee RITH row PEE nee ah)	abnormally reduced number of red blood cells
hem/o -lysis	r/cv s	blood dissolve	**hemolysis** (hee MALL ih siss)	rupture of the red blood cell membrane
hem/o -rrhag[e]	r/cv s	blood bleeding	**hemorrhage** (HEM eh rihj)	loss of blood from the circulation
macro- cyt -osis	p r s	large cell condition of	**macrocytosis** (MAK roh sigh TOH siss)	abnormally large-sized red blood cells
poikil/o cyt -osis	r/cv r s	irregular cell condition of	**poikilocytosis** (POY kih loh sigh TOH siss)	large, irregularly shaped red blood cells
poly- cyt -hemia	p r s	many cell condition of blood	**polycythemia** (pall ee sigh THEE mee ah)	abnormal increase in the number of erythrocytes in the blood
splen/o megal -y	r/cv r s	spleen abnormally large process of	**splenomegaly** (splee noh MEG ah lee)	abnormal enlargement of the spleen
tox -emia	r s	poison condition of blood	**toxemia** (tahk SEE mee ah)	presence of toxins in the bloodstream

SELF QUIZ 11.3

SAY IT—SPELL IT!

Review the terms of blood and the lymphatic system by speaking the phonetic pronunciation guides out loud, then writing in the correct spelling of the term.

1. bak teer EE mee ah _____

2. an EYE soh sigh TOH siss _____

3. ee RITH row PEE nee ah _____

4. splee noh MEG ah lee _____

5. tahk SEE mee ah _____

6. MAK roh sigh TOH siss _____

7. POY kih loh sigh TOH siss _____

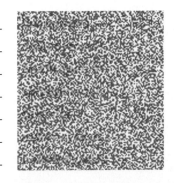

MATCH IT!

Match the term on the left with the correct definition on the right.

_____1. anisocytosis   a. presence of bacteria in the blood

_____2. bacteremia   b. abnormally reduced number of erythrocytes

_____3. splenomegaly   c. abnormally large red blood cells

11.8 _____4. toxemia   d. presence of red blood cells of unequal size

_____5. erythropenia   e. abnormal increase in red blood cells

_____6. macrocytosis   f. large, irregularly shaped red blood cells

_____7. poikilocytosis   g. presence of toxins in the blood

_____8. polycythemia   h. abnormal enlargement of the spleen

BREAK IT DOWN!

Analyze and separate each term into its word parts by labeling each word part using p = prefix, r = root, cv = combining vowel, and s = suffix.

1. erythropenia   _____

2. toxemia   _____

3. poikilocytosis   _____

4. splenomegaly   _____

5. polycythemia   _____

WORD BUILDING

Construct or recall medical terms from the following meanings.

1. The presence of bacteria in the blood   _____

2. Abnormal enlargement of the spleen   _____

3. Red blood cells that are abnormally large   _____

4. The presence of toxins in the blood   _____

5. Too many red blood cells in the blood   _____

6. Loss of blood, or bleeding   _____

7. The rupture of red blood cells   _____

8. Too few red blood cells in the blood   _____

FILL IT IN!

Fill in the blanks with the correct terms.

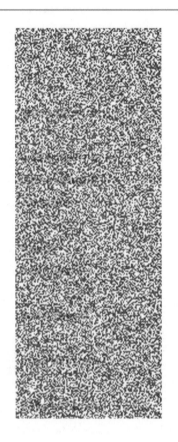

1. One form of anemia produces red blood cells that are of different shapes, a sign called _____, which leads to painful thrombosis and emboli. Anemia may also result from a reduced number of red blood cells, or

 ✛ 11.9   _____, which can be caused by the loss of blood from the circulation, or _____.

2. _____ is a series of signs and symptoms arising from infections that are caused by powerful molecules released by pathogens or

 ✛ 11.10   _____, which is the Greek word for poison.

3. In the symptom called _____, red blood cell membranes break open to result in the death of the cells. This symptom may accompany the presence of bacteria in the blood, or _____.

4. A sign in which red blood cells are abnormally large is an indication of disease, and is called _____. Another sign that indicates disease is the presence of too many red blood cells in the blood, known as

 ✛ 11.11   _____, which may increase blood thickness, or viscosity.

Diseases and Disorders

WORD PARTS (WHEN APPLICABLE)			TERM	DEFINITION
Part	Type	Meaning		
			AIDS (AYDZ)	the acronym for **acquired immune deficiency syndrome**, AIDS is caused by the human immunodeficiency virus (**HIV**), which disables the immune response by destroying mainly helper T cells (needed for activation of B cells); the loss of immune function allows opportunistic infections to proliferate, and eventually cause death
			allergy (AL er jee)	a response to an allergen, which is an antigen that produces a hypersensitivity reaction that includes immediate inflammation but does not elicit other immune responses; allergies are of many types, the most common of which are allergic rhinitis (hay fever) that affects the mucous membranes of the nasal cavity and throat, and allergic dermatitis, which affects the skin where it has made contact with the allergen (Figure 11.9::::)
ana-	p	up, toward	**anaphylaxis** (AN ah fih LAK siss)	an immediate reaction to an antigen that includes rapid inflammation and system-wide smooth muscle contractions
-phylaxis	s	protection		

WORD PARTS (WHEN APPLICABLE)			TERM	DEFINITION
Part	**Type**	**Meaning**		

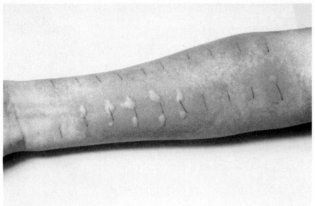

Figure 11.9 ::::

Results from an allergy skin test. The arm of the patient shows a reaction against the injected allergen, which has caused inflammation (swelling, redness, heat, and pain).
Source: Southern Illinois University/Photo Researchers, Inc.

WORD PARTS			TERM	DEFINITION
an- -emia	p s	without condition of blood	**anemia** (ah NEE mee ah)	a reduced ability of red blood cells to deliver oxygen to tissues resulting from a reduction of circulating RBCs, the amount of hemoglobin, or the volume of RBCs; common forms of anemia include **aplastic anemia, iron deficiency anemia, sickle cell anemia,** and **pernicious anemia**
a- -plastic	p s	without capable of being formed	**aplastic anemia** (ay PLASS tik ah NEE mee ah)	anemia characterized by the failure of red bone marrow to produce red blood cells
aut/o immun[e]	r/cv r	self exempt	**autoimmune disorder** (aw toh im YOON)	any one of several diseases that are caused by a person's own immune response attacking otherwise healthy tissues, including rheumatoid arthritis, systemic lupus erythematosus, and multiple sclerosis
			botulism (BAHT yoo lizm)	a form of poisoning caused by the ingestion of food contaminated with the toxin produced by the bacterium *Clostridium botulinum*
			diphtheria (diff THEER ee ah)	a disease caused by a bacterium and its toxin, resulting in inflammation of mucous membranes, primarily in the mouth and throat (Figure 11.10::::)

[FYI]

Diphtheria

Before the availability of antibiotics, diphtheria was a life-threatening scourge among children, killing thousands each year within the United States. It is caused by the toxins produced by the bacterium *Corynebacterium diphtheriae*, which produces inflammation of the throat and the formation of a thick secretion. Because the leather-like surface of the throat characterizes this disease, it was named after the Greek word for leather, *diphthera*.

WORD PARTS (WHEN APPLICABLE)			TERM	DEFINITION
Part	Type	Meaning		

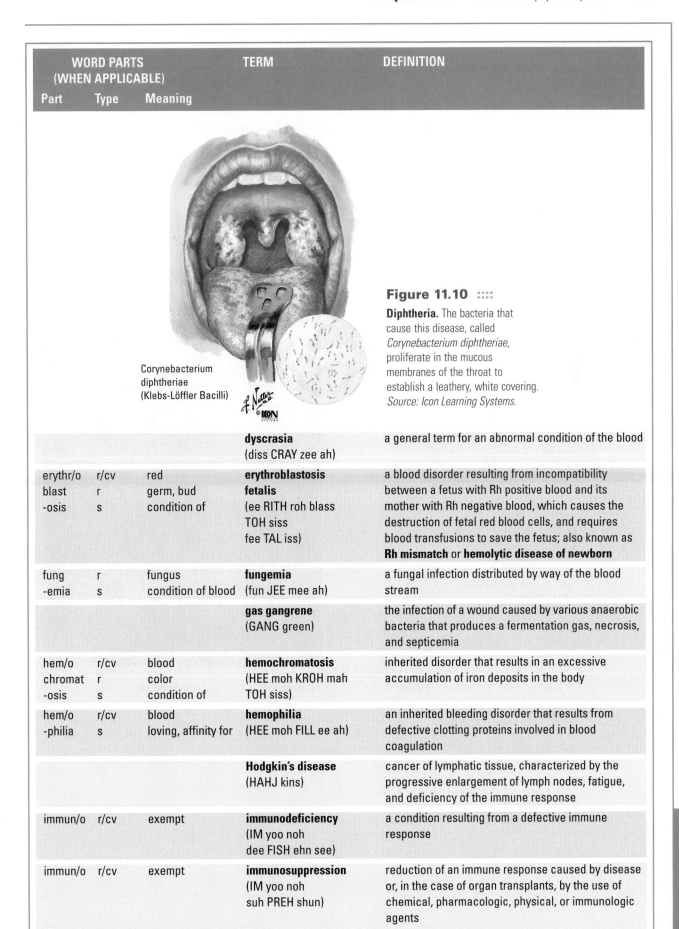

Corynebacterium diphtheriae (Klebs-Löffler Bacilli)

Figure 11.10

Diphtheria. The bacteria that cause this disease, called *Corynebacterium diphtheriae*, proliferate in the mucous membranes of the throat to establish a leathery, white covering. *Source: Icon Learning Systems.*

			dyscrasia (diss CRAY zee ah)	a general term for an abnormal condition of the blood
erythr/o blast -osis	r/cv r s	red germ, bud condition of	**erythroblastosis fetalis** (ee RITH roh blass TOH siss fee TAL iss)	a blood disorder resulting from incompatibility between a fetus with Rh positive blood and its mother with Rh negative blood, which causes the destruction of fetal red blood cells, and requires blood transfusions to save the fetus; also known as **Rh mismatch** or **hemolytic disease of newborn**
fung -emia	r s	fungus condition of blood	**fungemia** (fun JEE mee ah)	a fungal infection distributed by way of the blood stream
			gas gangrene (GANG green)	the infection of a wound caused by various anaerobic bacteria that produces a fermentation gas, necrosis, and septicemia
hem/o chromat -osis	r/cv r s	blood color condition of	**hemochromatosis** (HEE moh KROH mah TOH siss)	inherited disorder that results in an excessive accumulation of iron deposits in the body
hem/o -philia	r/cv s	blood loving, affinity for	**hemophilia** (HEE moh FILL ee ah)	an inherited bleeding disorder that results from defective clotting proteins involved in blood coagulation
			Hodgkin's disease (HAHJ kins)	cancer of lymphatic tissue, characterized by the progressive enlargement of lymph nodes, fatigue, and deficiency of the immune response
immun/o	r/cv	exempt	**immunodeficiency** (IM yoo noh dee FISH ehn see)	a condition resulting from a defective immune response
immun/o	r/cv	exempt	**immunosuppression** (IM yoo noh suh PREH shun)	reduction of an immune response caused by disease or, in the case of organ transplants, by the use of chemical, pharmacologic, physical, or immunologic agents

WORD PARTS (WHEN APPLICABLE)			TERM	DEFINITION
Part	**Type**	**Meaning**		
			infection (in FEK shun)	a multiplication of disease-causing microorganisms (Figure 11.11⣿)
			inflammation (in flah MAY shun)	a swelling of body tissue caused by the movement of plasma into the extracellular space to produce **edema** (eh DEE mah), or fluid accumulation in tissue; symptoms include swelling, redness, heat, and pain (Figure 11.12⣿)

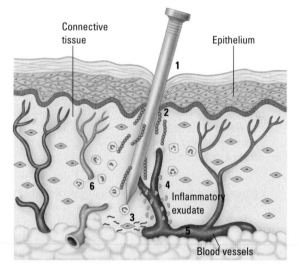

1. Dirty nail punctures skin.
2. Bacteria enter and multiply.
3. Injured cells release histamine.
4. Blood vessels dilate and become permeable, releasing inflammatory exudate.
5. Blood flow to the damaged site increases.
6. Neutrophils (polymorph) move toward bacteria (chemotaxis) and destroy them (phagocytosis).

Figure 11.11 ⣿ **Reaction against infection.**

Pathogens invade the body, in this example, by a pierce through the skin. The result of invasion is the proliferation of pathogens within body tissues, or infection. The body responds to the infection by mounting an attack that begins with inflammation, which promotes the movement of phagocytes to the site of the infection. Phagocytes localize the pathogens, and destroy them by phagocytosis. Pus is released, which is composed of dead bacteria and phagocytes.

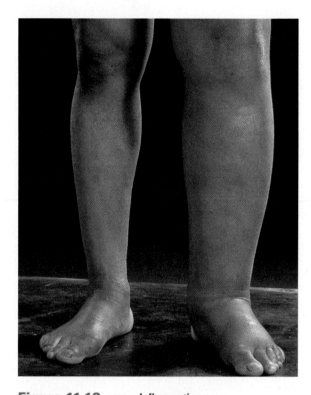

Figure 11.12 ⣿ **Inflammation.**

Inflammation is characterized by the presence of swelling, redness, heat, and pain. Swelling is caused by the accumulation of fluid in tissue spaces, and is also known as edema. In this photograph, the patient exhibits severe edema of the leg. *Source: MSNB/Custom Medical Stock Photo, Inc.*

WORD PARTS (WHEN APPLICABLE)			TERM	DEFINITION
Part	Type	Meaning		
			influenza (in floo EHN zah)	a viral disease characterized by a temporary inflammation of mucous membranes and fever. Commonly called "the flu," it is highly contagious and the virus is capable of mutating to escape detection by B and T memory cells
an- -emia	p s	without condition of blood	**iron deficiency anemia** (EYE ern dee FIH shen see ah NEE mee ah)	anemia that is caused by a lack of iron, which results in smaller red blood cells containing deficient levels of hemoglobin
leuk -emia	r s	white condition of blood	**leukemia** (loo KEE mee ah)	cancer of the red bone marrow, which is the blood-forming tissue (Figure 11.13)
lymph aden -itis	r r s	clear water or fluid gland inflammation	**lymphadenitis** (limm fad eh NYE tiss)	inflammation of the lymph nodes
lymph aden/o path -y	r r/cv r s	clear water or fluid gland disease process of	**lymphadenopathy** (limm FAD eh NOPP ah thee)	literally, disease of the lymph nodes; this general term is often applied to a syndrome, **lymphadenopathy syndrome** (**LAS**), which is a persistent swelling of the lymph nodes that often precedes the onset of AIDS
lymph -oma	r s	clear water or fluid tumor	**lymphoma** (limm FOH mah)	a tumor originating in lymphatic tissue
			malaria (mah LAIR ee ah)	a disease caused by a parasitic protozoan that infects red blood cells, which is carried by *Anopheles* mosquitoes; it is characterized by periodic fevers and fatigue (Figure 11.14)

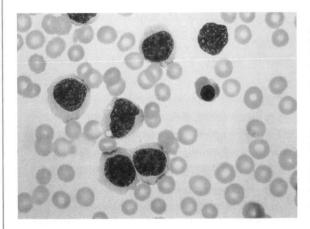

Figure 11.13 :::: **Leukemia.**

A blood smear from a patient suffering from leukemia demonstrates the abundance of enlarged, nonfunctional leukocytes that serve as a diagnostic characteristic of this disease.

Source: Getty Images, Inc./Stone Allstock

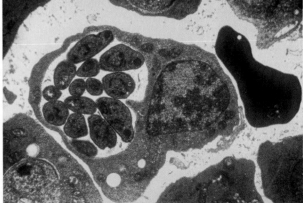

Figure 11.14 :::: **Malaria.**

Photograph of an infected white blood cell that has been sectioned, revealing the presence of malarial parasites (*Plasmodium*) within the cells.

Source: Photo Researchers, Inc.

WORD PARTS (WHEN APPLICABLE)			TERM	DEFINITION
Part	Type	Meaning		

Malaria
The word malaria is derived from combining the Italian words for bad, *mal,* with that of air, *aria.* It was first used during the Middle Ages, when malaria was believed to have been caused by breathing bad air near swamplands. We now know that this dreaded disease is caused by the bite of an *Anopheles* mosquito carrying the bacterium known as *Plasmodium.* Approximately 200,000 people die of this disease each year, mainly in tropical regions where the mosquitos flourish.

mon/o	r/cv	one	**mononucleosis**	a viral disease characterized by enlarged lymph
nucle	r	kernel	(MAHN oh noo	nodes, atypical lymphocytes, sore throat,
-osis	s	condition of	klee OH siss)	(pharyngitis), fever and fatigue (Figure 11.15)

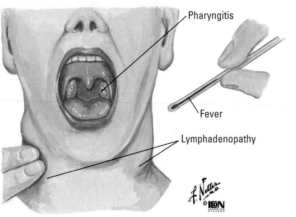

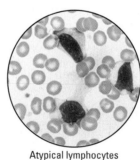
Atypical lymphocytes

Figure 11.15

Mononucleosis. Infectious mononucleosis is caused by the Epstein-Barr virus, and produces the symptoms of swollen palatine tonsils (pharyngitis), swollen cervical lymph nodes (lymphadenopathy), high fever, and a blood sample that reveals atypical lymphocytes.
Source: Icon Learning Systems.

myel/o	r/cv	bone marrow	**myelodysplasia**	bone marrow disorder characterized by the
dys-	p	bad, abnormal	(MY eh loh diss	proliferation of abnormal stem cells, which usually
plas	r	form	PLAY zee ah)	develops into a form of leukemia
-ia	s	condition of		
			nosocomial infections	a disorder, usually bacterial infections, contracted
			(noh soh KOH mee al	during a hospital stay; often due to antibiotic-
			in FEK shunz)	resistant strains of *Staphylococcus*
pernicious		destructive	**pernicious anemia**	anemia caused by an inadequate supply of folic acid
an-	p	without	(per NISH uss	(vitamin B$_{12}$), resulting in red blood cells that are
-emia	s	condition of blood	ah NEE mee ah)	large, varied in shape, and reduced in number
			plague	any infectious disease of wide prevalence or
			(PLAYG)	excessive mortality; it also refers specifically to an acute infectious disease caused by the bacterium *Yersinia pestis,* and characterized by high fever, skin eruptions, internal hemorrhage, and pneumonia; also called bubonic (boo BAHN ik) plague

WORD PARTS (WHEN APPLICABLE)			TERM	DEFINITION
Part	Type	Meaning		
			rabies (RAY beez)	a bacterial infection spread from the mouth of an infected animal, usually by way of a bite; the bacterium produces a neurotoxin that acts on the central nervous system, and is highly fatal
septic -emia	r s	putrefying condition of blood	**septicemia** (sep tih SEE mee ah)	a systemic disease caused by the presence of bacteria and their toxins in the circulating blood; a person suffering from this is referred to as "septic"
an- -emia	p s	without condition of blood	**sickle cell anemia** (SIH kl SELL ah NEE mee ah)	an inherited, chronic anemia that is characterized by defective hemoglobin that causes red blood cells to become misshapen (sickle-shaped), resulting in drowsiness, leg ulcerations, fever, joint and abdominal pain, and thrombosis (Figure 11.16)

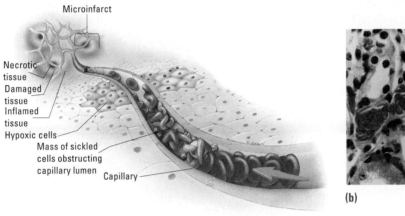

(a)

(b)

Figure 11.16

Sickle cell anemia.
(a) The presence of sickle-shaped red blood cells causes blockages within blood vessels, leading to reduced blood flow to tissues and, in some cases, necrosis (cell death). The inflammation and necrosis causes severe pain.
(b) Photograph of a section through a kidney, showing sickled cells that are clumped together due to their shape and sticky coat, causing a blockage.

			TERM	DEFINITION
			staphylococcemia (STAFF ih loh KOK SEE mee ah)	the presence of *Staphylococci* bacteria in the blood, which is the literal meaning of the term; commonly called a staph infection, it is a frequent complication to normal healing and also the most common cause of food poisoning, skin inflammation, osteomyelitus, and nosocomial infections
			tetanus (TETT ah nuss)	a disease caused by a powerful neurotoxin released by the common bacterium *Clostridium tetani;* the toxin acts upon the central nervous system to cause convulsions and paralysis
thym -oma	r s	wart-like; thymus gland tumor	**thymoma** (thigh MOH mah)	a tumor originating in the thymus gland

disease focus | HIV Mode of Infection

Most viruses have a very simple structure: a single coat of protein surrounds a small package of genetic material, ribonucleic acid (RNA) (or DNA for some viruses). Certain viruses, such as HIV, contain an added layer of fat molecules around the protein with receptor molecules that project outward. This structure is perfectly designed to allow viruses to do what they do: combine with a host cell using their receptor molecules as "landing gear," and inject virus RNA inside the host cell. Once within the host cell, the viral RNA redirects cell functions to make copies of the virus. Soon after large numbers of new viruses have been produced, they leave the host cell to infect other cells. The host cell is damaged or killed by the mass exodus of virus particles, or it is killed by the body's own antiviral immune response. In the case of HIV, viral particles may lie dormant for years. Once activated, they are capable of killing many types of cells, among them helper T cells.

HIV appears to prefer helper T cells to other cells in the body, although it attacks other T cells and monocytes as well (Figure 11.17::::). Helper T cells are the preferred victims because of the presence of receptors, known as CD-4 receptors, on the helper T cell membranes, with which HIV is able to form a chemical bond and gain entry into the cell. When HIV enters the body, its usual pattern is to infest helper T cells initially, which causes flu-like symptoms (fever, headache, fatigue, and swollen glands) that last for several weeks. The symptoms are caused by the body's immune response in an effort to "clear" the virus from the body. But in most documented cases, the body is unable to completely eliminate the virus. The surviving HIV particles enter a period of dormancy in which there is no active reproduction for about six months, although this time period is highly variable. Following the dormant phase, HIV begins its reproductive phase, invading primarily

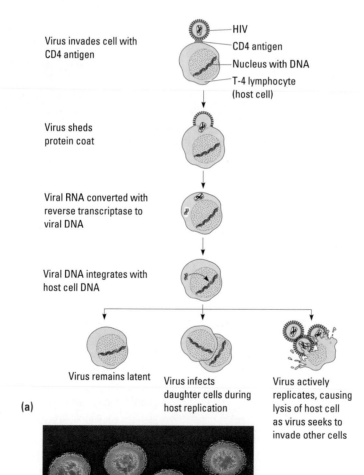

Virus invades cell with CD4 antigen

HIV
CD4 antigen
Nucleus with DNA
T-4 lymphocyte (host cell)

Virus sheds protein coat

Viral RNA converted with reverse transcriptase to viral DNA

Viral DNA integrates with host cell DNA

Virus remains latent

Virus infects daughter cells during host replication

Virus actively replicates, causing lysis of host cell as virus seeks to invade other cells

(a)

(b)

Figure 11.17 ::::

HIV, the virus that causes AIDS.
(a) HIV mode of infection, which targets helper T cells due to the presence of CD-4 receptors.
(b) Color enhanced photograph of HIV particles budding from a helper T cell, ready to infect additional helper T cells.
Source: Photo Researchers, Inc.

helper T cells and destroying them to produce new viruses. Although the immune response is mounted against the virus, in time the virus is able to decimate helper T cells. Eventually, HIV's reproductive phase destroys 60 to 90 percent of the helper T cells in the body. The result of helper T cell destruction is a suppression of acquired immunity, followed by the rise of opportunistic infections.

The opportunistic infections that usually arise as helper T cell populations are reduced during HIV infection have been documented and studied during the past 20 years. They include a very long list of infectious diseases, the most deadly of which are a fungal lung infection caused by *Pneumocystis carinii* that produces **pneumonia**, a primary lymphoma of the brain, and **tuberculosis**. Other less deadly diseases that are nonetheless painful and difficult to treat include a skin cancer called **Kaposi's sarcoma**, a protozoan infection called **toxoplasmosis**, **anorexia** caused by bacterial infection of the digestive tract, **squamous cell carcinoma**, infection by **Herpes** viruses types 1 and 2, and **candidiasis** (yeast infections caused by *Candida albicans*).

SELF QUIZ 11.4

SAY IT—SPELL IT!

Review the terms of blood and the lymphatic system by speaking the phonetic pronunciation guides out loud, then writing in the correct spelling of the term.

1. AL er jee _____
2. AN ah fih LAK siss _____
3. ay PLASS tik ah NEE mee ah _____
4. diff THEER ee ah _____
5. ee RITH roh blass TOH siss fee TAL iss _____
6. fun JEE mee ah _____
11.12 7. HEE moh FILL ee ah _____
8. HEE moh KROH mah TOH siss _____
9. IM yoo noh dee FISH ehn see _____
10. limm fad eh NYE tiss _____
11. limm FAD eh NOPP ah thee _____
12. limm FOH mah _____
13. loo KEE mee ah _____
14. MY eh loh diss PLAY zee ah _____
15. MAHN oh noo klee OH siss _____
16. aw toh im YOON _____
17. sep tih SEE mee ah _____
18. STAFF ih loh kok SEE mee ah _____
19. thigh MOH mah _____

MATCH IT!

Match the term on the left with the correct definition on the right.

_____ 1. sickle cell anemia   a. cancer of red bone marrow

_____ 2. erythroblastosis fetalis   b. anemia resulting from defective hemoglobin

_____ 3. aplastic anemia   c. inherited bleeding disorder

_____ 4. pernicious anemia   d. condition of abnormally small erythrocytes

_____ 5. hemochromatosis   e. proliferation of abnormal stem cells in bone marrow

_____ 6. hemophilia   f. reduced levels of RBCs due to a lack of folic acid

_____ 7. leukemia   g. result of incompatible blood between mother and baby

_____ 8. myelodysplasia   h. cancer of lymph nodes

_____ 9. septicemia   i. anemia caused by insufficiency of red bone marrow

_____10. thymoma   j. systemic bacterial infection

_____11. lymphadenitis   k. results in excessive iron deposits in the body

_____12. lymphoma   l. generalized disease of lymphatic tissue

_____13. lymphadenopathy   m. inflammation of lymph nodes

_____14. Hodgkin's disease   n. an immediate reaction that includes inflammation

_____15. mononucleosis   o. tumor originating in lymphatic tissue

_____16. anaphylaxis   p. viral disease that causes lymphadenitis

_____17. botulism   q. tumor originating in the thymus gland

_____18. fungemia   r. reduction of the immune response

_____19. immunodeficiency   s. presence of fungi in the blood

_____20. autoimmune   t. caused by *Clostridium botulinum*

_____21. immunosuppression   u. any infectious disease of wide prevalence

_____22. plague   v. results from a defective immune response

BREAK IT DOWN!

Analyze and separate each term into its word parts by labeling each word part using p = prefix, r = root, cv = combining vowel, and s = suffix.

1. leukemia   _____

2. hemophilia   _____

3. fungemia   _____

4. erythroblastosis   _____

11.13 5. mononucleosis _____

6. hemochromatosis _____

7. myelodysplasia _____

8. thymoma _____

FILL IT IN!

Fill in the blanks with the correct terms.

11.14 1. The general condition of _____ is an oxygen deficiency of blood.
There are four main types: _____ anemia occurs when the red

11.15 bone marrow fails to produce normal cells; _____
_____ occurs when there is an insufficient volume of
hemoglobin; _____ anemia results when there is a deficiency
of _____ _____ (vitamin B_{12}) in the diet; and a
chronic inherited form that results in misshapen cells called
_____ _____ anemia.

11.16 2. In _____ too many red blood cells are produced.

3. A generalized condition of blood is known as _____. One form
of this disease is an inherited condition in which iron deposits form, called
_____. In another inherited condition, hemostasis (the
stoppage of bleeding) is reduced. This disease is known as
_____. Finally, another blood condition arises due to bacterial

11.17 infection, and is known as _____.

4. An immunological response known as _____ may result from
exposure to an antigen that produces an allergic cascade of inflammation and
smooth muscle contractions. This response is an extreme form of
_____.

5. A disorder that results when the body's own immune response is turned against
otherwise healthy cells is called an _____ disorder.

6. The presence of *Staphylococci* bacteria in the blood, or _____,

11.18 is commonly known as a _____ infection. Another type of
bacterial infection that complicates healing is known as
_____ _____.

7. _____ _____ is a cancer of the lymph nodes,
with symptoms that include fatigue, enlargement of the lymph nodes, and a
reduction in the immune response. A _____ is a tumor
originating in the thymus gland, while a _____ originates in
lymphatic tissue in general.

8. _____ is caused by a virus, with symptoms that include fatigue, sore throat, and lymphadenitis.

9. Examples of toxemia include _____, which is often transmitted by an animal bite; _____, which causes muscular convulsions and paralysis; _____, which is caused by the bacterium *Clostridium botulinum;* and _____, in which the mucous membranes are targeted. Each of these conditions can be successfully treated by administering antibiotics.

10. The syndrome that is caused by HIV is known as _____ (acronym). HIV is a retrovirus that mutates frequently, making a cure very difficult to achieve. The common course of treatment is to administer combination therapy, or antiretroviral therapy, while treating the opportunistic infections that arise.

Treatments, Procedures, and Devices

WORD PARTS (WHEN APPLICABLE)			TERM	DEFINITION
Part	Type	Meaning		
anti- bi/o -tic	p r/cv s	against life pertaining to	**antibiotic** (AN tee bye OTT ik)	a therapeutic treatment in which a substance with known toxicity to bacteria, which may be obtained from a mold (fungus) or from other bacteria, is administered; it is effective only against bacteria, many types of which are capable developing resistance, especially when antibiotics are not administered properly
			anticoagulant (AN tye koh AG yoo lant)	a chemical agent that reduces the clotting process
			antiretroviral therapy (AN tye REH troh VYE ral THAIR ah pee)	application of drugs to battle against a class of viruses that tend to mutate quickly, known as retroviruses, of which HIV is a member; also known as combination therapy, the drugs form a cocktail that includes nucleotide analog reverse transcriptase inhibitors and protease inhibitors, all of which block HIV replication by a variety of means
			attenuation (ah TEN yoo AY shun)	a process in which pathogens are rendered less virulent, prior to their incorporation into a vaccine preparation
aut/o -log -ous	r/cv s s	self study pertaining to	**autologous transfusion** (aw TALL oh guss trans FYOO zhun)	transfusion of blood donated by a patient for personal use; this is a common procedure before a surgery to avoid potential incompatibility or contamination
			blood chemistry	a test or series of tests on plasma to measure the levels of particular components (glucose, albumin, cholesterol, etc.)
			blood culture	a test to determine infection in the blood by placing a blood sample on a nutritive media in an effort to grow populations of bacteria for analysis

WORD PARTS (WHEN APPLICABLE)			TERM	DEFINITION
Part	Type	Meaning		
			blood transfusion (trans FYOO zhun)	introduction of blood, blood products, or a blood substitute into a patient's circulation to restore blood volume to normal levels; the two main types of blood transfusions are **autologous transfusions** and **homologous transfusions** (Figure 11.18 ⸬⸬)

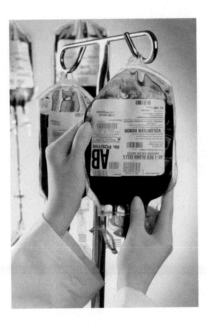

Figure 11.18 ⸬⸬

Blood transfusion. The photograph shows whole blood bags ready for transfusion to patients.
Source: Getty Images Inc./Image Bank.

			coagulation time (koh ahg yoo LAY shun)	a timed blood test to determine the time required for a blood clot to form; one type of this test, called **prothrombin time (PT),** measures the time required for prothrombin, a precursor protein, to form thrombin and is often used to monitor anticlotting therapy; another type of test is **partial thromboplastin time (PTT),** which is used to evaluate clotting ability
			complete blood count	a common laboratory blood test that provides diagnostic information of a patient's general health; abbreviated **CBC,** it includes several more specific tests including **hematocrit, hemoglobin, red blood count** and **white blood count**
			differential count (DIH fer EHN shal)	microscopic count of the number of each type of white blood cell using a stained blood smear
erythr/o -cyte	r/cv r	red cell	**erythrocyte sedimentation rate** (eh RITH roh sight SEH dih men TAY shun RAYT)	a timed test to measure the rate at which red blood cells fall through a volume of plasma to provide information on their hemoglobin content; abbreviated **ESR,** it is commonly used to evaluate nonspecific systemic inflammation
hemat/o -crit	r/cv s	blood to separate	**hematocrit** (hee MAT oh krit)	a test that measures the percentage of red blood cells in a volume of blood; abbreviated **HCT** or **Hct,** it is obtained from centrifuging a sample of blood to separate blood cells

WORD PARTS (WHEN APPLICABLE)			TERM	DEFINITION
Part	**Type**	**Meaning**		
hemat/o -logy	r/cv s	blood study of	**hematology** (HEE mah TALL oh jee)	the general field of medicine focusing on blood-related disease
hem/o -globin	r/cv s	blood globe-like protein	**hemoglobin** (HEE moh gloh binn)	a test that measures the level of hemoglobin in red blood cells (in grams); abbreviated **HGB** or **Hgb**
hem/o -stasis	r/cv s	blood standing still	**hemostasis** (HEE moh STAY siss)	stoppage of bleeding
hom/o log -ous	r/cv r s	same study pertaining to	**homologous transfusion** (hoh MALL oh gus trans FYOO zhun)	transfusion of blood that is voluntarily donated by another person; it requires blood type matching known as crossmatching to prevent incompatibility
			immunization (IM yoo nih ZAY shun)	a procedure that provides immunity against a particular antigen (Figure 11.19)

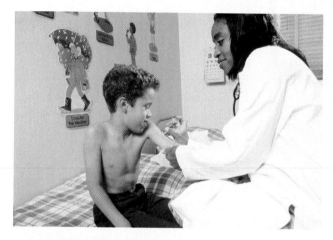

Figure 11.19 ::::

Immunization with a vaccine.
A physician is injecting a vaccine into the boy's arm to provide him with immunity against the influenza virus.
Source: PhotoEdit.

immun/o -logy	r/cv s	exempt, immunity study of	**immunology** (IM yoo NALL oh jee)	the study concerned with immunity and allergy
immun/o -therapy	r/cv s	exempt, immunity treatment	**immunotherapy** (IM yoo noh THAIR ah pee)	used in the treatment of infectious disease, it is the use of agents (serum, gamma globulin, treated antibodies, etc.) to activate or strengthen the immune response
			lymph node dissection (LIMF NOHD)	removal of lymph nodes for pathological study to assist in a diagnosis; also known as a **lymph node biopsy.**
lymph aden -ectomy	r r s	clear water, fluid gland excision	**lymphadenectomy** (limm fad eh NEK toh mee)	excision (surgical removal) of a lymph node
lymph aden/o -graphy	r r/cv s	clear water, fluid gland recording process	**lymphadenography** (limm FAD eh NOG rah fee)	the process of x-ray photography of the lymph nodes following injection of a contrast medium
lymph aden/o -tomy	r r/cv s	clear water, fluid; gland incision	**lymphadenotomy** (limm FAD eh NOTT oh mee)	incision into a lymph node

WORD PARTS (WHEN APPLICABLE)			TERM	DEFINITION
Part	**Type**	**Meaning**		
lymph angi/o -graphy	r r/cv s	clear water, fluid blood vessel recording process	**lymphangiography** (limm FAN jee OG rah fee)	the process of x-ray photography of lymphatic vessels following injection of a contrast medium; it produces an x-ray recording called a **lymphangiogram** (limm FAN jee oh gram)
			pheresis (fah REE sis)	removal of a donor's blood, which is then separated into blood components, with one portion retained for use and the remainder returned to the donor; it includes **plasmapheresis** (PLAZ mah fah REE siss), in which plasma is used, **leukapheresis** (LOO kah fah REE siss), in which white blood cells are used, and **plateletpheresis** (PLAYT let fah REE siss), in which platelets are used
			platelet count (PLAYT let)	calculation of the number of platelets in the blood; abbreviated **PLT**
pro- -phylaxis	p s	before protection	**prophylaxis** (proh fih LAK siss)	any treatment that tends to prevent the onset of an infection or other type of disease
			red blood count	measures the number of red blood cells per cubic centimeter (cc); abbreviated **RBC**
splen -ectomy	r s	spleen excision	**splenectomy** (splee NEK toh mee)	excision of the spleen
splen/o -pexy	r/cv s	spleen surgical fixation, suspension	**splenopexy** (SPLEE noh pek see)	surgical fixation of the spleen
thromb/o -lysis	r/cv s	clot to dissolve	**thrombolysis** (throm BALL ih siss)	the process of dissolving a blood clot
thym -ectomy	r s	wart-like; thymus gland excision	**thymectomy** (thigh MEK toh mee)	excision of the thymus gland
			vaccination (VAK sih NAY shun)	the inoculation of a culture that has reduced virulence as a means of providing a cure or a prophylaxis (prevention)
			vaccine (vak SEEN)	any preparation used to activate an immune response

[FYI]

Vaccines
Vaccines have been in use since the Middle Ages, when scrapings from smallpox sores were given to people as a prophylaxis against this deadly disease. The use of the term *vaccine* (derived from the Latin word *vaccinus*, which means *relating to a cow*) came about in 1796, when Edward Jenner discovered that scrapings from people infected with a related, mild form of the disease contracted from milking cows, known as *cowpox*, provided immunity against smallpox.

white blood count	measures the number of while blood cells per cubic centimeter; abbreviated **WBC**

SELF QUIZ 11.5

SAY IT—SPELL IT!

Review the terms of blood and the lymphatic system by speaking the phonetic pronunciation guides out loud, then writing in the correct spelling of the term.

1. koh ahg yoo LAY shun

2. AN tye koh AG yoo LANT

3. hee MAT oh krit

4. HEE moh STAY siss

5. PLAZ mah fah REE siss

6. limm fad eh NEK toh mee

7. thigh MEK toh mee

8. limm FAD eh NOG rah fee

9. vak SEEN

10. limm FAN jee OG rah fee

11. limm fad eh NOTT oh mee

12. splee NEK toh mee

13. VAK sih NAY shun

14. limm FAN jee oh gram

15. SPLEE noh pek see

MATCH IT!

Match the term on the left with the correct definition on the right.

_____ 1. hemostasis

_____ 2. hematocrit

_____ 3. plasmapheresis

_____ 4. thrombolysis

_____ 5. erythrocyte sedimentation rate

_____ 6. prothrombin time

_____ 7. autologous transfusion

_____ 8. lymphadenectomy

_____ 9. lymphangiogram

_____ 10. lymphadenotomy

_____ 11. splenectomy

_____ 12. vaccine

_____ 13. antibiotics

_____ 14. prophylaxis

_____ 15. antiretroviral

a. a timed test to evaluate RBC drop rates

b. process of dissolving a blood clot

c. stoppage of blood loss

d. donating blood for your own use

e. a timed test for coagulation rate

f. centrifugation of a blood sample

g. use of donated plasma

h. a preventative treatment

i. excision of a lymph node

j. incision into a lymph node

k. excision of the spleen

l. use of drugs to battle viruses

m. a preparation used to activate an immune response

n. x-ray of contrasted lymphatic vessels

o. a therapy against bacterial infections

BREAK IT DOWN!

Analyze and separate each term into its word parts by labeling each word part using p = prefix, r = root, cv = combining vowel, and s = suffix.

1. hematocrit   _____

2. hemostasis   _____

3. lymphangiography   _____

4. prophylaxis   _____

5. splenectomy   _____

FILL IT IN!

Fill in the blanks with the correct terms.

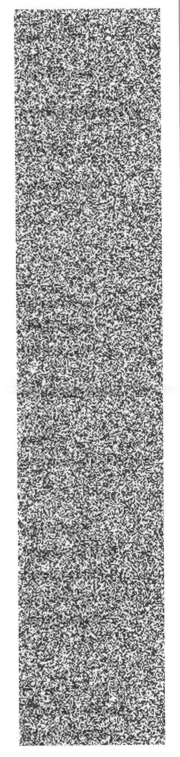

1. In cases of severe infection or trauma to the abdomen, enlargement of the

   11.19   spleen, or _____, may occur. A surgical fixation of the spleen,

   called a _____, may correct it. In other cases, the spleen must

   be removed by a _____ to avoid rupture.

2. A blood test or series of tests on blood to measure the levels of particular blood

   components is known as a _____ _____. A

   test for the source of an infection is a _____

   _____. A blood test that evaluates a patient's general health is

   11.20   a _____ _____ _____, or

   CBC.

3. A CBC may be focused on the percentage of red blood cells, known as a

   11.21   _____, on the oxygen-carrying protein content of blood, or

   _____, on the RBC volume, called a _____

   _____ _____, or on the WBC volume, called

   a _____ _____ _____.

4. The process of dissolving a blood clot is called _____. It may

   be required if a platelet count, abbreviated _____, is

   excessively high or the measured time for coagulation to occur, called a

   _____ _____, is too brief.

5. A _____ is frequently used as a sign to predict the onset of

   AIDS. Its most apparent characteristic is persistent _____, or

   inflammation of the lymph nodes.

6. If a lymphoma is suspected, a procedure in which a portion of a lymph node is removed for analysis, called a _____ _____ _____, often follows. The procedure is often accompanied by an x-ray process, called a _____. If the tests are positive for lymphoma, the affected nodes are removed in a _____ procedure.

7. In the disease influenza, commonly called the flu, a virus that is capable of mutating into different forms has made treatment and cure a challenge. However, _____ can be successful when the virus is identified early and the population provided with _____ created by inoculating viral particles that have been reduced in their virulence by _____.

8. The general field of medicine focusing on blood-related disease is called ₊-11.22 _____.

abbreviations of blood and the lymphatic system

The abbreviations that are associated with blood and the lymphatic system are summarized here. Study these abbreviations, and review them in the exercise that follows.

ABBREVIATION	DEFINITION	ABBREVIATION	DEFINITION
AIDS	acquired immune deficiency syndrome	LAS	lymphadenopathy syndrome
		PLT	platelet count
CBC	complete blood count	PT	prothrombin time
ESR	erythrocyte sedimentation rate	PTT	partial thromboplastin time
HCT, Hct	hematocrit	RBC	red blood cell or red blood count
HGB, Hgb	hemoglobin	WBC	white blood cell or white blood count
HIV	human immunodeficiency virus		
INR	international normalized ratio		

SELF QUIZ 11.6

Fill in the blanks with the abbreviation or the complete medical term.

Abbreviation	Medical Term
1. CBC	_____
2. _____	acquired immunodeficiency syndrome
3. RBC	_____
4. _____	erythrocyte sedimentation rate

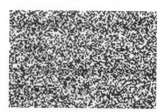

5. PT _____

6. _____ international normalized ratio

11.23 7. LAS _____

8. _____ partial thromboplastin time

9. WBC _____

10. _____ hemoglobin

11. HCT, Hct _____

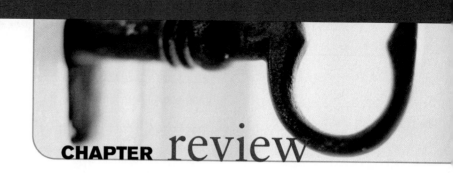

In this section, we will review all the word parts and medical terms from this chapter. As in earlier tables, the word roots are shown in **bold**.

Check each word part and medical term to be sure you understand the meaning. If any are not clear, please go back into the chapter and review that term. Then, complete the review exercises that follow.

[word parts **checklist**]

Prefixes

- ❑ ana-
- ❑ auto-
- ❑ homo-
- ❑ iso-
- ❑ macro-
- ❑ micro-
- ❑ pro-

Word Roots/Combining Vowels

- ❑ **aden**/o
- ❑ **aut**/o
- ❑ **bacter**/o
- ❑ **blast**/o

- ❑ **erythr**/o
- ❑ **hem**/o, **hemat**/o
- ❑ **immun**/o
- ❑ **leuk**/o
- ❑ **lymph**/o
- ❑ **mon**/o
- ❑ **path**/o
- ❑ **poikil**/o
- ❑ **splen**/o
- ❑ **staphyl**/o
- ❑ **strept**/o
- ❑ **therm**/o
- ❑ **thromb**/o

- ❑ **thym**/o
- ❑ **tox**/o

Suffixes

- ❑ -crit
- ❑ -cyte
- ❑ -emia, hemia
- ❑ -lysis
- ❑ -penia
- ❑ -pexy
- ❑ -phil, -philia
- ❑ -phylaxis
- ❑ -poiesis

[medical terminology **checklist**]

- ❑ acquired immune deficiency syndrome (AIDS)
- ❑ allergy
- ❑ anaphylaxis
- ❑ anemia
- ❑ aniso**cyt**osis
- ❑ anti**bi**otics
- ❑ antibody
- ❑ anticoagulant
- ❑ antigen
- ❑ antiretroviral therapy
- ❑ a**plast**ic anemia
- ❑ attenuation
- ❑ auto**immun**e disorder
- ❑ autologous transfusion red blood count
- ❑ B cell

- ❑ **bacter**emia
- ❑ basophil
- ❑ blood chemistry
- ❑ blood clot
- ❑ blood culture
- ❑ blood transfusion
- ❑ botulism
- ❑ coagulation
- ❑ coagulation time
- ❑ complete blood count (CBC)
- ❑ differential count
- ❑ diphtheria
- ❑ dyscrasia
- ❑ **erythr**o**blast**osis fetalis
- ❑ **erythr**o**cyt**e sedimentation rate (ESR)
- ❑ **erythr**ocytes

- ❑ **erythr**openia
- ❑ fibrinogen
- ❑ **fung**emia
- ❑ gas gangrene
- ❑ **hemat**ocrit (HCT, Hct)
- ❑ **hemat**opoiesis
- ❑ **hem**o**chromat**osis
- ❑ **hem**oglobin (HGB, Hgb)
- ❑ **hem**olysis
- ❑ **hem**ophilia
- ❑ **hem**orrhage
- ❑ **hem**ostasis
- ❑ Hodgkin's disease
- ❑ hom**olog**ous transfusion
- ❑ human **immun**odeficiency virus (HIV)
- ❑ **immun**ity

❑ **immun**ization
❑ **immun**odeficiency
❑ **immun**ology
❑ **immun**osuppression
❑ **immun**otherapy
❑ infection
❑ influenza
❑ international normalized ratio (INR)
❑ iron deficiency anemia
❑ **leuk**emia
❑ **leuk**ocytes
❑ **lymph**
❑ **lymph** node dissection
❑ **lymph** nodes
❑ **lymphaden**ectomy
❑ **lymphaden**itis
❑ **lymphaden**ography
❑ **lymphaden**opathy
❑ **lymphaden**opathy syndrome (LAS)
❑ **lymphaden**otomy
❑ **lymphangi**ography

❑ **lymph**atic capillaries
❑ **lymph**atic nodules
❑ **lymph**atic trunks
❑ **lymph**atic vessels
❑ **lymph**ocyte
❑ **lymph**oma
❑ macro**cyt**osis
❑ macrophage
❑ malaria
❑ mono**nucle**osis
❑ myelodys**plas**ia
❑ **neutr**ophil
❑ partial **thromb**oplastin time (PTT)
❑ **path**ogen
❑ pernicious anemia
❑ pheresis
❑ plague
❑ plasma
❑ platelet count (PLT)
❑ platelets
❑ poikilo**cyt**osis
❑ poly**cyth**emia

❑ pro**thromb**in time (PT)
❑ rabies
❑ **septic**emia
❑ serum
❑ sickle cell anemia
❑ spleen
❑ **splen**ectomy
❑ **splen**omegaly
❑ **splen**opexy
❑ **staphylo**coccemia
❑ T cell
❑ tetanus
❑ **thorac**ic duct
❑ **thromb**olysis
❑ **thym**ectomy
❑ **thym**oma
❑ **thym**us gland
❑ tonsils
❑ **tox**emia
❑ **tox**in
❑ vaccination
❑ vaccine
❑ white blood count (WBC)

[show what **you know!**]

BREAK IT DOWN!

Analyze and separate each term into its word parts by labeling each word part using p = prefix, r = root, cv = combining vowel, and s = suffix.

Example:	1.	erythrocyte	r cv s erythr/o/cyte
	2.	hematopoiesis	
	3.	leukocyte	
	4.	hematologist	
	5.	anisocytosis	
	6.	dyscrasia	
	7.	erythroblastosis	
	8.	erythropenia	
	9.	hemochromatosis	
	10.	hemolysis	
	11.	hemophilia	
	12.	leukemia	
	13.	macrocytosis	
	14.	myelodysplasia	

15. polycythemia _____

16. poikilocytosis _____

17. septicemia _____

18. hematocrit _____

19. hemostasis _____

20. plasmapheresis _____

21. thrombolysis _____

22. lymphadenitis _____

23. lymphadenopathy _____

24. splenomegaly _____

25. lymphadenectomy _____

26. lymphangiography _____

27. splenectomy _____

28. thymectomy _____

29. immunology _____

30. lymphocyte _____

31. macrophage _____

32. neutrophil _____

33. bacteremia _____

34. immunosuppression _____

35. staphylococcemia _____

36. toxemia _____

WORD BUILDING

Construct or recall medical terms from the following meanings.

Example: 1. reduced ability of blood to deliver oxygen _____ anemia _____

2. presence of red blood cells of unequal size _____

3. any abnormal condition of the blood _____

4. fetal blood incompatibility of Rh factor _____

5. abnormal reduction of red blood cells _____

6. excessive accumulation of iron deposits _____

7. inherited defect in blood coagulation _____

8. cancer originating in red bone marrow _____

9. abnormally large red blood cells _____

10. abnormally small red blood cells _____

11. development of abnormal stem cells _____

12. abnormal increase in red blood cells _____

13. red blood cells that are large and irregular _____

14. presence of bacteria and toxins in the blood _____

15. a chemical that reduces blood clotting _____

16. transfusion of blood donated by another person _____

17. measures percentage of red blood cells in a sample _____

18. stoppage of bleeding _____

19. calculation of the number of platelets in blood _____

20. cancer of lymphatic tissue _____

21. inflammation of the lymph nodes _____

22. any disease of the lymph nodes _____

23. a tumor originating in lymphatic tissue _____

24. abnormal enlargement of the spleen _____

25. a tumor originating in the thymus gland _____

26. excision of a lymph node _____

27. surgical fixation of the spleen _____

28. the spelled-out term for the AIDS acronym _____

29. a response to an allergen _____

30. rapid inflammation and smooth muscle contractions _____

31. disease caused by immune reaction against own tissues _____

32. presence of bacteria in the bloodstream _____

33. bacterial disease that causes mucous membrane inflammation _____

34. fungal infection spread by the bloodstream _____

35. a condition resulting from a defective immune response _____

36. viral disease known as the flu _____

37. a serious protozoan infection of red blood cells _____

38. an infectious disease of wide prevalence _____

39. a condition commonly called a staph infection _____

40. any preparation used to activate an immune response _____

41. renders a person immune to an antigen _____

CASE STUDIES

Fill in the blanks with the correct terms.

1. A 15-year-old male was seen by his personal physician after complaining of low energy and susceptibility to infections. Prior to being seen, the physician suspected a nonspecific blood disorder, or (a) _____, was the cause of the symptoms, and ordered tests to measure the levels of blood components, or a (b) _____ _____, including a test for the percentage of red blood cells, or (c) _____, and a timed test for the levels of hemoglobin in the blood by measuring the rate at which red blood cells fall through a volume of plasma, or a (d) _____ _____ _____. The tests showed normal hemoglobin content in red blood cells, but low numbers of red blood cells, suggesting (e) _____. Dietary supplements of iron and folic acid were administered. About two weeks later, the dietary supplements failed to correct the symptoms, ruling out (f) _____ anemia and (g) _____ _____ anemia. A microscopic evaluation of cells was then ordered, called a (h) _____ _____ This test revealed red blood cells were of unequal size, a condition known as (i) _____, and were irregularly shaped, a condition called (j) _____. Samples from bone marrow were then examined, which showed abnormal stem cells were producing the defective red blood cells, a condition known as (k) _____. Because the condition was identified early before the cells became cancerous (which would have resulted in the cancer known as (l) _____), treatment by irradiation was successful.

2. A 55-year-old female was admitted to the infectious disease wing of the clinic after having been referred by her personal physician, due to a prolonged inflammation of the lymph nodes, called (m) _____, in the armpit and groin regions. The doctor's initial diagnosis was an unspecified disease of the lymph nodes, or (n) _____, and he was concerned about a possible tumor originating in the lymph nodes, or (o) _____, which might include cancer of the nodes, or (p) _____ _____. Upon more thorough examinations that included x-ray photography of lymph nodes, or (q) _____, and excision of a lymph node for biopsy, or (r) _____ _____, no evidence of a tumor was found. However, an abnormal enlargement of the spleen, or (s) _____, was observed. Blood tests including a (t) _____ _____ were ordered to look for multiplication of pathogens, or an (u) _____. The tests were positive for bacteria, indicating the patient suffered from (v) _____, or bacterial infection of the blood. Further tests identified the common bacterium *Staphylococcus* as the causative pathogen, providing the diagnosis of (w) _____. The patient was administered (x) _____ therapy. However, after two weeks, the symptoms failed to lessen. The patient had developed a deficient immune response, or (y) _____. To combat this, (z) _____ was begun immediately that included antibody treatments in combination with antibiotic therapy. A complete recovery resulted after three months of treatment.

[piece it all **together!** 🧩]

CROSSWORD

From the chapter material, fill in the crossword puzzle with answers to the following clues.

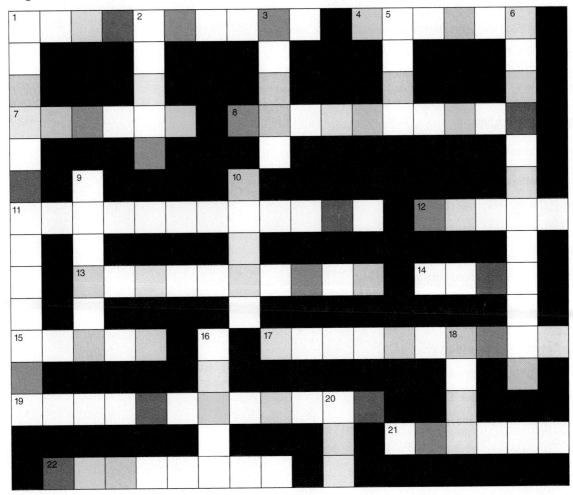

ACROSS

1. Where blood is the focus of evaluation or study. (Find puzzle piece 11.22)

4. To be exempt. (Find puzzle piece 11.6)

7. Low oxygen levels in the blood. (Find puzzle piece 11.14)

8. Abbreviated Hct. (Find puzzle piece 11.21)

11. Literally, "many cells in the blood." (Find puzzle piece 11.16)

12. The "B" word in "CBC." (Find puzzle piece 11.20)

13. Literally, a "blood condition of putrefaction." (Find puzzle piece 11.17)

14. Lymph is filtered as it flows through. (Find puzzle piece 11.4)

15. Shortened term for the bacterium *Staphylococcus*. (Find puzzle piece 11.18)

17. A disease characterized by reduced coagulation. (Find puzzle piece 11.12)

19. An abnormally enlarged spleen. (Find puzzle piece 11.19)

21. Includes the pharyngeal, palatine, and lingual. (Find puzzle piece 11.5)

22. A cell type that is involved in an allergic reaction. (Find puzzle piece 11.7)

DOWN

1. A continual process that occurs in the bone marrow. (Find puzzle piece 11.1)
2. A harmful molecule released by a pathogen. (Find puzzle piece 11.8)
3. The language in which "poison" means "toxin." (Find puzzle piece 11.10)
5. The prefix in mononucleosis. (Find puzzle piece 11.13)
6. A condition that may cause "pink" blood. (Find puzzle piece 11.9)
9. The fluid portion of blood. (Find puzzle piece 11.2)
10. A feature of blood with polycythemia. (Rhymes with "brick"; find puzzle piece 11.11)
16. The fluid found within the thoracic duct. (Find puzzle piece 11.3)
18. The metal that binds to oxygen in hemoglobin. (Find puzzle piece 11.15)
20. Abbreviation for lymphadenopathy syndrome. (Find puzzle piece 11.23)

WORD UNSCRAMBLE

From the completed crossword puzzle, unscramble:

1. All of the letters that appear in **red** squares __ __ ☐ __ __ __ __ __

   Clue: A protein that counters an antigen

2. All of the letters that appear in **purple** squares __ __ __ ☐ __ __ __ __ __ __

   Clue: An iron-containing protein in the blood

3. All of the letters that appear in **peach** squares __ __ __ __ __ __ __ __ ☐ __ __

   Clue: A body response to an antigen that includes inflammation

4. All of the letters that appear in **blue** squares __ ☐ __ __ __ __ __

   Clue: Caused by a toxin that attacks the CNS

5. All of the letters that appear in **yellow** squares ☐ __ __ __ __ __ __ __ __

   Clue: A phagocyte that is a "large eater"

6. All of the letters that appear in **green** squares __ __ __ __ __ ☐ __

   Clue: "Bad air"

7. All of the letters that appear in **gray** squares ☐ __ __ __ __ __

   Clue: "Without blood"

Now write down each of the letters that are boxed to find the hidden medical term: __ __ __ __ __ __ __ .

MEDmedia wrap-up

www.prenhall.com/wingerd

Before you go on to the next chapter, take advantage of the free CD-ROM and study guide website that accompany this book. Simply load the CD-ROM for additional activities, games, animations, videos, and quizzes linked to this chapter. Then visit www.prenhall.com/wingerd for even more!

CHAPTER 12

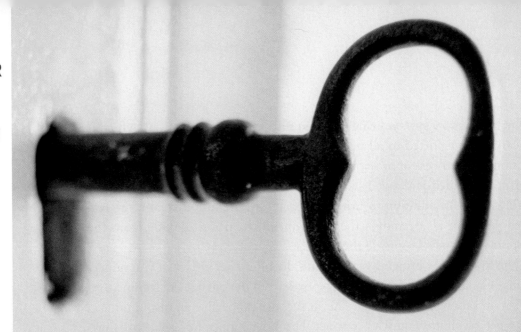

The Respiratory System

LEARNING OBJECTIVES

After completing this chapter, you will be able to:

- Define and spell the word parts used to create medical terms for the respiratory system

- Identify the organs of the respiratory system and describe their structure and function

- Define common medical terms used for the respiratory system

- Break down and define common medical terms used for symptoms, diseases, disorders, procedures, treatments, and devices for the respiratory system

MEDmedia

www.prenhall.com/wingerd

Enhance your study with the power of multimedia! Each chapter of this book links to activities, games, animations, videos, and quizzes that you'll find on your CD-ROM. Plus, you can click on www.prenhall.com/wingerd, to find a free chapter-specific companion website that's loaded with additional practice and resources.

CD-ROM

- Audio Glossary
- Exercises & Activities
- Flashcard Generator
- Animations
- Videos

 Companion Website

- Exercises & Activities
- Audio Glossary
- Drug Updates
- Current News Update

A secure distance learning course is available at www.prenhall.com/onekey.

The *respiratory system* brings oxygen into the bloodstream, by which it can be transported to all body cells. The system gets its name from its function: The process of providing cells with oxygen is commonly known as respiration, which is derived from the Latin word *respiratio*, meaning to breathe again. In addition to bringing oxygen to the bloodstream, the respiratory system also removes the waste product carbon dioxide from the blood and channels it outside the body.

The first step in bringing oxygen into the blood occurs when you inhale. During inhalation, or inspiration, air moves from the outside environment to the tiny air sacs within the lungs. The air sacs are called alveoli. Inspiration results when respiratory muscles contract. The most important respiratory muscle is the diaphragm, a sheet of muscle dividing the thoracic and abdominal cavities. Exhaling air results when the respiratory muscles relax, and is known as expiration. Together, inspiration and expiration are known as ventilation.

The second step of respiration begins when fresh air has filled the lungs. The air molecules diffuse between the alveoli and the capillaries surrounding them. Due to pressure differences, oxygen moves out of the alveoli and into the capillaries, and carbon dioxide moves in the opposite direction. This process is known as external respiration.

The third step of respiration is known as internal respiration. It occurs when oxygen carried in the bloodstream diffuses into surrounding body cells, and carbon dioxide moves from the cells into the bloodstream.

The final step of respiration occurs when the body exhales, or expires, pushing used air and carbon dioxide out of the body.

In this chapter, we will weave together the structural terms and the medical terminology of the respiratory system. Through a brief survey of the respiratory system structure, you will learn about its parts and how they work. Then, we will focus on the medical terms, including respiratory symptoms, diseases and disorders, and treatments, procedures, and devices.

word parts focus

Let's look at word parts. The following table contains a list of word parts that when combined build many of the terms of the respiratory system.

PREFIX	DEFINITION	PREFIX	DEFINITION
a-, an-	without, absence of (an is used when the word root begins with a vowel)	epi-	upon, over
		eu-	normal, good
dia-	through, between	pan-	all, entire
endo-	within	poly-	many

WORD ROOT	DEFINITION	WORD ROOT	DEFINITION
alveol	air sac, alveolus	pneum, pneumon,	
atel	imperfect, incomplete	pneumat	lung or air
bronch	airway, bronchus	pulmon	lung
glott, glottis	opening of the windpipe	py	pus
hem, hemat	blood	rhin	nose
laryng	voicebox, larynx	sept	wall, partition
lob	a rounded part, lobe	sinus	cavity
muc	mucus	somn	sleep
nas	nose	spir	to breathe
ox	oxygen	sten	narrowing, constriction
pharyng	throat, pharynx	thorac	chest, thorax
phragm, phragmat	partition	trache	wind pipe, trachea
pleur	rib, pleura	tubercul	little mass or swelling

SUFFIX	DEFINITION	SUFFIX	DEFINITION
-algia	pain	-oxia	oxygen
-ar, -ary	pertaining to	-pexy	surgical fixation, suspension
-capnia	carbon dioxide	-phonia	sound or voice
-cele	hernia, swelling, protrusion	-pnea	breathing
-centesis	puncture to aspirate, or remove, fluid	-ptysis	to spit out a fluid
-eal	pertaining to	-rrhagia	bleeding, hemorrhage
-ectasis	expansion, dilation	-spasm	sudden, involuntary muscle contraction
-emia	blood condition		
-metry	measurement	-stomy	surgical creation of an opening
-osis	condition of	-tomy	incision, or surgical cut into

[FYI]

-capnia
The suffix -capnia is derived from the Greek word *kapnos,* which means *smoke,* referring to exhaled air. It refers specifically to the gas, carbon dioxide.

SELF QUIZ 12.1

> **Success Hint:**   Once you get to the crossword puzzle at the end of the chapter, remember to check back here for clues! Your clues are indicated by the puzzle icon.

Review the word parts of respiratory system terminology by working carefully through the exercises that follow. Soon, we will apply this new information to build medical terms.

A.   Provide the definition of the following prefixes and suffixes.

1. a-, an-   _____

2. eu-   _____

3. poly-   _____

4. pan-   _____

5. -algia   _____

6. -capnia   _____

7. -ectasis   _____

8. -phonia   _____

9. -pnea   _____

10. -osis   _____

11. -cele   _____

12. -stomy   _____

B.   Provide the word root for each of the following terms.

1. larynx   _____

2. trachea   _____

3. epiglottis   _____

4. nose   _____

5. pleura   _____

6. cavity   _____

7. thorax   _____

8. lung   _____

9. alveolus   _____

12.1 10. mucus   _____

11. oxygen   _____

12. lung, air   _____

13. pus   _____

14. sleep   _____

15. wall, partition   _____

16. pharynx   _____

17. breathe   _____

18. sten   _____

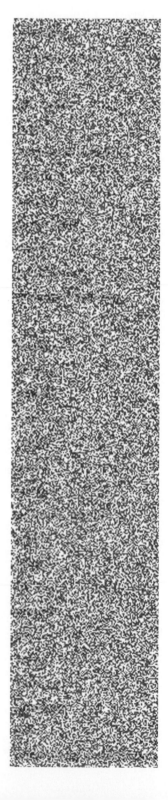

[anatomy and physiology overview]

The respiratory system consists of organs that support the activities of ventilation and external respiration. It includes a series of chambers and tubes that carry air to and from the lungs, and the alveoli within the lungs where external respiration takes place (Figure 12.1 ⁝⁝⁝⁝). Since the chambers and tubes conduct air, they are often

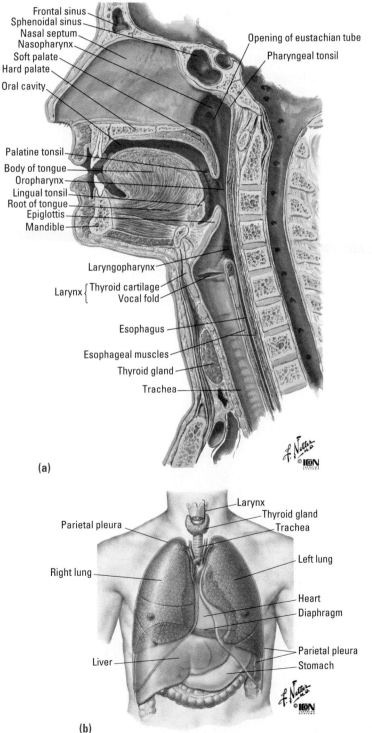

(a)

(b)

Figure 12.1 ⁝⁝⁝⁝

The respiratory system.
(a) Lateral view of the head and neck. The respiratory system includes the upper respiratory tract, which contains the nasal cavity, pharynx, larynx, and trachea.
(b) The lungs. The right and left lungs are shown with the rib cage superimposed over them.
Source: Icon Learning Systems.

called the **conducting portion** of the respiratory system. The alveoli within the lungs are known as the **respiratory portion,** since they are the sites of gas exchange with the bloodstream.

Conducting Portion

The organs of the conducting portion form the airway, extending from the nose down into the lungs. The organs that conduct air from the outside to the thoracic cavity are referred to as the **upper respiratory tract.** They include the **nose, pharynx, larynx,** and **trachea.** Each of these organs is internally lined with a moist mucous membrane, which serves to warm and humidify the air on its way to the lungs. The sticky mucus also traps foreign particles, and the cilia that line the mucous membrane beat in a rhythm to form a conveyor belt of motion that transports the foreign particles to the mouth or nose for elimination when you cough or sneeze (Figure 12.2::::). The expelled mucus is known as **sputum.**

Within the nose is the nasal cavity, which is divided by a central **nasal septum.** The **paranasal sinuses,** spaces within the bones of the face and skull, are connected to the nasal cavities. If an infection strikes the nasal cavities, it can travel into the paranasal sinuses to produce symptoms of swelling and headache. The pharynx, or throat, is surrounded by muscles and serves as a common chamber for swallowing food and for breathing air. Its muscles contract during swallowing. From the pharynx, inhaled air enters the larynx while swallowed food enters the esophagus (Figure 12.1a). The entry of food into the airway is prevented by a flap of cartilage that covers the opening into the larynx during swallowing. The opening is named after the Greek word for *opening of the windpipe,* the **glottis,** and the cartilage is the **epiglottis** (recall that the prefix *epi-* means *upon*). The larynx is frequently called the voice box, since it is a box-like structure that produces sound (Figure 12.3::::). Sound results when exhaled air squeezes between folds of membrane that partially block the airway. The trachea, or windpipe, is a foot-long tube that carries air between the larynx and the bronchi. It is prevented from collapsing by the presence of stiff cartilage rings, which strengthen its walls to form a rigid tube. Thus, the cartilage rings keep the tracheal airway patent (open).

The conducting organs within the chest form the **lower respiratory tract.** They include the **bronchi,** the **bronchial tree** within the lungs, and the tiny **bronchioles.**

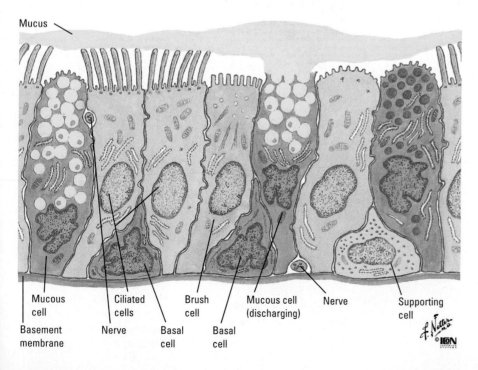

Mucus

| Mucous | Ciliated | Brush | Mucous cell | Nerve | Supporting |
| cell | cells | cell | (discharging) | | cell |

| Basement | Nerve | Basal | Basal | | |
| membrane | | cell | cell | | |

Figure 12.2 ::::

Ciliated respiratory lining.
The cilia beat in harmony to move the layer of mucus in a direction leading toward the mouth.
Source: Icon Learning Systems.

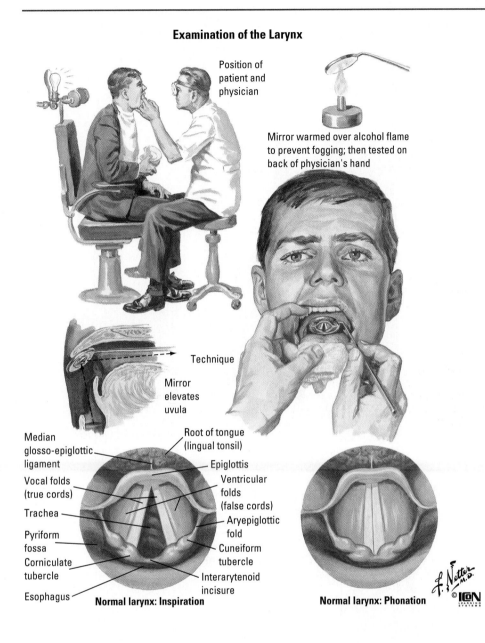

Examination of the Larynx

Position of patient and physician

Mirror warmed over alcohol flame to prevent fogging; then tested on back of physician's hand

Technique

Mirror elevates uvula

Median glosso-epiglottic ligament

Vocal folds (true cords)

Trachea

Pyriform fossa

Corniculate tubercle

Esophagus

Normal larynx: Inspiration

Root of tongue (lingual tonsil)

Epiglottis

Ventricular folds (false cords)

Aryepiglottic fold

Cuneiform tubercle

Interarytenoid incisure

Normal larynx: Phonation

Figure 12.3

Vocal cords. The series of illustrations shows a routine examination of the larynx, including the vocal cords.
Source: Icon Learning Systems.

The bronchi begin as two branches from the distal end of the trachea, forming the right and left primary bronchi. Similar to the trachea, the bronchi's walls are also kept rigid and open by the presence of cartilage rings. Soon after entering a lung, a bronchus divides into several smaller bronchi, which soon divide again and again to form the branching bronchial tree (Figure 12.4). Eventually, the branching leads to microscopic, thin-walled bronchioles. Bronchioles are not supported by rings of cartilage, so their walls may collapse during asthmatic attacks, infections, or coughing reflexes. The bronchioles lead into cul-de-sacs, each of which opens into a cluster of microscopic sac-like alveoli (Figure 12.5).

Respiratory Portion

Most people have about 300 million alveoli within each lung. If the alveoli of a lung were stretched out along a flat surface, they would cover an area the size of a tennis court! When combined with the capillaries that surround them and the bronchioles that carry air to and from them, the alveoli form the substance of the lung.

The wall of each alveolus is only one thin cell in thickness. Because adjacent capillary walls are also one cell thick, the barrier between the alveolus and the

thinking critically!

The trachea and bronchi are kept patent by cartilage rings, but bronchioles lack the cartilage support. Why do you suppose bronchioles do not contain cartilage in their walls?

Nomenclature of Bronchi: Schema

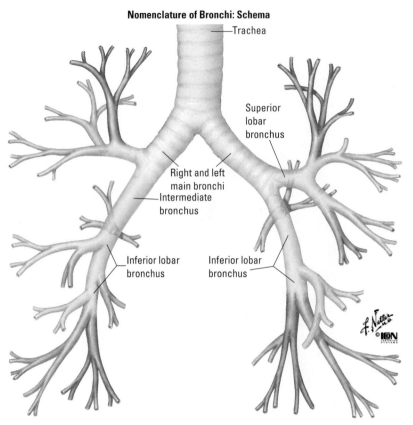

Trachea

Superior lobar bronchus

Right and left main bronchi

Intermediate bronchus

Inferior lobar bronchus

Inferior lobar bronchus

Figure 12.4 ::::

Bronchial tree. The bronchial tree resembles an upside-down olive tree.
Source: Icon Learning Systems.

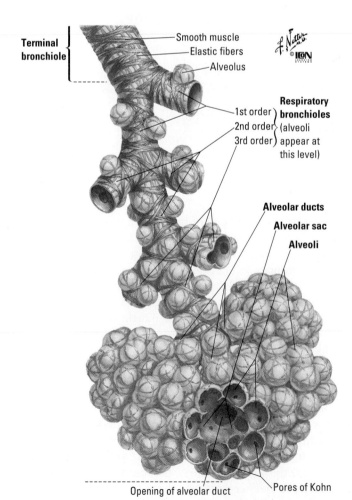

Terminal bronchiole

Smooth muscle
Elastic fibers
Alveolus

1st order
2nd order
3rd order

Respiratory bronchioles (alveoli appear at this level)

Alveolar ducts

Alveolar sac

Alveoli

Opening of alveolar duct

Pores of Kohn

Figure 12.5 ::::

Alveoli. The alveoli are located at the terminal end of the bronchioles, where they cluster like a bunch of grapes.
Source: Icon Learning Systems.

bloodstream is very thin. Known as the **respiratory membrane,** it represents the site of gas diffusion between the lungs and the blood (Figure 12.6::::).

During each inhalation, the alveoli swell with incoming air. Exhaling air causes them to shrink. The thin cells that form their walls are elastic, allowing them to stretch and recoil. In addition to the cells that form the walls, alveoli contain cells that secrete a waxy substance called surfactant that prevents the walls from sticking when they collapse during exhalation. Alveoli also contain a specialized type of

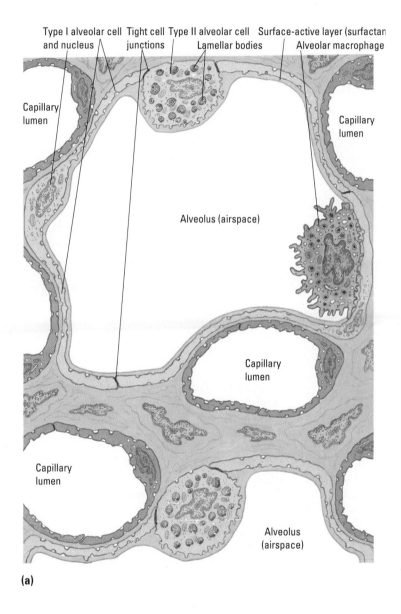

(a)

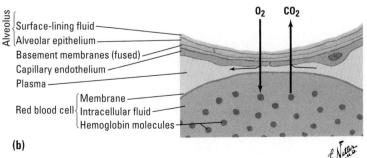

(b)

Figure 12.6 ::::

Alveoli and the respiratory membrane.

(a) A section through alveoli reveals the structure of the alveolar walls.
(b) Close-up of the alveolar wall, which consists of a single layer of flattened alveolar cells, a thin basement membrane, and the thin capillary wall.
Source: Icon Learning Systems.

white blood cell, known as an **alveolar macrophage,** which removes inhaled foreign particles like dust and pollen, and bacteria.

Each **lung** is a spongy, soft organ that fills half of the thoracic cavity. The lung is divided into compartments known as **lobes,** and further divides into smaller compartments called segments. The outer surface of the lung is a thin, almost transparent layer of serous membrane called the **visceral pleura.** An outer membrane layer is attached to the inside wall of the thorax, and is known as the **parietal pleura.** Between the two pleurae is a narrow space, the **pleural cavity.** The cavity contains a small amount of fluid, which reduces friction between the membranes during breathing.

[**thinking critically!**]

What is the advantage to respiration that is gained by alveolar walls containing only a single layer of cells?

getting to the root of it | anatomy and physiology terms

Many of the anatomy and physiology terms are formed from roots that are used to construct the more complex medical terms of the respiratory system, including symptoms, diseases, and treatments. In this section, we will review the terms that describe the structure and function of the respiratory system *in relation to their word roots,* which are shown in **bold.**

Study the word roots and terms in this list and complete the review exercises that follow.

Word Root (Meaning)	Terms Formed from the Word Root (Pronunciation)	Definition
alveol (air sac)	**alveol**ar macrophage (al VEE oh lahr MAK roh fayj)	a type of white blood cell housed inside alveoli that removes inhaled particles and bacteria; also called a dust cell
	alveoli (al VEE oh lye)	a terminal dilation branching from bronchioles and the site of gas exchange between lungs and blood; singular form is **alveolus** (al VEE oh luss)
bronch (airway)	**bronch**i (BRONG kye)	rigid air tubes that branch from the trachea and further divide to form extensive branching within the lungs; singular form is bronchus (BRONG kuss)
	bronchial tree (BRONG kee al)	the extensive branching network of the bronchi within the lungs
	bronchioles (BRONG kee ohlz)	microscopic tubes at the ends of the branching bronchial tree, which terminate at alveoli; bronchiole walls lack cartilage, and instead are composed of smooth muscle
phragm (partition)	dia**phragm** (DYE ah fram)	a sheet of muscle that divides the thoracic and abdominal cavities; it is the primary respiratory muscle, whose contraction and relaxation results in inspiration and expiration
glottis (opening of the windpipe)	**glottis** (GLAHT iss)	the opening into the larynx, at the junction between the pharynx and larynx
	epi**glottis** (ep ih GLAHT iss)	a flap of cartilage located above the glottis, which covers the opening to the larynx during swallowing

Word Root (Meaning)	Terms Formed from the Word Root (Pronunciation)	Definition
spir (to breathe)	external re**spir**ation (ress pih RAY shun)	the process of gas exchange between the alveoli and adjacent capillaries within the lungs
	in**spir**ation (in spih RAY shun)	the process of drawing air into the lungs, or inhaling
	internal re**spir**ation (ress pih RAY shun)	the process of gas exchange between the bloodstream and body cells
	lower re**spir**atory tract (RESS pih rah tor ee)	the segment of the respiratory system that lies within the thoracic cavity, including the bronchi, bronchial tree, and bronchioles
	re**spir**ation (ress pih RAY shun)	the process of oxygen delivery to cells
	re**spir**atory membrane (RESS pih rah tor ee MEHM brayn)	the thin barrier that is crossed during gas exchange within the lungs, which includes one alveolar cell, a thin region of connective tissue, and one capillary endothelial cell
	re**spir**atory portion (RESS pih rah tor ee)	the part of the respiratory system that includes the alveoli of the lungs
	upper re**spir**atory tract (RESS pih rah tor ee)	the segment of the respiratory system mainly located above the thoracic cavity, including the nose, pharynx, larynx, and trachea
laryng (voicebox)	**laryn**x (LAIR inks)	the part of the upper respiratory tract between the pharynx and trachea, which is also called the voicebox; it is composed of cartilage pieces that form a box-like structure containing vocal folds that produce sound and enable speech when vibrating
nas (nose)	**nas**al septum (NAY zl)	the partition within the nasal cavity, dividing it into right and left nasal chambers
	para**nas**al sinuses (pair ah NAY zl SIGH nuss ehz)	a series of membrane-lined chambers within the frontal bone and maxillary bones that connect with the nasal cavity
pharyng (throat)	**pharyn**x (FAIR inks)	the muscular chamber behind the mouth and above the larynx and esophagus; it is lined with mucous membrane and receives incoming air and food
pleur (rib)	**pleur**a (PLOO rah)	a serous membrane associated with the lungs
	visceral **pleur**a (VISS er al PLOO rah)	a serous membrane that forms the lungs' outer surface
	parietal **pleur**a (pah RYE eh tal PLOO rah)	a serous membrane attached to the inner thorax wall
	pleural cavity (PLOO ral CAV ih tee)	the cavity that lies between the visceral pleura and the parietal pleura
trache (windpipe)	**trache**a (TRAY kee ah)	a rigid tube about 12 inches long, extending from the larynx to the bronchi; also known as the windpipe, it is kept rigid by rings of cartilage in its wall, and is lined with mucous membrane

Trachea

The term *trachea* was first used by the ancient Greeks, who chose the term because the cartilage rings of the trachea form a rough series of ridges that one can feel along the surface of the neck. They referred to the organ as the *tracheia arteria,* or *rough artery,* because they wrongly believed at the time that arteries carried air, rather than blood.

OTHER IMPORTANT TERMS

The terms in this table are related to the structure and function of the respiratory system, but are not built from word roots.

conducting portion	the part of the respiratory system that conducts air between the outside environment and the alveoli. It includes the nose, pharynx, larynx, trachea, and bronchi
expiration (ek spih RAY shun)	the process of exhaling air
lung	a soft, spongy organ in the thoracic cavity composed of alveoli, capillaries, and the bronchial tree
nose	the facial appendage supported by the nasal bones and cartilage that encloses the nasal cavity
ventilation (vent ih LAY shun)	the process of breathing, which includes inhalation and exhalation

SELF QUIZ 12.2

SAY IT—SPELL IT!

Review the terms of the respiratory system by speaking the phonetic pronunciation guides out loud, then writing in the correct spelling of the term.

Success Hint: Use the audio glossary on the CD and CW for additional help with pronunciation of these terms.

1. al VEE oh lye _____

2. BRONG kye _____

3. BRONG kee ohlz _____

4. DYE ah fram _____

5. ek spih RAY shun _____

6. in spih RAY shun _____

7. LAIR inks _____

8. FAIR inks _____

9. ress pih RAY shun _____

10. TRAY kee ah _____

11. vent ih LAY shun _____

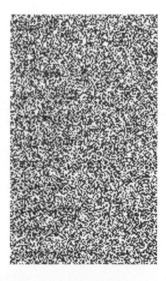

MATCH IT!

Match the term on the left with the correct definition on the right.

_____ 1. trachea   a. branches form the bronchial tree

_____ 2. nasal cavities   b. membranes of the lungs

_____ 3. larynx   c. nose, pharynx, larynx, trachea

_____ 4. epiglottis   d. air sacs within the lungs

_____ 5. bronchioles   e. within the nose

_____ 6. ventilation   f. the rigid wind pipe

_____ 7. pleura   g. inspiration and expiration

_____ 8. lung   h. prevents food from entering larynx

_____ 9. pharynx   i. its muscles perform swallowing

_____10. bronchi   j. the voicebox

_____11. upper respiratory tract   k. a soft, spongy organ in the chest

_____12. alveoli   l. microscopic tubes in the lungs

FILL IT IN!

Fill in the blanks with the correct terms.

1. The respiratory system is named after its primary function, _____, which is the delivery of _____ to the bloodstream.

2. The upper respiratory tract includes the nose, which includes an internal _____ _____ divided by a septum. All organs of the upper respiratory tract are internally lined with a moist _____ membrane.

3. The throat, or _____, is a chamber that receives both air and food.

4. The voicebox, or _____, is made of cartilages that form a box-like structure. It receives inhaled air from the pharynx through an opening known as the _____, which is protected from swallowed food by a flap of cartilage called the _____.

5. The windpipe, or _____, is kept open by rings of cartilage.

6. Within the chest, the trachea divides into the right and left primary _____. Soon after entering the lung, a bronchus divides again and again to form the _____ _____.

7. The branching bronchi eventually form microscopic tubes that are not supported by cartilage, called _____. They end at cul-de-sacs that are fringed with tiny air sacs, or _____.

12.2

8. The thin barrier that is the site of external respiration is the _____ membrane, which includes a single layer of _____ cells and a single layer of capillary cells.

12.3 9. The soft, spongy substance of each _____ is a combination of many alveoli, capillaries, and bronchioles. The _____ are two layers of serous membrane associated with the lungs.

10. The process that includes breathing in, or _____, and exhaling, or expiration, is known as _____.

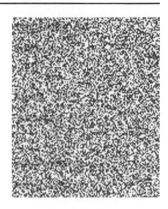

medical terms of the
respiratory system

Diseases of the respiratory system reduce the amount of oxygen that is normally supplied to body cells. Severe respiratory disease can lead to an inability to bring oxygen into the bloodstream, and may result in death. Breathing problems are reliable symptoms of respiratory disease, and may also lead to additional complications. In general, respiratory disease may be caused by congenital conditions, infections, allergies, tumors, a heart condition that results in a deficient circulation of blood, or injury.

The clinical treatment of a respiratory disease is performed by a physician with a specialization in treating the body region, the particular disorder, or a set of disorders. For example, a lung disease is treated by a **pulmonary** (lung) **specialist,** a disease of the pharynx is treated by a **nose and throat specialist,** and lung cancer is treated by an **oncologist** (cancer specialist). Often assisting the physician is a technician with special training in the treatment of breathing problems, called a **respiratory therapist.**

let's construct terms!

In this section, we will assemble all of the word parts to construct medical terminology related to the respiratory system. Abbreviations are used to indicate each word part: **p** = prefix, **r** = root, **cv** = combining vowel, and **s** = suffix. Note that some terms are not constructed from word parts, but they are included here to expand your vocabulary.

The medical terms of the respiratory system are listed in the following three sections:

■ Symptoms and Signs
■ Diseases and Disorders
■ Treatments, Procedures, and Devices

Each section is followed by review exercises. Study the lists in these tables and complete the review exercises that follow.

Symptoms and Signs

WORD PARTS (WHEN APPLICABLE)			TERM	DEFINITION
Part	Type	Meaning		
a- -capnia	p s	without carbon dioxide	**acapnia** (ah KAP nee ah)	absence of carbon dioxide
an- -oxia	p s	without oxygen	**anoxia** (ah NOK see ah)	absence of oxygen
a- -phonia	p s	without sound, voice	**aphonia** (ah FOH nee ah)	absence of voice
a- -pnea	p s	without breathing	**apnea** (AP nee ah)	inability to breathe
brady- -pnea	p s	slow breathing	**bradypnea** (brad ip NEE ah)	slow breathing
bronch/o -spasm	r/cv s	air way sudden, involuntary muscle spasm	**bronchospasm** (BRONG koh spazm)	narrowing of the airway caused by contraction of smooth muscles in the walls of the bronchioles
			Cheyne-Stokes respiration (CHAIN STOHKS ress pih RAY shun)	a pattern of breathing marked by a gradual increase of deep breathing, followed by shallow breathing that leads to apnea
dys- -phonia	p s	bad, abnormal sound, voice	**dysphonia** (diss FOH nee ah)	hoarseness of the voice
dys- -pnea	p s	bad, abnormal breathing	**dyspnea** (DISP nee ah)	difficulty breathing
epi- -staxis	p s	upon dripping	**epistaxis** (ep ih STAK siss)	a nosebleed
eu- -pnea	p s	good, normal breathing	**eupnea** (yoop NEE ah)	normal breathing
hem/o -ptysis	r/cv s	blood to spit out fluid	**hemoptysis** (hee MOP tih siss)	coughing up and spitting out blood originating from the lungs
hem/o thorax	r/cv r	blood chest	**hemothorax** (hee moh THOH raks)	blood in the pleural cavity
hyper- -capnia	p s	excessive carbon dioxide	**hypercapnia** (HIGH per KAP nee ah)	excessive carbon dioxide in the blood
hyper- -pnea	p s	excessive breathing	**hyperpnea** (HIGH per NEE ah)	deep breathing
			hyperventilation (HIGH per vent ih LAY shun)	excessive movement of air in and out of the lungs
hypo- -capnia	p s	below normal carbon dioxide	**hypocapnia** (HIGH poh KAP nee ah)	deficient levels of carbon dioxide in the blood

WORD PARTS (WHEN APPLICABLE)			TERM	DEFINITION
Part	**Type**	**Meaning**		
hypo- -pnea	p s	below normal breathing	**hypopnea** (high POPP nee ah)	shallow breathing
			hypoventilation (HIGH poh vent ih LAY shun)	breathing rhythm that fails to meet the body's gas exchange demands
hypo- ox -emia	p r s	below normal oxygen blood condtion	**hypoxemia** (high pahk SEE mee ah)	deficient levels of oxygen in the blood
hypo- ox -ia	p r s	below normal oxygen diseased state	**hypoxia** (high PAHK see ah)	deficient levels of oxygen in tissues throughout the body
laryng/o -spasm	r/cv s	voicebox or larynx sudden, involuntary muscle contraction	**laryngospasm** (lair ING goh spazm)	spasmodic closure of the glottis (the opening into the larynx)
orth/o -pnea	r/cv s	straight breathing	**orthopnea** (or THAHP nee ah)	ability to breathe is limited to an upright position
			paroxysm (PAIR ahk sizm)	a sudden sharp pain or convulsion
rhin/o -rrhagia	r/cv s	nose bleeding	**rhinorrhagia** (rye noh RAH jee ah)	rapid flow of blood from the nose; also called **epistaxis**
rhin/o -rrhea	r/cv s	nose excessive discharge	**rhinorrhea** (rye noh REE ah)	fluid discharge from the nose
			sputum (SPYOO tum)	expectorated (spit out) matter, usually containing mucus and sometimes pus
tachy- -pnea	p s	rapid, fast breathing	**tachypnea** (tak ihp NEE ah)	rapid breathing
thorac -algia	r s	chest pain	**thoracalgia** (thor ah KAL jee ah)	pain in the chest region

SELF QUIZ 12.3

SAY IT—SPELL IT!

Review the terms of the respiratory system by speaking the phonetic pronunciation guides out loud, then writing in the correct spelling of the term.

1. AP nee ah   _____

2. brad ip NEE ah   _____

3. BRONG koh spazm   _____

4. diss FOH nee ah   _____

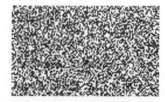

5. DISP nee ah _____

12.4 6. ep ih STAK siss _____

7. hee moh THOH raks _____

8. hee MOP tih siss _____

9. HIGH per KAP nee ah _____

10. HIGH per NEE ah _____

11. HIGH per vent ih LAY shun _____

12. high PAHK see ah _____

13. high pahk SEE mee ah _____

14. high POPP nee ah _____

15. lair ING goh spazm _____

16. or THAHP nee ah _____

17. rye noh RAH jee ah _____

18. thor ah KAL jee ah _____

19. yoop NEE ah _____

MATCH IT!

Match the term on the left with the correct definition on the right.

_____ 1. dyspnea

_____ 2. apnea

_____ 3. hypopnea

_____ 4. eupnea

_____ 5. bradypnea

_____ 6. hyperpnea

_____ 7. tachypnea

_____ 8. orthopnea

_____ 9. hemothorax

_____10. epistaxis

_____11. hypoxemia

_____12. rhinorrhagia

_____13. hypoxia

_____14. thoracalgia

_____15. hyperventilation

_____16. hemoptysis

_____17. dysphonia

_____18. hypercapnia

a. shallow breathing

b. deep breathing

c. difficulty breathing

d. can breathe only when upright

e. normal breathing

f. slow beathing

g. inability to breathe

h. rapid breathing

i. a hoarse voice

j. excessive carbon dioxide blood levels

k. pain in the chest region

l. blood in the pleural cavity

m. rapid flow of blood from the nose

n. deficient levels of oxygen in the blood

o. same as epistaxis

p. deficient levels of oxygen in body tissues

q. excessive movement of air in and out of lungs

r. coughing up and spitting blood

BREAK IT DOWN!

Analyze and separate each term into its word parts by labeling each word part using p = prefix, r = root, cv = combining vowel, and s = suffix.

1. bradypnea   _____

2. dysphonia   _____

3. dyspnea   _____

4. epistaxis   _____

5. hemoptysis   _____

6. hemothorax   _____

7. hypercapnia   _____

8. hyperpnea   _____

9. hypocapnea   _____

10. hypopnea   _____

11. hypoxemia   _____

12. hypoxia   _____

13. laryngospasm   _____

14. orthopnea   _____

15. rhinorrhagia   _____

16. thoracalgia   _____

Diseases and Disorders

WORD PARTS (WHEN APPLICABLE)			TERM	DEFINITION
Part	**Type**	**Meaning**		
a-	p	absence of	**asphyxia**	the absence of respiratory ventilation, or suffocation
sphyx	r	pulse	(ass FIK see ah)	
-ia	s	condition of		
			asthma (AZ mah)	a condition of the lungs characterized by widespread narrowing of the bronchioles and formation of mucus plugs, producing symptoms of wheezing, shortness of breath, and coughing; it is caused by the local release of factors during an allergic response (Figure 12.7⦂⦂⦂⦂)

[FYI]

Asthma

The term *asthma* is derived from the Greek word *astma,* which means *to pant.* This panting disease is on the rise in the U.S. for unknown reasons. There is no cure, and the most common treatment is the use of inhalers that dilate the bronchioles.

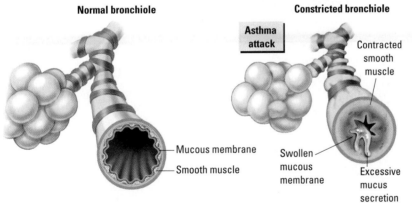

Normal bronchiole   **Constricted bronchiole**

Asthma attack

Contracted smooth muscle

Mucous membrane
Smooth muscle

Swollen mucous membrane

Excessive mucus secretion

Figure 12.7 ⦂⦂⦂⦂

Asthma.
(a) A normal bronchiole.
(b) An asthmatic bronchiole. During an asthma "attack," the bronchioles constrict to reduce the airway. Thickened mucus secretions form plugs that further reduce the airway.

WORD PARTS			TERM	DEFINITION
atel	r	incomplete	**atelectasis**	the absence of gas in the lungs due to a failure of
-ectasis	s	expansion, dilation	(at eh LEK tah siss)	alveolar expansion; also called collapsed lung
bronch/i	r/cv	airway	**bronchiectasis**	dilation of the bronchi
-ectasis	s	expansion, dilation	(BRONG kee EK tah siss)	
bronch	r	airway	**bronchitis**	inflammation of the bronchi
-itis	s	inflammation	(brong KYE tiss)	
bronch/o	r/cv	airway	**bronchogenic**	cancer originating in the bronchi (Figure 12.8⦂⦂⦂⦂)
-genic	s	pertaining to formation	**carcinoma** (brong koh JENN ik	
carcin	r	cancer	kar sih NOH mah)	
-oma	s	tumor		
bronch/o	r/cv	airway	**bronchopneumonia**	acute inflammation of the smaller bronchial tubes,
pneumon	r	lung or air	(BRONG koh noo MOH	bronchioles, and alveoli
-ia	s	diseased state	nee ah)	

WORD PARTS (WHEN APPLICABLE)			TERM	DEFINITION
Part	Type	Meaning		

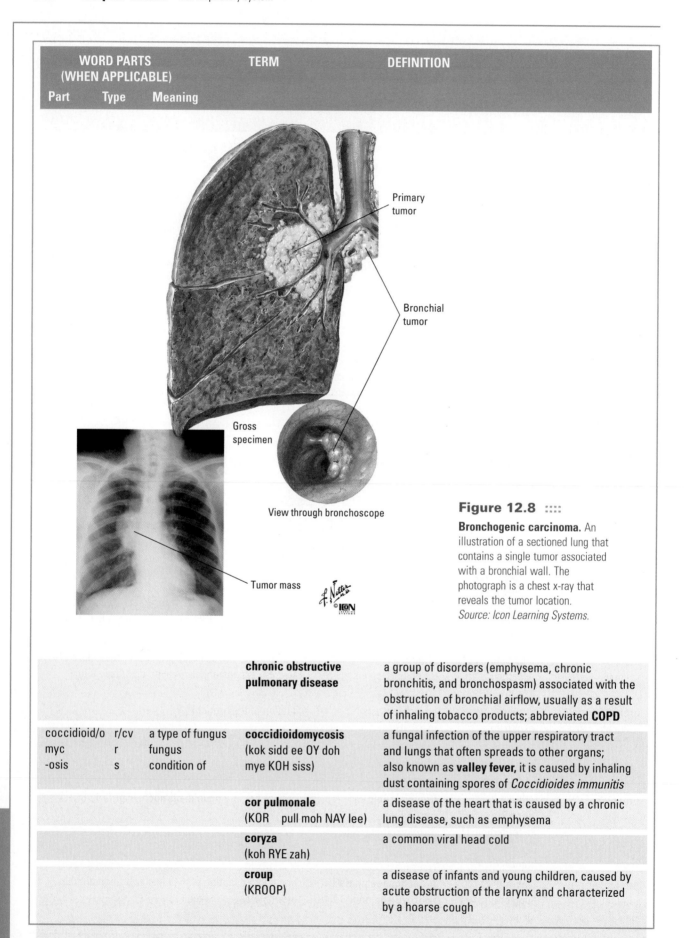

Primary tumor

Bronchial tumor

Gross specimen

View through bronchoscope

Tumor mass

Figure 12.8 ::::

Bronchogenic carcinoma. An illustration of a sectioned lung that contains a single tumor associated with a bronchial wall. The photograph is a chest x-ray that reveals the tumor location. *Source: Icon Learning Systems.*

Part	Type	Meaning	TERM	DEFINITION
			chronic obstructive pulmonary disease	a group of disorders (emphysema, chronic bronchitis, and bronchospasm) associated with the obstruction of bronchial airflow, usually as a result of inhaling tobacco products; abbreviated **COPD**
coccidioid/o	r/cv	a type of fungus	**coccidioidomycosis** (kok sidd ee OY doh mye KOH siss)	a fungal infection of the upper respiratory tract and lungs that often spreads to other organs; also known as **valley fever,** it is caused by inhaling dust containing spores of *Coccidioides immunitis*
myc	r	fungus		
-osis	s	condition of		
			cor pulmonale (KOR pull moh NAY lee)	a disease of the heart that is caused by a chronic lung disease, such as emphysema
			coryza (koh RYE zah)	a common viral head cold
			croup (KROOP)	a disease of infants and young children, caused by acute obstruction of the larynx and characterized by a hoarse cough

WORD PARTS (WHEN APPLICABLE)			TERM	DEFINITION
Part	Type	Meaning		
cyst -ic fibr -osis	r s r s	bladder, sac pertaining to fiber condition of	**cystic fibrosis** (SISS tik fye BROH siss)	a hereditary disease characterized by excess mucus production in the respiratory tract and elsewhere; abbreviated **CF**
			deviated septum (DEE vee ay ted SEHP tum)	the nasal septum dividing the two nasal cavities is not median, creating one cavity that is larger than the other
dia- phragmat/o -cele	p r/cv s	through, between partition hernia, swelling	**diaphragmatocele** (dye ah frag MAT oh seel)	hernia of the diaphragm
			emphysema (em fih SEE mah)	a chronic lung disease characterized by enlarged alveoli and damaged respiratory membrane; its symptoms include apnea, a barrel chest due to labored breathing, and gradual deterioration due to chronic hypoxemia (Figure 12.9▦)

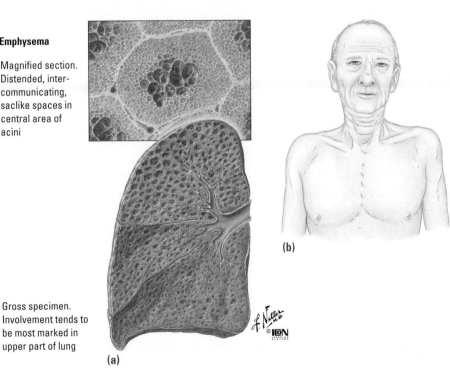

Emphysema

Magnified section. Distended, intercommunicating, saclike spaces in central area of acini

Gross specimen. Involvement tends to be most marked in upper part of lung

(a)

(b)

Figure 12.9 ▦

Emphysema. Alveolar walls lose their elasticity, making it difficult to push air out of the lungs. Also, the respiratory membrane becomes damaged, reducing the efficiency of gas exchange.

(a) In the upper view, a magnified section is shown that reveals saclike spaces which alveoli once occupied. In the lower image, a sectioned lung shows widespread replacement of alveoli by the spaces.
Source: Icon Learning Systems.

(b) Typical appearance of a patient with emphysema. Characteristic signs include reduced weight, a barrel chest, and a drawn facial appearance.
Source: Pearson Education.

epi- glottis -itis	p r s	upon mouth of the windpipe inflammation	**epiglottitis** (ep ih glah TYE tiss)	inflammation of the epiglottis
in- somn -ia	p r s	without sleep condition	**insomnia** (in SAHM nee ah)	inability to sleep
laryng -itis	r s	voicebox, larynx inflammation	**laryngitis** (LAIR in JYE tiss)	inflammation of the larynx

WORD PARTS (WHEN APPLICABLE)			TERM	DEFINITION
Part	**Type**	**Meaning**		
laryng/o	r/cv	voicebox, larynx	**laryngotracheobronchitis**	chronic inflammation of the larynx, trachea, and
trache/o	r/cv	windpipe, trachea	(lair RING goh TRAY	bronchi; the acute form that strikes infants and
bronch	r	airway, bronchus	kee oh brong KYE tiss)	children is called **croup**; abbreviated **LTB**
-itis	s	inflammation		
legionella		genus of bacteria	**legionellosis**	a form of pneumonia caused by the bacterium
-osis	s	condition	(lee juh nell OH siss)	*Legionella pneumophila;* also called Legionnaire's disease

[FYI]

Legionnaire's Disease

Legionellosis was first identified in 1976, when many members of a Legionnaire convention at a popular hotel became afflicted with an infection that caused 21 deaths. It took intensive research to reveal the bacterium and why it spread so quickly: It was delivered throughout the hotel via the hotel ventilation system under ideal conditions for the bacteria to proliferate.

nas/o	r/cv	nose	**nasopharyngitis**	inflammation of the nose and pharynx
pharyng	r	throat, pharynx	(nay zoh FAIR in JYE	
-itis	s	inflammation	tiss)	
a-	p	without	**obstructive sleep apnea**	collapse of the pharynx during sleep, resulting in
-pnea	s	sleep	(AP nee ah)	airway obstruction and the absence of breathing; abbreviated **OSA**
pan-	p	all, entire	**pansinusitis**	inflammation of all paranasal sinuses on one or both
sinus	r	cavity	(PAN sigh nuss EYE	sides of the face
-itis	s	inflammation	tiss)	
			pertussis	an acute infectious disease characterized by
			(per TUSS siss)	inflammation of the larynx, trachea, and bronchi that produces spasmodic coughing; also called whooping cough because of the noise produced during coughing when the larynx spasms
pharyng	r	throat, pharynx	**pharyngitis**	inflammation of the pharynx
-itis	s	inflammation	(FAIR in JYE tiss)	
pleur	r	rib, pleura	**pleural effusion**	escape of fluid into the pleural cavity during
-al	s	pertaining to	(PLOO ral	inflammation
effus	r	pouring out	eh FYOO zhun)	
-ion	s	pertaining to		
pleur	r	rib, pleura	**pleuritis**	inflammation of the pleurae; also called pleurisy
-itis	s	inflammation	(ploo RYE tiss)	(PLOOR ih see)
pneumat/o	r/cv	lung, air	**pneumatocele**	hernia of the lung, in which the lung protrudes
-cele	s	hernia, swelling	(noo MAT oh seel)	through an opening in the chest

WORD PARTS (WHEN APPLICABLE)			TERM	DEFINITION
Part	**Type**	**Meaning**		
pneum/o con/i -osis	r/cv r/cv s	lung, air dust condition	**pneumoconiosis** (noo moh KOH nee OH siss)	inflammation of the lungs caused by the chronic inhalation of fine particles, which leads to the formation of a fibrotic tissue around the alveoli that reduces their ability to stretch with incoming air; it includes asbestosis (az bess TOH siss), caused by asbestos inhalation, and silicosis (sill ih KOH siss), caused by fine silicon dust inhalation (Figure 12.10▦)

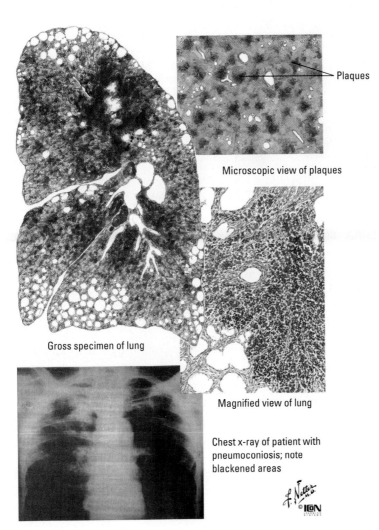

Microscopic view of plaques

Gross specimen of lung

Magnified view of lung

Chest x-ray of patient with pneumoconiosis; note blackened areas

Figure 12.10 ▦

Pneumoconiosus. Compared to a normal lung, the alveoli are surrounded by fibrotic plaques that prevent the alveoli from inflating, thereby restricting inspiration.
Source: Icon Learning Systems.

pneumon -ia	r s	lung, air condition	***Pneumocystis carinii* pneumonia** (noo moh SISS tiss kah RYE nee eye noo MOH nee ah)	a pneumonia caused by the fungus *P. carinii* that is a common opportunistic disease in patients with AIDS; abbreviated **PCP**
pneumon -ia	r s	lung, air condition	**pneumonia** (noo MOH nee ah)	inflammation of soft lung tissue (excluding the bronchi) caused by bacterial, viral, or fungal infection, in which the alveoli become filled with fluids (Figure 12.11▦)

WORD PARTS (WHEN APPLICABLE)			TERM	DEFINITION
Part	Type	Meaning		

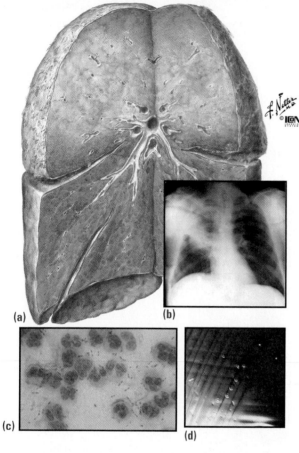

(a)   (b)

(c)   (d)

Figure 12.11 ::::
Pneumonia.

(a) A sectioned lung with lobar pneumonia, which is characterized by fluid accumulation and a fibrinous secretion.
(b) Pneumonia is often diagnosed with a chest x-ray, where it shows as a cloudy area in an otherwise dark field of the chest.
(c) A sputum sample often reveals the source of the infection, in this example, pneumococci (bacteria).
(d) A definitive test for the source of bacterial pneumonia can be made with a sputum sample on an agar plate, which grows the bacterial colonies for identification purposes.
Source: Icon Learning Systems.

Part	Type	Meaning	TERM	DEFINITION
pneumon	r	lung, air	**pneumonitis**	inflammation of the lungs, independent of a
-itis	s	inflammation	(NOO moh NYE tiss)	particular cause
pneum/o	r/cv	lung, air	**pneumothorax**	presence of air or gas in the pleural cavity
thorax	r	chest	(NOO moh THOH raks)	(Figure 12.12::::)
pulmon	r	lung	**pulmonary edema**	accumulation of fluid in the alveoli and bronchioles
-ary	s	pertaining to	(PULL mon air ee eh DEE mah)	
pulmon	r	lung	**pulmonary embolism**	blockage in the pulmonary circulation caused by a
-ary	s	pertaining to	(PULL mon air ee EM boh lizm)	moving blood clot; abbreviated **PE**
embol	r	a throwing in		
-ism	s	condition		
pulmon	r	lung	**pulmonary neoplasm**	tumor of the lung
-ary	s	pertaining to	(PULL mon air ee NEE oh plazm)	
neo-	p	new		
-plasm	s	something shaped		
pulmon	r	lung	**pulmonary tuberculosis**	infection of the lungs by the bacterium
-ary	s	pertaining to	(PULL mon air ee too ber kyoo LOH siss)	*Mycobacterium tuberculosis,* which includes
tubercul	r	a little swelling		tubercle formation, inflammation, and necrotic lesions;
-osis	s	condition		abbreviated **TB** (Figure 12.13::::)

WORD PARTS (WHEN APPLICABLE)			TERM	DEFINITION
Part	Type	Meaning		

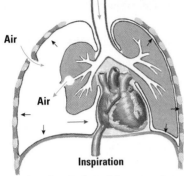

Air enters pleural cavity through lung wound or ruptured bleb (or occasionally via penetrating chest wound) with valvelike opening. Ipsilateral lung collapses and mediastinum shifts to opposite side, compressing contralateral lung and impairing its ventilating capacity

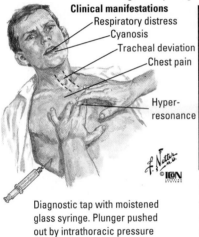

Clinical manifestations
- Respiratory distress
- Cyanosis
- Tracheal deviation
- Chest pain
- Hyper-resonance

Diagnostic tap with moistened glass syringe. Plunger pushed out by intrathoracic pressure

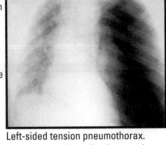

Left-sided tension pneumothorax. Lung collapsed, mediastinum and trachea deviated to opposite side, diaphragm depressed, intercostal spaces widened

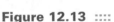

Primary plaque

Secondary plaque

Figure 12.12 ::::

Pneumothorax and atelectasis. Air entering a wound through the chest wall causes collapse of the lung. It often pushes the thoracic cavity contents to the opposite side, compressing the other lung. The chest x-ray confirms the diagnosis, which shows a left-sided pneumothorax and lung collapse.
Source: Icon Learning Systems.

Figure 12.13 ::::

Pulmonary tuberculosis. The figures show sectioned lungs that contain primary and secondary TB plaques.
Source: Icon Learning Systems.

py/o	r/cv	pus	**pyothorax**	a condition of pus in the pleural cavity; also called
thorax	r	chest	(pye oh THOH raks)	empyema (em pye EE mah)
			respiratory distress syndrome (RESS pih rah tor ee)	respiratory failure characterized by atelectasis, also called hyaline membrane disease or **HMD**; this condition occurs in two forms: ■ neonatal respiratory distress syndrome appears in infants and is caused by insufficient surfactant (a substance normally secreted by alveolar cells, which enables alveoli to reopen after expiration); abbreviated **NRDS** ■ adult (or acute) respiratory distress syndrome that affects adults and is caused by severe lung infections or injury; abbreviated **ARDS**

WORD PARTS (WHEN APPLICABLE)			TERM	DEFINITION
Part	Type	Meaning		
rhin	r	nose	**rhinitis**	inflammation of the nasal mucous membrane
-itis	s	inflammation	(rye NYE tiss)	
rhin/o	r/cv	nose	**rhinomycosis**	fungal infection of the nasal mucous membrane
myc	r	fungus	(RYE noh my KOH siss)	
-osis	s	condition		
sinus	r	cavity	**sinusitis**	inflammation of the sinus mucous membranes
-itis	s	inflammation	(sigh nuss EYE tiss)	
			severe acute respiratory syndrome (RESS pih rah tor ee)	a severe, rapidly onset viral infection resulting in respiratory distress that includes lung inflammation, alveolar damage, and atelectasis; abbreviated **SARS**
tonsil	r	almond	**tonsillitis**	inflammation of a tonsil, usually a palatine tonsil; an
-itis	s	inflammation	(TAHN sill EYE tiss)	inflamed pharyngeal tonsil is called an adenoid
trache	r	windpipe, trachea	**tracheitis**	inflammation of the trachea
-itis	s	inflammation	(tray kee EYE tiss)	
trache/o	r/cv	windpipe, trachea	**tracheostenosis**	narrowing of the trachea
sten	r	narrowing, constriction	(TRAY kee oh steh NOH siss)	
-osis	s	condition		
			upper respiratory infection (RESS pih rah tor ee in FEK shun)	infection of the upper respiratory tract (nose, pharynx, larynx, and trachea). Usually the result of a virus, it is abbreviated **URI**

disease focus | Tuberculosis

Tuberculosis, or TB, was the leading cause of death in the United States at the turn of the 20th century. At the time, it was a serious, widespread killer that led physicians to isolate TB sufferers in special hospitals known as sanatoriums. To protect healthy people, sanatoriums were often far from population centers, representing early efforts at medical quarantine. Treatments were limited to drastic measures that appear barbaric or foolish next to current treatments. For example, doctors would puncture and collapse a patient's infected lung in the hope of suffocating the microbes. Also, bright sunlight and fresh air were erroneously thought to help toward recovery. In some cases, TB would go into a state of remission (for reasons other than those believed at the time), but in most cases it resulted in a gradual deterioration until death. With the introduction of sulfa drugs in the early part of the 20th century, and antibiotics several decades later, TB incidence declined. For a time during the 1960s, the medical community believed complete eradication was possible. However, a resurgence of TB occurred in urban areas during the 1980s. Currently, TB continues to infect susceptible populations.

Tuberculosis is a contagious infection caused by the bacterium *Mycobacterium tuberculosis* (or tubercle bacillus). It is spread through the air in tiny droplets of sputum that are expelled when an infected person coughs or speaks. The bacteria then enter its next victim by way of the respiratory tract and usually establish in the lungs, although it can travel to almost any organ. (It has been found in the brain, kidneys, heart, liver, and bones.) Once established, the bacteria usually enter a dormant stage in the body, sometimes for decades, and is kept in check by the immune response. It is rarely detected early because its initial symptoms are very mild and the bacterium is in low concentrations. However, TB skin tests can reveal an antibody reaction to the bacterium, providing evidence of infection. TB becomes active when the immune system falters, which may be caused by an extended viral infection, increasing age, serious injury, or even substance abuse (alcohol or drugs). Once activated, TB establishes large colonies in the lungs and other organs. It destroys functional tissue by releasing toxins, and by replacing healthy tissue with fibrous plaques called tubercles.

Even when activated, TB tends to waste its victims slowly. Gradually, the patient loses weight, energy, and state of mind, until death comes. Nineteenth century doctors called this deadly disease "consumption" because of the way it ate away, or consumed, its victims.

TB is a difficult disease to treat and cure, because it requires a cocktail of antibiotic drugs that must be administered each day for as long as nine months. Many TB sufferers abandon the strict drug regimen as soon as they begin to feel better, thinking that they are cured. However, in these cases the symptoms return, and often with increased virulence. Also, the tubercle bacillus is particularly adept at mutating into forms that are resistant to drugs. These factors make TB very difficult to eradicate, or even to manage, in an urban population.

SELF QUIZ 12.4

SAY IT—SPELL IT!

Review the terms of the respiratory system by speaking the phonetic pronunciations out loud, then writing the correct spelling of the term.

12.5
1. at eh LEK tah siss _____
2. AZ mah _____
3. BRONG kee EK tah siss _____
4. brong KYE tiss _____
5. dye ah frag MAT oh seel _____
6. em fih SEE mah _____
7. ep ih glah TYE tiss _____
8. KOR pull moh NAY lee _____
9. koh RYE zah _____

12.6
10. KROOP _____
11. lair RING goh TRAY kee oh brong KYE tiss _____
12. LAIR in JYE tiss _____
13. lee juh nell OH siss _____
14. nay zoh FAIR in JYE tiss _____
15. noo MAT oh seel _____
16. noo moh KOH nee OH siss _____
17. noo MOH nee ah _____
18. NOO moh NYE tiss _____
19. PAN sigh nuss EYE tiss _____
20. per TUSS siss _____
21. pye oh THOH raks _____
22. ploo RI tis _____
23. rye NYE tiss _____

12.7
24. RYE noh my KOH siss _____
25. sigh nuss EYE tiss _____
26. SISS tik fye BROH siss _____
27. TAHN sill EYE tiss _____
28. TRAY kee oh steh NOH siss _____

MATCH IT!

Match the term on the left with the correct definition on the right.

_____ 1. epiglottitis

a. fungal infection in the nose

_____ 2. laryngitis

b. condition of pus in the chest

_____ 3. tuberculosis

c. inflammation of the trachea

_____ 4. rhinomycosis

d. collapsed lung

_____ 5. pulmonary neoplasm

e. cancer arising from lung tissue

_____ 6. atelectasis

f. inflammation of the nose and pharynx

_____ 7. tracheitis

g. a bacterial infection that primarily affects
   the lungs

_____ 8. pneumatocele

h. inflammation of the epiglottis

_____ 9. nasopharyngitis

i. inflammation of the larynx

_____10. bronchitis

j. herniation of a lung

_____11. pyothorax

k. also Legionaire's disease

_____12. croup

l. literally "a swelling"

_____13. legionellosis

m. inflammation of a bronchus

_____14. pertussis

n. caused by an acute obstruction in the larynx
   among children

_____15. emphysema

o. also known as whooping cough

BREAK IT DOWN!

Analyze and separate each term into its word parts by labeling each word part using p = prefix, r = root, cv = combining vowel, and s = suffix.

1. atelectasis   _____

2. diaphragmatocele   _____

3. epiglottitis   _____

4. tracheitis   _____

5. pneumatocele   _____

6. nasopharyngitis   _____

7. rhinomycosis   _____

8. bronchiectasis   _____

9. pansinusitis   _____

12.8 10. tracheostenosis   _____

12.9   11. pyothorax   _____

       12. tuberculosis   _____

FILL IT IN!

Fill in the blanks with the correct terms.

12.10   1. Adult respiratory distress syndrome, abbreviated _____, is respiratory failure characterized by atelectasis.

       2. The medical term for suffocation, or the absence of ventilation, is known as _____.

12.11   3. The shortness of breath and wheezing that characterizes _____ is caused by widespread bronchiole constriction and mucus plug formation.

       4. In Cheyne-Stokes respiration, a pattern of deep breathing gradually increases, followed by shallow breathing and eventually _____.

       5. COPD, or chronic _____ _____ disease, is a reduction in the bronchial airway that is mainly caused by _____.

       6. A chronic lung disease caused by enlarged alveoli and damaged respiratory membrane is characteristic of _____. It often leads to heart disease known as _____ _____.

12.12   7. A common head cold is also known as acute _____.

       8. Laryngitis in young children may lead to _____.

       9. _____ _____ is a hereditary disease that is characterized by excess mucus production in the respiratory tract and elsewhere.

12.13   10. An infectious disease of soft lung tissue is _____, which is characterized by the accumulation of fluids within alveoli, or _____ _____.

12.14   11. _____ is a bacterial form of pneumonia, whereas PCP, or _____ _____ pneumonia, is caused by a fungus. Due to excessive coughing, pneumonia may be complicated with the escape of fluids into the pleural cavity, known as _____ _____.

       12. An infectious disease characterized by an intense, spasmodic cough is known as _____, or "whooping cough."

       13. A generalized infection of the pharynx, larynx, and trachea is called a URI, or _____ _____ infection.

Treatments, Procedures, and Devices

WORD PARTS (WHEN APPLICABLE)			TERM	DEFINITION
Part	Type	Meaning		
			acid-fast bacilli smear (AH sihd FAST bah SILL eye smeer)	a clinical test performed on sputum to identify the presence of bacteria that react to acid, including *Mycobacterium tuberculosis;* abbreviated **AFB**
aden -oid -ectomy	r s s	gland condition surgical removal	**adenoidectomy** (ADD eh noyd EK toh mee)	excision of a swollen pharyngeal tonsil, known as an adenoid
anti- histamine	p r	against compounds that cause bronchoconstriction and vessel dilation	**antihistamine** (an tih HISS tah meen)	a therapeutic drug that inhibits the effects of histamines, which are compounds released by cells that cause bronchial constriction and blood vessel dilation
			arterial blood gases (ahr TEE ree al)	a clinical test on arterial blood to identify the levels of oxygen and carbon dioxide; abbreviated **ABGs**
			aspiration (ass pih RAY shun)	the removal of fluid with suction
auscultat -ion	r s	to listen to process	**auscultation** (aws kull TAY shun)	a physical examination that listens to sounds within the body, often with the aid of a stethoscope (Figure 12.14::::)

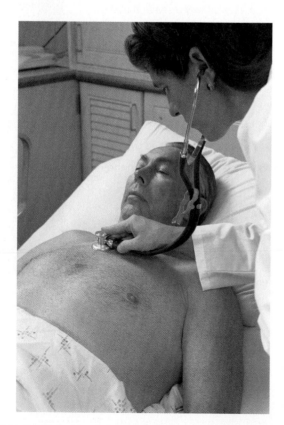

Figure 12.14 ::::

Auscultation. The stethoscope is pressed against the chest wall to listen for sound waves associated with breathing.

WORD PARTS (WHEN APPLICABLE)			TERM	DEFINITION
Part	**Type**	**Meaning**		
bronch/o dilat -ion	r/cv r s	airway, bronchus to widen process	**bronchodilation** (BRONG koh dye LAY shun)	use of a bronchodilating agent in an inhaler to reduce bronchial constriction and thereby improve breathing
bronch/o -gram	r/cv s	airway, bronchus recording	**bronchogram** (BRONG koh gram)	x-ray image of the bronchi
bronch/o -graphy	r/cv s	airway, bronchus recording procedure	**bronchography** (brong KOG rah fee)	the procedure of obtaining an x-ray of the bronchi
bronch/o -plasty	r/cv s	airway, bronchus surgical repair	**bronchoplasty** (BRONG koh plass tee)	surgical repair of a bronchus
bronch/o -scopy	r/cv s	airway, bronchus process of viewing	**bronchoscopy** (brong KOSS koh pee)	bronchi are examined with a **bronchoscope** (BRONG koh skope), a modified type of endoscope (Figure 12.15::::)
			chest CT **(computed tomography)** **scan** (toh MOG rah fee)	diagnostic imaging of the chest by a computed tomography (CT) scanning instrument; used to diagnose respiratory tumors, pleural effusion, pleurisy, and other diseases by providing 3-D imaging (Figure 12.16::::)

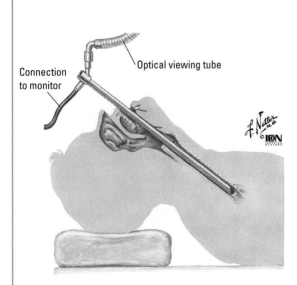

Connection to monitor

Optical viewing tube

Figure 12.15 ::::

Bronchoscopy. The bronchoscope is a modified endoscope that is inserted through the trachea for noninvasive visualization of the interior of the bronchi.
Source: Icon Learning Systems.

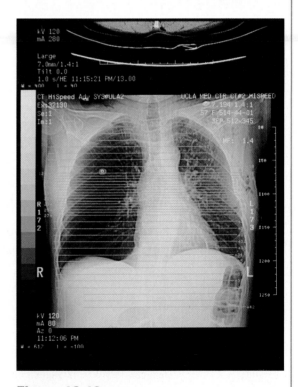

Figure 12.16 ::::

Chest CT scan.
Source: Getty Images Inc.-Stone Allstock

WORD PARTS (WHEN APPLICABLE)			TERM	DEFINITION
Part	Type	Meaning		
			chest x-ray	an x-ray photograph of the thoracic cavity used to diagnose tuberculosis, tumors, and other lung conditions; abbreviated **CXR**, it is also called a **chest radiograph** (Figure 12.17)

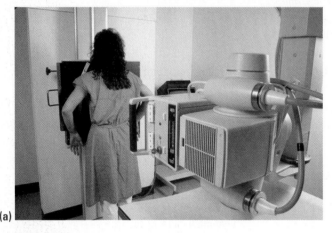

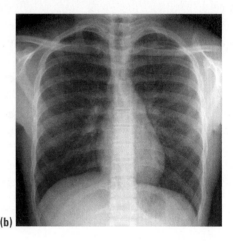

(a)   (b)

Figure 12.17

Chest x-ray.
(a) A patient undergoing the chest x-ray procedure. *Source: Bachman/Photo Researchers Inc.*
(b) An example of a normal chest x-ray. *Source: Icon Learning Systems.*

WORD PARTS (WHEN APPLICABLE)			TERM	DEFINITION
Part	Type	Meaning		
endo- -scopy	p s	within process of viewing	**endoscopy** (ehn DOSS koh pee)	visual examination of a body space with the use of an instrument with a flexible tube that contains mirrors or a camera, called an **endoscope** (EHN doh skope); it is a noninvasive technique for diagnostic and treatment purposes
endo- trache -al	p r s	within windpipe, trachea pertaining to	**endotracheal intubation** (EHN doh TRAY kee al in too BAY shun)	insertion of a tube into the trachea via the nose or mouth to open the airway
			expectorant (ek SPEK toh rant)	a drug that breaks up mucus and promotes coughing to remove the mucus
spir/o -metry	r/cv s	to breathe measurement	**incentive spirometry** (in SEHN tiv spy RAH meh tree)	a postoperative breathing therapy in which a portable spirometer is used by a patient to encourage lung exercise; it reduces pulmonary complications (Figure 12.18)
laryng -ectomy	r s	voicebox, larynx surgical removal	**laryngectomy** (lair in JEK toh mee)	surgical removal or excision of the larynx
laryng/o -centesis	r/cv s	voicebox, larynx surgical puncture	**laryngocentesis** (lair RING goh sehn TEE siss)	surgical puncture and aspiration of fluid from the larynx

WORD PARTS (WHEN APPLICABLE)			TERM	DEFINITION
Part	Type	Meaning		

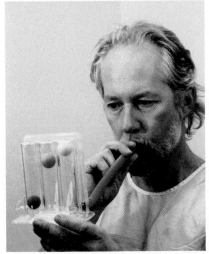 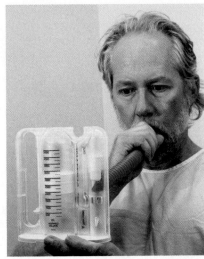

Figure 12.18 ::::

Incentive spirometer. A portable incentive spirometer is useful in encouraging patients to exercise their breathing function following an operation. Two alternate types of incentive spirometers are shown.

Part	Type	Meaning	TERM	DEFINITION
laryng/o	r/cv	voicebox, larynx	**laryngoplasty**	surgical repair of the larynx
-plasty	s	surgical repair	(lair RING goh plass tee)	
laryng/o	r/cv	voicebox, larynx	**laryngoscopy**	procedure that examines the larynx with a
-scopy	s	examine	(lair ring GOSS koh pee)	**laryngoscope** (lair RING goh skope)
laryng/o	r/cv	voicebox, larynx	**laryngostomy**	surgical creation of an opening into the larynx
-stomy	s	surgical creation of an opening	(lair ring GOSS toh mee)	
laryng/o	r/cv	voicebox, larynx	**laryngotracheotomy**	incision into the larynx and trachea
trache/o	r/cv	windpipe, trachea	(lair ring goh TRAY kee OTT oh mee)	
-tomy	s	incision		
lob	r	rounded part, lobe	**lobectomy**	excision of a section or lobe of a lung
-ectomy	s	surgical removal	(loh BEK toh mee)	
			magnetic resonance imaging (mag NETT ik REZ oh nenns)	noninvasive diagnostic imaging of the body with the use of magnetic fields and computer imaging equipment; abbreviated **MRI**
			mechanical ventilation (meh KAN ih kal vent ih LAY shun)	a technique used by a respiratory therapist or EMT to provide assisted breathing using a **ventilator,** which pushes air into the patient's airway (Figure 12.19::::)
			nebulizer (NEBB yoo lye zer)	a device used to convert a liquid medication to a mist and deliver it to the lungs with the aid of a deep inhalation
			nose and throat specialist	a physician specializing in the treatment of nose and throat conditions

WORD PARTS (WHEN APPLICABLE)			TERM	DEFINITION
Part	Type	Meaning		

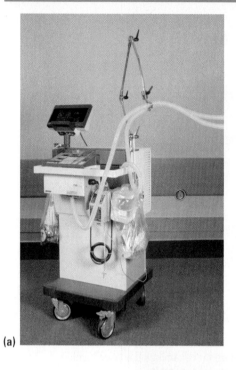

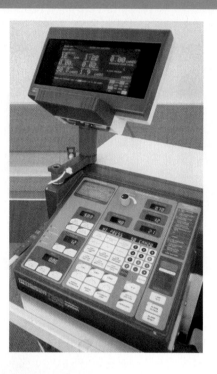

(a)

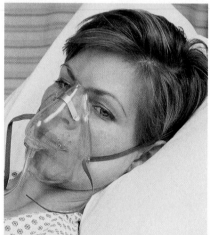

(b)

Figure 12.19 ::::

Mechanical ventilation. The ventilator is an instrument that pushes air through a tube that is connected to the airway, providing an artificial source of ventilation. **(a)** A positive pressure ventilator. *Source: Pearson Education* **(b)** A patient fitted with a face mask, which is connected to a positive pressure ventilator.

Part	Type	Meaning	TERM	DEFINITION
ox/i	r/cv	oxygen	**oximetry**	measurement of oxygen levels in the blood using an
-metry	s	measurement	(ok SIM eh tree)	instrument called an **oximeter** (ok SIM eh ter); a **pulse oximeter** is a noninvasive procedure using an oximeter that is pressed against the fingertip (Figure 12.20::::)
pleur/o	r/cv	rib, pleura	**pleurocentesis**	surgical puncture and aspiration of fluid from the
-centesis	s	surgical puncture	(ploor oh sehn TEE siss)	pleural cavity
pneum/o	r/cv	lung, air	**pneumobronchotomy**	incision of the lung and bronchus
bronch/o	r/cv	airway, bronchus	(NOO moh brong	
-tomy	s	incision	KOTT oh mee)	

WORD PARTS (WHEN APPLICABLE)			TERM	DEFINITION
Part	Type	Meaning		

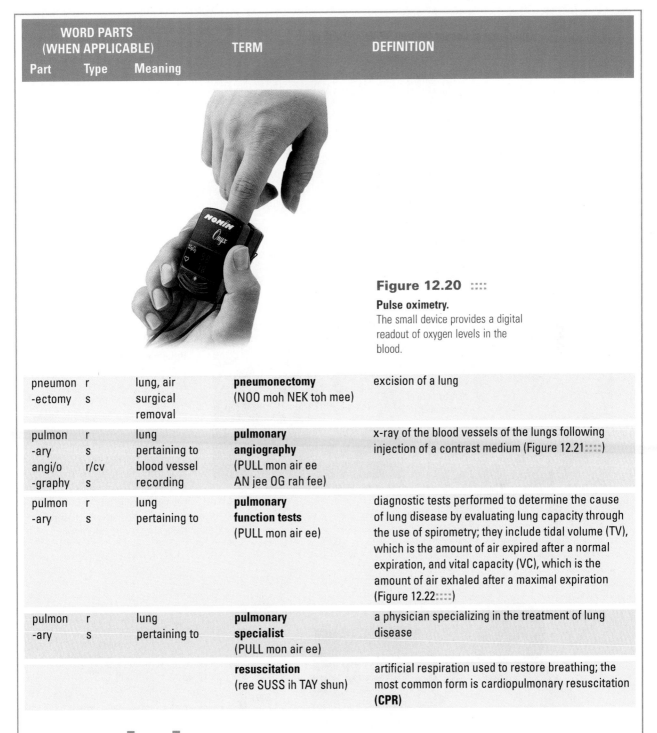

Figure 12.20 ⁝⁝⁝⁝

Pulse oximetry.
The small device provides a digital readout of oxygen levels in the blood.

Part	Type	Meaning	TERM	DEFINITION
pneumon	r	lung, air	**pneumonectomy** (NOO moh NEK toh mee)	excision of a lung
-ectomy	s	surgical removal		
pulmon	r	lung	**pulmonary angiography** (PULL mon air ee AN jee OG rah fee)	x-ray of the blood vessels of the lungs following injection of a contrast medium (Figure 12.21⁝⁝⁝⁝)
-ary	s	pertaining to		
angi/o	r/cv	blood vessel		
-graphy	s	recording		
pulmon	r	lung	**pulmonary function tests** (PULL mon air ee)	diagnostic tests performed to determine the cause of lung disease by evaluating lung capacity through the use of spirometry; they include tidal volume (TV), which is the amount of air expired after a normal expiration, and vital capacity (VC), which is the amount of air exhaled after a maximal expiration (Figure 12.22⁝⁝⁝⁝)
-ary	s	pertaining to		
pulmon	r	lung	**pulmonary specialist** (PULL mon air ee)	a physician specializing in the treatment of lung disease
-ary	s	pertaining to		
			resuscitation (ree SUSS ih TAY shun)	artificial respiration used to restore breathing; the most common form is cardiopulmonary resuscitation **(CPR)**

[FYI]

Resuscitation
The word *resuscitation* is derived from the Latin word *resuscito,* which means *to rise up again* or *revive.* Its present meaning refers to any procedure that involves a restoration of breathing, and includes the popular technique of massaging the chest and heart called cardiopulmonary resuscitation (CPR). It also includes mouth-to-mouth resuscitation, in which air is blown into the patient's mouth while holding the nose, and the Heimlich maneuver, during which an obstruction (usually food) may be dislodged by elevating the patient from behind and pushing on the diaphragm to force an expulsion of air.

Embolism of Lesser Degree Without Infarction

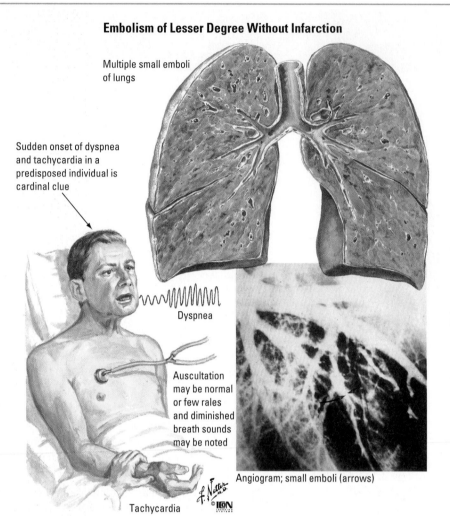

Multiple small emboli of lungs

Sudden onset of dyspnea and tachycardia in a predisposed individual is cardinal clue

Dyspnea

Auscultation may be normal or few rales and diminished breath sounds may be noted

Tachycardia

Angiogram; small emboli (arrows)

Figure 12.21 ::::

Pulmonary embolism and pulmonary angiography.
An angiogram is used to reveal pulmonary emboli that may obstruct pulmonary blood flow. In this figure, the lungs are sectioned to show the numerous emboli (darkened areas), which are revealed by the angiogram. The patient is shown expressing the symptoms of pulmonary embolism, which include shortness of breath and chest pain. *Source: Icon Learning Systems.*

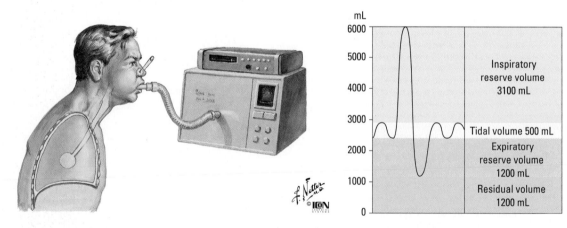

mL

6000	
5000	Inspiratory reserve volume 3100 mL
4000	
3000	Tidal volume 500 mL
2000	Expiratory reserve volume 1200 mL
1000	Residual volume 1200 mL
0	

Figure 12.22 ::::

Pulmonary function test: spirometry
(a) Illustration of a patient expiring into a spirometer, which measures air volume. *Source: Icon Learning Systems.*
(b) Normal respiratory volumes, as measured during spirometry. A patient's spirometry data is compared to this chart to identify breathing deficiencies.

WORD PARTS (WHEN APPLICABLE)			TERM	DEFINITION
Part	**Type**	**Meaning**		
rhin/o	r/cv	nose	**rhinoplasty**	surgical repair of the nose
-plasty	s	surgical repair	(RYE noh plass tee)	
sept/o	r/cv	partition	**septoplasty**	surgical repair of the nasal septum
-plasty	s	surgical repair	(SEPP toh plass tee)	
sept/o	r/cv	parition	**septotomy**	incision of the nasal septum
-tomy	s	incision	(sepp TOTT oh mee)	
sinus/o	r/cv	cavity	**sinusotomy**	incision of a paranasal sinus
-tomy	s	incision	(SIGH nuss OTT oh mee)	
spir/o	r/cv	breathe	**spirometry**	a procedure measuring breathing volumes using a
-metry	s	measurement	(spy ROM eh tree)	spirometer (Figure 12.22)
spir/o	r/cv	breathe	**spirometer**	an instrument used to measure breathing volume;
-meter	s	measuring instrument	(spy ROM eh ter)	the patient exhales into a tube that carries air to a measuring drum (Figure 12.22)
steth/o	r/cv	chest	**stethoscope**	a diagnostic instrument used to hear sounds in the
-scope	s	viewing instrument	(STETH oh skope)	body, such as breathing (Figure 12.14)
			TB skin test	a test to determine the presence of a TB infection, in which a purified protein derivative (PPD) sample of the TB bacillus is injected beneath the epidermis (intradermal); also called PPD skin test or Mantoux skin test (Figure 12.23:::::)
thorac/o	r/cv	chest, thorax	**thoracocentesis**	surgical puncture into the chest cavity to aspirate
-centesis	s	surgical puncture	(THOR ah koh sehn TEE siss)	fluid; also called thoracentesis (THOR ah sehn TEE siss)
thorac/o	r/cv	chest, thorac	**thoracoscopy**	examination of the thoracic cavity using a
-scopy	s	process of viewing	(THOR ah KOSS koh pee)	thoracoscope (thor RAH koh skope)
thorac/o	r/cv	chest, thorax	**thoracostomy**	surgical puncture into the chest cavity, usually for
-stomy	s	surgical creation of an opening	(THOR ah KOSS toh mee)	the insertion of a tube. The procedure is often termed "placing a chest tube"
thorac/o	r/cv	chest, thorac	**thoracotomy**	incision into the chest (Figure 12.24:::::)
-tomy	s	incision	(THOR ah KOTT oh mee)	
tonsil	r	almond	**tonsillectomy**	excision of one or more tonsils, usually palatine
-ectomy	s	surgical removal	(TAHN sill EK toh mee)	
trache/o	r/cv	windpipe, trachea	**tracheoplasty**	surgical repair of the trachea
-plasty	s	surgical repair	(TRAY kee oh PLASS tee)	
trache/o	r/cv	windpipe, trachea	**tracheostomy**	surgical creation of an opening into the trachea,
-stomy	s	surgical creation of an opening	(TRAY kee OSS toh mee)	usually for the insertion of a tube (Figure 12.25:::::)
trache/o	r/cv	windpipe, trachea	**tracheotomy**	incision into the trachea (Figure 12.25)
-tomy	s	incision	(TRAY kee OTT oh mee)	

Tuberculin Testing

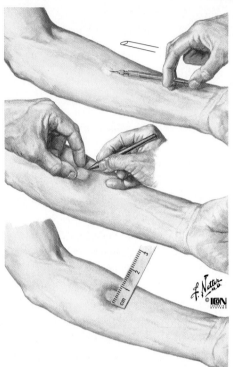

0.1 ml tuberculin (5 TU) injected just under skin surface of forearm. Pale elevation results. Needle bevel directed upward to prevent too deep penetration.

Test read in 48 to 72 hr. Extent of induration determined by direct observation and palpation; limits marked. Area of erythema has no significance.

Diameter of marked indurated area measured in transverse plane. Reactions over 9 mm in diameter are regarded as positive; those 5 to 9 mm are questionable, and test may be repeated after 7 or more days to obtain booster effect. Less than 5 mm of induration is regarded as negative.

Figure 12.23

TB skin test.
Source: Icon Learning Systems.

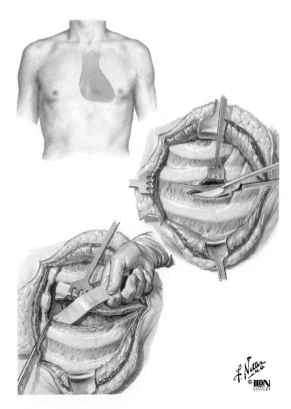

Figure 12.24

Thoracotomy. In this procedure, which is often performed to treat pleural effusion, an incision is made through the skin and intercostal muscles to enter the pleural cavity.
Source: Icon Learning Systems.

WORD PARTS (WHEN APPLICABLE)			TERM	DEFINITION
Part	Type	Meaning		
			ventilation-perfusion scanning	a diagnostic tool of nuclear medicine that is used to evaluate pulmonary function, it can identify pulmonary embolism and pulmonary edema; abbreviated **VPS**, it is also called lung scan and V/Q scan (Figure 12.26::::)

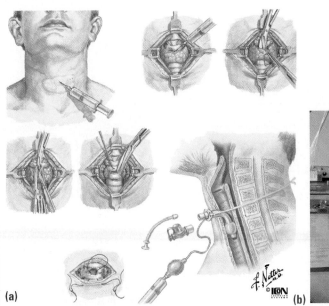
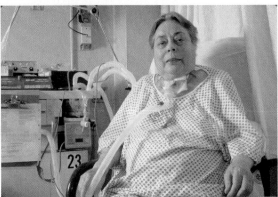

(a)   (b)

Figure 12.25 ::::

Tracheostomy.

(a) A tracheotomy, or incision through the trachea, is performed to create an opening through the trachea, or tracheostomy, as shown in this series of illustrations. *Source: Icon Learning Systems.*

(b) A patient with a tracheostomy attached to a breathing tube, which is connected to a mechanical ventilator. *Source: (Ansell Horn/Phototake NYC)*

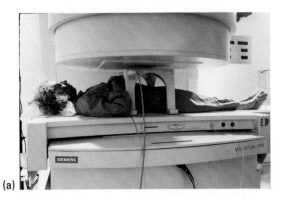
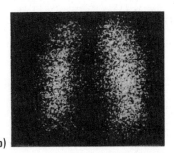

(a)   (b)

Figure 12.26 ::::

Ventilation-perfusion scanning.

(a) A lung scan instrument, which utilizes radioactive material to reveal pulmonary function. *Source: Science Photo Library/Photo Researchers, Inc.*

(b) A lung scan. *Source: Icon Learning Systems.*

SELF QUIZ 12.5

SAY IT—SPELL IT!

Review the terms of the respiratory system by speaking the phonetic pronunciation guides out loud, then writing in the correct spelling of the term.

1. an tih HISS tah meen   _____
2. BRONG koh dye LAY shun   _____
3. BRONG koh gram   _____
4. brong KOG rah fee   _____
5. BRONG koh plass tee   _____
6. ehn DOSS koh pee   _____
7. lair ring GOSS koh pee   _____
8. EHN doh TRAY kee al
   in too BAY shun   _____
9. lair in JEK toh mee   _____
10. lair RING goh sehn TEE siss   _____
11. lair RING goh plass tee   _____
12. lair ring goh TRAY kee OTT oh mee   _____
13. loh BEK toh mee   _____
14. ok SIM eh tree   _____
15. ploor oh sehn TEE siss   _____
16. NOO moh brong KOTT oh mee   _____
17. NOO moh NEK toh mee   _____
18. RYE noh plass tee   _____
19. SEPP toh plass tee   _____
20. sepp TOTT oh mee   _____
21. SIGH nuss OTT oh mee   _____
22. spy ROM eh tree   _____
23. THOR ah koh sehn TEE siss   _____
24. TRAY kee oh PLASS tee   _____
25. TRAY kee OSS toh mee   _____
12.15 26. TRAY kee OTT oh mee   _____

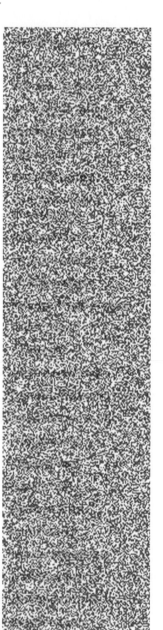

MATCH IT!

Match the term on the left with the correct definition on the right.

_____ 1. rhinoplasty   a. endoscopic evaluation of a bronchus

_____ 2. pulse oximeter   b. excision of a lung

_____ 3. bronchodilation   c. oxygen and carbon dioxide blood levels

_____ 4. bronchoscopy   d. puncture and aspiration of pleural fluid

_____ 5. thoracotomy   e. use of a flexible tube with mirrors or a camera

_____ 6. pneumonectomy   f. a blood oxygen measuring device

_____ 7. septoplasty   g. drug that reduces bronchial constriction

_____ 8. endoscopy   h. x-ray of lung blood vessels

_____ 9. pulmonary angiography   i. surgical repair of a deviated septum

_____10. pleurocentesis   j. incision into the thoracic cavity

_____11. pulmonary function tests   k. surgical repair of the nose

_____12. mechanical ventilation   l. breaks up mucus and promotes coughing

_____13. arterial blood gases   m. CPR is one example

_____14. expectorant   n. use of spirometry to evaluate lung function

_____15. resuscitation   o. assisted breathing using a ventilator

BREAK IT DOWN!

Analyze and separate each term into its word parts by labeling each word part using p = prefix, r = root, cv = combining vowel, and s = suffix.

1. antihistamine   _____

12.16 2. bronchogram   _____

3. endotracheal   _____

4. spirometry   _____

5. layngectomy   _____

6. lobectomy   _____

7. oximetry   _____

8. pleurocentesis   _____

9. pneumobronchotomy   _____

10. septotomy   _____

11. thoracocentesis _____

12. tracheoplasty _____

WORD BUILDING

Construct or recall medical terms from the following meanings.

1. A skin test for tuberculosis _____

2. An emergency procedure that
   restores breathing _____

3. A physical exam that listens for sounds _____

4. A clinical measurement of blood gases _____

5. 3-D imaging of the thoracic cavity _____

6. Assisted breathing with the use of a
   ventilator _____

7. A clinical test for acid-producing
   bacteria _____

8. An x-ray of the thoracic cavity _____

9. Tests that determine lung capacity _____

FILL IT IN!

Fill in the blanks with the correct terms.

1. A clinical test that identifies the presence of acidic secretions, such as those

   released by the bacterium that causes the disease tuberculosis, is an

   _____ _____ _____ smear.

2. A physical exam that is named after the Latin word for "listen" is

   12.17 _____.

3. A series of diagnostic tests that evaluate lung capacity with the use of a

   _____ is known as _____

   _____ tests.

4. A clinical test that identifies blood gases from an arterial blood sample is known as

   an _____ _____ _____, or ABG.

5. A diagnostic imaging tool that is commonly used to view the chest without relying

   on invasive surgery is called a _____ _____

   _____.

6. A diagnostic x-ray of the thoracic cavity is known as a _____

   _____.

7. Assisted breathing uses a device that pushes air into the lungs in a technique

   known as _____ _____.

8. A lung scan is also called _____ _____ scanning,

   or VPS.

9. A test that uses a protein purified derivative of *Mycobacterium tuberculosis* is called the _____ _____ _____.

10. A technique that restores breathing to a patient in respiratory distress is commonly called _____.

abbreviations of the respiratory system

The abbreviations that are associated with the respiratory system are summarized here. Study these abbreviations, and review them in the exercise that follows.

ABBREVIATION	DEFINITION	ABBREVIATION	DEFINITION
ABGs	arterial blood gases	MRI	magnetic resonance imaging
ARDS	adult (acute) respiratory distress syndrome	OSA	obstructive sleep apnea
		PCP	*Pneumocystis carinii* pneumonia
AFB	acid-fast bacilli	PE	pulmonary embolism
CF	cystic fibrosis	PPD	purified protein derivative
COPD	chronic obstructive pulmonary disease	RDS	respiratory distress syndrome
		SARS	severe acute respiratory syndrome
CPR	cardiopulmonary resuscitation		
CXR	chest x-ray	TB	tuberculosis
HMD	hyaline membrane disease	TV	tidal volume
LTB	laryngotracheobronchitis	URI	upper respiratory infection
NRDS	neonatal respiratory distress syndrome	VC	vital capacity
		VPS or V/Q scan	ventilation-perfusion scanning

SELF QUIZ 12.6

Fill in the blanks with the abbreviation or the complete medical term.

Abbreviation   **Medical Term**

1. VC   _____

2. _____   laryngotracheobronchitis

3. HMD   _____

4. _____   tuberculosis

5. TV   _____

6. _____   adult respiratory distress syndrome

12.18 7. CPR   _____

8. _____   purified protein derivative

9. CXR   _____

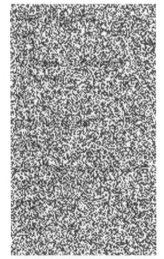

10. _____   cystic fibrosis

11. RDS   _____

12. _____   chronic obstructive pulmonary disease

13. ABGs   _____

12.19 14. _____   obstructive sleep apnea

15. PE   _____

12.20 16. _____   *Pneumocystis carinii* pneumonia

17. URI   _____

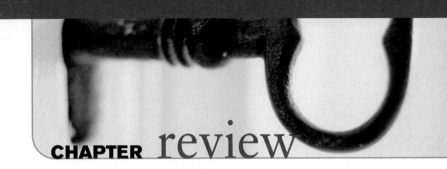

In this section, we will review all the word parts and medical terms from this chapter. As in earlier tables, the word roots are shown in **bold**.

Check each word part and medical term to be sure you understand the meaning. If any are not clear, please go back into the chapter and review that term. Then, complete the review exercises that follow.

[word parts **checklist**]

Prefixes

- ❑ a-, an-
- ❑ dia-
- ❑ endo-
- ❑ epi-
- ❑ eu-
- ❑ pan-
- ❑ poly-

Word Roots/Combining Vowels

- ❑ **alveol**/o
- ❑ **atel**/o
- ❑ **bronch**/i, **bronch**/o
- ❑ **glottis**/o
- ❑ **hem**/o, **hemat**/o
- ❑ **laryng**/o
- ❑ **lob**/o
- ❑ **muc**/o
- ❑ **nas**/o
- ❑ **ox**/i

- ❑ **pharyng**/o
- ❑ **phragm**/o, **phragmat**/o
- ❑ **pleur**/o
- ❑ **pneum**/o, **pneumon**/o, **pneumat**/o
- ❑ **pulmon**/o
- ❑ **py**/o
- ❑ **rhin**/o
- ❑ **sept**/o
- ❑ **sinus**/o
- ❑ **somn**/o
- ❑ **spir**/o
- ❑ **sten**/o
- ❑ **thorac**/o
- ❑ **trache**/o
- ❑ **tubercul**/o

Suffixes

- ❑ -algia
- ❑ -ar, -ary

- ❑ -capnia
- ❑ -cele
- ❑ -centesis
- ❑ -eal
- ❑ -ectasis
- ❑ -emia
- ❑ -metry
- ❑ -osis
- ❑ -oxia
- ❑ -pexy
- ❑ -phonia
- ❑ -pnea
- ❑ -ptysis
- ❑ -rrhagia
- ❑ -spasm
- ❑ -stomy
- ❑ -tomy

[medical terminology **checklist**]

- ❑ acapnia
- ❑ acid-fast bacilli smear
- ❑ **alveol**i
- ❑ an**ox**ia
- ❑ antihistamine
- ❑ a**phon**ia
- ❑ apnea
- ❑ ARDS
- ❑ arterial blood gases (ABGs)
- ❑ a**sphyx**ia
- ❑ asthma
- ❑ atelectasis
- ❑ **auscultat**ion

- ❑ bradypnea
- ❑ **bronch**i
- ❑ **bronch**ial tree
- ❑ **bronch**iectasis
- ❑ **bronch**ioles
- ❑ **bronch**itis
- ❑ **bronch**odilation
- ❑ **bronch**ogenic **carcin**oma
- ❑ **bronch**ogram
- ❑ **bronch**ography
- ❑ **bronch**oplasty
- ❑ **bronch**o**pneumon**ia
- ❑ **bronch**oscopy

- ❑ **cardi**o**pulmon**ary resuscitation (CPR)
- ❑ chest CT scan
- ❑ chest x-ray (CXR)
- ❑ Cheyne-Stokes re**spir**ation
- ❑ chronic obstructive **pulmon**ary disease (COPD)
- ❑ **coccidioid**o**myc**osis
- ❑ conducting portion
- ❑ cor pulmonale
- ❑ coryza
- ❑ croup
- ❑ **cyst**ic **fibr**osis (CF)

❑ deviated septum
❑ dia**phragm**atocele
❑ dia**phragm**
❑ dust macrophage
❑ dys**phon**ia
❑ dyspnea
❑ emphysema
❑ endoscopy
❑ endo**trache**al intubation
❑ epi**glott**itis
❑ epistaxis
❑ eupnea
❑ expectorant
❑ expiration
❑ external re**spir**ation
❑ **glottis**
❑ **hem**optysis
❑ **hem**o**thorax**
❑ HMD
❑ hypercapnia
❑ hyperpnea
❑ hyperventilation
❑ hypocapnia
❑ hypoventilation
❑ hypopnea
❑ hyp**ox**emia
❑ hyp**ox**ia
❑ incentive **spir**ometry
❑ in**somn**ia
❑ in**spir**ation
❑ internal re**spir**ation
❑ **laryng**ectomy
❑ **laryng**ocentesis
❑ **laryng**oplasty
❑ **laryng**oscopy
❑ **laryng**ostomy
❑ **laryngotrache**o**bronch**itis (LTB)
❑ **laryngotrache**otomy

❑ **larynx**
❑ legionellosis
❑ **lob**ectomy
❑ lower re**spir**atory tract
❑ lung
❑ lung scan
❑ mechanical ventilation
❑ **nas**al cavity
❑ **nas**o**pharyng**itis
❑ nose
❑ NRDS
❑ obstructive sleep apnea (OSA)
❑ **orth**opnea
❑ **ox**imetry
❑ pan**sinus**itis
❑ PCP
❑ PE
❑ pertussis
❑ **pharyng**itis
❑ **pharynx**
❑ **pleur**a
❑ **pleur**al effusion
❑ **pleur**itis
❑ **pleur**ocentesis
❑ **pneumat**ocele
❑ **pneum**o**bronch**otomy
❑ **pneum**o**coni**osus
❑ *Pneumocystis carinii*
❑ **pneumon**ia
❑ **pneumon**ectomy
❑ **pneumon**ia
❑ **pneumon**itis
❑ **pneum**o**thorax**
❑ PPD
❑ **pulmon**ary **angi**ography
❑ **pulmon**ary edema
❑ **pulmon**ary **embol**ism
❑ **pulmon**ary function tests
❑ **pulmon**ary neoplasm

❑ **pulmon**ary **tubercu**losis (TB)
❑ **py**o**thorax**
❑ re**spir**ation
❑ respiratory distress syndrome (RDS)
❑ re**spir**atory membrane
❑ resuscitation
❑ **rhin**itis
❑ **rhin**o**myc**osis
❑ **rhin**oplasty
❑ **rhin**orrhagia
❑ **rhin**orrhea
❑ **sept**oplasty
❑ **sept**otomy
❑ severe acute re**spir**atory syndrome (SARS)
❑ **sinus**otomy
❑ **spir**ometry
❑ tachypnea
❑ TB skin test
❑ **thorac**algia
❑ **thorac**ocentesis
❑ **thorac**oplasty
❑ **thorac**otomy
❑ **trache**a
❑ **trache**itis
❑ **trache**oplasty
❑ **trache**ostenosis
❑ **trache**ostomy
❑ **trache**otomy
❑ TV
❑ upper re**spir**atory infection (URI)
❑ upper re**spir**atory tract
❑ VC
❑ ventilation
❑ ventilation-perfusion scanning

[show what **you know!**]

BREAK IT DOWN!

Analyze and separate each term into its word parts by labeling each word part using p = prefix, r = root, cv = combining vowel, and s = suffix.

Example:
1. laryngitis

                                                         r   s
                                              laryng/itis

2. tracheitis

3. bronchoscope

4. hypopnea _____

5. hypercapnia _____

6. hemothorax _____

7. apnea _____

8. dyspnea _____

9. rhinorrhagia _____

10. dysphonia _____

11. thoracalgia _____

12. hyperventilation _____

13. bronchitis _____

14. hypoxia _____

15. bronchiectasis _____

16. coccidioidomycosis _____

17. rhinomycosis _____

18. nasopharyngitis _____

19. sinusitis _____

20. septoplasty _____

21. thoracocentesis _____

22. laryngotracheotomy _____

23. oximetry _____

24. spirometry _____

25. tracheotomy _____

26. laryngectomy _____

WORD BUILDING

Construct or recall medical terms from the following meanings.

Example: 1. inflammation of the larynx _____ laryngitis _____

2. absence of oxygen _____

3. inflammation of the bronchi _____

4. normal breathing _____

5. inability to breathe _____

6. deficient oxygen levels in the blood _____

7. difficulty breathing _____

8. excessive carbon dioxide levels in the blood _____

9. dilation of the bronchi _____

10. hernia of a lung _____

11. lung inflammation due to dust inhalation _____

12. excessive air movement in and out of the lungs _____

13. a group of disorders that obstruct bronchial
    air flow   _____

14. an inherited disease of excessive mucus
    production   _____

15. inflammation of the trachea   _____

16. infection of the upper respiratory tract   _____

17. the absence of respiratory ventilation   _____

18. x-ray image of the bronchi   _____

19. surgical puncture and aspiration of fluid
    from the pleural cavity   _____

20. respiratory failure characterized by atelectasis   _____

21. surgical repair of the nose   _____

22. measurement of oxygen levels in the blood   _____

23. surgical repair of the trachea   _____

24. tumor of the lung   _____

25. physical exam that listens to body sounds   _____

26. respiratory failure characterized by atelectasis   _____

CASE STUDIES

Fill in the blanks with the correct terms.

1. A 65-year-old female complained of difficulty breathing and chest pain. Her personal physician began with a chest

   (a) _____ using a stethoscope, followed by fingertip measurement of oxygen levels in the blood using

   a (b) _____ _____ and a measurement of breathing volumes, including

   (c) _____ _____ _____ using a

   (d) _____. The tests indicated reduced oxygen levels in the blood, or

   (e) _____, in combination with reduced lung capacity. Breathing sounds suggested labored breathing

   with some gurgling sounds. The physician diagnosed the condition as a lung inflammation with alveolar fluids, or

   (f) _____, caused by an unknown infectious agent. To identify the source of the infection, blood tests

   were performed that included (g) _____ _____ bacilli. The blood tests showed

   the source of the infection as a fungus that is an opportunistic pathogen in immune-suppressed patients, known as

   (h) _____ _____ This disease is a common diagnostic indicator of patients

   suffering from HIV infection, known as (i) _____. The patient was admitted for continual monitoring

   during antibiotic treatments and kept within an oxygen tent to improve oxygen blood levels. After the treatment, blood tests

   and radiographic images of blood vessels in the thoracic cavity, called (j) _____

   _____, indicated the pathogen had been defeated.

2. A 6-year-old boy with a healthy history was admitted into an emergency clinic when his mother became concerned about his

   respiratory function. She explained that he had come home from school three weeks ago with a common cold, or

(k) _____, which progressed into an inflammation of the nasal mucous membranes, a condition

known as (l) _____. He began coughing violently shortly afterward, preventing him from sleep.

Physical exams showed an acute inflammation of the larynx, trachea, and bronchi, indicating the acute condition known as

(m) _____, which was bacterial in origin. Following the prescribed use of antibiotic therapy and the

use of inhaled (n) _____ agents to reduce bronchial constriction, the patient recovered initially. But

several months later, coughing returned and the boy complained of low energy. Following a (o) _____

skin test and a blood test that included (p) _____ _____ bacilli, positive results

indicated an active lung infection known as (q) _____. TB was confirmed with the use of

radiographic images of the thorax, or (r) _____ _____. The course of treatment

included a cocktail of antibiotics administered over a six-month period.

3. A 50-year-old male with a history of heavy smoking was admitted into a clinic when he complained of shortness of breath, or

(s) _____, and blood in the sputum, or (t) _____. Radiographic images

showed no evidence of lung cancer, or (u) _____ _____, but did suggest

alveolar enlargement. To examine the respiratory tract lining, a flexible tube was inserted into the bronchi, known as a

(v) _____. The visual images it provided showed a chronic inflammation of the bronchi, or

(w) _____. The diagnosis was (x) _____ and (y)

_____. Because of the chronic, progressed status of the two conditions, the patient was identified

with (z) _____ _____ _____

_____, or COPD. A prognosis was provided that indicated 2–3 years of life expected, assuming the pa-

tient stopped smoking and committed to using an oxygen breathing apparatus.

[piece it all **together!**]

CROSSWORD

From the chapter material, fill in the crossword puzzle with answers to the following clues.

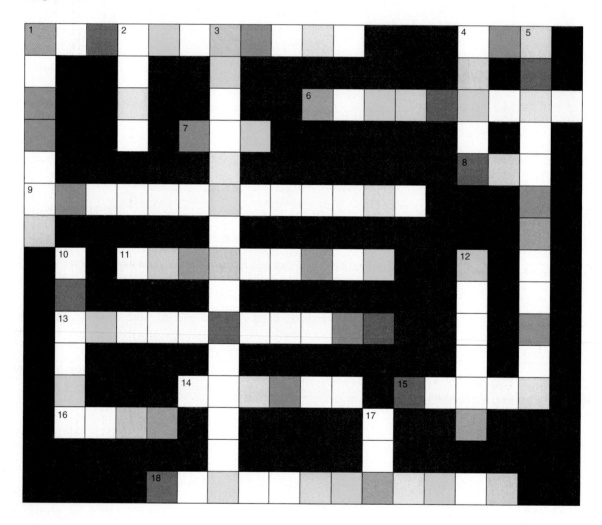

ACROSS

1. The term for a collapsed lung. (Find puzzle piece 12.5)

4. Cardiopulmonary resuscitation. (Find puzzle piece 12.18)

6. An infection of the lungs resulting in fluid accumulation. (Find puzzle piece 12.13)

7. Abbreviation for an opportunistic infection of AIDS. (Find puzzle piece 12.20)

8. A word root that means *pus*. (Find puzzle piece 12.9)

9. Legionnaire's disease. (Find puzzle piece 12.14)

11. A nosebleed. (Find puzzle piece 12.4)

13. Incision through the windpipe. (Find puzzle piece 12.15)

14. The technical term for a common cold. (Find puzzle piece 12.12)

15. A sticky substance that is overproduced in CF. (Find puzzle piece 12.1)

16. Adult respiratory distress syndrome. (Find puzzle piece 12.10)

18. A physical exam that "listens." (Find puzzle piece 12.17)

DOWN

1. Microscopic air sacs in the lungs. (Find puzzle piece 12.2)

2. A sponge-like organ in the thoracic cavity. (Find puzzle piece 12.3)

3. A narrowed windpipe. (Find puzzle piece 12.8)

4. A swollen voice box that causes a loud cough. (Find puzzle piece 12.6)

5. A fungal infection of the nasal mucosa. (Find puzzle piece 12.7)

10. Produces symptoms of wheezing due to airway constriction. (Find puzzle piece 12.11)

12. A word root within the term "bronchodilation." (Find puzzle piece 12.16)

17. Obstructive sleep apnea. (Find puzzle piece 12.19)

WORD UNSCRAMBLE

From the completed crossword puzzle, unscramble:

1. All of the letters that appear in **red** squares __ __ ☐ __ __ __ __ __ __

   Clue: A lung disease characterized by enlarged and damaged alveoli

2. All of the letters that appear in **purple** squares ☐ __ __ __ __ __ __

   Clue: Also known as pyothorax

3. All of the letters that appear in **peach** squares ☐ __ __ __ __ __ __ __

   Clue: Inflammation of the nasal mucous membranes

4. All of the letters that appear in **blue** squares ☐ __

   Clue: A bacterial lung infection that was formerly called "consumption"

5. All of the letters that appear in **yellow** squares __ __ __ ☐ __ __ __ __

   Clue: Inflammation of the membrane surrounding the lungs

6. All of the letters that appear in **green** squares ☐ __ __ __ __ __ __ __ __

   Clue: An instrument used to measure VC and TV

7. All of the letters that appear in **gray** squares __ __ __ ☐

   Clue: Neonatal respiratory distress syndrome

8. All of the letters that appear in **pink** squares __ __ __ __ __ __ ☐ __

   Clue: An inability to breathe, or suffocation

9. All of the letters that appear in **brown** squares __ __ ☐

   Clue: A lung scanning procedure (abbreviation)

Now write down each of the letters that are boxed to find the hidden medical term, which is a severe disease that was common among children before vaccinations became available: __ __ __ __ __ __ __ __ __

MEDmedia wrap-up

www.prenhall.com/wingerd

Before you go on to the next chapter, take advantage of the free CD-ROM and study guide website that accompany this book. Simply load the CD-ROM for additional activities, games, animations, videos, and quizzes linked to this chapter. Then visit www.prenhall.com/wingerd for even more!

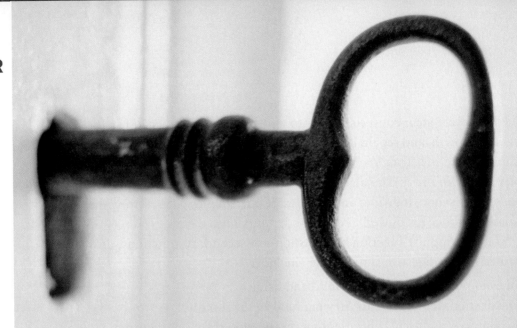

CHAPTER
13

The Digestive System

After completing this chapter, you will be able to:

- Define and spell the word parts used to create medical terms for the digestive system

- Identify the organs of the digestive system and describe their structure and function

- Define common medical terms used for the digestive system

- Break down and define common medical terms used for symptoms, diseases, disorders, procedures, treatments, and devices for the digestive system

MEDmedia

www.prenhall.com/wingerd
Enhance your study with the power of multimedia! Each chapter of this book links to activities, games, animations, videos, and quizzes that you'll find on your CD-ROM. Plus, you can click on www.prenhall.com/wingerd, to find a free chapter-specific companion website that's loaded with additional practice and resources.

CD-ROM
- Audio Glossary
- Exercises & Activities
- Flashcard Generator
- Animations
- Videos

 Companion Website
- Exercises & Activities
- Audio Glossary
- Drug Updates
- Current News Update

A secure distance learning course is available at www.prenhall.com/onekey.

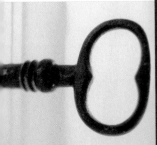

The digestive system converts food into a form that the body can use for energy, growth, and repair. It derives its name from its primary function, digestion. The term is from the Latin word *digestus*, which means *to divide, dissolve, or set in order.* The digestive system actually does all three: When the body digests food, it divides and dissolves it into simpler parts, setting the food parts in order for powering other body functions.

Accompanying the function of digestion are secondary functions, also performed by the digestive system. They include:

- Ingestion, the introduction of food and drink
- Mastication, the process of chewing food in the mouth
- Swallowing, a muscular process that moves food through the throat
- Absorption, the transport of nutrient and water molecules from the digestive tract to the bloodstream
- Defecation, the release of solid waste, or feces

These functions are important steps in the processing of food for your body's use. As you will soon discover, each function is performed by a specialized organ that is part of the digestive system.

We will begin this chapter with a study of word parts and then move on to an exploration of the basic structure and function of the digestive system. This introductory study will prepare you for the chapter's emphasis: medical terminology of digestive disorders and their symptoms. We will also study the terminology of treatments and procedures that are in common use in clinics and hospitals.

word parts focus

Let's look at word parts. The following table contains a list of word parts that when combined build many of the terms of the digestive system.

PREFIX	DEFINITION	PREFIX	DEFINITION
a-, an-	without	pan-	all, entire
ad-	toward	peri-	around
dys-	bad, abnormal	re-, retro-	back

WORD ROOT	DEFINITION	WORD ROOT	DEFINITION
abdomin	abdomen, abdominal cavity	ile	to roll (ileum)
an	anus	jejun	empty (jejunum)
append	to hang onto (appendix)	lapar	abdomen, abdominal cavity
bil	bile	lingu	tongue
cec	blind intestine (cecum)	lith	stone
celi	abdomen, abdominal cavity	or	mouth
cheil	lip	palat	roof of the mouth (palate)
chol	bile, gall	pancreat	sweetbread (pancreas)
choledoch	common bile duct	peps, pept	digestion
cirrh	orange, tawny	periton	to stretch over (peritoneum)
col, colon	colon	phag	eat or swallow
dent	teeth	polyp	a small growth
diverticul	a small blind pouch (diverticulum)	proct	anus
duoden	twelve (duodenum)	pylor	gatekeeper (pylorus)
enter	small intestine	rect	straight, erect (rectum)
esophag	gullet (esophagus)	sial	saliva
gastr	stomach	sigm	the letter S (sigmoid)
gingiv	gums	steat	fat
gloss	tongue	stomat	mouth
halat	breath	uvul	a grape (uvula)
hepat	liver		
hern, herni	a rupture, or protrusion through a weakened membrane or wall (hernia)		

SUFFIX	DEFINITION	SUFFIX	DEFINITION
-centesis	puncture	-pepsia	digestion
-emesis, -emetic	vomiting	-rraphy	suturing
-iasis	condition		

SELF QUIZ 13.1

Review the word parts of digestive system terminology by working carefully through the exercises that follow. Soon, we will apply this new information to build medical terms.

Success Hint: Once you get to the crossword puzzle at the end of the chapter, remember to check back here for clues! Your clues are indicated by the puzzle icon.

A. Provide the definition of the following prefixes and suffixes.

1. -centesis _____
2. -emesis, -emetic _____
13.1 3. -pepsia _____
4. ad- _____
5. dys- _____
6. pan- _____
7. peri- _____
8. re- _____

B. Provide the word root for each of the following terms.

1. abdomen _____
2. anus _____
3. appendix _____
4. bile _____
5. colon _____
6. common bile duct _____
7. diverticulum _____
8. duodenum _____
9. gums _____
10. hernia _____
11. ileum _____
12. jejunum _____
13. lip _____
14. liver _____
15. mouth _____
16. palate _____
17. pancreas _____
18. peritoneum _____
13.2 19. a small growth _____
20. pylorus _____
21. rectum _____
22. saliva _____

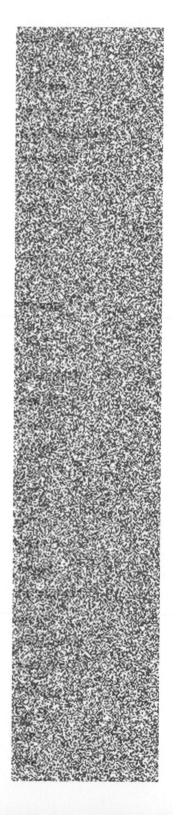

23. letter S   _____

24. small intestine   _____

25. stomach   _____

26. teeth   _____

27. to eat or swallow _____

28. tongue   _____

29. uvula   _____

30. vomiting   _____

[anatomy and physiology overview]

The digestive system is structurally divided into two main parts: a long, winding tube that carries food through its length, and a series of supportive organs outside of the tube (Figure 13.1⸭⸭⸭⸭). The long tube is called the **gastrointestinal (GI) tract.** An older term that is still occasionally used is **alimentary canal,** which is derived from the Latin word *alimentarius,* which means *nourishment.* The GI tract extends from the mouth to the anus, and consists of the mouth, or oral cavity, the pharynx, the esophagus, the stomach, the small intestine, and the large intestine. The supportive organs that lie outside the GI tract are known as **accessory organs,** and include the salivary glands, liver, gallbladder, and pancreas.

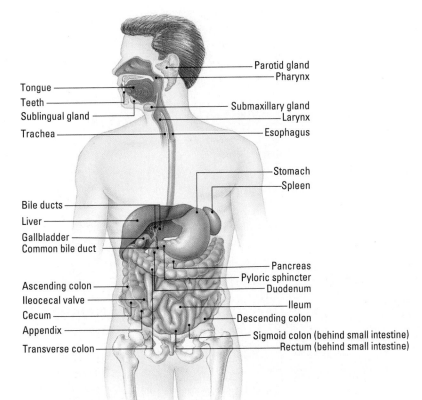

Figure 13.1 ⸭⸭⸭⸭

Organs of the digestive system.

Source: Pearson Education.

Organs of the GI Tract

The processing of food begins in the mouth, or **oral cavity**, where food initially enters (Figure 13.2::::). The roof of the oral cavity is the **palate**, which includes an anterior bony portion called the **hard palate** and a posterior boneless portion called the **soft palate.** The soft palate ends as a projection that hangs downward like a grape, known as the **uvula.** Derived from the Latin word for grape, the uvula triggers the swallow reflex when it receives contact. The floor of the oral cavity is dominated by the **tongue,** which assists in swallowing and in speech. The **teeth** border the front and sides of the oral cavity, providing hard surfaces for mastication.

From the oral cavity, food passes through the opening at the back of the mouth to enter the **pharynx** (throat). Moving the masticated ball of food is accomplished by a series of muscular movements of the pharynx, in which the soft palate elevates, the walls of the pharynx close, and the larynx is pushed upward against the epiglottis. These movements are collectively called the swallowing reflex. As a result, food is pushed down the pharynx and into the next organ, the esophagus.

The **esophagus** is a muscle-walled tube that carries food from the pharynx to the stomach. The term is derived from the Greek word for *gullet*. It is internally

[**thinking critically!**]

What opening is guarded by the epiglottis during swallowing to prevent food from "passing down the wrong tube"?

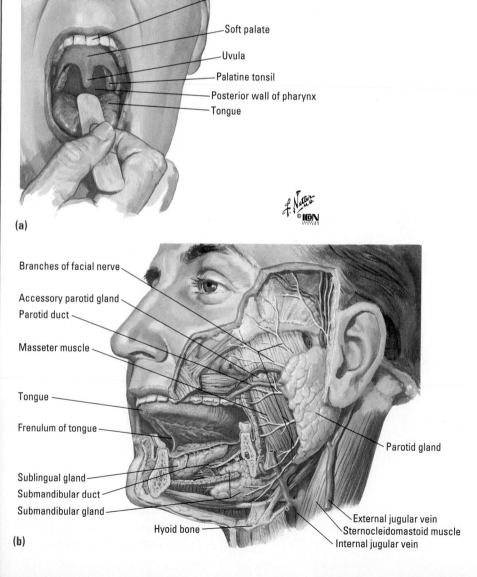

(a)

(b)

Teeth

Soft palate

Uvula

Palatine tonsil

Posterior wall of pharynx

Tongue

Branches of facial nerve

Accessory parotid gland

Parotid duct

Masseter muscle

Tongue

Frenulum of tongue

Sublingual gland

Submandibular duct

Submandibular gland

Hyoid bone

Parotid gland

External jugular vein

Sternocleidomastoid muscle

Internal jugular vein

Figure 13.2 ::::

The oral cavity.

(a) Anterior view of the open mouth.

(b) Lateral view of the sectioned head.

Source: Icon Learning Systems.

enrichment module enrichment module **enrichment module** enrichment module enrichment module **enrichment module** enrichment module **enrichment module**

lined with a protective mucosa, which includes layers of epithelial cells and a coating of mucus. The esophagus moves food to the stomach by muscular contractions that move like the waves of the ocean, known as **peristalsis.** Peristalsis is not unique to the esophagus: it occurs throughout the GI tract. The distal end of the esophagus penetrates through an opening in the diaphragm to enter the abdominal cavity, which is lined with a membrane called the **peritoneum.**

From the esophagus, swallowed food is pushed into the **stomach.** The stomach is divided into four regions: the **cardia,** near the esophagus; the **fundus,** an upper, domed part; the **body,** the central area of the stomach; and the **pylorus,** the lower area that joins the small intestine (Figure 13.3::::). The ring of muscle that borders the stomach and small intestine is the **pyloric valve.** Internally, the stomach is lined with a mucosa that contains many one-celled glands. The glands secrete a mixture known as **gastric juice,** made up of hydrochloric acid (HCl), a protein called pepsinogen, and mucus. The pepsinogen is converted to pepsin, a powerful protein-cleaving enzyme, in the acid environment created by HCl. Thus, the stomach begins the chemical digestion of proteins. The mucus protects the stomach lining from damage that would otherwise be caused by HCl and pepsin. A reduction of mucus or excessive HCl production can upset the protective balance, resulting in damage to the stomach mucosa known as peptic (or gastric) ulcers.

Contractions of the muscular stomach wall push the partially digested food into the next organ of the GI tract, the **small intestine.** About 20 feet in length, it is a coiled tube that extends between the stomach and the large intestine (Figure 13.4::::). The small intestine includes three sections: a **duodenum,** a **jejunum,** and an **ileum.** Each section is lined with a mucosa that includes tiny fingerlike projections, known as **villi.** The villi improve the small intestine's ability to absorb nutrients, which is its primary function. The small intestine is also the organ that completes chemical digestion. Peristaltic contractions of the small intestine move

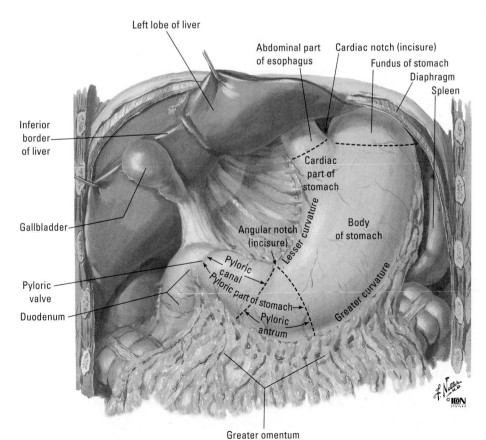

Figure 13.3 ::::

The stomach in its normal shape and location within the abdominal cavity.

The liver is shown pulled upward, to reveal the entire stomach and the underside of the liver.
Source: Icon Learning Systems.

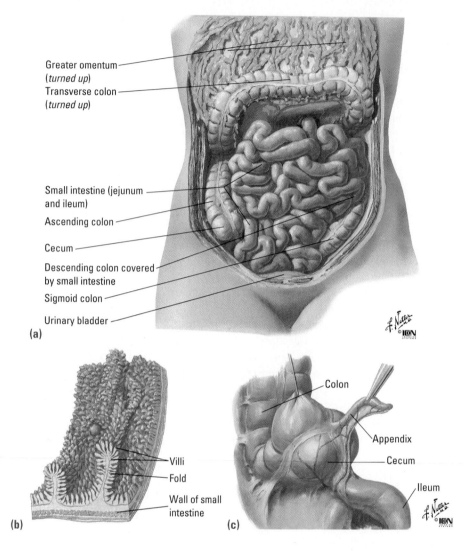

(a)

(b) (c)

Figure 13.4 ::::

The small and large intestines.
(a) The small and large intestines, shown with the greater omentum pulled upward.
(b) A section of the small intestinal wall reveals the presence of villi.
(c) The cecum and appendix of the large intestine.
Source: Icon Learning Systems.

food slowly to maximize absorption, eventually pushing the watery indigestible waste into the large intestine.

[FYI]

Duodenum, Jejunum, and Ileum
The term *duodenum* is derived from the Medieval Latin word, *duodeni*, which means *twelve*. This word first appeared in the anatomical texts in 1050 AD, taken from a monk's description of it as the "first part of the small intestine, about 12 fingerbreadths in length." *Ileum* means *to roll* in Greek, and is named after its peristaltic waves of muscle contraction that roll through the organ like an ocean wave. The term *jejunum* is named from the Latin word *jejunus,* meaning *empty,* because it was usually found empty during a dissection.

The large intestine forms the waste into a solid material, known as **feces,** by absorbing water as it moves the material in slow, peristaltic contractions. The three segments of the large intestine are the **cecum,** the **colon,** and the **rectum.** The short, pouch-like cecum receives material from the small intestine, and includes a 2-to-5-inch-long dead-ended appendage known as the **appendix.** The long colon extends from the cecum for about eight feet, and includes ascending, transverse, descending, and sigmoid segments. The rectum is the terminal end of the large intestine, which opens to the body's exterior by way of the **anus.**

[thinking critically!]

In addition to the esophagus, what organs of the GI tract propel material by peristalsis?

Accessory Organs

Each of the digestive accessory organs manufactures materials that benefit the process of digestion. The **salivary glands** begin the process of chemical digestion in the mouth by secreting **saliva.** The saliva enters the oral cavity through small ducts. It includes an enzyme, known as amylase, that breaks down polysaccharides (complex carbohydrates) to begin the process of chemical digestion. There are three pairs of salivary glands: the large **parotid glands** in the cheeks, the **submandibular glands** behind the chin, and the **sublingual glands** below the tongue (Figure 13.2).

The **liver** is the largest visceral organ in the body (Figure 13.3). Its cells, known as hepatic cells, perform many functions that include the production of **bile,** the interconversion of nutrients, the recycling of red blood cell components, and the removal of toxins from the blood. Bile is a greenish fluid delivered to the small intestine by way of **biliary ducts,** where it aids in the digestion of fats. The main biliary duct is the **common bile duct** (Figure 13.5::::). Bile obtains its color from pigments resulting from the recycling process of red blood cells. When liver function is affected by disease, one of the first signs is the accumulation of bile pigments in the skin and sclera of the eyes, producing the yellowing symptom of jaundice.

The **gallbladder** is a small sac located in a small depression on the posterior side of the liver (Figures 13.3 and 13.5). It receives bile from the liver, which it stores until a meal is ingested. The bile leaves the gallbladder and is delivered into the small intestine by way of a duct, where it aids in fat digestion.

The **pancreas** is an oblong organ located behind the stomach (Figure 13.5). Most of its cells produce digestive enzymes, which are delivered to the small intestine by way of a duct. The digestive enzymes, collectively called **pancreatic juice,** enable the small intestine to complete the process of chemical digestion. Other cells of the pancreas secrete the hormones insulin and glucagon, which regulate sugar levels in the blood.

[FYI]

Liver Failure
The leading cause of acute liver failure in the United States is acetaminophen overdose. This drug has been sold over the counter since its discovery as a "safe" analgesic in 1970. Its most popular market name is Tylenol.

[thinking critically!]

Why does the small intestine receive most of the digestive enzymes produced by accessory organs?

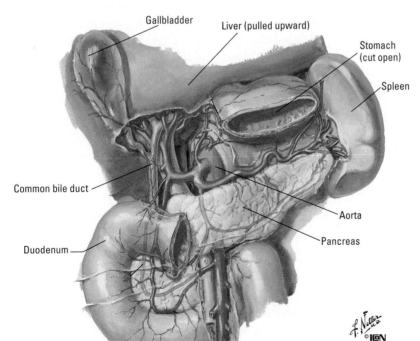

Figure 13.5 ::::

The pancreas, gallbladder, and bile ducts.

In this view of the upper abdomen, the stomach has been removed to reveal the pancreas behind it. Also, the liver is reflected upward to reveal the gallbladder and bile ducts.
Source: Icon Learning Systems.

getting to the root of it | anatomy and physiology terms

Many of the anatomy and physiology terms are formed from roots that are used to construct the more complex medical terms of the digestive system, including symptoms, diseases, and treatments. In this section, we will review the terms that describe the structure and function of the digestive system *in relation to their word roots,* which are shown in **bold.**

Study the word roots and terms in this list and complete the review exercises that follow.

Word Root (Meaning)	Terms Formed from the Word Root (Pronunciation)	Definition
bil (bile)	**bil**e	a greenish fluid produced by liver cells that aids in the digestion of fats in the small intestine
card (heart)	**card**ia (KAR dee ah)	the area of the stomach that receives food from the esophagus; it is named after the heart because it is the part nearest to the heart
cec (blind intestine)	**cec**um (SEE kum)	the proximal segment of the large intestine, it is short and pouch-like and contains a short, narrow appendage known as the appendix
col (colon)	**col**on (KOH lunn)	the largest segment of the large intestine, it extends from the cecum to the rectum and includes the ascending colon, transverse colon, descending colon, and sigmoid colon
duoden (twelve)	**duoden**um (doo ODD eh num)	the first segment of the small intestine, it receives material from the stomach via the pyloric valve. It also receives pancreatic juice from the pancreas and bile from the liver and gallbladder
esophag (gullet)	**esophag**us (eh SOFF ah guss)	the muscular tube that moves food by peristalsis from the pharynx to the stomach
	lower **esophag**eal sphincter (eh SOFF ah JEE al SFINGK ter)	a ring-shaped muscle at the border of the esophagus and the stomach; abbreviated **LES**
gastr (stomach)	**gastr**ointestinal tract (GAS troh in TESS tih nal)	the digestive tube extending from the mouth to the anus; abbreviated **GI tract**, it is also called the alimentary canal.
ile (to roll)	**ile**um (ILL ee um)	the third segment of the small intestine that delivers digestive waste material to the cecum of the large intestine
jejun (empty)	**jejun**um (jee JOO num)	the middle segment of the small intestine
or (mouth)	**or**al cavity	the mouth, which receives food for digestion; it contains the palate, tongue, and uvula
palat (roof of the mouth)	**palat**e (PAHL aht)	the roof of the mouth, including an anterior hard palate and a posterior soft palate
pancreat (sweetbread)	**pancrea**s (PAN kree ass)	an organ that secretes pancreatic juice (a mixture of digestive enzymes) into the small intestine. It also secretes the hormones insulin and glucagon, which regulate blood sugar levels.
periton (to stretch over)	**periton**eum (PAIR ih toh NEE um)	a serous membrane that lines the abdominal cavity and covers most of the abdominal organs

Word Root (Meaning)	Terms Formed from the Word Root (Pronunciation)	Definition
pylor (gatekeeper)	**pylor**us (pye LOR uss)	the constricted, distal area of the stomach terminating at the pyloric valve
	pyloric valve (pye LOR ik)	a ring of muscle that functions as the gatekeeper between the stomach and small intestine by controlling the passage of materials between them
rect (straight, erect)	**rect**um (REK tum)	the distal, straight segment of the large intestine; its terminal opening is the anus
uvul (a grape)	**uvul**a (YOO vyoo lah)	a small projection at the posterior end of the soft palate in the oral cavity

OTHER IMPORTANT TERMS
The terms in this table are related to the structure and function of the digestive system, but are not built from word roots.

feces (FEE seez)	digestive waste material, usually solid, released by the process of defecation
body	the main central area of the stomach
fundus (FUN duss)	the dome-shaped, lateral portion of the stomach
gallbladder (GAWL blahd der)	a sac-like organ behind the liver that stores bile
large intestine	the segment of the GI tract, including the cecum, colon, and rectum, that forms the feces through absorbing water and peristalsis and eliminates the feces by the process of defecation
liver	the large organ at the right side of the abdomen that produces bile and manages the interconversion of nutrients, removal of toxins from the blood, and recycling of red blood cell components
peristalsis (pair ih STALL siss)	movement of the esophagus and lower GI tract produced by waves of smooth muscle contraction, resulting in propulsion of GI tract contents
pharynx (FAIR inks)	the throat, which functions as a passageway for food on its way to the esophagus and air to and from the larynx
salivary glands (SAHL ih vair ee)	three pairs of glands around the mouth that secrete saliva to lubricate food and begin the process of chemical digestion, which include the large parotid glands in the cheeks, the submandibular glands below the jaw, and the sublingual glands below the tongue
small intestine	a long, twisting tube between the stomach and the large intestine that is the final site of chemical digestion, and is the primary site of nutrient absorption; it includes three segments: the duodenum, the jejunum, and the ileum
stomach (STUM ahk)	the J-shaped segment of the GI tract between the esophagus and the small intestine that includes four areas: the cardia, the fundus, the body, and the pylorus; it contains one-celled glands that produce gastric juice, a mixture of HCl, pepsinogen, and mucus to begin the process of protein digestion
tongue (TUNG)	the muscular organ at the floor of the mouth, which aids in swallowing and in speech

SELF QUIZ 13.2

SAY IT—SPELL IT!

Review the terms of the digestive system by speaking the phonetic pronunciation guides out loud, then writing in the correct spelling of the term.

Success Hint: Use the audio glossary on the CD and CW for additional help with pronunciation of these terms.

1. eh SOFF ah guss _____
2. GAWL blahd er _____
3. GAS troh in TESS tih nal _____
4. SEE kum _____
5. KOH lunn _____
6. TUNG _____
7. YOO vyoo lah _____
8. PAN kree ass _____
9. doo ODD eh num _____
10. jee JOO num _____
11. pye LOR uss _____

MATCH IT!

Match the term on the left with the correct definition on the right.

_____ 1. tongue   a. the third segment of the small intestine

_____ 2. uvula   b. a mixture of enzymes

_____ 3. pharynx   c. begins chemical digestion in the mouth

_____ 4. esophagus   d. the largest salivary gland

_____ 5. peristalsis   e. the dome-shaped area of the stomach

_____ 6. parotid gland   f. a downward projection of the soft palate

_____ 7. saliva   g. dominates the floor of the oral cavity

_____ 8. fundus   h. produces bile

_____ 9. pyloric valve   i. the first segment of the small intestine

_____ 10. gastric juice   j. the longest segment of the large intestine

_____ 11. bile   k. wave-like muscular contractions

_____ 12. pancreatic juice   l. a mixture of HCl, pepsinogen, and mucus

_____ 13. pepsin   m. borders the stomach and small intestine

_____ 14. liver   n. the first segment of the large intestine

_____ 15. duodenum   o. enzyme in the stomach that digests protein

_____ 16. ileum   p. a fluid produced by liver cells

_____ 17. cecum   q. provides the swallowing function

_____ 18. colon   r. located in the thoracic and abdominal cavities

FILL IT IN!

Fill in the blanks with the correct terms.

1. The posterior roof of the _____ _____, or mouth, is not supported by bone and is known as the _____ _____. At its posterior margin is a downward projection called the _____, which triggers the swallowing reflex.

2. Contractions of the wall of the _____ allow food to be swallowed. In the muscular tube called the _____, wave-like contractions known as _____ push food to the stomach. Before the esophagus joins the stomach, it penetrates into the _____ cavity, which is lined with a membrane known as the _____.

3. The stomach is lined with a mucosa that is filled with small glands, which secrete a mixture known as _____ juice. It includes HCl, pepsinogen, and mucus. The pepsinogen is converted to _____, which digests proteins. The _____ forms a protective coating on the stomach mucosa. The stomach includes four areas: the cardia, fundus, body, and _____.

4. The small intestine completes the process of chemical _____ and is the primary site of nutrient _____. Its tiny projections known as _____ improve the efficiency of absorption. The first segment, the _____, receives material from the stomach via a circular muscle called the _____ _____. The middle segment is known as the _____. The final segment, called the ileum, pushes undigestible waste into the first part of the large intestine, called the _____.

5. In addition to the cecum, the large intestine includes the long _____, and its final segment is the _____. During the process of waste elimination or _____, feces are pushed out of the terminal opening called the _____.

6. The cells of the liver produce a greenish fluid known as _____, which aids the small intestine in the digestion of _____. Once produced, the fluid is usually stored in the _____ before it enters the duodenum. Other fluids that aid in digestion include _____ released into the mouth and _____ _____ that is produced by cells of the pancreas.

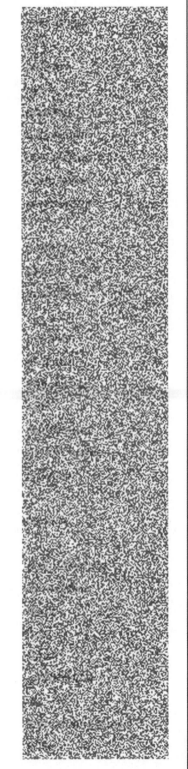

[medical terms of the

digestive system]

The digestive system is under a constant risk of infection, since food and other substances that often contain pathogens are introduced into the body through the mouth every day. To make matters even more risky, the GI tract normally contains an enormous number of bacteria. Known as the digestive flora, most of these organisms are beneficial, when their populations are contained within the tract. For example, *E. coli* assists in the breakdown of indigestible plant materials and synthesizes vitamin K. But if the flora is allowed to increase in density or spread to other body areas, severe infections can result.

In addition to infections, the GI tract organs are also susceptible to inherited defects and the development of tumors. In each case, the result of the disease may be a reduction of the body's ability to digest food, eliminate wastes, absorb and conserve water, or perform other specific functions. Most digestive disorders affect overall health rather than remain localized, due to the abundance of blood vessels associated with GI tract organs and the functional importance of the accessory organs like the liver and pancreas.

The clinical treatment of a digestive disorder is performed by a physician with a specialization in treating the body region or organ, the particular disorder, or a set of disorders. For example, a disease of the mouth or throat is treated by a **head and neck specialist,** stomach or intestinal disease is treated by a **gastroenterologist,** a disease of the rectum is treated by a **proctologist,** and a disease of the liver is treated by a **hepatobiliary specialist.** Cancer is treated by an **oncologist,** often in association with a regional specialist. The area within a hospital that treats digestive disorders is often called **internal medicine.**

Since most digestive organs are deep within the body, the diagnosis of digestive disorders often requires a noninvasive imaging procedure, such as magnetic resonance imaging (MRI), a computed axial tomography (CAT) scan, or a specialized x-ray technique. Once diagnosed, most disorders may be treated with therapeutic agents or by surgery. Some disorders, such as eating disorders, are treated with psychological counseling and a strict diet regimen.

let's construct terms!

In this section, we will assemble all of the word parts to construct medical terminology related to the digestive system. Abbreviations are used to indicate each word part: **p** = prefix, **r** = root, **cv** = combining vowel, and **s** = suffix. Note that some terms are not constructed from word parts, but they are included here to expand your vocabulary.

The medical terms of the digestive system are listed in the following three sections:

- Symptoms and Signs
- Diseases and Disorders
- Treatments, Procedures, and Devices

Each section is followed by review exercises. Study the lists in these tables and complete the review exercises that follow.

Symptoms and Signs

WORD PARTS (WHEN APPLICABLE)			TERM	DEFINITION
Part	Type	Meaning		
a- phag -ia	p r s	without eat, swallow diseased state	**aphagia** (ah FAY jee ah)	inability to swallow
			ascites (ah SIGH teez)	an accumulation of fluid within the peritoneal cavity; a symptom of liver dysfunction
			constipation (kon stih PAY shun)	reduced peristalsis in the large intestine, resulting in infrequent or incomplete defecation
dia- rrhea	p r	through excessive discharge	**diarrhea** (dye ah REE ah)	a frequent discharge of watery fecal material which may be caused by an improper diet, but more commonly by infection of virus, bacteria, or protozoa; it can lead to severe dehydration

[FYI]

Diarrhea

In the United States, the most common cause of diarrhea is bacteria-contaminated food, usually by *E. coli*, through the fecal-to-oral route. It can be fatal to the young, old, and those who are immunosuppressed.

WORD PARTS (WHEN APPLICABLE)			TERM	DEFINITION
dys- peps -ia	p r s	bad, abnormal digestion diseased state	**dyspepsia** (diss PEPP see ah)	indigestion
dys- phag -ia	p r s	bad, abnormal eat, swallow diseased state	**dysphagia** (diss FAY jee ah)	difficulty in swallowing
			flatus (FLAY tuss)	a condition of gas trapped in the GI tract or released through the anus
gastr/o -dynia	r/cv s	stomach pain	**gastrodynia** (GAS troh DINN ee ah)	pain in the stomach
halit -osis	r s	breath condition of	**halitosis** (hall ih TOH siss)	bad breath
hemat -emesis	r s	blood vomiting	**hematemesis** (hee mah TEM eh siss)	vomiting blood
hepat/o megal -y	r/cv r s	liver large process of	**hepatomegaly** (HEPP ah toh MEG ah lee)	enlargement of the liver
hyper- bil/i rubin -emia	p r/cv r s	excessive bile red pigment blood	**hyperbilirubinemia** (HIGH per BILL ih roo bih NEE mee ah)	excessive levels of the bile pigment, bilirubin, in the blood
			jaundice (JAWN diss)	a yellowish staining of the skin, sclera of the eyes, and deeper tissues caused by the accumulation of bile pigments in the bloodstream that are normally removed by the liver and thus, a symptom of liver dysfunction; it may also be a symptom of red blood cell destruction

WORD PARTS (WHEN APPLICABLE)			TERM	DEFINITION
Part	Type	Meaning		

[FYI]

Jaundice
The term *jaundice* is derived from the old French word for yellow, *jain,* to describe the yellowing appearance of the skin and sclera. An alternate term for this symptom is *icterus,* which is the Greek work for *yellow bird.*

Part	Type	Meaning	TERM	DEFINITION
			nausea (NAW see ah)	from the Latin and Greek word for seasickness, it is a symptomatic urge to vomit; when accompanied by vomiting, it may be abbreviated **N&V**
re- flux	p r	back flow	**reflux** (REE fluks)	a backward flow of material in the GI tract, or regurgitation
steat/o -rrhea	r/cv s	fat excessive discharge	**steatorrhea** (STEE at oh REE ah)	abnormal fat levels in the feces

SELF QUIZ 13.3

SAY IT—SPELL IT!

Review the terms of the digestive system by speaking the phonetic pronunciation guides out loud, then writing in the correct spelling of the term.

1. ah FAY jee ah _____

13.3 2. diss PEPP see ah _____

3. hee mah TEM eh siss _____

4. HIGH per BILL ih roo bih NEE mee ah _____

5. GAS troh DINN ee ah _____

13.4 6. STEE at oh REE ah _____

7. HEPP ah toh MEG ah lee _____

8. diss FAY jee ah _____

9. NAW see ah _____

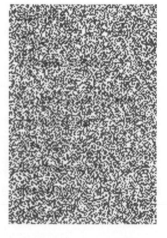

MATCH IT!

Match the term on the left with the correct definition on the right.

_____ 1. dysphagia

_____ 2. dyspepsia

_____ 3. hematemesis

_____ 4. hepatomegaly

_____ 5. hyperbilirubinemia

_____ 6. steatorrhea

_____ 7. flatus

_____ 8. vomit

_____ 9. ascites

_____10. diarrhea

_____11. nausea

_____12. constipation

_____13. jaundice

a. excessive bilirubin levels in the blood

b. enlargement of the liver

c. difficulty in swallowing

d. abnormal fat levels in the feces

e. indigestion

f. vomiting blood

g. from the Old French for "yellow"

h. reduced peristalsis in the large intestine

i. a symptomatic urge to vomit

j. accumulation of fluid in the peritoneal cavity

k. frequent discharge of watery fecal material

l. expelled from the stomach out the mouth

m. gas trapped in the GI tract

BREAK IT DOWN!

Analyze and separate each term into its word part by labeling each word part using p = prefix, r = root, cv = combining vowel, and s = suffix.

1. aphagia _____

2. dyspepsia _____

3. gastrodynia _____

4. hyperbilirubinemia _____

5. hematemesis _____

Diseases and Disorders

WORD PARTS (WHEN APPLICABLE)			TERM	DEFINITION
Part	Type	Meaning		
			adhesion (add HEE zhun)	an abnormal growth connecting two surfaces, which may arise as a complication to healing after surgery
an-	p	without	**anorexia nervosa** (an oh REK see ah	a personality disorder characterized by an extreme aversion to food that results in weight loss and
or	r	mouth	ner VOH sah)	malnourishment
ex-	p	outside, away from		
-ia	s	diseased state		
nerv	r	nerve		
-osa	s	condition of		

WORD PARTS (WHEN APPLICABLE)			TERM	DEFINITION
Part	Type	Meaning		
append	r	to hang onto, appendix	**appendicitis** (ah pen dih SIGH tiss)	inflammation of the appendix (Figure 13.6::::)
-ic	s	pertaining to		
-itis	s	inflammation		

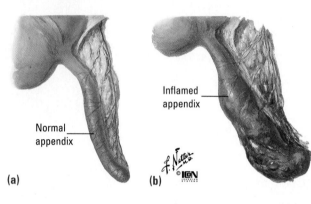

Normal appendix

(a)

Inflamed appendix

(b)

Figure 13.6 ::::

Appendicitis.
(a) A normal appendix.
(b) An inflamed appendix in appendicitis.
Source: Icon Learning Systems.

			bulimia (boo LIHM ee ah)	an eating disorder involving repeated gorging with food that is followed by induced vomiting or laxative abuse; commonly known as "binging and purging"
cheil	r	lip	**cheilitis** (kye LYE tiss)	inflammation of the lip
-itis	s	inflammation		
chol	r	bile, gall	**cholangioma** (koh LAHN jee OH mah)	a tumor originating from a bile duct, usually from within the liver
angi	r	blood vessel		
-oma	s	tumor		
chol/e	r/cv	bile, gall	**cholecystitis** (koh lee siss TYE tiss)	inflammation of the gallbladder
cyst	r	bladder		
-itis	s	inflammation		

[FYI]

Cholecystitis

Chol is the Greek word for *bile*. Cholecystitis, which literally means *inflammation of the bile-filled bladder*, afflicts more than 20 million people in the United States. It is usually caused by gallstones, which block the bile ducts to produce symptoms of pain and jaundice.

choledoch/o	r/cv	common bile duct	**choledocholithiasis** (koh LEH doh koh lith EYE ah siss)	presence of mineralized masses, called gallstones or stones, in the common bile duct where they block bile flow (Figure 13.7::::)
lith	r	stone		
-iasis	s	condition		
chol/e	r/cv	bile, gall	**cholelithiasis** (KOH lee lith EYE ah siss)	generalized condition of gallstones (Figure 13.7)
lith	r	stone		
-iasis	s	condition		
cirrh	r	orange, tawny	**cirrhosis** (ser ROH siss)	a chronic, progressive liver disease resulting from hepatic cell failure, which may be caused by chronic alcoholism or viral infection (Figure 13.8::::)
-osis	s	condition		

WORD PARTS (WHEN APPLICABLE)			TERM	DEFINITION
Part	Type	Meaning		

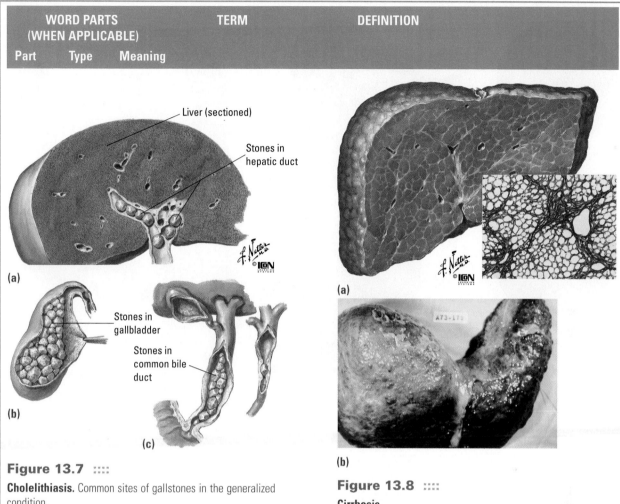

Figure 13.7 ::::

Cholelithiasis. Common sites of gallstones in the generalized condition.
(a) Stones in the hepatic duct.
(b) Stones in the gallbladder.
(c) Stones in the common bile duct.
Source: Icon Learning Systems.

Figure 13.8 ::::

Cirrhosis.
(a) Cirrhosis is characterized by a chronic deterioration of the liver, replacing healthy cells with connective tissue that causes a mottled appearance. *Source: Icon Learning Systems.*
(b) In this photograph, the liver was removed from a deceased patient in an advanced state of cirrhosis. *Source: Pearson Education.*

Part	Type	Meaning	TERM	DEFINITION
col -itis	r s	colon inflammation	**colitis** (koh LYE tiss)	inflammation of the colon; when the condition is chronic and results in the formation of colonic ulcers, it is called **ulcerative colitis,** the main symptom of which is severe and sometimes bloody diarrhea (Figure 13.9::::)
col/o rect -al	r/cv r s	colon straight, erect, colon pertaining to	**colorectal cancer** (koh loh REK tall)	cancer of the colon and rectum, which often originates as a polyp to become an aggressive, metastatic tumor (Figure 13.10::::)
			Crohn's disease (KROHNZ)	chronic inflammation of any part of the GI tract, most commonly of the ileum, that involves small ulcerations of the intestinal wall, resulting in scar tissue formation and intestinal obstruction; also called regional ileitis or regional enteritis, it is usually an inherited condition (Figure 13.11::::)

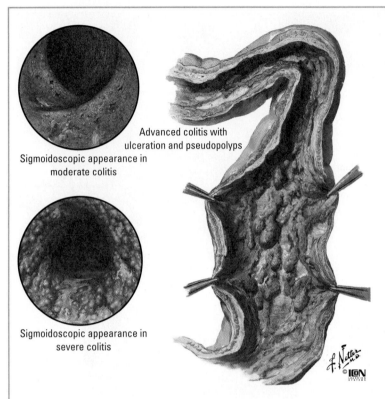

Sigmoidoscopic appearance in
moderate colitis

Advanced colitis with
ulceration and pseudopolyps

Sigmoidoscopic appearance in
severe colitis

Figure 13.9 ::::

Colitis. In this chronic disease, the inner lining of the colon is inflamed. In severe
cases, open sores or ulcers develop. *Source: Icon Learning Systems.*

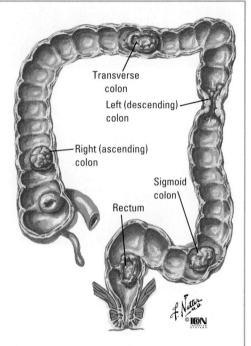

Transverse
colon

Left (descending)
colon

Right (ascending)
colon

Sigmoid
colon

Rectum

Figure 13.10 ::::

Colorectal cancer. The most common sites of
tumor development are shown.
Source: Icon Learning Systems.

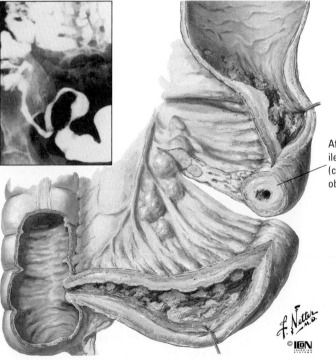

Affected
ileum
(cut to show
obstruction)

Figure 13.11 ::::

Crohn's disease.
This chronic disease is
characterized by a thickening of the
intestinal wall and a gradual
erosion of the inner lining. The
ileum of the small intestine is
shown affected in this illustration,
and the insert is a barium enema
x-ray that reveals obstructions.
Source: Icon Learning Systems.

WORD PARTS (WHEN APPLICABLE)			TERM	DEFINITION
Part	Type	Meaning		

Crohn's Disease
Dr. B. B. Crohn first described the disease that bears his name in 1932. At the time, he believed it was caused by a pathogen. New evidence suggests that he may have been correct, although the causative organism has not yet been identified.

| diverticul | r | a small blind pouch | **diverticulitis** (DYE ver tik yoo LYE tiss) | inflammation of abnormal small pouches in the wall of the colon (called **diverticula**) (Figure 13.12::::) |
| -itis | s | inflammation | | |

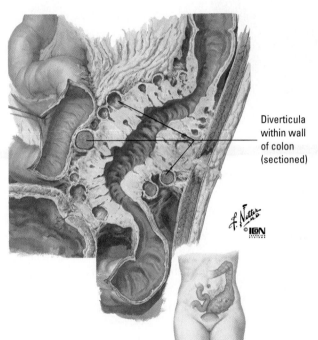

Diverticula within wall of colon (sectioned)

Figure 13.12 ::::
Diverticulitis.
Source: Icon Learning Systems.

diverticul	r	a small blind pouch	**diverticulosis** (DYE ver tik yoo LOH siss)	condition of diverticula in the colon
-osis	s	condition		
duoden	r	twelve, duodenum	**duodenal ulcer** (doo ODD eh nal)	an ulcer in the wall of the duodenum
-al	s	pertaining to		
dys-	p	bad, abnormal	**dysentery** (DISS in tair ee)	severe inflammation of the intestine marked by frequent diarrhea, abdominal pain, fever, and dehydration; it is usually caused by infection by bacteria or protozoa
enter	r	small intestine		
-y	s	process of		
enter	r	small intestine	**enteritis** (ehn ter EYE tiss)	inflammation of the small intestine
-itis	s	inflammation		
esophag	r	gullet, esophagus	**esophagitis** (eh soff ah JYE tiss)	inflammation of the esophagus
-itis	s	inflammation		

WORD PARTS (WHEN APPLICABLE)			TERM	DEFINITION
Part	**Type**	**Meaning**		
gastr	r	stomach	**gastric cancer**	cancer of the stomach, also called stomach
-ic	s	pertaining to	(GAS trik KANN ser)	carcinoma (Figure 13.13::::)

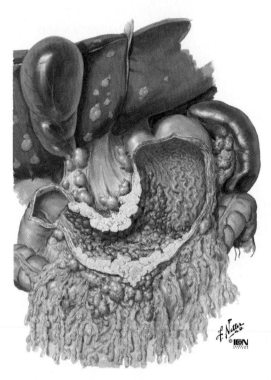

Figure 13.13 ::::

Gastric cancer.
Advanced stomach carcinoma
includes the spread of malignant
cells to form tumors in the lymph
nodes, liver, omentum, pancreas,
and bile ducts.
Source: Icon Learning Systems.

WORD PARTS			TERM	DEFINITION
gastr	r	stomach	**gastric ulcer**	an ulcer in the wall of the stomach
-ic	s	pertaining to	(GAS trik ULL ser)	
gastr	r	stomach	**gastritis**	inflammation of the stomach
-itis	s	inflammation	(gas TRY tiss)	
gastr/o	r/cv	stomach	**gastroenteritis**	inflammation of the stomach and small intestine
enter	r	small intestine	(GAS troh ehn ter EYE tiss)	
-itis	s	inflammation		
gastr/o	r/cv	stomach	**gastroenterocolitis**	inflammation of the stomach, small intestine, and
enter/o	r/cv	small intestine	(GAS troh EHN ter oh	colon
col	r	colon	koh LYE tiss)	
-itis	s	inflammation		
gastr/o	r/cv	stomach	**gastroesophageal**	recurring backflow of stomach contents into the
esophag/e	r/cv	gullet, esophagus	**reflux disease**	esophagus as a result of a weakened lower
-al	s	pertaining to	(GAS troh eh	esophageal sphincter, producing burning pain;
re-	p	back	SOFF ah JEE al)	abbreviated GERD
flux	r	flow		
gastr/o	r/cv	stomach	**gastromalacia**	softening of the stomach wall
-malacia	s	softening	(GAS troh mah LAY she ah)	
giardia	r	genus of protozoa	**giardiasis**	infection of the intestinal protozoa *Giardia*
-sis	s	state of	(jee ahr DYE ah siss)	*intestinalis* or *G. lambia,* producing symptoms of diarrhea, cramps, nausea, and vomiting

WORD PARTS (WHEN APPLICABLE)			TERM	DEFINITION
Part	Type	Meaning		
gingiv	r	gums	**gingivitis**	inflammation of the gums
-itis	s	inflammation	(jin jih VYE tiss)	
gloss	r	tongue	**glossitis**	inflammation of the tongue (Figure 13.14::::)
-itis	s	inflammation	(gloss EYE tiss)	

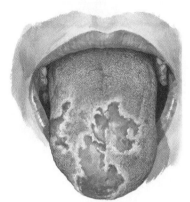

Geographic tongue

Hairy tongue

Figure 13.14 ::::

Glossitis.

Two common forms of glossitis are illustrated: geographic tongue, so-called because the inflammation forms a map-like appearance, and hairy tongue, named after the false appearance of hair on the tongue surface.
Source: Icon Learning Systems.

gloss/o	r/cv	tongue	**glossopathy**	generalized disease of the tongue (Figure 13.14)
-pathy	s	disease	(gloss OPP ah thee)	
hemorrh	r	likely to bleed	**hemorrhoids**	a varicose (swollen) condition of veins in the anus
-oid	s	condition	(HEM oh roydz)	that results in painful swellings
hepat	r	liver	**hepatitis**	inflammation of the liver
-itis	s	inflammation	(hepp ah TYE tiss)	

[FYI]

Hepatitis Types

There are five main categories of hepatitis, all caused by related forms of a virus: Type A (infectious hepatitis) is transmitted by eating contaminated food; type B (serum hepatitis) is transmitted via body fluids, such as blood or semen; type C is mainly transmitted through the blood and often causes permanent liver damage; type D is similar to type B and may combine with it to severely damage the liver; and type E is similar to type A and is the most common form worldwide.

hepat	r	liver	**hepatoma**	tumor of the liver (Figure 13.15::::)
-oma	s	tumor	(hepp ah TOH mah)	
hiatal	r	pertaining to an opening	**hiatal hernia** (high AY tal HER nee ah)	protrusion of part of the stomach upward through an opening in the diaphragm normally penetrated by
hern	r	a rupture		the esophagus, known as the esophageal hiatus
-ia	s	diseased state		(Figure 13.16::::)
ile	r	to roll, ileum	**ileitis**	inflammation of the ileum
-itis	s	inflammation	(ILL ee EYE tiss)	

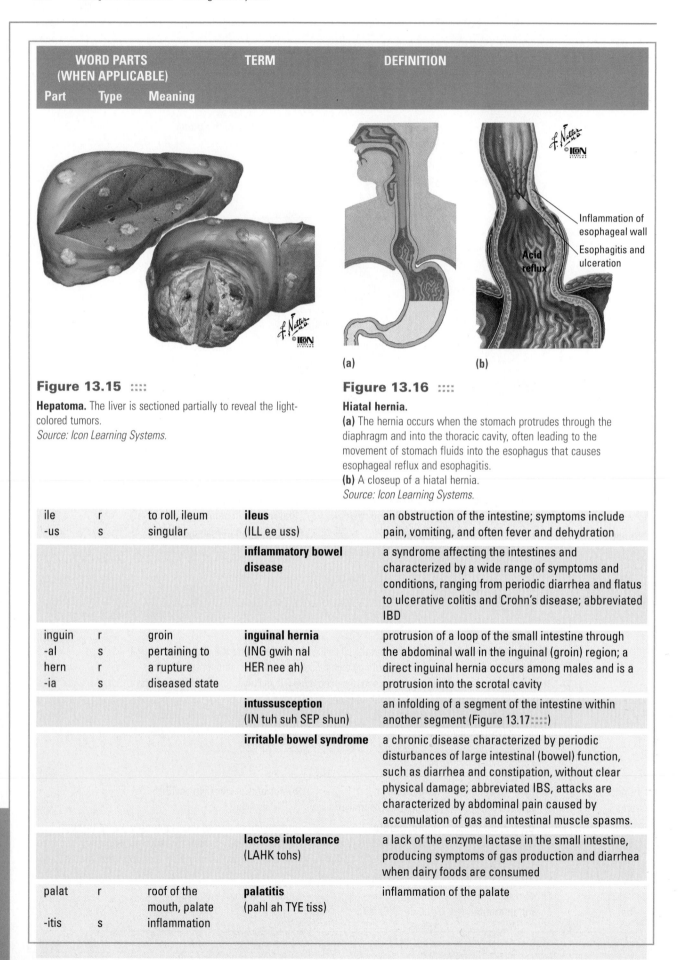

WORD PARTS (WHEN APPLICABLE)			TERM	DEFINITION
Part	Type	Meaning		

Figure 13.15 ::::

Hepatoma. The liver is sectioned partially to reveal the light-colored tumors.
Source: Icon Learning Systems.

Figure 13.16 ::::

Hiatal hernia.
(a) The hernia occurs when the stomach protrudes through the diaphragm and into the thoracic cavity, often leading to the movement of stomach fluids into the esophagus that causes esophageal reflux and esophagitis.
(b) A closeup of a hiatal hernia.
Source: Icon Learning Systems.

Part	Type	Meaning	TERM	DEFINITION
ile	r	to roll, ileum	**ileus** (ILL ee uss)	an obstruction of the intestine; symptoms include pain, vomiting, and often fever and dehydration
-us	s	singular		
			inflammatory bowel disease	a syndrome affecting the intestines and characterized by a wide range of symptoms and conditions, ranging from periodic diarrhea and flatus to ulcerative colitis and Crohn's disease; abbreviated IBD
inguin	r	groin	**inguinal hernia** (ING gwih nal HER nee ah)	protrusion of a loop of the small intestine through the abdominal wall in the inguinal (groin) region; a direct inguinal hernia occurs among males and is a protrusion into the scrotal cavity
-al	s	pertaining to		
hern	r	a rupture		
-ia	s	diseased state		
			intussusception (IN tuh suh SEP shun)	an infolding of a segment of the intestine within another segment (Figure 13.17 ::::)
			irritable bowel syndrome	a chronic disease characterized by periodic disturbances of large intestinal (bowel) function, such as diarrhea and constipation, without clear physical damage; abbreviated IBS, attacks are characterized by abdominal pain caused by accumulation of gas and intestinal muscle spasms.
			lactose intolerance (LAHK tohs)	a lack of the enzyme lactase in the small intestine, producing symptoms of gas production and diarrhea when dairy foods are consumed
palat	r	roof of the mouth, palate	**palatitis** (pahl ah TYE tiss)	inflammation of the palate
-itis	s	inflammation		

Inflammation of esophageal wall

Esophagitis and ulceration

Acid reflux

(a)　　(b)

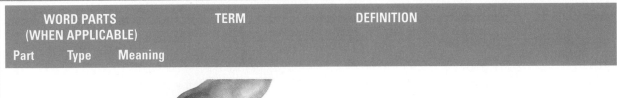

WORD PARTS (WHEN APPLICABLE)			TERM	DEFINITION
Part	Type	Meaning		

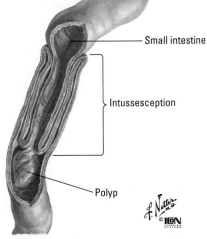

— Small intestine

} Intussesception

— Polyp

Figure 13.17 ::::

Intussusception.
The condition is caused by an infolding of the small intestine, which often causes a reduction of intestinal motility and is often associated with polyp formation.
Source: Icon Learning Systems.

Part	Type	Meaning	TERM	DEFINITION
pancreat	r	sweetbread, pancreas	**pancreatitis** (PAN kree ah TYE tiss)	inflammation of the pancreas
-itis	s	inflammation		
parot	r	parotid gland	**parotitis** (pahr oh TYE tiss)	inflammation of the parotid gland; also called mumps
-itis	s	inflammation		
pept	r	digestion	**peptic ulcer** (PEPP tik ULL ser)	an erosion in the wall of the stomach (gastric ulcer), duodenum (duodenal ulcer), or any other part of the GI tract that may be exposed to gastric juice, that is usually due to a reduction of the protective mucus layer; about 80 percent of peptic ulcers are correlated to an infection from *Helicobacter pylori* (Figure 13.18::::)
-ic	s	pertaining to		

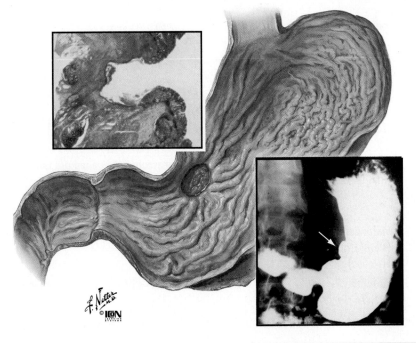

Figure 13.18 ::::

Peptic ulcer.
A gastric (stomach) ulcer is shown, which includes a histology section (upper left), an illustration of a sectioned stomach with one ulcer (middle), and an upper GI with the arrow pointing to the ulcer (lower right).
Source: Icon Learning Systems.

WORD PARTS (WHEN APPLICABLE)			TERM	DEFINITION
Part	Type	Meaning		
periton	r	to stretch over, peritoneum	**peritonitis** (pair ih toh NYE tiss)	inflammation of the peritoneum
-itis	s	inflammation		
polyp	r	a small growth	**polyp** (PALL ip)	any abnormal mass of tissue that projects outward from a wall; usually a benign growth that may occur in the nose, throat, and intestines
polyp	r	a small growth	**polyposis** (pall ee POH siss)	presence of many polyps, usually in the colon or rectum, which poses a high level of risk for malignancy (Figure 13.19▪▪▪▪)
-osis	s	condition of		

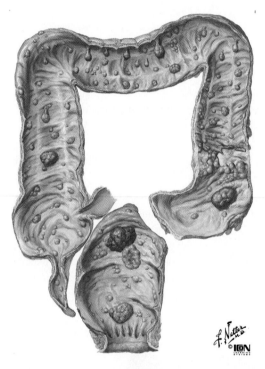

Figure 13.19 ▪▪▪▪

Polyps and polyposis.
A polyp is a protruding growth from a mucous membrane. In the disease polyposis, multiple polyps develop, usually along the inner wall of the large intestine.
Source: Icon Learning Systems.

proct	r	anus	**proctitis** (prok TYE tiss)	inflammation of the rectum and anus
-itis	s	inflammation		
proct/o	r/cv	anus	**proctoptosis** (PROK top TOH siss)	prolapse of the rectum
-ptosis	s	condition of falling downward		
rect/o	r/cv	straight, erect, rectum	**rectocele** (REK toh seel)	protrusion of the rectum, also called proctocele (PROK toh seel)
-cele	s	hernia, swelling, protrusion		
sial/o	r/cv	saliva	**sialoadenitis** (sigh AL oh add eh NYE tiss)	inflammation of a salivary gland
aden	r	gland		
-itis	s	inflammation		
sial/o	r/cv	saliva	**sialolith** (sigh AL oh lith)	mineralized object, or stone, in a salivary gland
lith	r	stone		

WORD PARTS (WHEN APPLICABLE)			TERM	DEFINITION
Part	Type	Meaning		
stomat	r	mouth	**stomatitis**	inflammation of the mouth
-itis	s	inflammation	(stoh mah TYE tiss)	
hern	r	a rupture	**strangulated hernia**	a hernia that is constricted, which reduces blood
-ia	s	diseased state	(STRANG yoo lay ted HER nee ah)	flow to the organ; if early intervention does not occur, the organ may develop gangrene
umbilic	r	the navel	**umbilical hernia**	a protrusion of a loop of the intestine through the
-al	s	pertaining to	(um BILL ih kal	abdominal wall in the umbilical region (the area
hern	r	a rupture	HER nee ah)	surrounding the umbilicus, or navel)
-ia	s	diseased state		
uvul	r	a grape, uvula	**uvulitis**	inflammation of the uvula
-itis	s	inflammation	(yoo vyoo LYE tiss)	
volvul	r	to roll	**volvulus**	a twisting of the intestine that leads to obstruction
-us	s	pertaining to	(VOLL vyoo luss)	(Figure 13.20)

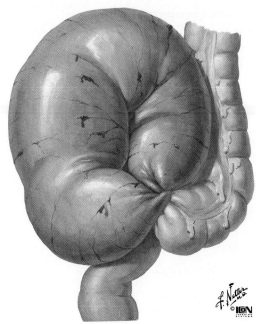

Figure 13.20

Volvulus.

A volvulus results when the small intestine twists, causing an obstruction that can lead to severe complications.
Source: Icon Learning Systems.

disease focus | The Common Cause of GI Ulcers

Ulcers are a common disease. About three to eight percent of the Third World suffers from them, and about 0.5 percent of the population in developed countries is afflicted with this disease. Approximately 300 million people have ulcers worldwide. Until recently, ulcers were thought to be caused by anxiety, an acidic diet, or heredity. Physicians often treated them by recommending antacid medicines and milk, and warning patients to stay away from spicy foods. In severe cases, surgery was needed to repair holes or remove damaged portions of the stomach, including operations such as **gastrectomy, pyloroplasty,** or **vagotomy.**

During the 1980s, an Australian physician, Dr. Barry Marshall, suspected that the damage wrought by ulcers might begin with an infectious microorganism. His idea was initially rejected because it was largely believed that microorganisms could not survive the hostile, acid environment within the stomach. By the end of the decade, however, Marshall and others had identified a bacterium found in nearly all patients with ulcers.

Amazingly, in an effort to further prove his point, Dr. Marshall infected himself with the bacterium after he was tested to be clear of it. About a week later he began to feel sick, and an examination revealed the beginnings of an ulcer with a growing population of the bacterium in the same location. Treatment with antibiotics knocked out the bacterial population and the ulcer healed soon thereafter.

The bacterium that Dr. Marshall had identified is called *Helicobacter pylori,* or *H. pylori.* Subsequent studies found that *H. pylori* is able to survive the acid of the stomach for moments, allowing it enough time to burrow through the protective mucus coating and into the safe environment of the cells lining the stomach wall. Once infected, the cells release signals to phagocytic white blood cells, which respond by mounting an attack against the bacteria and the infected cells. However, *H. pylori* divide rapidly, often staying ahead of the white blood cell attacks. The combination of the destructive chemicals released by the white blood cells and the damage caused by *H. pylori* injures the stomach lining, resulting in the erosion of tissue that characterizes peptic ulcers.

It is now widely recognized that *H. pylori* is an extremely widespread pathogen. About 80 percent of people in Third World countries are infected, and the incidence in developed countries increases with age by 1 percent for each year of life. Thus, about 30 percent of 30-year-old Americans are infected with *H. pylori.* The medical community believes that this germ is the cause for at least 80 percent of all peptic ulcers. The germ is easily passed from person to person by the fecal-to-oral route (usually due to poor hand washing), and it is suspected to be transmittable by the oral-to-oral route as well (usually by kissing or sharing food or drinks). Currently, researchers suspect that *H. pylori*-induced gastritis may not stop with ulcers, but may also initiate stomach cancers. Fortunately, *H. pylori* infections can be effectively treated with antibiotic therapy (Figure 13.21 ::::).

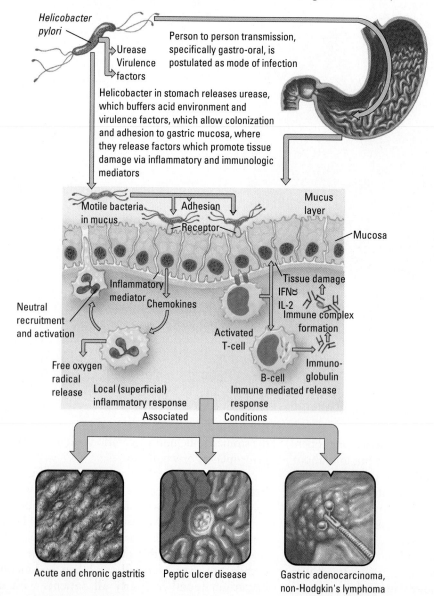

Acute and chronic gastritis   Peptic ulcer disease   Gastric adenocarcinoma, non-Hodgkin's lymphoma

Figure 13.21 ::::

Diagnosis and management of *Helicobacter pylori.*

SELF QUIZ 13.4

SAY IT—SPELL IT!

Review the terms of the digestive system by speaking the phonetic pronunciation guides out loud, then writing in the correct spelling of the term.

1. add HEE zhun _____

2. an oh REK see ah   ner VOH sah _____

3. boo LIHM ee ah _____

13.5 4. DISS in tair ee _____

5. DYE ver tik yoo LOH siss _____

13.6 6. GAS troh EHN ter oh koh LYE tiss _____

13.7 7. GAS troh mah LAY she ah _____

8. gloss EYE tiss _____

9. hepp ah TYE tiss _____

10. HER nee ah _____

11. ILL ee EYE tiss _____

12. IN tuh suh SEP shun _____

13. jin jih VYE tiss _____

14. kye LYE tiss _____

15. koh LAHN jee OH mah _____

16. koh LEE doh koh lith EYE ah siss _____

13.8 17. koh lee siss TYE tiss _____

18. koh LYE tiss _____

19. koh loh REK tall KANN ser _____

20. PAN kree ah TYE tiss _____

21. pair ih toh NYE tiss _____

22. PALL ip _____

23. PROK top TOH siss _____

24. REK toh seel _____

25. ser ROH siss _____

13.9 26. sigh AL oh add eh NYE tiss _____

27. sigh AL oh lith _____

28. stoh mah TYE tiss _____

29. VOLL vyoo luss _____

30. yoo vyoo LYE tiss _____

MATCH IT!

Match the term on the left with the correct definition on the right.

_____ 1. adhesion

_____ 2. polyp

_____ 3. anorexia nervosa

_____ 4. ileus

_____ 5. bulimia

_____ 6. ulcer

_____ 7. volvulus

_____ 8. intussesception

_____ 9. cirrhosis

_____10. Crohn's disease

_____11. irritable bowel syndrome

_____12. hernia

_____13. appendicitis

_____14. cheilitis

_____15. choledocholithiasis

_____16. colitis

_____17. diverticulitis

_____18. gastroesophageal reflux disease

_____19. gastroenterocolitis

_____20. gingivitis

a. infolding of a small intestinal segment

b. a chronic inflammation, usually of the ileum

c. general term for intestinal obstruction

d. an extreme aversion to food

e. twisting of the intestine causing an obstruction

f. a rupture

g. characterized by periodic bowel disturbances

h. a chronic liver disease

i. post-surgical growths between body walls

j. an abnormal mass projecting outward

k. an eating disorder of binging and purging

l. a lesion through a tissue or organ wall

m. inflammation of the colon

n. inflammation of the gums

o. inflammation of the stomach and intestines

p. inflammation of the appendix

q. recurring backflow of stomach contents

r. inflammation of the lips

s. inflammation of abnormal pouches in the colon

t. presence of stones in the common bile duct

BREAK IT DOWN!

Analyze and separate each term into its word parts, by labeling each word part using p = prefix, r = root, cv = combining vowel, and s = suffix.

1. appendicitis   _____

2. cheilitis   _____

3. cholelithiasis   _____

4. colitis   _____

5. diverticulitis   _____

6. enteritis   _____

7. esophagitis   _____

8. gastroenteritis _____

9. gingivitis _____

10. glossitis _____

11. hepatoma _____

12. ileitis _____

13. pancreatitis _____

14. polyposis _____

15. proctitis _____

FILL IT IN!

Fill in the blanks with the correct terms.

1. After abdominal surgery, two surfaces may grow together to form an

   _____.

2. A personality disorder characterized by an adversion to food that results in

   malnourishment and severe weight loss is known as _____

   _____. It mainly strikes young women, similar to the eating

   disorder that involves a cycle of gorging and purging, known as

   _____.

3. The accumulation of fluid in the peritoneal cavity causes a distension of the

   abdomen, a condition known as _____. It is a symptom of liver

   dysfunction, similar to a yellowing of the skin, or _____. Both

   symptoms can indicate a chronic condition of the liver known as

   _____.

4. A chronic inflammation of the GI tract, usually the ileum, that results in scarring

   and bowel obstruction is known as _____ disease, or regional

   _____.

5. A frequent and uncomfortable discharge of watery fecal material is a condition

   known as _____. It is often accompanied by the discharge of

   gas, or _____, and abdominal pain. In the chronic condition

   known as irritable _____ _____, or IBS, the

   two conditions are common symptoms.

6. A painful condition arises when an intestinal obstruction occurs. A general term for intestinal obstruction is _____. One particular type of obstruction occurs when a segment of the small intestine folds into another segment. This condition is known as _____. Another type of obstruction arises when the small intestine twists, and is called a _____.

7. A sensation of an urge to regurgitate stomach contents, or _____, is known as _____.

8. A rupture through the diaphragm resulting in the stomach extending into the thoracic cavity is a condition called _____ _____. When a loop of the small intestine drops into the scrotal cavity, it is a _____ _____ hernia.

9. A lesion resulting from erosion through the inner wall of the duodenum is known
13.13 as a _____ _____. When this occurs through the stomach wall, it is called a _____ _____.

10. An aggressive cancer that originates in the colon or rectum is called
13.14 _____ _____. A cancer of the liver, which is also
13.15 often aggressive, is called a _____.

Treatments, Procedures, and Devices

WORD PARTS (WHEN APPLICABLE)			TERM	DEFINITION
Part	**Type**	**Meaning**		
abdomin/o	r/cv	abdomen	**abdominocentesis** (ab DOM ih noh sehn TEE siss)	a surgical puncture through the abdominal wall to remove fluid; also called paracentesis (pair ah sehn TEE siss)
-centesis	s	surgical puncture		
abdomin/o	r/cv	abdomen	**abdominoperineal resection** (ab DOM ih noh PAIR ih NEE al)	surgical removal of the colon and rectum that includes entry through both the abdomen and perineum (the area in front of the anus); it includes a colostomy, and is performed to treat colorectal cancer and severe IBD; abbreviated **A&P resection**
perine	r	area of evacuation		
-al	s	pertaining to		
re-	p	back		
sect	r	to cut		
-ion	s	pertaining to		
abdomin/o	r/cv	abdomen	**abdominoplasty** (ab DOM ih noh plass tee)	surgical repair of the abdomen
-plasty	s	surgical repair		
an/o	r/cv	anus	**anoplasty** (AY noh plass tee)	surgical repair of the anus (Figure 13.22 ▦)
plasty	s	surgical repair		
ant-	p	against	**antacid** (ant ASS ihd)	a drug that neutralizes stomach acid
acid	r	sour		
anti-	p	against	**antiemetic** (an tye ee MEH tik)	a drug that prevents or stops vomiting
-emetic	s	vomiting		

Thrombosed External Hemorrhoid

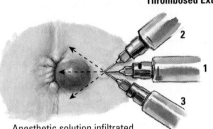

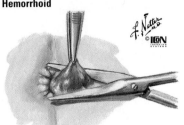

Anesthetic solution infiltrated subcutaneously over thrombotic hemorrhoid (1) and slightly deeper around it (2 and 3)

Skin over hemorrhoid drawn up by forceps and elliptical segment of skin excised

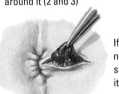

If thrombus does not pop out spontaneously, it is extracted

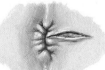

Elliptical incision partially falls together, ready for cotton dressing

Figure 13.22 ::::

Anoplasty.
The surgical repair of a hemorrhoid is illustrated.
Source: Icon Learning Systems.

Part	Type	Meaning	Term	Definition
anti- spasm	p r	against involuntary muscle contraction	**antispasmodic** (an tye spaz MAH dik)	a drug that decreases peristalsis in the GI tract to arrest spasm or diarrhea
-odic	s	pertaining to		
append	r	to hang onto, appendix	**appendectomy** (app ehn DEK toh mee)	surgical removal, or excision, of the appendix
-ectomy	s	surgical removal		
			barium enema (BAH ree um EHN eh mah)	an enema containing barium (a contrast medium used for x-ray) administered for a **lower GI series** diagnostic test; abbreviated **BE** (Figure 13.23::::)

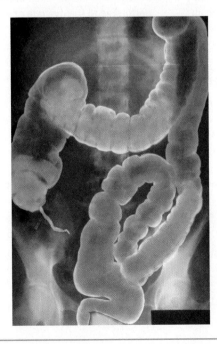

Figure 13.23 ::::

Barium enema.
Enhanced color x-ray of the large and small intestines during a barium enema exam.
Source: CNRI/Science Photo Library/Photo Researchers, Inc.

Part	Type	Meaning	TERM	DEFINITION
			cathartic (kah THAHR tik)	drug that stimulates peristalsis of the colon; also called a **laxative**
celi/o	r/cv	abdomen, abdominal cavity	**celiotomy** (see lee OTT oh mee)	incision into the abdominal cavity
-tomy	s	incision		
cheil/o	r/cv	lip	**cheilorrhaphy** (kye LOR ah fee)	suture of the lip
-rraphy	s	suture		
chol	r	bile, gall	**cholangiogram** (koh LAHN jee oh gram)	x-ray image of the bile ducts between the liver, gallbladder, and duodenum
angi/o	r/cv	blood vessel		
-gram	s	recording		
chol/e	r/cv	bile, gall	**cholecystectomy** (KOH lee siss TEK toh mee)	excision of the gallbladder
cyst	r	bladder		
-ectomy	s	surgical removal		

[FYI]

Cholecystectomy

Due to the prevalence of cholecystitis, cholecystectomy is the most common surgery of the abdomen performed in the United States, numbering about 500,000 each year. To reduce the invasiveness of the procedure, laparoscopic surgery is increasing in popularity, replacing the more traditional laparotomy.

Part	Type	Meaning	TERM	DEFINITION
chol/e	r/cv	bile, gall	**cholecystogram** (KOH lee SISS toh gram)	x-ray image of the gallbladder, which is used to confirm diagnosis of cholelithiasis
cyst/o	r/cv	bladder		
-gram	s	recording		
choledoch/o	r/cv	common bile duct	**choledocholithotomy** (koh LEH doh koh lih THOTT oh mee)	incision into the common bile duct, which is performed to remove one or more obstructive stones
lith/o	r/cv	stone		
-tomy	s	incision		
col	r	colon	**colectomy** (koh LEK toh mee)	excision of the colon
-ectomy	s	surgical removal		
colon/o	r/cv	colon	**colonoscopy** (koh lunn OSS koh pee)	visual examination of the colon, using a colonoscope (Figure 13.24▒▒▒▒)
-scopy	s	viewing process		
col/o	r/cv	colon	**colostomy** (koh LOSS toh mee)	surgical creation of an opening into the colon by way of the abdominal wall, which establishes an artificial anus, and may be temporary or permanent as a treatment for cancer, obstructions, or ulcerative colitis (Figure 13.25▒▒▒▒)
-stomy	s	surgical creation of an opening		
diverticul	r	a small blind pouch	**diverticulectomy** (DYE ver tik yoo LEK toh mee)	excision of a diverticulum
-ectomy	s	surgical removal		

WORD PARTS (WHEN APPLICABLE)			TERM	DEFINITION
Part	Type	Meaning		

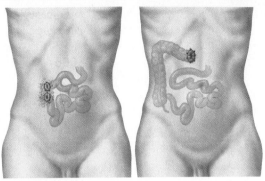

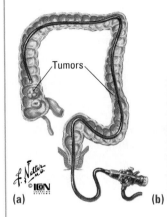

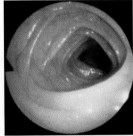

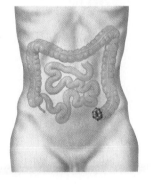

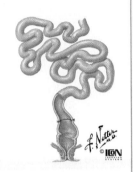

Figure 13.24 ::::

Colonoscopy.

(a) Colonoscopy involves the insertion of a flexible tube into the colon, primarily to detect colon cancers and diverticulitis. In a sigmoidoscopy, the instrument is inserted only as far as the sigmoid colon. *Source: Icon Learning Systems.*
(b) Colonoscope photograph of the transverse colon. *Source: CNRI/Science Photo Library/Photo Researchers, Inc.*

Figure 13.25 ::::

Colostomy.
Alternate versions of colostomy, each of which creates one or more new openings that serve as an artificial anus. *Source: Icon Learning Systems.*

Part	Type	Meaning	TERM	DEFINITION
endo-	p	within	**endoscopic retrograde cholangiopancreatography** (ehn doh SKOPP ik RET roh grayd koh LAHN jee oh pan kree ah TOG rah fee)	endoscopic procedure that includes x-ray fluoroscopy to visualize the ducts of the liver, gallbladder, and pancreas; abbreviated **ERCP**
-scop[e]	s	viewing instrument		
-ic	s	pertaining to		
retro-	p	back		
grade	r	to go		
chol	r	bile, gall		
angi/o	r/cv	blood vessel		
pancreat/o	r/cv	sweetbread, pancreas		
-graphy	s	recording process		
endo-	p	within	**endoscopic ultrasound** (ehn doh SKOPP ik ULL trah sound)	a diagnostic procedure that combines the use of an endoscope and an ultrasound probe to generate images of the intestinal wall to evaluate tumor progression; abbreviated **EUS**
-scop[e]	s	viewing instrument		
-ic	s	pertaining to		

WORD PARTS (WHEN APPLICABLE)			TERM	DEFINITION
Part	**Type**	**Meaning**		
esophag/o	r/cv	gullet, esophagus	**esophagogastro-duodenoscopy** (eh SOFF ah goh GAS troh DOO oh dehn OSS koh pee)	visual examination of the esophagus, stomach, and duodenum with an endoscope; abbreviated **EGD**
gastr/o	r/cv	stomach		
duoden/o	r/cv	twelve, duodenum		
-scopy	s	viewing process		
esophag/o	r/cv	gullet, esophagus	**esophagoscopy** (eh SOFF ah GOSS koh pee)	visual examination of the esophagus with an esophagoscope (eh SOFF ah goh skope), a specialized form of endoscope
-scopy	s	viewing process		
			fecal occult blood test (FEE kal uh CULT)	a lab test performed to detect blood in the feces
gastr	r	stomach	**gastrectomy** (gas TREK toh mee)	surgical removal of any part of the stomach, or in extreme cases, the entire organ
-ectomy	s	surgical removal		
gastr	r	stomach	**gastric lavage** (GAS trik lah VAHZH)	a cleansing procedure in which the stomach is rinsed with a saline solution
-ic	s	pertaining to		
gastr/o	r/cv	stomach	**gastroscopy** (gas TROSS koh pee)	visual examination of the stomach with a gastroscope (GAS troh skope), a specialized type of endoscope (Figure 13.26 ⦂⦂⦂)
-scopy	s	viewing process		

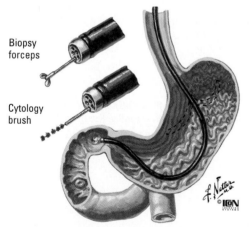

Biopsy forceps

Cytology brush

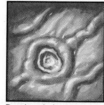

Duodenal ulcers

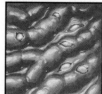

Gastritis with erosions

Figure 13.26 ⦂⦂⦂

Gastroscopy.
The flexible endoscope provides many diagnostic advantages over surgery.
Source: Icon Learning Systems.

WORD PARTS			TERM	DEFINITION
gastr/o	r/cv	stomach	**gastrostomy** (gas TROSS toh mee)	surgical creation of a new opening into the stomach
-stomy	s	surgical creation of an opening		
			gavage (gah VAHZH)	the process of feeding a patient through a tube inserted into the nose that drops into the stomach, called a nasogastric tube

WORD PARTS (WHEN APPLICABLE)			TERM	DEFINITION
Part	**Type**	**Meaning**		
endo -scopy	p s	within viewing process	**GI endoscopy** (ehn DOSS koh pee)	visual examination of the GI tract using an endoscope, which includes a camera, fiber optics, and long flexible tube; endoscopic procedures used in GI tract diagnostics (each using slight variations of endoscopes) include colonoscopy, esophago-gastroduodenoscopy, esophagoscopy, gastroscopy, laparoscopy, proctoscopy, and sigmoidoscopy (Figure 13.26)
gingiv -ectomy	r s	gums surgical removal	**gingivectomy** (JIN jih VEK toh mee)	surgical removal of diseased tissue in the gums
gloss/o -rrhaphy	r/cv s	tongue suture	**glossorrhaphy** (gloss OR ah fee)	suture of the tongue
hemi- col -ectomy	p r s	one-half colon surgical removal	**hemicolectomy** (HEM ee koh LEK toh mee)	excision of approximately one-half of the colon
hemorrh -oid -ectomy	r s s	likely to bleed condition surgical removal	**hemorrhoidectomy** (HEM oh royd EK toh mee)	excision of hemorrhoids (Figure 13.22)
herni/o -rrhaphy	r/cv s	a rupture surgical repair	**herniorrhaphy** (HER nee OR ah fee)	surgical repair of a hernia
ile/o -stomy	r/cv s	to roll, ileum surgical creation of an opening	**ileostomy** (ILL ee OSS toh mee)	surgical opening through the abdominal wall and into the ileum, to establish a secondary anus for the passage of feces (Figure 13.27⋮⋮)

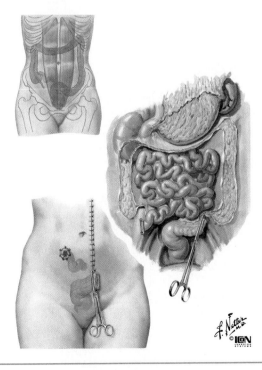

Figure 13.27 ⋮⋮

Ileostomy.

An ileostomy provides a bypass of the large intestine, establishing the opening of the ileum as the artificial anus. In this example, the cecum and colon have been completely removed in surgery.
Source: Icon Learning Systems.

WORD PARTS (WHEN APPLICABLE)			TERM	DEFINITION
Part	Type	Meaning		
lapar/o	r/cv	abdomen, abdominal cavity	**laparoscopy** (lap ahr OSS koh pee)	visual examination of the abdominal cavity with a laparoscope (LAP ah roh skope), which often replaces open abdominal surgery (**laparotomy**) when an invasive procedure should be avoided (Figure 13.28)
-scopy	s	viewing process		

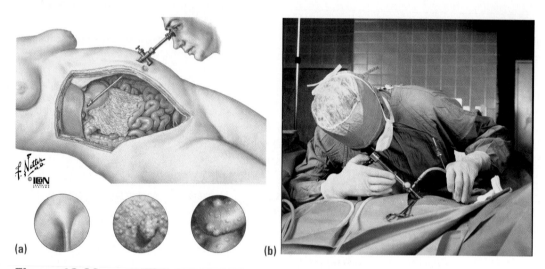

(a) (b)

Figure 13.28

Laparoscopy.
(a) Laparoscopy involves the insertion of a laparoscope through the abdominal wall by way of a small incision. The three circled images are views through the laparoscope. *Source: Icon Learning Systems.*
(b) Photograph of the laparoscopic procedure. *Source: Southern Illinois University/Photo Researchers, Inc.*

lapar/o	r/cv	abdomen, abdominal cavity	**laparotomy** (lap ah ROTT oh mee)	incision into the abdomen
-tomy	s	incision		
palat/o	r/cv	roof of mouth, palate	**palatoplasty** (PAHL ah toh PLASS tee)	surgical repair of the palate, usually as a treatment for cleft palate, an inherited defect
-plasty	s	surgical repair		
polyp	r	a small growth	**polypectomy** (pall ih PEK toh mee)	excision of a polyp
-ectomy	s	surgical removal		
proct/o	r/cv	anus	**proctoscopy** (prok TOSS koh pee)	visual examination of the rectum with a proctoscope (PROK toh skope), a specialized type of endoscope
-scopy	s	viewing process		
pylor/o	r/cv	gatekeeper, pylorus	**pyloroplasty** (pye LOR oh plass tee)	surgical repair of the pylorus region of the stomach or the pyloric valve
-plasty	s	surgical repair		

WORD PARTS (WHEN APPLICABLE)			TERM	DEFINITION
Part	**Type**	**Meaning**		
sigmoid/o -scopy	r/cv s	S-shape, sigmoid colon viewing process	**sigmoidoscopy** (sig moyd OSS koh pee)	visual examination of the sigmoid colon with a sigmoidoscope (sig MOYD oh skope), a specialized type of endoscope
			stool culture and sensitivity	collection of a fecal (stool) sample and growth of microorganisms from it in a culture to identify a pathogenic cause of disease
			upper GI series	diagnostic x-ray images of the stomach and duodenum following the administration of barium as a radiopaque contrast medium; abbreviated **UGI** (Figure 13.29▫▫▫▫)

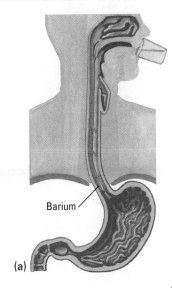
Barium

(a)

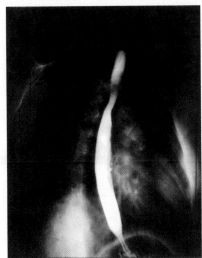

(b) Barium contrast study shows normal esophagus at esophagogastic junction

(c) Deformed duodenal bulb

Figure 13.29 ▫▫▫▫

Upper GI.
(a) In this procedure, a liquid shake with barium is swallowed, which produces a contrast in an x-ray photograph that highlights interior structures.
(b) Upper GI of the esophagus.
(c) Upper GI of the stomach.
Source: Icon Learning System.

uvul -ectomy	r s	a grape, uvula surgical removal	**uvulectomy** (YOO vyoo LEK toh mee)	excision of the uvula
uvul/o palat/o pharyng/o -plasty	r/cv r/cv r/cv s	a grape, uvula roof of mouth, palate throat, pharynx surgical repair	**uvulopalatopharyn- goplasty** (YOO vyoo loh PAHL ah toh FAIR in GOH plass tee)	surgical repair of uvula, palate, and pharynx, which is usually performed to correct obstructive sleep apnea; abbreviated **UPPP**
vag/o -tomy	r/cv s	vagus nerve incision	**vagotomy** (vah GOTT oh mee)	surgical dissection of branches of the vagus nerve, which innervates much of the GI tract; it is performed to reduce gastric juice secretion to treat chronic gastric ulcers

SELF QUIZ 13.5

SAY IT—SPELL IT!

Review the terms of the digestive system by speaking the phonetic pronunciation out loud, then writing the correct spelling of the term.

1. ab DOM ih noh PAIR ih NEE al _____

2. ab DOM ih noh plass tee _____

3. ab DOM ih noh sehn TEE siss _____

4. AY noh plass tee _____

5. an tye ee MEH tik _____

6. an tye spaz MAH dik _____

7. eh SOFF ah goh GAS troh
   DOO oh dehn OSS koh pee _____

8. HEM oh royd EK toh mee _____

9. HER nee OR ah fee _____

10. JIN jih VEK toh mee _____

11. kye LOR ah fee _____

12. koh LAHN jee oh
    pan kree ah TOG rah fee _____

13. koh LEH doh koh lih THOTT oh mee _____

14. KOH lee siss TEK toh mee _____

15. koh lunn OSS koh pee _____

16. koh LOSS toh mee _____

17. lap ahr OSS koh pee _____

13.16 18. lap ah ROTT oh mee _____

19. pall ih PEK toh mee _____

20. prok TOSS koh pee _____

21. see lee OTT oh mee _____

22. sig moyd OSS koh pee _____

23. vah GOTT oh mee _____

24. YOO vyoo loh PAHL ah toh
    FAIR in GOH plass tee _____

MATCH IT!

Match the term on the left with the correct definition on the right.

_____ 1. cheilorrhaphy

_____ 2. esophagogastroduo-
       denoscopy

_____ 3. antacid

_____ 4. abdominoperineal
       resection

_____ 5. choledocholithotomy

_____ 6. antispasmodic

_____ 7. celiotomy

_____ 8. antiemetic

_____ 9. cholangiogram

_____ 10. abdominoplasty

_____ 11. herniorrhaphy

_____ 12. cholecystectomy

_____ 13. endoscopic retrograde
       cholangiopancreatography

_____ 14. colonoscopy

_____ 15. sigmoidoscopy

_____ 16. colectomy

_____ 17. abdominocentesis

_____ 18. endoscopic ultrasound

_____ 19. hemorrhoidectomy

_____ 20. appendectomy

a. endoscopy of the colon

b. x-ray image of the bile ducts

c. incision into the common bile duct

d. endoscopy of the sigmoid colon

e. surgical repair of a hernia

f. suture of the lip

g. surgical repair of the abdomen

h. evaluation using an endoscope and ultrasound

i. a drug that neutralizes stomach acid

j. excision of a diseased appendix

k. surgical removal of hemorrhoids

l. endoscopy of three GI tract organs

m. excision of the colon

n. A&P resection

o. a procedure combining endoscopy and fluroscopy

p. a drug that decreases peristalsis

q. incision into the abdominal cavity

r. excision of the gallbladder

s. drug that prevents or stops vomiting

t. also known as paracentesis

BREAK IT DOWN!

Analyze and separate each term into its word parts, by labeling each word part using p = prefix, r = root, cv = combining vowel, and s = suffix.

1. abdominocentesis   _____

2. anoplasty   _____

3. antiemetic   _____

4. appendectomy   _____

13.17 5. cheilorrhaphy   _____

6. cholangiogram   _____

7. choledocholithotomy   _____

8. cholangiopancreatography   _____

9. colonoscopy   _____

10. esophagogastroduodenoscopy _____

11. glossorrhaphy   _____

12. laparoscopy   _____

13. sigmoidoscopy   _____

14. hemorrhoidectomy   _____

15. herniorrhaphy   _____

WORD BUILDING

Construct or recall medical terms from the following meanings.

13.18 1. a drug that evacuates the large
          intestine   _____

2. a lab test that evaluates a stool
    sample for blood   _____

3. use of x-rays and a barium shake to
    visualize the stomach and duodenum   _____

4. cleansing procedure of the stomach
    contents   _____

5. evaluation of a stool sample for
    pathogenic bacteria   _____

6. process of feeding a patient through
    a nasogastric tube   _____

7. x-rays of the large intestine using a
    barium contrast   _____

FILL IT IN!

Fill in the blanks with the correct terms.

1. The diagnostic procedure in which barium is administered, known as a barium

    _____, to evacuate the bowel prior to x-rays. It is also called a

    _____ _____ series. When the barium is

    administered by ingestion to visualize the stomach and duodenum, the procedure

    is called an _____ _____ series.

2. A drug that is administered to increase peristalsis of the large intestine, often as a treatment for constipation, is called a _____, or laxative.

3. When a patient requires feeding through a tube, a _____ tube is usually used in the procedure called a _____.

4. A cleansing procedure of the stomach is a _____ _____.

5. A lab test that is performed to determine if blood is present in the stool, which is symptomatic of diverticulosis and colorectal cancer, is called a _____ _____ blood test.

13.19 6. If a pathogenic disease is suspected, a _____ _____ and sensitivity test may be performed to identify the bacterial populations.

abbreviations of the digestive system

The abbreviations that are associated with the digestive system are summarized here. Study these abbreviations, and review them in the exercise that follows.

ABBREVIATION	DEFINITION	ABBREVIATION	DEFINITION
A&P resection	abdominoperineal resection	GI	gastrointestinal
BE	barium enema	IBD	inflammatory bowel disease
EGD	esophagogastroduodenoscopy	IBS	irritable bowel syndrome
ERCP	endoscopic retrograde cholangiopancreatography	N&V	nausea and vomiting
		UGI	upper GI series
EUS	endoscopic ultrasound	UPPP	uvulopalatopharyngoplasty
GERD	gastroesophageal reflux disease		

SELF QUIZ 13.6

Fill in the blanks with the abbreviation or the complete medical term.

Abbreviation   **Medical Term**

1. _____   esophagogastroduodenoscopy
2. BE   _____
3. _____   inflammatory bowel disease
4. UGI   _____
5. _____   uvulopalatopharyngoplasty
6. N&V   _____
7. _____   endoscopic retrograde cholangiopancreatography
8. IBS   _____

13.20 9. _____   endoscopic ultrasound
10. A&P resection   _____
11. _____   gastroesophageal reflux disease

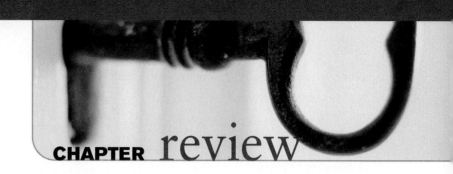

CHAPTER review

In this section, we will review all the word parts and medical terms from this chapter. As in earlier tables, the word roots are shown in **bold.**

Check each word part and medical term to be sure you understand the meaning. If any are not clear, please go back into the chapter and review that term. Then, complete the review exercises that follow.

[word parts **checklist**]

Prefixes

- ❑ a-, an-
- ❑ ad-
- ❑ dys-
- ❑ pan-
- ❑ peri-
- ❑ re-, retro-

Word Roots/Combining Vowels

- ❑ **abdomin**/o
- ❑ **an**/o
- ❑ **append**/o
- ❑ **bil**/i
- ❑ **cec**/o
- ❑ **celi**/o
- ❑ **cheil**/o
- ❑ **chol**/e
- ❑ **choledoch**/o
- ❑ **cirrh**/o

- ❑ **col**/o, **colon**/o
- ❑ **dent**/i
- ❑ **diverticul**/o
- ❑ **duoden**/o
- ❑ **enter**/o
- ❑ **esophag**/o
- ❑ **gastr**/o
- ❑ **gingiv**/o
- ❑ **gloss**/o
- ❑ **halat**/o
- ❑ **hepat**/o
- ❑ **hern**/o, **herni**/o
- ❑ **ile**/o
- ❑ **jejnun**/o
- ❑ **lapar**/o
- ❑ **lingu**/o
- ❑ **lith**/o
- ❑ **or**/o,
- ❑ **palat**/o

- ❑ **pancreat**/o
- ❑ **peps**/o, **pept**/o
- ❑ **periton**/o
- ❑ **phag**/o
- ❑ **polyp**/o
- ❑ **proct**/o
- ❑ **rect**/o
- ❑ **sial**/o
- ❑ **sigm**/o
- ❑ **steat**/o
- ❑ **stomat**/o
- ❑ **uvul**/o

Suffixes

- ❑ -centesis
- ❑ -emesis, -emetic
- ❑ -iasis
- ❑ -pepsia
- ❑ -rrhaphy

[medical terminology **checklist**]

- ❑ **abdomin**ocentesis
- ❑ **abdomin**operineal resection (A&P resection)
- ❑ **abdomin**oplasty
- ❑ acites
- ❑ adhesion
- ❑ **an**oplasty
- ❑ an**orex**ia nervosa
- ❑ ant**acid**
- ❑ antiemetic
- ❑ antispasmodic
- ❑ **an**us
- ❑ a**phag**ia
- ❑ **append**ectomy

- ❑ **append**icitis
- ❑ **append**ix
- ❑ barium enema (BE)
- ❑ bile
- ❑ body (of stomach)
- ❑ bulimia
- ❑ cardia
- ❑ cathartic
- ❑ **cec**um
- ❑ **celi**otomy
- ❑ **cheil**itis
- ❑ **cheil**orrhaphy
- ❑ **chol**angiogram
- ❑ **chol**angioma

- ❑ **cholecyst**ectomy
- ❑ **cholecyst**itis
- ❑ **cholecyst**ogram
- ❑ **choledoch**olithiasis
- ❑ **choledoch**olithotomy
- ❑ **cirrh**osis
- ❑ **col**ectomy
- ❑ **col**itis
- ❑ **colon**
- ❑ **colon**oscopy
- ❑ **colorect**al cancer
- ❑ constipation
- ❑ Crohn's disease
- ❑ diarrhea

- ❑ **diverticul**itis
- ❑ **diverticul**osis
- ❑ **duoden**al ulcer
- ❑ **duoden**um
- ❑ dys**entery**
- ❑ dys**peps**ia
- ❑ dys**phag**ia
- ❑ endoscopic retrograde **cholangiopancreat**ography (ERCP)
- ❑ endoscopic ultrasound (EUS)
- ❑ **enter**itis
- ❑ **esophag**itis
- ❑ **esophagogastroduoden**o scopy (EGD)
- ❑ **esophag**oscopy
- ❑ **esophag**us
- ❑ fecal occult blood test
- ❑ feces
- ❑ flatus
- ❑ fundus
- ❑ gallbladder
- ❑ **gastr**ectomy
- ❑ **gastr**ic cancer
- ❑ **gastr**ic juice
- ❑ **gastr**ic lavage
- ❑ **gastr**ic ulcer
- ❑ **gastr**itis
- ❑ **gastr**odynia
- ❑ **gastroenter**itis
- ❑ **gastroenter**ocolitis
- ❑ **gastr**ointestinal (GI)
- ❑ **gastr**omalacia
- ❑ **gastr**oscopy
- ❑ **gastroesophag**eal reflux disease (GERD)
- ❑ gavage
- ❑ giardiasis

- ❑ **gingiv**ectomy
- ❑ **gingiv**itis
- ❑ **gloss**itis
- ❑ **gloss**opathy
- ❑ **gloss**orrhaphy
- ❑ **halat**osis
- ❑ hard palate
- ❑ **hemat**emesis
- ❑ **hemicol**ectomy
- ❑ **hemorrh**oids
- ❑ **hepat**itis
- ❑ **hepat**omegaly
- ❑ **herni**orrhaphy
- ❑ hiatal **hernia**
- ❑ hyper**bilirub**inemia
- ❑ **ile**itis
- ❑ **ile**ostomy
- ❑ **ile**um
- ❑ **ile**us
- ❑ inflammatory bowel disease (IBD)
- ❑ intussesception
- ❑ irritable bowel syndrome (IBS)
- ❑ jaundice
- ❑ **jejun**um
- ❑ lactose intolerance
- ❑ **lapar**oscopy
- ❑ **lapar**otomy
- ❑ large **intestine**
- ❑ liver
- ❑ lower **esophag**eal sphincter
- ❑ nausea
- ❑ **or**al cavity
- ❑ **palat**e
- ❑ **palat**itis
- ❑ **palat**oplasty
- ❑ **pancrea**s
- ❑ **pancreat**ic juice

- ❑ **pancreat**itis
- ❑ **pept**ic ulcer
- ❑ **periton**eum
- ❑ **periton**itis
- ❑ **pharynx**
- ❑ **polyp**
- ❑ **polyp**ectomy
- ❑ **polyp**osis
- ❑ **proct**itis
- ❑ **proct**optosis
- ❑ **proct**oscopy
- ❑ **pylor**ic valve
- ❑ **pylor**oplasty
- ❑ **pylor**us
- ❑ **rect**ocele
- ❑ **rect**um
- ❑ salivary glands
- ❑ **sial**oadenitis
- ❑ **sial**olith
- ❑ **sigm**oidoscopy
- ❑ small **intestine**
- ❑ soft **palate**
- ❑ **steat**orrhea
- ❑ stomach
- ❑ **stomat**itis
- ❑ stool culture and sensitivity
- ❑ tongue
- ❑ upper GI series (UGI)
- ❑ **uvulopalatopharyng**oplasty (UPPP)
- ❑ **uvul**a
- ❑ **uvul**ectomy
- ❑ **uvul**itis
- ❑ **vag**otomy
- ❑ volvulus
- ❑ vomit

[show what **you know!**]

BREAK IT DOWN!

Analyze and separate each term into its word parts by labeling each word part using p = prefix, r = root, cv = combining vowel, and s = suffix.

				p r s
Example:	1.	aphagia		a/phag/ia
	2.	dyspepsia		_____
	3.	hyperbilirubinemia		_____
	4.	appendicitis		_____
	5.	choledocholithiasis		_____

6. colitis   _____

7. diverticulosis   _____

8. enteritis   _____

9. gastromalacia   _____

10. glossopathy   _____

11. hepatoma   _____

12. peritonitis   _____

13. bronchiectasis   _____

14. polyposis   _____

15. abdominocentesis   _____

16. anoplasty   _____

17. antiemetic   _____

18. cheilorrhaphy   _____

19. cholecystogram   _____

20. laryngotracheotomy   _____

21. gastrectomy   _____

22. esophagogastroduodenoscopy   _____

23. gingivectomy   _____

24. hemorrhoidectomy   _____

25. uvulopalatopharyngoplasty   _____

26. dyspepsia   _____

27. hepatomegaly   _____

WORD BUILDING

Construct or recall medical terms from the following meanings.

Example: 1. indigestion   _____dyspepsia_____

2. enlargement of the liver   _____

3. difficulty swallowing   _____

4. inflammation of the lip   _____

5. tumor originating from the bile duct   _____

6. inflammation of the gallbladder   _____

7. condition of gallstones   _____

8. inflammation of the colon   _____

9. cancer of the colon and rectum   _____

10. inflammation of the small intestine   _____

11. softening of the stomach wall   _____

12. inflammation of the ileum   _____

13. tumor of the liver   _____

14. inflammation of a salivary gland _____

15. inflammation of the mouth _____

16. surgical repair of the abdomen _____

17. excision of the appendix _____

18. x-ray image of the bile ducts _____

19. surgical creation of an opening into the colon _____

20. surgical removal of part of the stomach _____

21. endoscopic evaluation of the rectum _____

22. endoscopic evaluation of the abdominal cavity _____

23. suture of the tongue _____

24. excision of a polyp _____

25. repair of the uvula, palate, and pharynx _____

CASE STUDIES

Fill in the blanks with the correct terms.

1. A 60-year-old female was checked in to the emergency clinic with a two-week history of N&V, or (a) _____

   and vomiting, which also included frequent watery stools, or (b) _____, trapped gas, or

   (c) _____, and abdominal pain. A review of her medical history revealed erosion of the stomach wall,

   or peptic (d) _____ disease, about 25 years ago, but symptoms lessened after treatment with acid-

   reducing agents, or (e) _____, and a change in diet. She had no history of gallstones, or

   (f) _____. GI endoscopy was performed to evaluate the rectum first, called a

   (g) _____, followed with visualization of the sigmoid colon in a (h) _____,

   then the stomach in a (i) _____. In addition, barium was administered prior to x-rays in a barium

   (j) _____ procedure to visualize the large intestine. This was repeated to visualize the stomach and

   duodenum in an (k) _____ _____ series. Following the endoscopy procedures, a

   biopsy was taken from the stomach and the tissue cultured for bacteria. In addition, a collection of fecal material was

   cultured using a (l) _____ _____ and sensitivity test. The BE and stool culture

   tests were negative for lower GI disease, but the UGI was positive for ulceration of the stomach wall, and thereby diagnosed

   as a (m) _____ _____. Ulceration was almost complete, justifying the need for

   a partial (n) _____, in which a section of the stomach is excised. Also, the stomach biopsy was

   positive for the primary causative organism of peptic ulcers, (o) _____ _____.

   Immediately following surgery, the patient was treated with antibiotic therapy to eliminate further tissue damage.

2. A 10-year-old male was admitted following a history of four weeks of intermittent watery stools, or

   (p) _____, accompanied with trapped gas, or (q) _____, occasional reduced

   peristalsis of the large intestine, or (r) _____, abdominal pain, and vomiting. Initial diagnosis by his

   personal GP was the lack of the digestive enzyme lactase, known as (s) _____

_____, although IBS, or (t) _____ _____

_____, was ruled as another possibility. With time, symptoms of pain and irregularity increased,

raising the concern that the child might be suffering from a chronic inflammation of the ileum, or

(u) _____ _____, a type of IBD, or (v) _____

_____ disease. Once admitted, thorough testing including a lactase enzyme test, BE (also known as

(w) _____ _____), a UGI series, and an endoscopy into the abdomen, called a

(x) _____ ensued. The BE revealed the presence of inflamed diverticula, leading to the diagnosis of

(y) _____. The laparoscopy indicated an infolding of a segment of the small intestine into another

segment, a condition known as (z) _____, which had led to intestinal obstruction, or

(aa) _____. Due to the severe damage of the ileum, its removal in the (bb)

_____ procedure was recommended.

[piece it all **together!**]

CROSSWORD

From the chapter material, fill in the crossword puzzle with answers to the following clues.

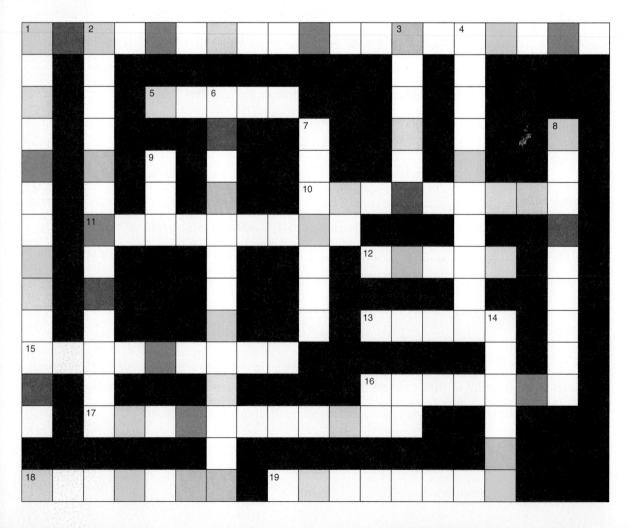

ACROSS

1. Inflammation of the stomach, small intestine, and colon. (Find puzzle piece 13.6)
5. An erosion, which is often associated with *H. pylori*. (Find puzzle piece 13.13)
10. A chronic, progressive liver disease. (Find puzzle piece 13.11)
11. Indigestion. (Find puzzle piece 13.3)
12. A synonym for feces. (Find puzzle piece 13.19)
13. A small growth from the wall of an organ. (Find puzzle piece 13.2)
15. A synonym for laxative. (Find puzzle piece 13.18)
16. A suffix that means surgical correction by suturing. (Find puzzle piece 13.17)
17. Abnormal levels of fat in the feces. (Find puzzle piece 13.4)
18. A chronic form is known as Crohn's disease. (Find puzzle piece 13.12)
19. Cancer originating from the liver. (Find puzzle piece 13.15)

DOWN

1. Softening of the stomach wall. (Find puzzle piece 13.7)
2. Also known as the mumps. (Find puzzle piece 13.9)
3. Arises from a mutation that develops into a tumor. (Find puzzle piece 13.14)
4. Incision into the abdomen. (Find puzzle piece 13.16)
6. Inflammation of the gallbladder. (Find puzzle piece 13.8)
7. Accumulation of fluid in the peritoneal cavity. (Find puzzle piece 13.10)
8. Intestinal infection resulting in severe diarrhea. (Find puzzle piece 13.5)
9. Endoscopic ultrasound. (Find puzzle piece 13.20)
14. A suffix that means digestion, referring to the enzyme pepsin. (Find puzzle piece 13.1)

WORD UNSCRAMBLE

From the completed crossword puzzle, unscramble:

1. All of the letters that appear in **red** squares __ __ __ ☐ __ __

   Clue: A word root that means *rupture* in Latin

2. All of the letters that appear in **purple** squares __ __ ☐ __ __ __ __ __

   Clue: A frequent release of watery stools

3. All of the letters that appear in **peach** squares __ __ __ ☐ __

   Clue: An obstruction of the intestine

4. All of the letters that appear in **blue** squares __ __ __ __ __ __ ☐

   Clue: Inflammation of the colon

5. All of the letters that appear in **yellow** squares __ __ ☐ __ __ __ __ __ __

   Clue: Inflammation of the lip

6. All of the letters that appear in **green** squares __ __ ☐ __ __ __ __ __ __ __

   Clue: Intestinal inflammation caused by a protozoan infection

Now write down each of the letters that are boxed to find the hidden medical term, which is a word derived from a nautical term: __ __ __ __ __ __.

MEDmedia wrap-up

www.prenhall.com/wingerd

Before you go on to the next chapter, take advantage of the free CD-ROM and study guide website that accompany this book. Simply load the CD-ROM for additional activities, games, animations, videos, and quizzes linked to this chapter. Then visit www.prenhall.com/wingerd for even more!

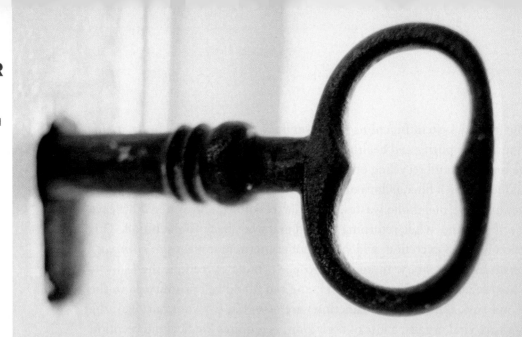

The Urinary System

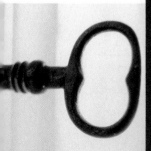

The urinary system functions as the sanitary engineer of the body, maintaining the purity and health of the body's fluids by removing unwanted waste materials and recycling other materials. Its most important organs are the kidneys, which filter gallons of fluids from the bloodstream every day. The kidneys remove metabolic wastes, toxins, excess ions, and water that leave the body as urine, while returning needed materials back to the blood. This function is called excretion, which is a modern term that means *to eliminate as waste from the body.* In addition to performing excretion, the kidneys also help regulate blood pressure, pH, and red blood cell production in the bone marrow. Because these functions are essential for your survival, the kidneys are vital organs; a loss of both kidneys requires medical intervention in order to sustain life.

word parts focus

Let's look at word parts. The following table contains a list of word parts that when combined build many of the terms of the urinary system.

PREFIX	DEFINITION	PREFIX	DEFINITION
a-, an-	without, absence of	epi-	on top of
dia-	passing through	hypo-	under
en-	within		

WORD ROOT	DEFINITION	WORD ROOT	DEFINITION
albumin	protein	noct	night
azot	urea, nitrogen	olig	few in number
blast	developing cell, germ cell, bud	py	pus
cyst	bladder, sac	pyel	renal pelvis
glomerul	little ball, glomerulus	ren	kidney
gluc, glyc, glycos	sweet, sugar	spadias	rip, tear
hydr	water	tom	cut, section
keton	ketone	ureter	ureter
lith	stone	urethr	urethra
meat	opening, passage	urin, ur	urine
nephr	kidney	vesic	bladder, sac

SUFFIX	DEFINITION	SUFFIX	DEFINITION
-cele	hernia, swelling, protrusion	-trophy	nourishment, development
-ptosis	falling downward (condition of)	-uresis	urination
-tripsy	surgical crushing	-uria	urine, urination

SELF QUIZ 14.1

Review the word parts of urinary system terminology by working carefully through the exercises that follow. Soon, we will apply this new information to build medical terms.

A. Provide the definition of the following prefixes and suffixes.

1. a-, an-   _____

2. epi-   _____

3. -tripsy   _____

4. -trophy   _____

5. -uria   _____

6. hypo-   _____

B. Provide the word root for each of the following terms.

1. urea or nitrogen   _____

2. protein   _____

3. developing cell   _____

4. bladder   _____

5. glomerulus   _____

6. sugar   _____

7. water   _____

8. stone   _____

9. opening   _____

10. kidney   _____

11. few in number   _____

14.1 12. renal pelvis _____

13. pus   _____

14. kidney   _____

15. urine   _____

16. urethra   _____

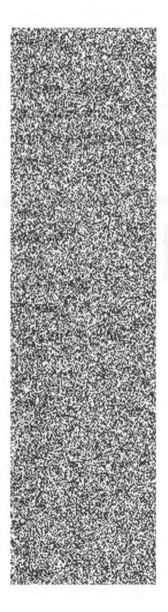

[anatomy and physiology overview]

Kidneys

The kidneys are a pair of soft organs located against the posterior abdominal wall, one to the right and one to the left of the body's midline (Figure 14.1::::). Each kidney is about the size of your clenched fist and in the shape of a kidney bean, with the concave margin facing the midline.

The concave margin is called the **hilum,** and is where the renal artery, renal vein, nerves, and **ureter** join the kidney (Figure 14.2::::). The structure of a kidney is unlike that of any other organ. Externally, it is covered with a protective layer of fat and a fibrous membrane. Internally, the kidney is divided into three regions: the **renal pelvis,** a membrane-lined basin that collects urine in the center, the **renal medulla,** which lies external to the pelvis, and the outermost **renal cortex.**

[FYI]

The Kidney

All of the three parts of the kidney are named for their structure or location. The term *pelvis* is the Latin word for washbasin. The renal pelvis is a bowl-shaped basin that collects newly formed urine. The term *medulla* is from the Latin word for *marrow,* and refers to any inner soft part. The renal medulla is the inner soft tissue of the kidney. The term *cortex* is from the Latin word for *tree bark* and refers to any outer covering; the renal cortex forms the outer margin of the kidney.

The renal medulla and renal cortex are composed of about one million subunits, known as **nephrons** (Figure 14.3::::). Each nephron is a tube that consists of a hollow ball at one end, called **Bowman's capsule (BC),** and a long twisting por-

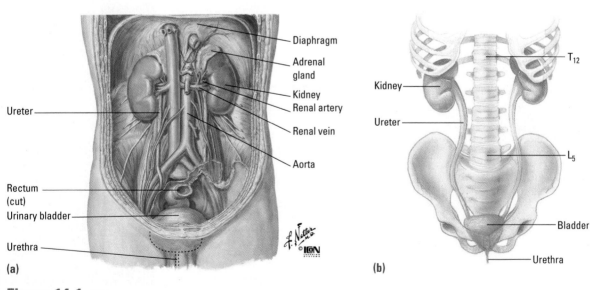

(a)

(b)

Figure 14.1 ::::

Organs of the urinary system.

(a) This illustration is an anterior view of a male with the abdominal wall and digestive organs removed. *Source: Icon Learning Systems.*

(b) Position of urinary organs. *Source: Pearson Education.*

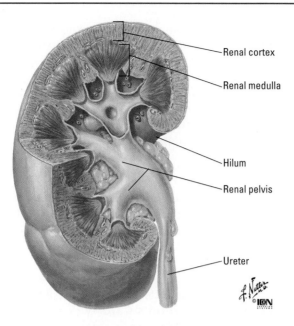

- Renal cortex
- Renal medulla
- Hilum
- Renal pelvis
- Ureter

Figure 14.2 ::::

The kidney.

Illustration of a sectioned kidney, which reveals its internal features. *Source: Icon Learning Systems.*

tion at the other, called the **renal tubule.** The BC contains a tightly coiled capillary, called the **glomerulus.** Together, the BC and thread-like glomerulus make up the **renal corpuscle.**

The kidneys participate in excretion by forming urine, which is done in a three-stage process within each of the nephrons. It begins with blood **filtration.** The filter is a very thin membrane between the wall of the glomerulus and the inner wall of the Bowman's capsule. As blood pressure pushes blood through the glomerulus, some of the blood's plasma is forced through tiny openings in the membrane, filling the Bowman's capsule with fluid. As the fluid flows through the adjoining renal

[FYI]

Glomerulus

The term *glomerulus* is derived from the Latin word *glomus,* which means *a ball of thread.*

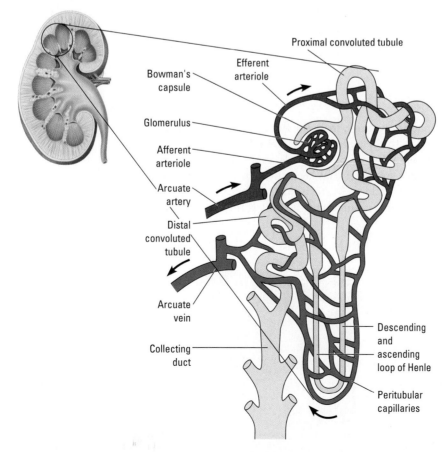

- Proximal convoluted tubule
- Efferent arteriole
- Bowman's capsule
- Glomerulus
- Afferent arteriole
- Arcuate artery
- Distal convoluted tubule
- Arcuate vein
- Collecting duct
- Descending and ascending loop of Henle
- Peritubular capillaries

Figure 14.3 ::::

The nephron.

The glomerulus is a twisted capillary within the hollow Bowman's capsule. The renal tubule includes a proximal convoluted tubule, descending and ascending loops of Henle, and a distal convoluted tubule.

enrichment module enrichment module **enrichment module** enrichment module **enrichment module** enrichment module **enrichment module**

tubule, most of the water is reabsorbed into the bloodstream, achieving the second stage of urine formation, commonly referred to as **reabsorption.** In the third and final stage, excess electrolytes (salts in an ionic form) and other wastes are transported into the renal tubule. This last stage is called **secretion.**

The result of all three stages is the formation of urine. Urine is mostly water, but also includes excess electrolytes and the metabolic waste materials, urea and ammonia. By forming urine, the kidneys help maintain the water and electrolyte balance in body fluids. They also regulate pH by removing excess hydrogen ions.

Ureters

After urine is formed, it drains into the renal pelvis and then enters the **ureter.** The paired ureters are spaghetti-sized, tubular organs that transport urine from the kidneys to the **urinary bladder** (Figure 14.4). After arising from the renal pelvis of each kidney, the ureters extend downward along each side of the vertebral column until they unite with the urinary bladder.

The wall of each ureter consists of an inner mucous membrane and an outer layer of smooth muscle. The mucous membrane protects the ureter from potentially damaging effects of urine. The smooth muscle provides waves of peristalsis that help propel the urine along its way to the next urinary organ, the urinary bladder.

Urinary Bladder

The urinary bladder is a hollow, muscular organ located at the floor of the pelvic cavity (Figure 14.4⁛) that temporarily stores urine. In many ways its features are like that of a latex balloon: Its walls are extremely elastic, so that when it is empty, it shrivels in shape and its inner wall contains many wrinkles. As it fills with urine, its walls become smoother, expanding dramatically into a pear-shaped dome that often presses against nearby organs. When full, its capacity averages about 500 ml (one pint), although it can hold more than twice that amount if necessary.

The interior of the urinary bladder has openings for the two ureters and the single **urethra.** The openings form a triangular region known as the **trigone,** which is a frequent site of urinary infections. The bladder is lined with an elastic mucous membrane, and its outer wall is composed of involuntary muscle that contracts during urination.

Urethra

The urethra is a muscular tube that drains urine from the floor of the urinary bladder and transports it out of the body to the exterior (Figure 14.4). At the junction between the bladder and the urethra is a thickening of muscle, called the **internal urethral sphincter.** This is an involuntary sphincter that keeps urine from entering the urethra while it is being stored in the bladder. As the urethra extends through the floor of the pelvic cavity, a second sphincter surrounds it. This is the **external ure-**

[**thinking critically!**]

Excessively high blood pressure can damage the filtration membranes in a kidney. If the membranes tear, what do you suppose would be a symptom that is noticeable in a urine sample?

[**FYI**]

Ureter
The term *ureter* is derived from the Greek word *oureter,* which means *urinary canal.*

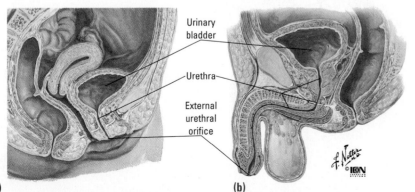

(a)   (b)

Urinary bladder

Urethra

External urethral orifice

Figure 14.4 ⁛

Urinary bladder and urethra.
Section through the pelvic region reveals the urinary bladder, urethra, and associated structures.
(a) Female.
(b) Male.
Source: Icon Learning Systems.

thral sphincter, which is composed of muscle that is under voluntary control. Like the ureters and the urinary bladder, the urethra is lined internally with a protective mucous membrane. The opening to the exterior is called the **external urethral orifice,** also called the **urinary meatus.** The release of urine to the exterior is called **micturition,** from the Latin word that means *a making of water.* It is also called **voiding.**

The urethra differs considerably between males and females. In females it is about 3-4 cm (1.5 inches) long and is tightly bound to the anterior wall of the vagina by connective tissue. The urinary meatus lies between the vaginal opening and the clitoris. In males the urethra is about 20 cm (8 inches) long and extends from the urinary bladder to the end of the penis, where it opens as the urinary meatus. Near its emergence from the bladder, the male urethra passes through the prostrate gland that surrounds it. Later in life, it is common for the prostate gland to enlarge, resulting in difficulty urinating. In addition to carrying urine, the male urethra also carries reproductive fluids.

> **[thinking critically!]**
>
> The external urethral sphincter takes about a year after birth to become functional. During the first year of an infant's life, what behavior characterizes this developmental requirement?

getting to the root of it | anatomy and physiology terms

Many of the anatomy and physiology terms are formed from roots that are used to construct the more complex medical terms of the urinary system, including symptoms, diseases, and treatments. In this section, we will review the terms that describe the structure and function of the urinary system *in relation to their word roots,* which are shown in **bold**.

Study the word roots and terms in this list and complete the review exercises that follow.

Word Root (Meaning)	Terms Formed from the Word Root (Pronunciation)	Definition
glomerul (little ball)	**glomerul**us (gloh MAIR yoo luss)	a coiled capillary tucked within the space of a Bowman's capsule through which blood passes, leaking fluids through openings in its wall during the process of filtration
meat (opening)	urinary **meat**us (YOO rih nair ee mee AY tuss)	the external opening of the urethra
nephr (kidney)	**nephr**on (NEFF rahn)	the subunits of each kidney, composed of a renal corpuscle (Bowman's capsule and glomerulus) and a renal tubule
ren (kidney)	**ren**al pelvis (REE nal PELL viss)	a membrane-enclosed basin that collects urine in the interior of a kidney
	renal cortex (REE nal KOR teks)	the outer portion of the interior of a kidney
	renal medulla (REE nal meh DULL lah)	the inner portion of the interior of a kidney
	renal corpuscle (REE nal KOR puss el)	composed of the Bowman's capsule and the glomerulus
	renal tubule (REE nal TOO byool)	the long, twisting part of a nephron
ureter (ureter)	**ureter**s (yoo REE terz)	paired, narrow tubes that conduct urine from each kidney to the posterior part of the urinary bladder

Word Root (Meaning)	Terms Formed from the Word Root (Pronunciation)	Definition
urethr (urethra)	**urethr**a (yoo REE thrah)	a tube that conveys urine from the urinary bladder to the exterior, through the external urethral orifice (urinary meatus)
	internal **urethr**al sphincter (IN ter nal yoo REE thral SFINK ter)	an involuntary muscle that keeps urine from entering the urethra while it is stored in the bladder
	external **urethr**al sphincter (EKS ter nal yoo REE thral SFINK ter)	a voluntary muscle that prevents or allows urine to be released
urin, ur (urine)	**urin**ary bladder (YOO rih nair ee BLAHD der)	a hollow, muscular organ located at the base of the pelvic cavity that serves as a temporary reservoir for urine
	urine (YOO rin)	a yellowish liquid waste, normally about 95 percent water and 5 percent electrolytes and nitrogenous waste, produced through filtration, reabsorption, and secretion in the kidneys

OTHER IMPORTANT TERMS

The terms in this table are related to the structure and function of the urinary system, but are not built from multiple word roots.

Bowman's capsule	named for its 18th century discoverer, Sir William Bowman, the Bowman's capsule is a hollow, ball-shaped structure located at one end of a nephron that includes an internal membrane, which filters fluid passing out of the glomerulus; abbreviated **BC**
hilum (HIGH lum)	the concave side of a kidney, which receives the renal artery, renal vein, nerves, and a ureter
kidneys (kid neez)	a pair of organs located against the posterior abdominal wall on each side of the vertebral column, which form urine through filtration of the blood and also help regulate blood pressure and maintain water and electrolyte balance
micturition (mik too RIH shun)	the release of urine; also called voiding

---

SELF QUIZ 14.2

Success Hint: Once you get to the crossword puzzle at the end of the chapter, remember to check back here for clues! Your clues are indicated by the puzzle icon.

SAY IT—SPELL IT!

Review the terms of the urinary system by speaking the phonetic pronunciation out loud, then writing the correct spelling of the term.

1. gloh MAIR yoo luss   _____

2. YOO rih nair ee   mee AY tuss   _____

3. NEFF rahn   _____

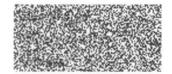

4. REE nal   KOR puss el   _____

5. yoo REE terz   _____

6. yoo REE thrah   _____

7. IN ter nal   yoo REE thral
   SFINK ter   _____

8. EKS ter nal   yoo REE thral
   SFINK ter   _____

9. YOO rin   _____

10. YOO rih nair ee   BLAHD der   _____

11. HIGH lum   _____

12. mik too RIH shun   _____

MATCH IT!

Match the term on the left with the correct definition on the right.

_____ 1. kidneys   a. nitrogenous waste material in urine

_____ 2. renal cortex   b. composed of a renal corpuscle and renal
                                         tubule

_____ 3. renal medulla   c. performs the function of excretion in three
                                         stages

_____ 4. renal pelvis   d. liquid waste formed within the kidneys

_____ 5. nephron   e. the long, twisting part of a nephron

_____ 6. Bowman's capsule   f. the exterior opening of the urethra

_____ 7. glomerulus   g. a membrane-lined basin in a kidney

_____ 8. urea   h. an involuntary muscle

_____ 9. renal tubule   i. a coiled capillary in a renal corpuscle

_____ 10. ureter   j. a hollow muscular organ that stores urine

_____ 11. urine   k. the outer part of a kidney

_____ 12. urethra   l. a hollow ball in a renal corpuscle

_____ 13. urinary bladder   m. a thin tube between a kidney and the bladder

_____ 14. internal urethral sphincter   n. considerably different between females and
                                         males

_____ 15. urinary meatus   o. the inner part of a kidney

FILL IT IN!

Fill in the blanks with the correct terms.

1. The pair of organs that perform the function of excretion are the

   _____. Each organ is internally divided into an outer area,

   called the _____ _____, an inner area known

   as the _____ _____, and a membrane-lined

   basin that collects newly formed urine, called the _____

   _____.

2. The cortex and medulla of each kidney contain approximately one million subunits known as _____. Each contains two main parts, a ball-shaped _____ _____ and a long, twisting renal tubule. The ball-shaped part is also composed of two portions, a hollow ball known as the _____ _____ and a coiled capillary called the _____. The process of filtration occurs within the renal corpuscle.

3. Once urine is formed, it drains into a narrow tube called the _____, which conducts urine to the hollow muscular organ at the base of the pelvic cavity, the _____ _____. During urination, urine flows through the next organ, the _____, to the exterior. This final tube differs in size between females and males. Its opening to the exterior is called the external _____ orifice or the _____ _____. Near its union with the bladder, it is encircled by two muscles that control the release of urine. Control of the inner muscle is involuntary but control of the outer muscle, called the _____ _____ _____, is voluntary.

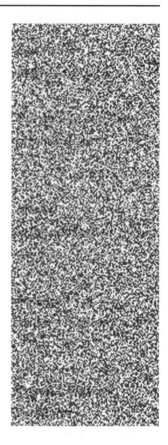

[medical terms of the]

urinary system

The urinary system is subject to infections, since it communicates to the exterior by way of the urinary meatus. Although the urethra, urinary bladder, and ureters are each protected by a mucous membrane, bacteria and viruses are sometimes able to gain entry into the tissue. Once established, they are capable of spreading through the urinary tract, bringing disease to the kidneys and beyond. Also, the close location of the urinary meatus to the anus in females enables some bacterial populations that normally form the intestinal flora to infect the urinary tract. In addition to infections, other sources of disease may afflict the urinary system, including tumors, inherited disorders, and cardiovascular disease.

Because urine originates from the bloodstream and the urinary system releases urine on a regular basis, urine testing provides a convenient means for testing general health. Many diseases can be diagnosed from a urine sample that contains abnormal contents, such as blood cells, bacteria, albumin (a protein normally found in blood), glucose, and high levels of **creatinine** (a protein product of metabolism).

The clinical treatment of urinary disease is a medical discipline known as **urology.** This is a constructed word that can be written as:

ur/o/logy

in which ur/o is a combining form derived from the Greek word for urine, *ouron*. The suffix -logy means *a study of.* In most hospitals and clinics, the ward specializing in the treatment of urinary disease is simply called *urology.* A physician specializing in this

[**thinking critically!**]

If you are experiencing pain during urination, what specialist may be the best choice to visit?

field of medicine is called a **urologist.** The field specializing in the treatment of kidney disease is known as **nephrology,** which can be written as:

nephr/o/logy

in which nephr/o is a combining form derived from the Greek word *nephros,* which means *kidney.* A physician specializing in this field is called a **nephrologist.**

let's construct terms!

In this section, we will assemble all of the word parts to construct medical terminology related to the urinary system. Abbreviations are used to indicate each word part: **p** = prefix, **r** = root, **cv** = combining vowel, and **s** = suffix. Recall from chapter one that the addition of a combining vowel to the word root creates the combining form for the term. Note that some terms are not constructed from word parts, but they are included here to expand your vocabulary.

The medical terms of the urinary system are listed in the following three sections:

- Symptoms and Signs
- Diseases and Disorders
- Treatments, Procedures, and Devices

Each section is followed by review exercises. Study the lists in these tables and complete the review exercises that follow.

Symptoms and Signs

WORD PARTS (WHEN APPLICABLE)			TERM	DEFINITION
Part	**Type**	**Meaning**		
albumin	r	protein	**albuminuria**	presence of albumin, a protein normally in the blood, in the urine
-uria	s	urine, urination	(AL byoo men YOO ree ah)	
an-	p	without	**anuresis**	inability to pass urine
-uresis	s	urination	(an yoo REE siss)	
an-	p	without	**anuria**	absence of urine
-uria	s	urine, urination	(an YOO ree ah)	
azot	r	urea, nitrogen	**azotemia**	abnormally high urea and other nitrogenous compounds in the blood
-emia	s	blood condition	(az oh TEE mee ah)	
bacter/i	r/cv	bacteria	**bacteriuria**	presence of bacteria in the urine
-uria	s	urine, urination	(bak ter ee YOO ree ah)	
di[a]-	p	passing through	**diuresis**	condition of urine passing (usually refers to excessive urine discharge)
-uresis	s	urine	(DYE yoo REE siss)	
dys-	p	bad, abnormal	**dysuria**	difficulty or pain in urination
-uria	s	urine, urination	(diss YOO ree ah)	
en-	p	within	**enuresis**	to void urine (refers to an involuntary release of urine, usually due to a lack of bladder control); nocturnal enuresis is also known as bed-wetting
-uresis	s	urination	(ehn yoo REE siss)	
glycos	r	sweet, sugar	**glycosuria**	presence of glucose (sugar) in the urine
-uria	s	urine, urination	(glye kohs YOO ree ah)	

WORD PARTS (WHEN APPLICABLE)			TERM	DEFINITION
Part	**Type**	**Meaning**		
hemat	r	blood	**hematuria**	presence of blood in the urine (Figure 14.5 ::::)
-uria	s	urine, urination	(HEE mah TOO ree ah)	

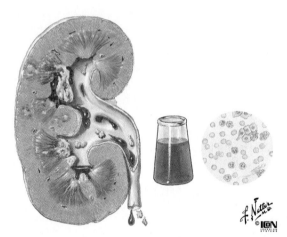

Figure 14.5 ::::

Hematuria and pyuria.
An analysis of urine is performed to evaluate kidney function. In this illustration, the beaker contains urine that is red, indicating the symptom of hematuria. It is confirmed in the microscopic specimen (in circle), which also shows the presence of white blood cells, indicating the symptom of pyuria.
Source: Icon Learning Systems.

keton	r	ketone	**ketonuria**	presence of ketone bodies in the urine, which is a common sign of acidosis among patients suffering from diabetes mellitus
-uria	s	urine, urination	(kee tohn YOO ree ah)	
noct	r	night	**nocturia**	urination at night
-uria	s	urine, urination	(nok TOO ree ah)	
olig	r	few in number	**oliguria**	reduced urination
-uria	s	urine, urination	(all ig YOO ree ah)	
poly	p	many	**polyuria**	excessive urination
-uria	s	urine, urination	(pall ee YOO ree ah)	
protein	r	protein	**proteinuria**	presence of protein in the urine
-uria	s	urine, urination	(proh tee NYOO ree ah)	
py	r	pus	**pyuria**	presence of pus (white blood cells) in the urine (Figure 14.5)
-uria	s	urine, urination	(pye YOO ree ah)	

SELF QUIZ 14.3

SAY IT—SPELL IT!

Review the terms of the urinary system by speaking the phonetic pronunciation out loud, then writing the correct spelling of the term.

> **Success Hint:** Use the audio glossary on the CD and CW for additional help with pronunciation of these terms.

1. AL byoo men YOO ree ah   _____

2. an yoo REE siss   _____

3. an YOO ree ah   _____

14.2 4. az oh TEE mee ah   _____

5. bak ter ee YOO ree ah _____

6. DYE yoo REE siss _____

7. diss YOO ree ah _____

14.3 8. ehn yoo REE siss _____

9. glye kohs YOO ree ah _____

10. HEE mah TOO ree ah _____

11. nok TOO ree ah _____

12. all ig YOO ree ah _____

14.4 13. pall ee YOO ree ah _____

14. proh tee NYOO ree ah _____

15. pye YOO ree ah _____

14.5 16. kee tohn YOO ree ah _____

MATCH IT!

Match the term on the left with the correct definition on the right.

_____1. albuminuria

_____2. anuria

_____3. anuresis

_____4. azotemia

_____5. bacteriuria

_____6. diuresis

_____7. dysuria

_____8. nocturnal enuresis

_____9. glycosuria

_____10. hematuria

_____11. ketonuria

_____12. nocturia

_____13. oligouria

_____14. polyuria

_____15. proteinuria

_____16. pyuria

a. urination at night

b. wetting the bed

c. presence of blood in the urine

d. the absence of urine

e. presence of bacteria in the urine

f. excessive urination

g. ketone bodies in the urine

h. high urea levels in the blood

i. inability to pass urine

j. presence of sugar in the urine

k. presence of albumin in the urine

l. presence of pus in the urine

m. reduced urination

n. presence of protein in the urine

o. difficulty or pain in urination

p. flowing through of urine

BREAK IT DOWN!

Analyze and separate each term into its word part by labeling each word part using p = prefix, r = root, cv = combining vowel, and s = suffix.

1. albuminuria _____

2. anuresis _____

3. azotemia _____

4. bacteriuria _____

5. dysuria _____

6. enuresis _____

7. glycosuria _____

8. ketonuria _____

WORD BUILDING

Construct or recall medical terms from the following meanings.

1. urination at night _____

2. presence of bacteria in the urine _____

3. presence of glucose (sugar) in the urine _____

4. absence of urine _____

5. difficulty or pain in urination _____

6. an involuntary release of urine _____

7. abnormally high urea and other nitrogenous compounds in the blood _____

8. excessive urine discharge _____

Diseases and Disorders

WORD PARTS (WHEN APPLICABLE)			TERM	DEFINITION
Part	Type	Meaning		
cyst	r	bladder	**cystitis**	inflammation of the urinary bladder
-itis	s	inflammation	(siss TYE tiss)	
cyst/o	r/cv	bladder	**cystocele**	protrusion of the urinary bladder
-cele	s	hernia, swelling	(SISS toh seel)	
cyst/o	r/cv	bladder	**cystolith**	a stone in the urinary bladder
-lith	s	stone	(SISS toh lith)	
epi-	p	upon	**epispadias**	a congenital defect resulting in the urinary meatus positioned on the dorsal surface of the penis; in the female, the meatus opens dorsal to the clitoris (Figure 14.6▪▪▪▪)
spadias	r	rip, tear	(EP ih SPAY dee ass)	
glomerul/o	r/cv	glomerulus	**glomerulonephritis**	inflammation of the glomeruli within a kidney
nephr	r	kidney	(gloh MAIR yoo loh neh	
-itis	s	inflammation	FRYE tiss)	

WORD PARTS (WHEN APPLICABLE)			TERM	DEFINITION
Part	**Type**	**Meaning**		
hydro-	p	water	**hydronephrosis**	condition of water in a kidney, usually caused by
nephr	r	kidney	(HIGH droh neh FROH siss)	obstruction and backup of urine leading to
-osis	s	condition of		distension of the renal pelvis (Figure 14.7 :::)

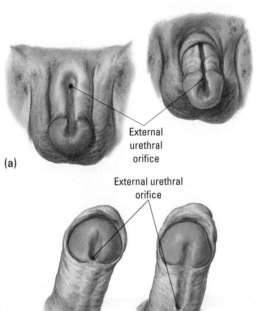

External urethral orifice

(a)

External urethral orifice

(b)

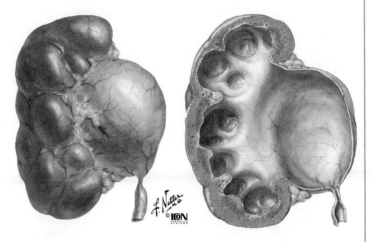

Figure 14.6 ::::

Epispadias and hypospadias.
Congenital defects can result in the abnormal location of the external urethral orifice (urinary meatus).
(a) In male epispadias, the orifice opens on the dorsal side of the penis. Two alternative locations of the orifice are shown.
(b) In male hypospadias, the orifice opens on the ventral side of the penis, as shown in the two alternate locations illustrated.
Source: Icon Learning Systems.

Figure 14.7 ::::

Hydronephrosis.
External (left) and internal (right) views of a kidney with hydronephrosis. Note the distension (swelling) of the renal pelvis. In this illustration, the distension was caused by the constriction of the ureter, causing urine to back up in the pelvis. *Source: Icon Learning Systems.*

hypo-	p	under	**hypospadias**	a congenital defect in which the urinary meatus
spadias	r	rip, tear	(HIGH poh SPAY dee ass)	opens on the underside of the penis; in the female, the opening is within the vagina (Figure 14.6)
			incontinence (in KON tih nens)	the involuntary discharge of urine, which may also refer to the inability to prevent the discharge of feces; **stress incontinence** is the involuntary discharge of urine due to a cough, sneeze, or strained movement

WORD PARTS (WHEN APPLICABLE)			TERM	DEFINITION
Part	**Type**	**Meaning**		

Incontinence

The Latin meaning of *continent* is *to hold together*, and *in* means *not*. The term was first applied during the 16th century, when *incontinently* was used by Shakespeare's contemporaries to mean *immediately*. Today's use of *incontinence* is limited to mean *the inability to prevent discharge of urine and/or feces*. As Shakespeare might say, "a most tragic limitation of a word."

WORD PARTS			TERM	DEFINITION
nephr	r	kidney	**nephritis**	inflammation of a kidney
-itis	s	inflammation	(neh FRYE tiss)	
nephr/o	r/cv	kidney	**nephroblastoma**	tumor originating from a kidney that includes
blast	r	germ, bud	(NEFF roh blass TOH mah)	developing embryonic cells; also called **Wilms'**
-oma	s	tumor		**tumor** (Figure 14.8::::)

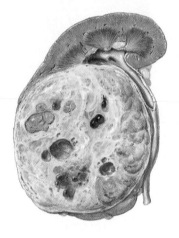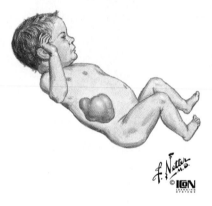

Figure 14.8 ::::

Nephroblastoma.
A sectioned kidney reveals the presence of a very large tumor, which arose from fetal cells during development. A newborn with nephroblastoma is illustrated to show the location and relative size of the tumor.
Source: Icon Learning Systems.

WORD PARTS			TERM	DEFINITION
nephr/o	r/cv	kidney	**nephrohypertrophy**	excessive development of a kidney, resulting in an
hyper-	p	excessive	(NEFF roh high	abnormal growth in size
-trophy	s	development	PER troh fee)	
nephr/o	r/cv	kidney	**nephrolithiasis**	presence of one or more stones in a kidney
lith	r	stone	(NEFF roh lith EYE ah siss)	(Figure 14.9::::)
-ia	s	condition of		
-sis	s	state of		
nephr	r	kidney	**nephroma**	tumor originating from a kidney
-oma	s	tumor	(neff ROH mah)	
nephr/o	r/v	kidney	**nephromegaly**	enlargement of a kidney
megal	r	large	(neff roh MEG ah lee)	
-y	s	process of		
nephr/o	r/v	kidney	**nephroptosis**	condition of a drooped kidney position, which occurs
-ptosis	s	condition of	(neff ropp TOH siss)	when the kidney is no longer held in its proper
		falling		position; also called **floating kidney**
		downward		

WORD PARTS (WHEN APPLICABLE)			TERM	DEFINITION
Part	**Type**	**Meaning**		

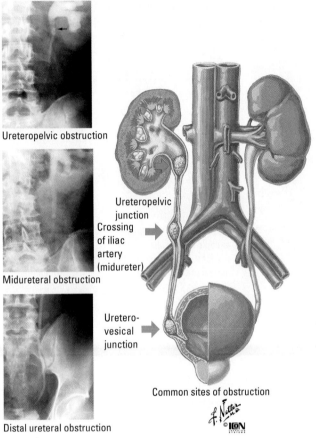

Ureteropelvic obstruction

Midureteral obstruction

Distal ureteral obstruction

Ureteropelvic junction

Crossing of iliac artery (midureter)

Uretero-vesical junction

Common sites of obstruction

Figure 14.9 ⁝⁝⁝⁝

Nephrolithiasis.
Stones, or renal calculi, may form in several areas within the urinary tract. When they form in the kidney, they usually arise within the renal pelvis to form the condition nephrolithiasis. Kidney stones may dislocate to form obstructions in the ureter, bladder, or urethra, usually at their junctions. The images to the left of the illustration are x-rays; the arrows point to obstructions, which are caused by stones.
Source: Icon Learning Systems.

Part	Type	Meaning	Term	Definition
poly-	p	many	**polycystic kidney**	a kidney condition characterized by the presence of
cyst	r	bladder	(PALL ee SISS tik	many polyps, resulting in the loss of functional
-ic	s	pertaining to	KID nee)	tissue (Figure 14.10⁝⁝⁝⁝)
pyel	r	renal pelvis	**pyelitis**	inflammation of the renal pelvis
-itis	s	inflammation	(PYE eh LYE tiss)	
pyel/o	r/cv	renal pelvis	**pyelonephritis**	inflammation of the renal pelvis and nephrons
nephr	r	kidney	(PYE eh loh neh FRYE tiss)	(Figure 14.11⁝⁝⁝⁝)
-itis	s	inflammation		
ren	r	kidney	**renal calculi**	stones in the kidney (in the renal pelvis) (Figure 14.9)
-al	s	pertaining to	(REE nal	
calcul	r	small calcium	KAL kyoo lye)	
-i	s	plural		
ren	r	kidney	**renal hypertension**	elevated blood pressure caused by kidney disease
-al	s	pertaining to	(REE nal	
hyper-	p	excessive	high per TEN shun)	
tens	r	pressure		
-ion	s	process of		
			stricture	abnormal narrowing, as in urethral stricture
			(STRIK cher)	

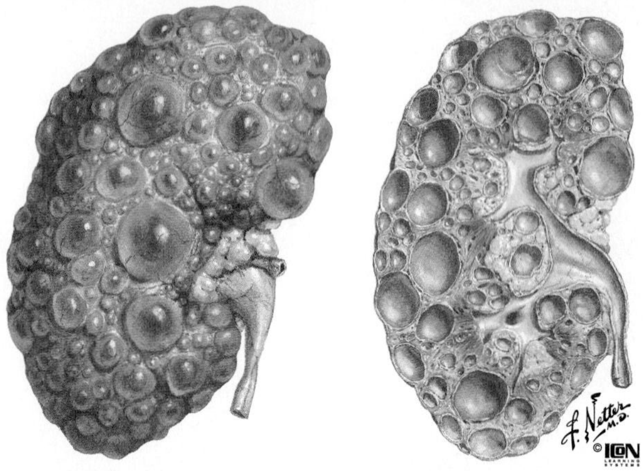

WORD PARTS (WHEN APPLICABLE)			TERM	DEFINITION
Part	Type	Meaning		

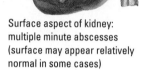

Surface aspect of kidney: multiple fluid-filled cysts

Cut section: fluid-filled cysts crowd out functional tissue

Figure 14.10 ::::

Polycystic kidney.
The condition is characterized by the presence of multiple polyps, which form a bubble-like pattern.
Source: Icon Learning Systems.

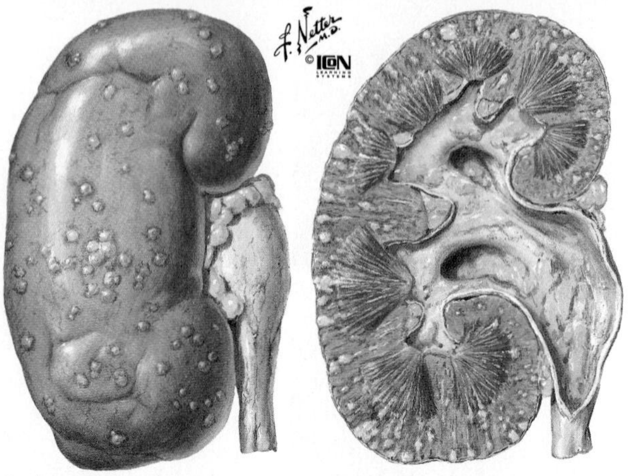

Surface aspect of kidney: multiple minute abscesses (surface may appear relatively normal in some cases)

Cut section: radiating yellowish gray streaks in pyramids and abscesses in cortex; moderate hydronephrosis with infection; blunting of calyces (ascending infection)

Figure 14.11 ::::

Pyelonephritis.
The condition is characterized by the presence of numerous sites of infection, or abscesses, on the surface (left) and within (right) the kidney. The most common cause of pyelonephritis is a bacterial infection that has traveled through the urinary tract (a urinary tract infection, or UTI).
Source: Icon Learning Systems.

Part	Type	Meaning	TERM	DEFINITION
ur -emia	r s	urine condition of blood	**uremia** (yoo REE mee ah)	an excess of urea and other nitrogenous wastes in the blood, caused by failure of the kidneys to remove urea during urine formation
ureter -itis	r s	ureter inflammation	**ureteritis** (yoo REE ter EYE tiss)	inflammation of a ureter
ureter/o -cele	r/cv s	ureter hernia, swelling	**ureterocele** (yoo REE ter oh seel)	protrusion of a ureter
ureter/o lith -ia -sis	r/cv r s s	ureter stone condition of state of	**ureterolithiasis** (yoo REE ter oh lith EYE ah siss)	presence of stone(s) in a ureter (Figure 14.9)
ureter/o -stenosis	r/cv s	ureter condition of narrowing	**ureterostenosis** (yoo REE ter oh sten OH siss)	condition of a narrowed ureter
urethr/o cyst -itis	r/cv r s	urethra bladder inflammation	**urethrocystitis** (yoo REE throh siss TYE tiss)	inflammation of the urethra and urinary bladder

WORD PARTS (WHEN APPLICABLE)			TERM	DEFINITION
Part	Type	Meaning		
			urinary retention (YOO rih nair ee ree TEN shun)	abnormal accumulation of urine in the urinary bladder resulting from an inability to void (urinate)
			urinary suppression (YOO rih nair ee suh PREH shun)	an acute stoppage of urine formation by the kidneys
			urinary tract infection (YOO rih nair ee TRAKT in FEK shun)	infection of urinary organs, usually the urethra and bladder, in which symptoms often include fever, dysuria, and lumbar or abdominal pain; abbreviated **UTI** (Figure 14.12 ::::)

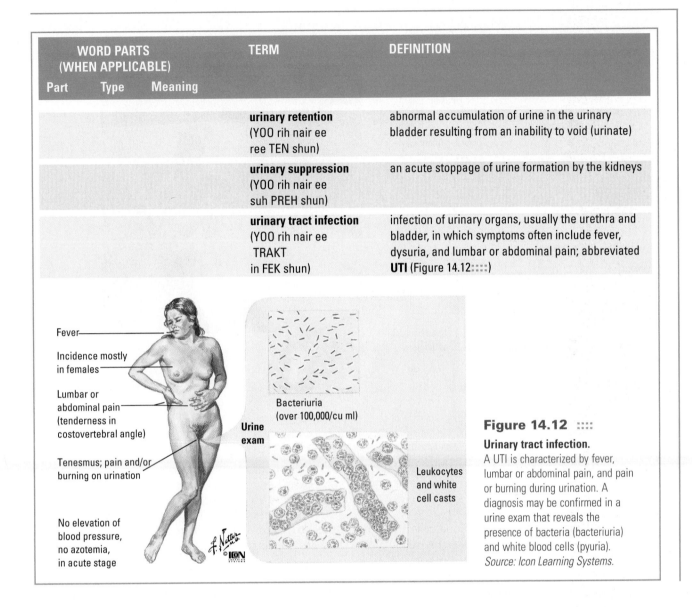

Fever

Incidence mostly in females

Lumbar or abdominal pain (tenderness in costovertebral angle)

Tenesmus; pain and/or burning on urination

No elevation of blood pressure, no azotemia, in acute stage

Urine exam

Bacteriuria (over 100,000/cu ml)

Leukocytes and white cell casts

Figure 14.12 ::::

Urinary tract infection.
A UTI is characterized by fever, lumbar or abdominal pain, and pain or burning during urination. A diagnosis may be confirmed in a urine exam that reveals the presence of bacteria (bacteriuria) and white blood cells (pyuria). *Source: Icon Learning Systems.*

disease focus | Renal Failure and Dialysis

Renal failure is the loss of the kidneys' abilities to respond to the changing conditions of the body, resulting in the rapid loss of body fluid maintenance, electrolyte balance, and pH regulation. It also leads to the accumulation of toxic metabolic waste products in tissues. The loss of kidney function can be acute or chronic.

Acute renal failure, also called **glomerulonephritis,** is the abrupt stoppage of kidney function. It is usually recoverable and temporarily results in a reduced urine output, an increase in urea in the blood, and sometimes local pain. It can be caused by a loss of body fluids, such as occurs in excessive bleeding, diarrhea, and heavy use of diuretics. It can also be caused by damage to the nephrons by injury, infectious microorganisms, hypertension, or toxic chemicals and drugs.

Chronic renal failure is the progressive loss of functioning nephrons and is manifested by reduced glomeru-

lar filtration rates, accumulation of urea in the blood, electrolyte imbalances, and acid-base imbalances. It can be caused by metabolic disorders, accumulation of toxins, inherited connective tissue disorders, and hypertensive vascular diseases. If not treated by **hemodialysis** or **kidney transplant,** chronic renal failure usually results in death.

During total kidney failure, the formation of urine stops completely. This results in a rapid accumulation of toxic wastes and a progressively acidic pH of body fluids, which can lead to death in about eight to twelve days. In order to remove the toxic wastes that build up in the blood, hemodialysis or peritoneal dialysis may be performed if kidney transplantation is not possible. In hemodialysis, the patient's blood is channeled through cellophane-like tubing whose walls are permeable only to certain substances, such as nitrogenous

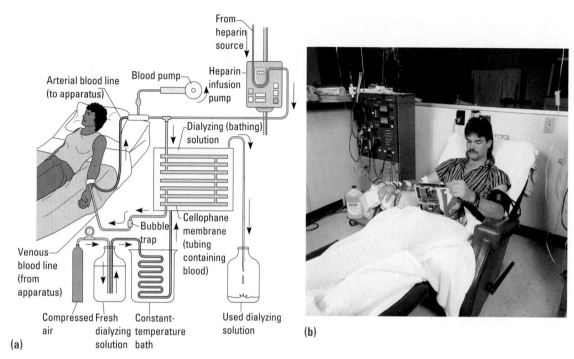

Figure 14.13 ::::

Hemodialysis.
(a) The process of hemodialysis replaces the kidney function of blood filtration by forcing blood from the patient through cellophane membranes, as shown in this schematic. *Source: Pearson Education.*
(b) A patient undergoing hemodialysis. *Source: Southern Illinois University/Photo Researchers Inc.*

wastes and potassium, but not to blood cells and proteins (Figure 14.13::::). The tubing is immersed in a solution similar to normal, waste-free plasma. As the blood circulates through the tubing, nitrogenous wastes and excess ions diffuse from the blood to the dialyzing solution across the tubing walls. Patients are usually dialyzed three times a week, and they can often undergo

this procedure at home. The main drawbacks to dialysis are the constant risk of infection and hemorrhage during dialysis, the development of uremia between periods of dialysis, and its high cost. Dialysis is, however, the only way of keeping chronic kidney patients alive and functioning until the only present cure for this disease, a kidney transplant, becomes available.

SELF QUIZ 14.4

SAY IT—SPELL IT!

Review the terms of the urinary system by speaking the phonetic pronunciation out loud, then writing the correct spelling of the term.

1. EP ih SPAY dee ass _____

■14.6 2. gloh MAIR yoo loh neh FRYE tiss _____

3. HIGH droh neh FROH siss _____

4. HIGH poh SPAY dee ass _____

5. in KON tih nens _____

6. neh FRYE tiss _____

7. NEFF roh blass TOH mah _____

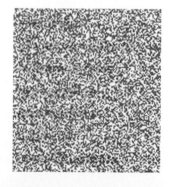

8. NEFF roh high PER troh fee _____

9. NEFF roh lith EYE ah siss _____

10. neff ROH mah _____

11. neff roh MEG ah lee _____

12. neff ropp TOH siss _____

13. PYE eh LYE tiss _____

14. PYE eh loh neh FRYE tiss _____

15. PALL ee SISS tik   KID nee _____

16. REE nal   KAL kyoo lye _____

17. REE nal   high per TEN shun _____

18. siss TYE tiss _____

19. SISS toh lith _____

20. SISS toh seel _____

14.7 21. yoo REE mee ah _____

22. yoo REE ter EYE tiss _____

23. yoo REE ter oh lith EYE ah siss _____

24. yoo REE ter oh seel _____

25. yoo REE ter oh sten OH siss _____

26. yoo REE throh siss TYE tiss _____

27. YOO rih nair ee   ree TEN shun _____

28. YOO rih nair ee   suh PREH shun _____

MATCH IT!

Match the term on the left with the correct definition on the right.

_____ 1. cystitis

_____ 2. cystocele

_____ 3. cystolith

_____ 4. glomerulonephritis

_____ 5. hydronephrosis

_____ 6. nephritis

_____ 7. nephroblastoma

_____ 8. nephrohypertrophy

_____ 9. nephrolithiasis

_____10. nephroma

_____11. nephromegaly

_____12. nephroptosis

_____13. pyelitis

_____14. pyelonephritis

_____15. uremia

_____16. ureteritis

_____17. ureterocele

_____18. ureterostenosis

_____19. urethrocystitis

_____20. epispadias

_____21. hypospadias

_____22. polycystic disease

_____23. renal calculi

_____24. renal hypertension

_____25. urinary retention

_____26. urinary suppression

a. a tumor arising from a kidney

b. inflammation of a ureter

c. condition of excess urea in the blood

d. a drooping kidney

e. inflammation of the urinary bladder

f. condition of stone(s) in a kidney

g. protrusion of the urinary bladder

h. inflammation of the renal pelvis and nephrons

i. protrusion of a ureter

j. inflammation of the glomeruli in a kidney

k. inflammation of the renal pelvis

l. a kidney tumor containing developing cells

m. stone(s) in the urinary bladder

n. inflammation of the urethra and urinary bladder

o. condition of a narrowed ureter

p. enlargement of a kidney

q. abnormal growth of a kidney

r. distension of the renal pelvis due to an obstruction

s. inflammation of a kidney

t. urinary meatus opens on the penis underside

u. a condition of stones in the kidneys

v. an acute stoppage of urine formation

w. urinary meatus opens on the dorsal penis

x. high blood pressure resulting from kidney disease

y. a condition of many polyps within a kidney

z. abnormal accumulation of urine in the bladder

BREAK IT DOWN!

Analyze and separate each term into its word parts by labeling each word part using p = prefix, r = root, cv = combining vowel, and s = suffix.

1. cystitis   _____

2. cystocele   _____

3. cystolith   _____

4. glomerulonephritis _____

5. hydronephrosis _____

6. nephroblastoma _____

7. nephromegaly _____

8. pyelonephritis _____

14.8 9. hypospadias _____

FILL IT IN!

Fill in the blanks with the correct terms.

1. A congenital defect in which the urinary meatus is incorrectly positioned occurs in both males and females. When the urinary meatus opens on the dorsal side of the penis in males or on the dorsal side of the clitoris in females, it is called an _____. When the meatus opens on the underside of the penis or into the vagina, it is called a _____.

2. The inability to prevent urine discharge is commonly called _____.

3. A kidney disease that is characterized by the presence of many polyps within a
14.9   kidney is called _____ _____.

4. A common term for the condition of stones in a kidney is _____ _____.

5. Kidney disease often leads to an imbalance of water and electrolytes in all body fluids, causing elevated blood pressure. This type of high blood pressure is
14.10   termed _____ _____. A kidney disease that can lead to this condition is an acute failure to form urine, known as _____ _____.

6. An infection of the urinary tract is usually bacterial in origin. The condition is called _____ _____ _____. In some cases, it leads to inflammation that can obstruct urine discharge, leading to
14.11   the abnormal accumulation of urine (which prevents _____) in the bladder known as _____ _____.

Treatments, Procedures, and Devices

WORD PARTS (WHEN APPLICABLE)			TERM	DEFINITION
Part	Type	Meaning		
			blood urea nitrogen (yoo REE ah NIGH troh jenn)	a clinical lab test that measures urea concentration in a sample of blood as an indicator of kidney function; an elevated value indicates kidney disease; abbreviated **BUN**
			creatinine (kree ATT ih neen)	a protein that is a normal component of urine, as a result of muscle metabolism; elevated levels in a urine sample indicate kidney disease
cyst -ectomy	r s	bladder excision	**cystectomy** (siss TEK toh mee)	excision of the urinary bladder
cyst/o -graphy	r/cv s	bladder recording process	**cystography** (siss TOG rah fee)	x-ray technique of imaging the urinary bladder; the resulting x-ray image is called a cystogram (SISS toh gram)
cyst/o lith/o -tomy	r/cv r/cv s	bladder stone incision	**cystolithotomy** (siss toh lith OTT oh mee)	incision into the urinary bladder to remove a stone
cyst/o -plasty	r/cv s	bladder surgical repair	**cystoplasty** (SISS toh plass tee)	surgical repair of the urinary bladder
cyst/o pyel/o -graphy	r/cv r/cv s	bladder renal pelvis recording process	**cystopyelography** (SISS toh pye ell OG rah fee)	x-ray technique that images the urinary bladder and renal pelvis; the resulting x-ray image is called a cystopyelogram (siss toh pye ELL oh gram)
cyst/o -rrhaphy	r/cv s	bladder suturing	**cystorrhaphy** (sist OR ah fee)	suturing of the urinary bladder wall
cyst/o -scopy	r/cv s	bladder process of viewing	**cystoscopy** (siss TOSS koh pee)	use of a modified endoscope, known as a cystoscope (SISS toh skope) to visually examine the urinary bladder (Figure 14.14::::)
cyst/o -stomy	r/cv s	bladder surgical creation of an opening	**cystostomy** (siss TOSS toh mee)	surgical creation of an artificial opening into the urinary bladder to provide an alternate exit pathway for urine (Figure 14.15::::)
cyst/o -tomy	r/cv s	bladder incision	**cystotomy** (siss TOTT oh mee)	incision into the urinary bladder; also called **vesicotomy** (VESS ih KOTT oh mee) (Figure 14.15)
cyst/o ureter/o -graphy	r/cv r/cv s	bladder ureter recording process	**cystoureterography** (SISS toh yoo REE ter OG rah fee)	x-ray technique imaging the urinary bladder and ureters; the x-ray image is called a cystoureterogram (SISS toh yoo REE ter oh gram)
cyst/o urethr/o -graphy	r/cv r/cv s	bladder urethra recording process	**cystourethrography** (SISS toh YOO ree THROG rah fee)	x-ray technique imaging the urinary bladder and the urethra; the x-ray image is called a cystourethrogram (siss toh yoo REE throh gram); in a voiding cystourethrogram (VOY ding siss toh yoo REE throh gram), the x-ray image is taken after the bladder is emptied of urine; abbreviated **VCUG**
			fulguration (full guh RAY shun)	a surgical procedure that destroys living tissue with an electric spark; commonly used to remove tumors or polyps from the interior bladder wall

WORD PARTS (WHEN APPLICABLE)			TERM	DEFINITION
Part	**Type**	**Meaning**		

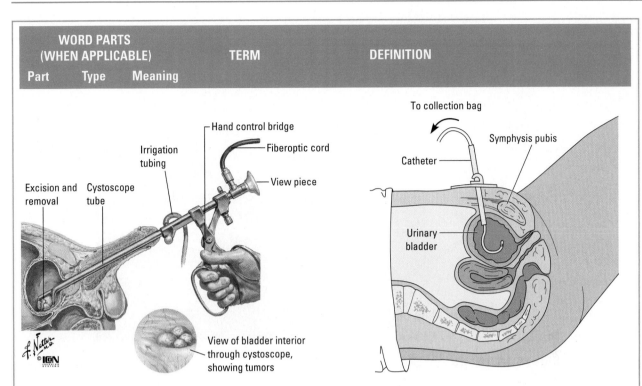

Figure 14.14 ::::

Cystoscopy.
In this procedure, a specialized endoscope with a rigid tube, known as a cystoscope, is used to view the internal environment of the urinary bladder. As shown, the cystoscope may be outfitted to include surgical devices to remove tumors or stones.
Source: Icon Learning Systems.

Figure 14.15 ::::

Cystostomy.
An artificial opening is made through the urinary bladder wall during this procedure. As the illustration suggests, it is often performed to enable a patient to bypass obstructions for voiding.

WORD PARTS (WHEN APPLICABLE)			TERM	DEFINITION
Part	**Type**	**Meaning**		
hem/o	r/cv	blood	**hemodialysis**	procedure that removes nitrogenous wastes and
dia-	p	passing through	(HEE moh dye AL ih siss)	excess ions from the blood, replacing the normal function of the kidneys as an intervention for kidney
lys	r	dissolution		failure, using the process of dialysis, in which blood
-is	s	pertaining to		is pushed through a semipermeable membrane filter to separate substances based on their molecular size; abbreviated **HD** (Figure 14.13)
			kidney, ureter, and bladder x-ray	an x-ray procedure that images the abdomen; used as a gross (large-scale) view of the urinary organs to assess their positions, and to identify possible locations of calculi or other obstructions; abbreviated **KUB**
lith/o	r/cv	stone	**lithotripsy**	surgical technique that crushes stones (Figure
-tripsy	s	surgical crushing	(LITH oh trip see)	14.16::::)
lys	r	dissolution	**lysis**	a gradual reduction of symptoms of an acute disease,
-is	s	pertaining to	(LYE siss)	or the destruction of red blood cells or bacteria

[FYI]

Lysis
The term lysis is derived from the Greek word, *lusis,* which means *a loosening.*

WORD PARTS (WHEN APPLICABLE)			TERM	DEFINITION
Part	Type	Meaning		

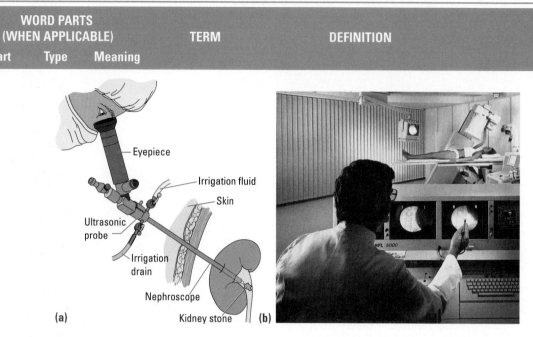

Figure 14.16 ::::

Lithotripsy. The direction of a sound pulse crushes the stones into smaller fragments that can be passed with urine. It includes invasive and noninvasive procedures.
(a) During the invasive procedure known as intracorporeal shock wave lithotripsy, or ISWL, the ultrasound device is surgically inserted near the stone. *Source: Pearson Education.*
(b) When applied through the skin, the noninvasive procedure is called extracorporeal shock wave lithotripsy, or ESWL. *Source: Courtesy of Dormier Medical Products.*

Part	Type	Meaning	TERM	DEFINITION
meat/o -scopy	r/cv s	opening process of viewing	**meatoscopy** (mee ah TOSS koh pee)	use of a modified endoscope, known as a meatoscope (mee ATT oh skope), to visually examine the urinary meatus
meat/o -tomy	r/cv s	opening incision	**meatotomy** (mee ah TOTT oh mee)	an incision made to enlarge the urinary meatus
nephr -ectomy	r s	kidney excision	**nephrectomy** (neh FREK toh mee)	excision of a kidney
nephr/o -graphy	r/cv s	kidney recording process	**nephrography** (neh FROG rah fee)	an x-ray technique imaging a kidney; the x-ray image is called a **nephrogram** (NEFF roh gram)
nephr/o lys -is	r/cv r s	kidney dissolution pertaining to	**nephrolysis** (neh FRALL ih siss)	freeing of the kidney from inflammatory adhesions
nephr/o -pexy	r/cv s	kidney surgical fixation	**nephropexy** (NEFF roh pek see)	surgical fixation of an abnormally mobile kidney
nephr/o -scopy	r/cv s	kidney process of viewing	**nephroscopy** (neh FROSS koh pee)	use of a modified endoscope, known as a **nephroscope** (NEFF roh skope) to visually examine the kidney

WORD PARTS (WHEN APPLICABLE)			TERM	DEFINITION
Part	Type	Meaning		
nephr/o son/o -graphy	r/cv r/cv s	kidney sound recording process	**nephrosonography** (NEFF roh son OG rah fee)	an ultrasound procedure in which a kidney is imaged with the use of sound waves
nephr/o -stomy	r/cv s	kidney surgical creation of an opening	**nephrostomy** (neff ROSS toh mee)	surgical creation of an artificial opening into the kidney, between the renal pelvis and the kidney exterior
nephr/o tom/o -graphy	r/cv r s	kidney cut, section recording process	**nephrotomography** (NEH froh toh MOG rah fee)	x-ray technique imaging the kidney using sectional x-ray exposures; the image is called a nephrotomogram (NEH froh tohm MOH gram)
periton/e -al dia- lys -is	r/cv s p r s	peritoneum pertaining to passing through dissolution pertaining to	**peritoneal dialysis** (pair ih TOH nee al dye AL ih siss)	a procedure in which toxic wastes are removed from the peritoneal cavity reservoir by artificial filtration as a cleansing treatment to compensate for kidney failure
pyel lith/o -tomy	r r/cv s	renal pelvis stone incision	**pyelithotomy** (pye eh lith OTT oh mee)	incision into the renal pelvis to remove a stone
pyel/o -gram	r/cv s	renal pelvis recording	**pyelogram** (PYE ell oh gram)	x-ray image of the renal pelvis; in a retrograde pyelogram (REH troh grayd PYE ell oh gram), a contrast medium is injected into the urethra using a cystoscope and the x-ray moves in a direction opposite from the norm, in an effort to detect the presence of stones or other obstructions; abbreviated **RP** (Figure 14.17▓▓▓); in an intravenous pyelogram (in trah VEE nuss PYE ell oh gram), iodine is used as the contrast medium and is injected into the bloodstream; abbreviated **IVP**
pyel/o -plasty	r/cv s	renal pelvis surgical repair	**pyeloplasty** (PYE ell oh PLASS tee)	surgical repair of the renal pelvis, usually involving the removal of an obstruction
pyel/o -stomy	r/cv s	renal pelvis surgical creation of an opening	**pyelostomy** (PYE ell OSS toh mee)	surgical creation of an artificial opening into the renal pelvis to provide an alternate exit route for urine
ren -al	r s	kidney pertaining to	**renal transplant** (REE nal)	a surgical procedure in which a donor kidney, usually obtained from a close relative, is implanted to replace a nonfunctional kidney (Figure 14.18▓▓▓)
ren/o -graphy	r/cv s	kidney recording process	**renography** (ree NOG rah fee)	a nuclear medicine test using a radioactive substance to highlight internal aspects of a kidney; the recording is called a renogram (REE noh gram)

WORD PARTS (WHEN APPLICABLE)			TERM	DEFINITION
Part	**Type**	**Meaning**		

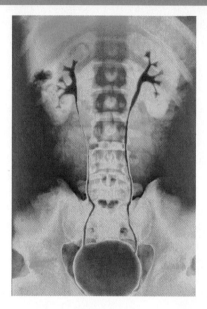

Figure 14.17 ::::

Retrograde pyelogram.
A contrast medium is injected into the urethra using a cystoscope and the x-ray moves in a direction opposite from the norm, producing the image that is shown. It serves to highlight the internal features of the renal pelvis and ureters. *Source: Clinique Ste. Catherine/ CNRI/Science Photo Library/Photo Researchers Inc.*

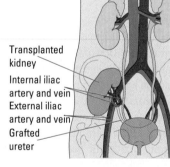

Transplanted kidney

Internal iliac artery and vein

External iliac artery and vein

Grafted ureter

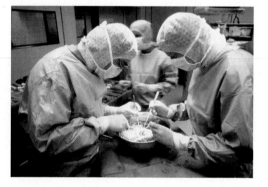

Figure 14.18 ::::

Renal transplant.
(a) A transplanted kidney is placed within the pelvic cavity below the location of the kidney requiring replacement. *Source: Pearson Education.*
(b) Two nephrologists examine a donated kidney prior to its insertion into the recipient during a renal transplant.

			specific gravity	the relative concentration of water molecules in a liquid sample; abbreviated **SG**; the clinical lab test that measures specific gravity in a sample of urine evaluates filtration and water reasborption in the kidneys using a urinometer (Figure 14.19::::)
ureter -ectomy	r s	ureter excision	**ureterectomy** (yoo REE ter EK toh mee)	excision of a ureter
ureter/o -gram	r/cv s	ureter recording	**ureterogram** (yoo REE ter oh gram)	x-ray image of the ureters

WORD PARTS (WHEN APPLICABLE)			TERM	DEFINITION
Part	Type	Meaning		

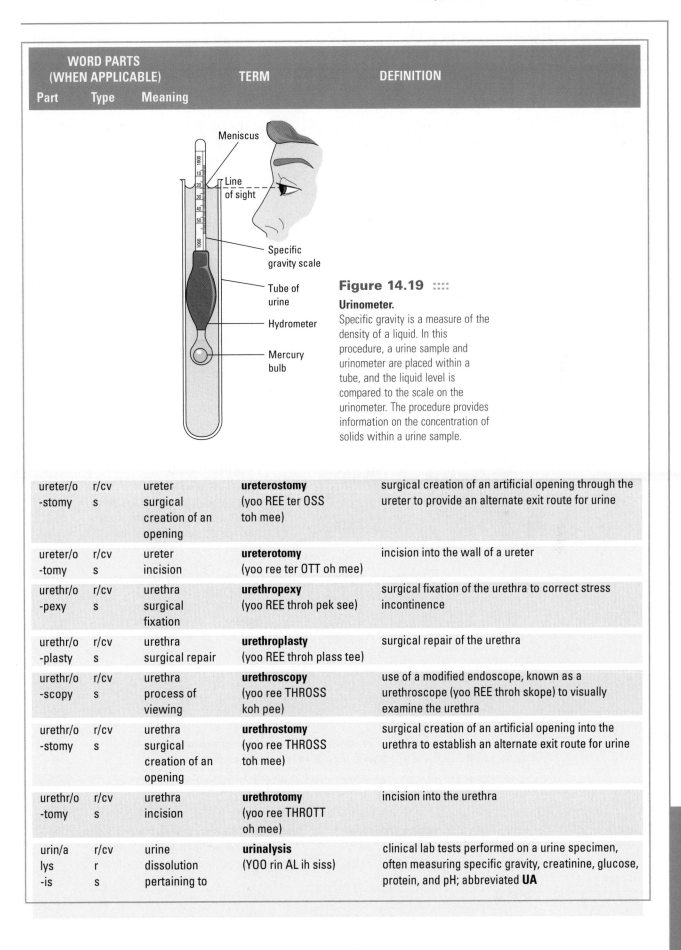

Meniscus

Line of sight

Specific gravity scale

Tube of urine

Hydrometer

Mercury bulb

Figure 14.19 ::::

Urinometer.
Specific gravity is a measure of the density of a liquid. In this procedure, a urine sample and urinometer are placed within a tube, and the liquid level is compared to the scale on the urinometer. The procedure provides information on the concentration of solids within a urine sample.

Part	Type	Meaning	TERM	DEFINITION
ureter/o -stomy	r/cv s	ureter surgical creation of an opening	**ureterostomy** (yoo REE ter OSS toh mee)	surgical creation of an artificial opening through the ureter to provide an alternate exit route for urine
ureter/o -tomy	r/cv s	ureter incision	**ureterotomy** (yoo ree ter OTT oh mee)	incision into the wall of a ureter
urethr/o -pexy	r/cv s	urethra surgical fixation	**urethropexy** (yoo REE throh pek see)	surgical fixation of the urethra to correct stress incontinence
urethr/o -plasty	r/cv s	urethra surgical repair	**urethroplasty** (yoo REE throh plass tee)	surgical repair of the urethra
urethr/o -scopy	r/cv s	urethra process of viewing	**urethroscopy** (yoo ree THROSS koh pee)	use of a modified endoscope, known as a urethroscope (yoo REE throh skope) to visually examine the urethra
urethr/o -stomy	r/cv s	urethra surgical creation of an opening	**urethrostomy** (yoo ree THROSS toh mee)	surgical creation of an artificial opening into the urethra to establish an alternate exit route for urine
urethr/o -tomy	r/cv s	urethra incision	**urethrotomy** (yoo ree THROTT oh mee)	incision into the urethra
urin/a lys -is	r/cv r s	urine dissolution pertaining to	**urinalysis** (YOO rin AL ih siss)	clinical lab tests performed on a urine specimen, often measuring specific gravity, creatinine, glucose, protein, and pH; abbreviated **UA**

WORD PARTS (WHEN APPLICABLE)			TERM	DEFINITION
Part	Type	Meaning		
urin	r	urine	**urinary**	insertion of a catheter (or cath), a flexible tube for
-ary	s	pertaining to	**catheterization**	channeling fluids into the urinary bladder to drain
catheter	r	flexible tube	(YOO rih nair ee	urine (Figure 14.20▫▫▫▫)
-ization	s	process of	KATH eh ter ih ZAY shun)	

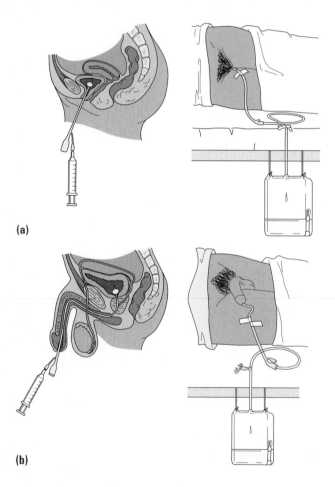

(a)

(b)

Figure 14.20 ▫▫▫▫

Urinary catheterization.
The procedure involves the insertion of a flexible tube, or catheter, through the urethra and into the urinary bladder. Voiding occurs through the catheter and is collected in a plastic bag adjacent to the patient.
(a) Catheterization of a female patient.
(b) Catheterization of a male patient.

Catheter
The term *catheter* is from the Greek word, *katheter,* which means *a thing let down,* so named because it is a flexible tube that lets urine down from the urinary bladder.

urin	r	urine	**urinary endoscopy**	use of an endoscope to view internal structures of
-ary	s	pertaining to	(YOO rih nair ee	the urinary system; includes: cystoscopy,
endo	p	within	ehn DOSS koh pee)	meatoscopy, nephroscopy, and urethroscopy
-scopy	s	process of viewing		

WORD PARTS (WHEN APPLICABLE)			TERM	DEFINITION
Part	**Type**	**Meaning**		
urin/o -meter	r/cv s	urine measuring instrument	**urinometer** (yoo rih NOM eh ter)	instrument that measures the water density of urine, a value known as specific gravity (Figure 14.19)
vesic/o urethr -al	r/cv r s	bladder, sac urethra pertaining to	**vesicourethral suspension** (vess ih koh yoo REE thral)	a surgery performed to stabilize the urinary bladder position as a treatment for stress incontinence

---

SELF QUIZ 14.5

SAY IT—SPELL IT!

Review the terms of the urinary system by speaking the phonetic pronunciation guides out loud, then writing in the correct spelling of the term.

1. siss TOG rah fee _____
2. sist OR ah fee _____
3. SISS toh yoo REE ter oh gram _____
4. SISS toh yoo REE ter OG rah fee _____
5. siss toh yoo REE throh gram _____
6. SISS toh YOO ree THROG rah fee _____
7. HEE moh dye AL ih siss _____
14.12 8. LITH oh trip see _____
9. neh FREK toh mee _____
10. NEFF roh gram _____
11. neh FROG rah fee _____
12. neh FRALL ih siss _____
13. NEFF roh pek see _____
14. NEFF roh son OG rah fee _____
15. neff ROSS toh mee _____
16. NEH froh TOH moh gram _____
14.13 17. pye eh lith OTT oh mee _____
14.14 18. yoo REE ter OSS toh mee _____
19. yoo REE ter oh gram _____
14.15 20. PYE ell oh gram _____
21. yoo REE throh pek see _____
22. yoo REE throh plass tee _____
23. yoo ree THROSS koh pee _____
24. yoo ree THROSS toh mee _____

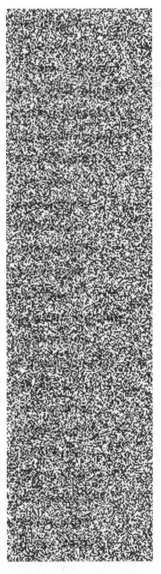

25. yoo rih NOM eh ter   _____

26. yoo REE ter EK toh mee   _____

27. vess ih koh yoo REE thral _____

MATCH IT!

Match the term on the left with the correct definition on the right.

_____ 1. cystectomy   a. surgical repair of the urethra

_____ 2. cystolithotomy   b. suture of the urinary bladder

_____ 3. cystoplasty   c. creates a new opening through the kidney

_____ 4. cystorrhaphy   d. incision to enlarge the urinary meatus

_____ 5. cystotomy   e. removal of a stone from the urinary bladder

_____ 6. lithotripsy   f. stabilizes the position of the urinary bladder

_____ 7. meatotomy   g. removal of a stone from the renal pelvis

_____ 8. nephrectomy   h. surgical repair of the urinary bladder

_____ 9. nephropexy   i. incision to enter the urethra

_____10. pyelithotomy   j. removal of a ureter

_____11. pyelostomy   k. surgical fixation of a mobile kidney

_____12. pyeloplasty   l. removal of a kidney

_____13. ureterectomy   m. surgical repair of a renal pelvis

_____14. ureterotomy   n. incision into the urinary bladder

_____15. urethroplasty   o. incision into a ureter

_____16. urethrotomy   p. removal of the urinary bladder

_____17. vesicourethal suspension   q. technique that crushes stones

_____18. fulguration   r. test for protein levels in a urine sample

_____19. renal transplant   s. test for water concentration in urine

_____20. kidney, ureter, and   t. spark that kills unwanted tissue
         bladder x-ray

_____21. blood urea nitrogen   u. test for urea in the blood

_____22. peritoneal dialysis   v. insertion of a tube to drain urine

_____23. creatinine   w. general x-ray of the abdomen

_____24. specific gravity   x. surgical procedure replacing a diseased kidney

_____25. urinary catheter   y. a collection of clinical tests on a urine specimen

_____26. urinalysis   z. blood filtration using the peritoneal cavity

BREAK IT DOWN!

Analyze and separate each term into its word parts by labeling each word part using p = prefix, r = root, cv = combining vowel, and s = suffix.

1. cystolithotomy _____

14.16 2. cystopyelography _____

3. cystoureterogram _____

14.17 4. meatotomy _____

5. nephrosonography _____

6. nephrolysis _____

7. nephrotomogram _____

8. renography _____

9. ureterogram _____

10. urethrostomy _____

11. urethroscope _____

12. ureterostomy _____

13. urethrotomy _____

14. vesicourethral _____

WORD BUILDING

Construct or recall medical terms from the following meanings.

1. a flexible tube inserted into the urinary bladder _____

2. a measure of water concentration in a urine sample _____

3. surgical replacement of a diseased kidney _____

4. procedure that destroys unwanted growths with a spark _____

5. clinical test for characteristics of a urine specimen _____

6. x-ray of the abdomen to identify urinary obstructions _____

7. artificial filtration of blood using the peritoneum as a reservoir _____

8. endoscope modified to view the kidneys

   _____

9. procedure that replaces kidney filtration

   _____

10. produces a cystourethrogram

    _____

11. imaging the kidney by taking sectional x-rays

    _____

12. use of iodine injected into the bloodstream

    _____

13. x-ray technique to image the bladder and renal pelvis

    _____

14. endoscope modified to view the urinary meatus

    _____

15. endoscopic evaluation of the urinary bladder

    _____

FILL IT IN!

Fill in the blanks with the correct terms.

1. A clinical lab test that measures the amount of a protein normally released during skeletal muscle metabolism, known as _____, is an evaluation of kidney function. It is often combined with a measurement of water density in a urine sample, or _____ _____, and often glucose and pH, in a comprehensive exam known as a _____.

2. Kidney function may be evaluated from a sample of blood during a _____ _____ _____ test.

3. If kidney failure occurs, toxins from the bloodstream can be periodically removed through the procedure known as _____ _____, in which the peritoneal cavity is used as a reservoir for fluid during artificial filtration. If failure is permanent, the patient may be considered for _____ _____, during which a diseased kidney is surgically replaced by a donated organ.

4. A general diagnostic x-ray of the abdomen often precedes further procedures, and is called a _____, _____, and bladder x-ray. If the cause of symptoms is identified as an obstruction in the urethra due to a tumor or polyp, urine from the bladder may be drained by insertion of a _____ _____. In many cases, the obstruction can be removed by an instrument that generates an electric spark to destroy the unwanted tissue in a procedure called a _____.

abbreviations of the urinary system

The abbreviations that are associated with the urinary system are summarized here.
Study these abbreviations, and review them in the exercise that follows.

ABBREVIATION	DEFINITION	ABBREVIATION	DEFINITION
BC	Bowman's capsule	RP	retrograde pyelogram
BUN	blood urea nitrogen	SG	specific gravity
cath	catheter, catheterization	UA	urinalysis
HD	hemodialysis	UTI	urinary tract infection
IVP	intravenous pyelogram	VCUG	voiding cystourethrogram
KUB	kidney, ureter, and bladder x-ray		

SELF QUIZ 14.6

Fill in the blanks with the abbreviation or the complete medical term.

	Abbreviation	Medical Term
14.18	1. UA	_____
14.19	2. _____	retrograde pyelogram
	3. BC	_____
	4. _____	voiding cystourethrogram
14.20	5. IVP	_____
	6. _____	kidney, ureter, and bladder x-ray
	7. HD	_____
14.21	8. _____	urinary tract infection
	9. cath	_____

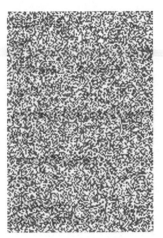

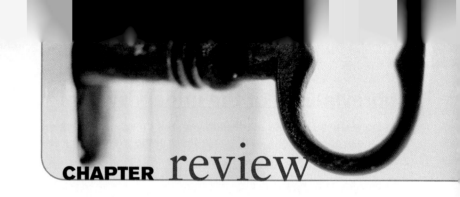

In this section, we will review all the word parts and medical terms from this chapter. As in earlier tables, the word roots are shown in **bold**.

Check each word part and medical term to be sure you understand the meaning. If any are not clear, please go back into the chapter and review that term. Then, complete the review exercises that follow.

[word parts **checklist**]

Prefixes

❏ a-, an-
❏ dia-
❏ en-
❏ epi-
❏ hypo-

Word Roots/Combining Vowels

❏ **albumin**/o
❏ **azot**/o
❏ **blast**/o
❏ **cyst**/o
❏ **glomerul**/o

❏ **gluc**/o, **glyc**/o, **glycos**/o
❏ **hydr**/o
❏ **keton**/o
❏ **lith**/o
❏ **meat**/o
❏ **nephr**/o
❏ **noct**/i
❏ **olig**/o
❏ **py**/o
❏ **pyel**/o
❏ **ren**/o
❏ **spadias**/o
❏ **tom**/o

❏ **ureter**/o
❏ **urethr**/o
❏ **urin**/o, **ur**/o
❏ **vesic**/o

Suffixes

❏ -cele
❏ -ptosis
❏ -tripsy
❏ -trophy
❏ -uresis
❏ -uria

[medical terminology **checklist**]

❏ **albumin**uria
❏ an**ur**esis
❏ an**ur**ia
❏ **azot**emia
❏ **bacter**iuria
❏ blood urea nitrogen (BUN)
❏ Bowman's capsule (BC)
❏ catheter (cath)
❏ catheterization (cath)
❏ creatinine
❏ **cyst**ectomy
❏ **cyst**itis
❏ **cyst**ocele
❏ **cyst**ogram
❏ **cyst**ography
❏ **cyst**olith
❏ **cyst**olithotomy
❏ **cyst**oplasty
❏ **cyst**opyelography
❏ **cyst**opyelogram

❏ **cyst**orrhaphy
❏ **cyst**oscope
❏ **cyst**oscopy
❏ **cyst**ostomy
❏ **cyst**oureterogram
❏ **cyst**oureterography
❏ di**ur**esis
❏ dys**ur**ia
❏ en**ur**esis
❏ external **urin**ary orifice
❏ fulguration
❏ **glomerul**o**nephr**itis
❏ **glomerul**us
❏ **glycos**uria
❏ **hemat**uria
❏ **hem**odialysis (HD)
❏ hilum
❏ **hydr**o**nephr**osis
❏ intravenous **pyel**ogram (IVP)
❏ **keton**uria

❏ kidney
❏ kidney, ureter, and bladder x-ray (KUB)
❏ **lith**otripsy
❏ **meat**oscope
❏ **meat**oscopy
❏ **meat**otomy
❏ **nephr**ectomy
❏ **nephr**itis
❏ **nephr**o**blast**oma
❏ **nephr**ogram
❏ **nephr**ography
❏ **nephr**ohypertrophy
❏ **nephr**o**lith**iasis
❏ **nephr**o**lysis**
❏ **nephr**oma
❏ **nephr**omegaly
❏ **nephr**on
❏ **nephr**oplexy
❏ **nephr**optosis

❑ **nephr**oscope
❑ **nephr**oscopy
❑ **nephr**o**son**ography
❑ **nephr**ostomy
❑ **nephr**o**tom**ogram
❑ **nephr**o**tom**ography
❑ **noct**uria
❑ **olig**uria
❑ **periton**eal dia**lys**is
❑ **poly**uria
❑ **protein**uria
❑ **pyel**i**thot**omy
❑ **pyel**itis
❑ **pyel**ogram
❑ **pyel**onephritis
❑ **pyel**oplasty
❑ **pyel**ostomy
❑ **py**uria
❑ **ren**al capsule

❑ **ren**al cortex
❑ **ren**al medulla
❑ **ren**al pelvis
❑ **ren**al transplant
❑ **ren**al tubule
❑ **ren**ogram
❑ **ren**ography
❑ retrograde **pyel**ogram (RP)
❑ specific gravity (SG)
❑ trigone
❑ **ur**emia
❑ **ur**eter
❑ **ureter**ectomy
❑ **ureter**itis
❑ **ureter**ocele
❑ **ureter**o**lith**iasis
❑ **ureter**ostenosis
❑ **ureter**ostomy
❑ **ureter**otomy

❑ **urethr**a
❑ **urethr**o**cystitis**
❑ **urethr**opexy
❑ **urethr**oplasty
❑ **urethr**oscopy
❑ **urethr**ostomy
❑ **urethr**otomy
❑ **urin**alysis (UA)
❑ **urin**ary bladder
❑ **urin**ary catheterization
❑ **urin**ary endoscopy
❑ **urin**ary **meat**us
❑ **urin**ary tract infection (UTI)
❑ **urin**e
❑ **urin**ometer
❑ **vesic**o**urethr**al suspension
❑ voiding **cyst**o**urethr**ogram (VCUG)

[show what **you know!**]

BREAK IT DOWN!

Analyze and separate each term into its word parts by labeling each word part using p = prefix, r = root, cv = combining vowel, and s = suffix.

			r cv s ur/o/logy
Example:	1.	urology	
	2.	nephrologist	_____
	3.	albuminuria	_____
	4.	anuria	_____
	5.	azotemia	_____
	6.	dysuria	_____
	7.	enuresis	_____
	8.	hematuria	_____
	9.	cystitis	_____
	10.	glomerulonephritis	_____
	11.	nephrolithiasis	_____
	12.	uterostenosis	_____
	13.	urethrocystitis	_____
	14.	cystectomy	_____
	15.	meatotomy	_____
	16.	nephroplexy	_____
	17.	pyelostomy	_____

18. ureterotomy _____

19. urethroplasty _____

20. urethrotomy _____

21. vesicourethral _____

22. cystopyelography _____

23. cystoureterogram _____

24. hemodialysis _____

25. nephrography _____

26. pyelogram _____

27. renography _____

28. meatoscope _____

WORD BUILDING

Construct or recall medical terms from the following meanings.

Example:

1. inability to pass urine _____ anuresis _____

2. absence of urine _____

3. presence of bacteria in the urine _____

4. presence of a stone in the bladder _____

5. inflammation of a kidney _____

6. excess of urea in the blood _____

7. protrusion of a ureter _____

8. involuntary discharge of urine _____

9. presence of stones in the kidney _____

10. infection of the urinary tract _____

11. fixation of an abnormally mobile kidney _____

12. surgical creation of an opening into the renal pelvis _____

13. surgical repair of the urethra _____

14. incision into the ureter wall _____

15. x-ray image of the urinary bladder _____

16. x-ray technique imaging a kidney _____

17. ultrasound technique imaging a kidney _____

18. x-ray image of the renal pelvis with iodine _____

19. endoscopy examining the urinary meatus _____

20. an endoscope modified to view a kidney _____

21. lab test measuring urea in the blood _____

22. instrument measuring water concentration in urine _____

23. urine test that includes multiple parameters _____

24. insertion of a flexible tube to drain urine _____

CASE STUDIES

Fill in the blanks with the correct terms.

1. A 45-year-old male was admitted to the hospital after presenting himself to the emergency department in acute distress. He complained of intermittent pain in the left posterior lumbar region, radiating to the left flank. He also complained of pain and difficulty in voiding, a symptom known as (a) _____, with the sensation of the need to void at night, or (b) _____, that interrupts his sleep. A generalized lab test of his urine sample, or (c) _____, revealed no abnormalities. A review of his family history revealed stones in the renal pelvis, called (d) _____ _____, and in the ureter, or (e) _____. The attending physican referred the patient to (f) _____. The specialist in treating urinary disorders, or (g) _____, immediately prepared the patient for diagnostics that included an x-ray technique that images the renal pelvis with a contrast medium injected into the (h) _____, known as a (i) _____ _____, followed with an endoscopic evaluation of the kidney called a (j) _____. Both exams revealed the presence of stones in the renal pelvis, or (k) _____ _____. The stones were pulverized successfully using the extracorporeal (l) _____ procedure, and passed the next day.

2. A 60-year-old female was admitted to urology by her general practitioner following a physical exam that included blood tests revealing abnormally high levels of urea in the blood. A generalized test of urine composition, or (m) _____, revealed elevated levels of albumin, a symptom known as (n) _____, and the presence of red blood cells in the urine, or (o) _____. Following diagnostics exams that included an x-ray technique evaluating the urinary bladder and renal pelvis, or (p) _____; an x-ray technique imaging the kidney by sections called (q) _____; and an endoscopic evaluation of the kidney known as (r) _____, the attending physician concluded a diagnosis of enlargement of the left kidney, or (s) _____, caused by multiple polyps, or (t) _____ _____, which had resulted in inflammation of the renal pelvis and nephrons, or (u) _____ and renal failure. Artificial filtration of the blood, or (v) _____, was ordered, due to a growing insufficiency of the right kidney in addition. Surgical removal of the left kidney was scheduled immediately and the patient was placed on a waiting list for a replacement kidney as a (w) _____ _____.

[piece it all **together!**]

CROSSWORD

From the chapter material, fill in the crossword puzzle with answers to the following clues.

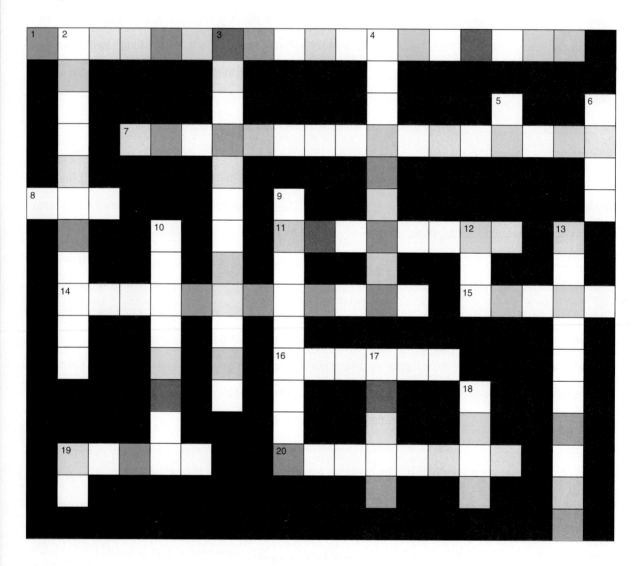

ACROSS

1. Inflammation of the glomeruli within a kidney. (Find puzzle piece 14.6)
7. Procedure that takes x-rays of the bladder and renal pelvis. (Find puzzle piece 14.16)
8. Abbreviation for an infection of the urinary tract. (Find puzzle piece 14.21)
11. If it occurs at night, it is commonly called "bed-wetting." (Find puzzle piece 14.3)
14. Removal of a stone within the renal pelvis. (Find puzzle piece 14.13)
15. A word root with combining vowel that means "renal pelvis." (Find puzzle piece 14.1)
16. Too much urea in the blood. (Find puzzle piece 14.7)
19. Pertaining to the kidneys. (Find puzzle piece 14.10)
20. High nitrogenous compounds in the blood. (Find puzzle piece 14.2)

DOWN

2. Procedure that crushes stones. (Find puzzle piece 14.12)

3. A treatment that provides an alternate exit route for urine. (Find puzzle piece 14.14)

4. An x-ray image of the renal pelvis. (Find puzzle piece 14.15)

5. Abbreviation for urinalysis. (Find puzzle piece 14.18)

6. The prefix in the term hypospadias. (Find puzzle piece 14.8)

9. Excessive ketone bodies in the urine. (Find puzzle piece 14.5)

10. The symptom of excessive urination. (Find puzzle piece 14.4)

12. Abbreviation for a treatment where iodine is injected to highlight this kidney x-ray. (Find puzzle piece 14.20)

13. A kidney with multiple polyps. (Find puzzle piece 14.9)

17. A word root and combining vowel that means "opening." (Find puzzle piece 14.17)

18. Literally "to empty." it is a synonym for micturition. (Find puzzle piece 14.11)

19. An abbreviation for an x-ray image of a kidney that is taken from an opposite direction. (Find puzzle piece 14.19)

WORD UNSCRAMBLE

From the completed crossword puzzle, unscramble:

1. All of the letters that appear in **red** squares ☐ __ __ __ __

   Clue: A fluid that is normally clear and yellowish, pH about 6.2

2. All of the letters that appear in **purple** squares ☐ __ __ __ __ __ __ __

   Clue: Image of a kidney from a nuclear medicine procedure

3. All of the letters that appear in **peach** squares __ __ __ __ ☐ __ __ __ __

   Clue: X-ray image of the urinary bladder

4. All of the letters that appear in **blue** squares __ __ __ __ __ __ __ ☐ __ __ __ __

   Clue: A procedure that artificially filters blood

5. All of the letters that appear in **yellow** squares __ __ __ __ __ ☐ __ __

   Clue: A tumor that arises from a kidney

6. All of the letters that appear in **green** squares __ __ __ ☐ __ __ __ __

   Clue: Reduced urination

7. All of the letters that appear in **pink** squares __ ☐ __ __ __ __ __ __ __

   Clue: Is often treated with lithotripsy

Now write down each of the letters that are boxed and unscramble them to find the hidden medical term of the urinary system: __ __ __ __ __ __ __.

MEDmedia **wrap-up**

www.prenhall.com/wingerd
Before you go on to the next chapter, take advantage of the free CD-ROM and study guide website that accompany this book. Simply load the CD-ROM for additional activities, games, animations, videos, and quizzes linked to this chapter. Then visit www.prenhall.com/wingerd for even more!

CHAPTER
15

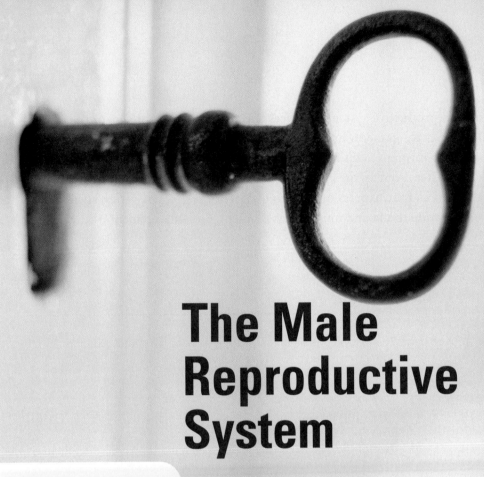

The Male Reproductive System

LEARNING OBJECTIVES

After completing this chapter, you will be able to:

- Define and spell the word parts used to create terms for the male reproductive system

- Identify the major organs of the male reproductive system and describe their structure and function

- Break down and define common medical terms used for symptoms, diseases, disorders, procedures, treatments, and devices associated with the male reproductive system

- Build medical terms from the word parts associated with the male reproductive system

- Pronounce and spell common medical terms associated with the male reproductive system

MEDmedia

www.prenhall.com/wingerd

Enhance your study with the power of multimedia! Each chapter of this book links to activities, games, animations, videos, and quizzes that you'll find on your CD-ROM. Plus, you can click on www.prenhall.com/wingerd, to find a free chapter-specific companion website that's loaded with additional practice and resources.

CD-ROM
- Audio Glossary
- Exercises & Activities
- Flashcard Generator
- Animations
- Videos

 Companion Website
- Exercises & Activities
- Audio Glossary
- Drug Updates
- Current News Update

A secure distance learning course is available at www.prenhall.com/onekey.

The male reproductive system produces the sex cells, or gametes, of the male. The male gametes are called spermatozoa, or sperm cells. The male system also sustains and transports the sperm cells. In addition, the male reproductive system secretes the hormone testosterone, which regulates sperm cell production and the expression of secondary sexual characteristics, such as hair distribution, bone and muscle development, and enlargement of the larynx.

word parts focus

Let's look at word parts. The following table contains a list of word parts that when combined build many of the terms of the male reproductive system.

PREFIX	DEFINITION	PREFIX	DEFINITION
im-	not	trans-	through, across, beyond

WORD ROOT	DEFINITION	WORD ROOT	DEFINITION
andr	male	semin	seed, sperm
balan	glans penis	sperm, spermat	seed, sperm
epididym	epididymis	test, testicul	testis or testicle
orch, orchid, orchi	testis or testicle	vas	vessel, duct
pen	penis	vesicul	vesicle (as in seminal vesicle)
prostat	prostate gland		

> **[FYI]**
>
> **Orchi/o**
> The combining form *orchi/o* is derived from the Greek word for testis. Early Greek scholars noted the resemblance of a testis to the bulb of the orchid plant, which shares the root word. Due to this resemblance, they believed the orchid bulb had medicinal value and used it to treat diseases of the testes, including sterility.

SUFFIX	DEFINITION	SUFFIX	DEFINITION
-pexy	surgical fixation	-rrhea	excessive discharge

SELF QUIZ 15.1

Review the word parts of male reproductive system terminology by working carefully through the exercises that follow. Soon, we will apply this new information to build medical terms.

A. Provide the definition of the following prefixes and suffixes.

1. im- _____

2. trans- _____

3. -pexy _____

4. -rrhea _____

B. Provide the word root for each of the following terms.

1. epididymus _____

2. testis _____

3. glans penis _____

4. prostate gland _____

5. male _____

6. sperm _____

7. vessel or duct _____

8. vesicle _____

9. penis _____

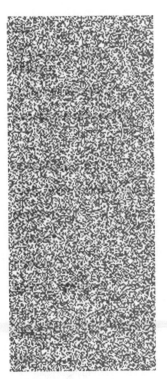

[anatomy and physiology overview]

A properly functioning male reproductive system has the capability to transmit sperm cells to a female during sexual intercourse, or **coitus,** which is Latin for *a sexual union.* The release of sperm cells is called **ejaculation,** and it usually accompanies **sexual climax,** or **orgasm.**

The primary organs of the male reproductive system are the paired **testes,** which produce sperm cells and secrete testosterone (Figure 15.1⋮⋮⋮). Other organs either transport the sperm cells or produce substances that support the sperm. The organs that transport sperm are tubules that include the **epididymis, vas deferens,** and **urethra,** and the male glands that provide supportive secretions are the **seminal vesicles,** the **prostate gland,** and the **bulbourethral glands.**

The Testes

The **testes** (singular form is **testis**) are the male gonads, and they produce the male gametes (sperm cells). They are paired, oval organs located within a skin-covered sac known as the **scrotum** (Figure 15.1). The scrotum hangs below the pelvic wall, enclosing each testis within a small compartment. The testes initially develop within the pelvic cavity, then descend into the scrotum shortly before birth. The scrotum provides an environment that is more favorable to sperm development because it has a cooler temperature than the 98°F of the pelvic cavity.

[FYI]

Testis
The Latin word *testis* means *a witness* or *one who testifies.* In Roman courts, no man was allowed to act as a witness unless he could prove his testes were intact. He was required to take an oath with his hand on his testes.

enrichment module **enrichment mod**

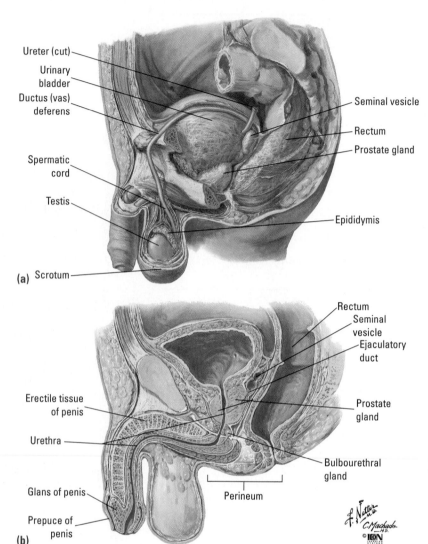

Ureter (cut)
Urinary bladder
Ductus (vas) deferens
Spermatic cord
Testis
(a) Scrotum

Seminal vesicle
Rectum
Prostate gland
Epididymis

Rectum
Seminal vesicle
Ejaculatory duct

Erectile tissue of penis
Urethra
Glans of penis
Prepuce of penis
(b)

Prostate gland
Bulbourethral gland
Perineum

Figure 15.1 ::::

Male reproductive organs.
(a) Partial section through the pelvic cavity.
(b) Complete section through the pelvic cavity.
Source: Icon Learning Systems.

Male Tubules

The testes are each composed of about 900 small, tightly coiled tubules, which are known as **seminiferous tubules** and are the sites of sperm cell production (Figure 15.2::::). The process of sperm cell production is known as **spermatogenesis.** Clusters of cells between the seminiferous tubules, called **interstitial cells,** produce testosterone. Both sperm cell production and testosterone production begin at puberty, under the direction of the pituitary gland.

The male tubules transport sperm cells from the testes to the outside environment. They begin when the seminiferous tubules within each testis merge to form larger tubules, which eventually merge again to form a single tubule. The tubule emerges from the testis as the **ductus epididymidis,** which coils to form an elongated structure attached to the posterior side of the testis called the **epididymis** (Figures 15.1 and 15.2)

The ductus epididymidis terminates when it unites with a thick-walled tubule, the **vas deferens** (Figure 15.2). Also known as the **ductus deferens** or **seminal duct,** the wall of the vas deferens includes smooth muscle, enabling the tube to form peristaltic waves that push the sperm along their route. A vas deferens extends from each testis upward through the scrotum, emerging from it to enter the pelvic cavity. The route through the scrotum is joined by arteries, veins, and nerves and wrapped by a layer of connective tissue, forming the **spermatic cord.** After entering

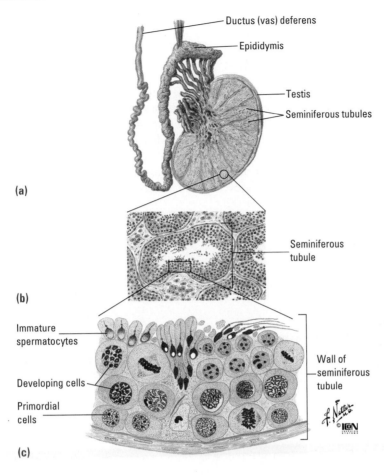

(a)

(b)

Immature spermatocytes

Developing cells

Primordial cells

(c)

Ductus (vas) deferens

Epididymis

Testis

Seminiferous tubules

Seminiferous tubule

Wall of seminiferous tubule

Figure 15.2 ::::

The testis.

(a) A sectioned testis reveals the coiled seminferous tubules. Note that the tubules unite to form the coiled tube within the epididymus, which then enlarges to form the ductus (vas) deferens.
(b) A magnified cross section through a testis shows a seminiferous tubule (center).
(c) Under high magnification, the wall of a seminiferous tubule reveals several cell layers. Sperm cells are produced from meiotic divisions of the outer cells.
Source: Icon Learning Systems.

the pelvic cavity, the two vas deferens pass through a pair of glands, the **seminal vesicles,** to form the **ejaculatory duct** before uniting with the next tubule, the **urethra** (Figure 15.1).

The male urethra is the final tubule, extending from the bladder to its opening at the **urinary meatus** (or external urethral orifice). As it emerges from the bladder, it receives the two vas deferens. The urethra then passes through the **prostate gland** before entering the **penis.** At the base of the penis, the urethra receives secretions from another pair of glands, called **bulbourethral glands.**

Male Glands

The male glands include the seminal vesicles, the prostate gland, and the bulbourethral glands (Figure 15.1). The seminal vesicles are a pair of sac-like structures at the base of the urinary bladder that secrete fluids into the vas deferens. The prostate gland is a single, walnut-sized gland that surrounds the urethra near its emergence from the bladder and releases secretions directly into the urethra. The paired bulbourethral glands are small, pea-shaped glands located at the base of the penis, which also release secretions into the urethra.

Together, the male glands contribute to the formation of **semen,** which is released during ejaculation. Semen normally includes sperm cells, fluid from the seminal vesicles that is rich in sugar (fructose) for nourishing sperm cells, a thick, milky, alkaline fluid released by the prostate gland, and a clear mucus released by the bulbourethral glands.

[thinking critically!]

If the vas deferens were cut, what do you suppose would happen to the sperm cells during an ejaculation?

enrichment module enrichment module **enrichment module** enrichment module **enrichment module** enrichment module **enrichment module** *enrichment module* enrichment module *enrichment module* enrichment module *enrichment module* enrichment module *enrichment module* enrichment module *enrichment module* enrichment modu

Male External Genitals

The external organs, or **external genitalia,** of the male are the scrotum and the penis. The scrotum is a skin-covered sac that hangs below the pelvic cavity wall and contains the testes.

The penis is an external cylindrical organ that contains the distal part of the urethra (Figure 15.3 ::::). The penis also contains three cylindrical masses of erectile tissue that enable it to enlarge and harden during the physiological response known as erection. An erection enables the penis to be inserted into the female vagina during sexual intercourse. The distal end of the penis is soft and spongy, and is called the **glans penis.** A fold of skin covers most or all of the glans penis, and is known as the **prepuce,** or foreskin. The prepuce may be removed by an elective surgical procedure called a **circumcision,** usually soon after birth.

[**thinking critically!**]

In a fertile male, what glands contribute to the formation of semen?

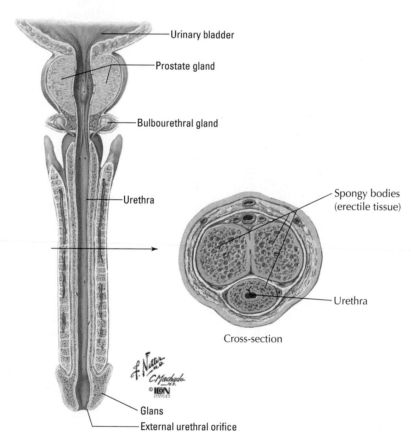

Figure 15.3 ::::

The penis.
A longitudinal section (left) through a penis and its associated structures, and a cross section (right) through the penis at the shaft.
Source: Icon Learning Systems.

getting to the root of it | anatomy and physiology terms

Many of the anatomy and physiology terms are formed from roots that are used to construct the more complex medical terms of the male reproductive system, including symptoms, diseases, and treatments. In this section, we will review the terms that describe the structure and function of the male reproductive system *in relation to their word roots,* which are shown in **bold.**

Study the word roots and terms in this list and complete the review exercises that follow.

Word Root (Meaning)	Terms Formed from the Word Root (Pronunciation)	Definition
epididym (epididymis)	**epididym**is (ep ih DID ih miss)	an elongated organ on the posterior surface of each testis and composed of a single, tightly coiled tubule that transports sperm from the testis to the vas deferens; the literal meaning is "upon a twin," due to its location on each of the two testes, and the plural form is epididymides (ep ih did ih MY des)
pen (penis)	**pen**is (PEE niss)	the male external genital organ that conveys semen to the female during sexual intercourse; it consists of the glans penis, which is covered by the prepuce, and a shaft
prostat (prostate gland)	**prostat**e gland (PROSS tayt)	a walnut-sized gland that surrounds the urethra as it emerges from the urinary bladder, it secretes a milky alkaline fluid that contributes to semen
semin (seed)	**semen** (SEE men)	the ejaculatory fluid, which normally consists of sperm cells and secretions from the seminal vesicles, prostate gland, and bulbourethral glands
	seminiferous tubules (SEM ih NIF er uss TOO byoolz)	approximately 900 tightly coiled tubules, forming the substance of the testes, with walls made up of cells that produce sperm cells by the process of spermatogenesis
sperm, spermat (seed)	**sperm** cells	male gametes, which are produced within the seminiferous tubules of the testes; also called **sperm**atozoon (singular) or **sperm**atozoa (plural)
	spermatic cord (sper MAT ik KORD)	a combination of tissues extending from each testis upward through the scrotum, which includes a vas deferens, arteries, veins, and nerves that are enclosed within a connective tissue covering
test (testis, testicle)	**test**is (TESS tiss)	the male gonad, also called **test**icle, which contains cells that undergo spermatogenesis to produce sperm cells and other cells that secrete testosterone; the plural form is **test**es
	testosterone (tess TOSS ter ohn)	the male sex hormone, which is produced by interstitial cells within the testes
vas (vessel, duct)	**vas** deferens (VAS DEFF er enz)	the male tubule that conveys sperm cells from the epididymis to the urethra; also called the ductus deferens or seminal duct
vesicul (vesicle)	seminal **vesicl**es (SEM ih nal VESS ih klz)	paired glands at the base of the urinary bladder that secrete fluid into the vas deferens, which contributes to semen

OTHER IMPORTANT TERMS
The terms in this table are related to the structure and function of the male reproductive system, but are not built from multiple word roots.

bulbourethral glands (BUHL boh yoo REE thral)	paired, pea-shaped glands at the base of the penis that contribute a mucus product to semen; also called Cowper's glands
ejaculation (ee JAK yoo LAY shun)	the release of semen during sexual climax, or orgasm
ejaculatory duct (ee JAK yoo lah tor ee)	the duct formed by the union of the vas deferens and the seminal vesicle ducts

perineum (pair ih NEE um)	the external region between the scrotum and anus in the male (and between the vulva and anus in the female)
scrotum (SKROH tum)	a skin-covered pouch that hangs below the wall of the pelvic cavity, containing the two testes and spermatic cords

SELF QUIZ 15.2

SAY IT—SPELL IT!

Review the terms of the male reproductive system by speaking the phonetic pronunciations out loud, then writing the correct spelling of the term.

> **Success Hint:** Once you get to the crossword puzzle at the end of the chapter, remember to check back here for clues! Your clues are indicated by the puzzle icon.

1. BUHL boh yoo REE thral _____

2. ee JAK yoo LAY shun _____

3. ep ih DID ih miss _____

4. PEE niss _____

5. pair ih NEE um _____

6. PROSS tayt _____

7. SKROH tum _____

8. SEE men _____

9. SEM ih nal   VESS ih klz _____

10. SEM ih NIF er uss TOO byoolz _____

11. sper MAT ik   KORD _____

12. TESS tiss _____

13. tess TOSS ter ohn _____

14. VAS   DEF er enz _____

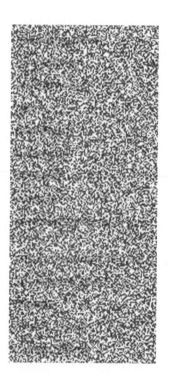

MATCH IT!

Match the term on the left with the correct definition on the right.

_____ 1. testis   a. contains the ductus epididymidis

_____ 2. spermatic cord   b. also called spermatozoa

_____ 3. seminiferous tubules   c. forms part of the spermatic cord

_____ 4. testosterone   d. a male external genital organ

_____ 5. sperm cells   e. the distal end of the penis

_____ 6. scrotum   f. a gland that surrounds the urethra

_____ 7. epididymis   g. a fold of skin removed during a circumcision

_____ 8. vas deferens   h. carries urine and semen

_____ 9. urethra   i. coiled tubules that produce sperm cells

_____ 10. seminal vesicles   j. the male sex hormone

_____ 11. prostate gland   k. pea-sized glands that secrete mucus

_____ 12. bulbourethral glands   l. a cord of tissues within the scrotum

_____ 13. glans penis   m. the male gonad

_____ 14. prepuce   n. a pair of glands that secrete sugar-rich fluid

FILL IT IN!

Fill in the blanks with the correct terms.

1. The male gonads are the paired _____, which are located within the skin-covered _____. During the process of spermatogenesis, _____ _____ are produced by cells located within the walls of the _____ _____. The male sex hormone, called _____, is produced by cells between the tubules.

2. Sperm cells are transported by a series of tubules. The elongated organ that carries sperm from each testis is called the _____, which consists of a single, coiled tubule. From here, sperm enters the

15.1   _____ _____, which is enclosed within the

15.2   cord of tissue known as the _____ _____ as it passes through the scrotum. After entering the pelvic cavity, it forms the _____ _____ before it unites with the _____.

15.3

3. The male glands that are the first to contribute to the ejaculatory fluid, known as

   _____, secrete a fluid rich in sugar. The glands are the paired

   _____ _____. Soon after the urethra

   emerges from the bladder, it is surrounded by a walnut-sized gland called the

   _____ _____, which secretes a milky alkaline

   fluid. At the base of the penis are the paired _____

   _____, which secrete a clear mucus.

4. The male external genital organ that is cylindrical is the _____.

   Its distal end is called the _____ _____, which

   is covered by a fold of skin called the _____.

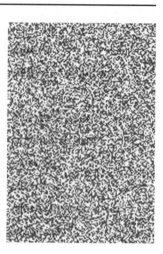

[medical terms of the

male reproductive system]

Because the urethra is responsible for transporting both urine and semen, diseases of the male reproductive system are usually treated within the field of **urology** by an **urologist.** Some large hospitals may also include an area that specializes in **reproductive medicine,** where sexual function disorders may receive special treatment.

Because the body's interior connects to the exterior by way of the urinary meatus, the urinary tract is subject to infections that might travel from the meatus into the body's interior. Although a protective mucous membrane lines the meatus and the urethra, bacteria and viruses may still gain entry into the bloodstream by way of breaks in the mucosal lining. Once established, these pathogens may spread throughout the body. **Sexually transmitted diseases (STDs),** or venereal diseases, often enter the body this way. STDs are usually acquired during intimate physical contact that occurs during coitus or other sexual activities. They may be caused by a variety of viruses, bacteria, and protozoans, the most common of which are described in this chapter. In addition to infections, the male reproductive system is afflicted with other diseases, including tumors and inherited disorders.

Diseases of the male reproductive system are often diagnosed during a physical examination. For example, most STDs diseases receive an initial diagnosis during a simple office exam, and **benign prostatic hyperplasia** is usually diagnosed by a routine rectal exam. The disorders that require confirmation or an internal evaluation may be assessed by the noninvasive procedures of MRI, CAT scan, or ultrasound imaging.

[**thinking critically!**]

Why are STDs usually obtained through sexual intercourse?

let's construct terms!

In this section, we will assemble all of the word parts to construct medical terminology related to the male reproductive system. Abbreviations are used to indicate each word part: **p** = prefix, **r** = root, **cv** = combining vowel, and **s** = suffix. Recall from chapter one that the addition of a combining vowel to the word root creates the combining form for the term. Note that some terms are not constructed from word parts, but they are included here to expand your vocabulary.

The medical terms of the male reproductive system are listed in the following three sections:

- Symptoms and Signs
- Diseases and Disorders
- Treatments, Procedures, and Devices

Each section is followed by review exercises. Study the lists in these tables and complete the review exercises that follow.

Symptoms and Signs

WORD PARTS (WHEN APPLICABLE)			TERM	DEFINITION
Part	Type	Meaning		
a- sperm -ia	p r s	without seed, sperm condition of	**aspermia** (ah SPER mee ah)	inability to produce or ejaculate sperm, as a symptom of male infertility
a- zo/o sperm -ia	p r/cv r s	without animal seed, sperm condition of	**azoospermia** (AY zoh oh SPER mee ah)	absence of living sperm in semen, which is a sign of male infertility
balan/o -rrhea	r/cv s	glans penis excessive discharge	**balanorrhea** (BALL ah noh REE ah)	excessive discharge from the glans penis
			chancres (SHANG kerz)	small ulcers on the skin, a symptom of the sexually transmitted disease **syphilis**
olig/o sperm -ia	r/cv r s	few in number seed, sperm condition of	**oligospermia** (all ih goh SPER mee ah)	abnormally low sperm count, as a sign of male infertility
			papillomas (pap ih LOH mahz)	wart-like lesions on the skin and mucous membranes, a sign of the sexually transmitted **human papilloma virus;** commonly known as genital warts
proct -itis	r s	anus inflammation	**proctitis** (prok TYE tiss)	inflammation of the rectal area, a symptom of the sexually transmitted diseases **chlamydia** and **trichomoniasis**
prostat/o -rrhea	r/cv s	prostate gland excessive discharge	**prostatorrhea** (PROSS tah toh REE ah)	abnormal, excessive discharge from the prostate gland
urethr -itis	r s	urethra inflammation	**urethritis** (yoo ree THRYE tiss)	inflammation of the urethra, a symptom of the sexually transmitted diseases **chlamydia** and **trichomoniasis**

SELF QUIZ 15.3

SAY IT—SPELL IT!

Review the terms of the male reproductive system by speaking the phonetic pronunciation guides out loud, then writing in the correct spelling of the term.

> **Success Hint:** Use the audio glossary on the CD and CW for additional help with pronunciation of these terms.

1. AY zoh oh SPER mee ah _____

2. BALL ah noh REE ah _____

3. PROSS tah toh REE ah _____

4. SHANG kerz _____

15.4   5. ah SPER mee ah _____

15.5   6. all ih goh SPER mee ah _____

7. yoo ree THRYE tiss _____

8. prok TYE tiss _____

9. pap ih LOH mahz _____

MATCH IT!

Match the term on the left with the correct definition on the right.

_____1. azoospermia   a. excessive discharge from the prostate gland

_____2. balanorrhea   b. absence of living sperm in semen

_____3. prostatorrhea   c. excessive discharge from the glans penis

_____4. proctitis   d. inflammation of the urethra

_____5. aspermia   e. inflammation of the rectal area

_____6. urethritis   f. inability to produce or ejaculate sperm

BREAK IT DOWN!

Analyze and separate each term into its word parts by labeling each word part using p = prefix, r = root, cv = combining vowel, and s = suffix.

1. azoospermia _____

2. balanorrhea _____

3. prostatorrhea _____

4. oligospermia _____

5. proctitis _____

WORD BUILDING

Construct or recall medical terms from the following meanings.

1. absence of living sperm in semen _____

2. excessive discharge from the glans penis _____

3. abnormal discharge from the prostate gland _____

4. wart-like lesion on the skin _____

5. abnormally low sperm count _____

6. inability to produce sperm _____

7. small ulcers on the skin _____

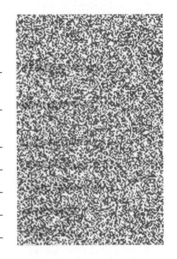

Diseases and Disorders

Part	Type	Meaning	TERM	DEFINITION
			acquired immunodeficiency syndrome (IM yoo noh dee FISH ehn see SIN drohm)	a syndrome caused by infection of the human immunodeficiency virus (**HIV**), mainly through the exchange of body fluids during sex or by the use of contaminated IV needles; abbreviated **AIDS**
andr/o	r/cv	male	**andropathy**	diseases that afflict only males
-pathy	s	disease	(an DROPP ah thee)	
an-	p	without, absence of	**anorchism** (an OR kizm)	absence of one or both testes
orch	r	testis		
-ism	s	condition of		
balan	r	glans penis	**balanitis**	inflammation of the glans penis
-itis	s	inflammation	(bal ah NYE tiss)	
benign	r	mild	**benign prostatic hyperplasia** (bee NINE pross TAT ik HIGH per PLAY zee ah)	nonmalignant, excessive growth of the prostate gland resulting in constriction of the urethra; symptoms include nocturia (nighttime urination), urinary retention, and a frequent need to void; also called benign prostatic hypertrophy; abbreviated **BPH** (Figure 15.4)
prostat	r	prostate gland		
-ic	s	pertaining to		
hyper-	p	excessive		
-plasia	s	shape, formation		
			chlamydia (klah MID ee ah)	the most common bacteria-caused STD in North America; symptoms include urethritis, proctitis, and inflammation of the eye's conjunctiva (Figure 15.5)
crypt	r	hidden	**cryptorchidism** (kript OR kid izm)	condition of an undescended testis; also called cryptorchism (kript OR kizm) (Figure 15.6)
orchid	r	testis		
-ism	s	condition of		

Cryptorchidism
Cryptorchidism is derived from the Greek word *kruptorkhos* which literally means *a condition of a hidden testis*. It is named this way because an undescended testis is in a location that is hidden from view.

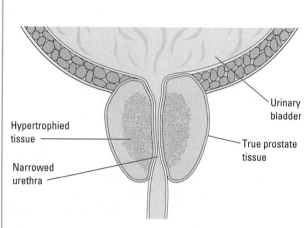

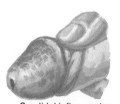

Candidal inflammation
of glans and prepuce

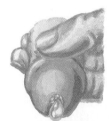

Urethral discharge of
chlamydial infection

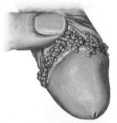

Papillomas
(genital warts)

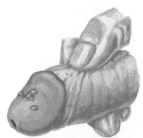

Marked edema and vesicle
formation in primary herpes

Figure 15.4 ::::

Benign prostatic hyperplasia.
The condition results when an inner capsule of nonfunctional
prostate tissue swells, pushing against the walls of the urethra to
cause a restriction of urine flow.
Source: Pearson Education.

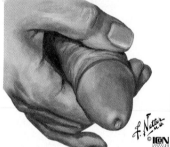

Urethral discharge of gonorrheal
infection

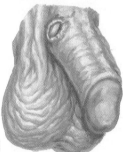

Syphilitic chancre of penile
shaft above level of condom
protection

Figure 15.5 ::::

Signs of sexually transmitted diseases.
Source: Icon Learning Systems.

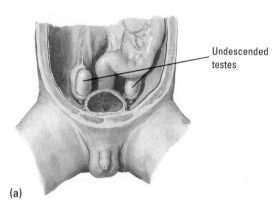

(a)

(b)

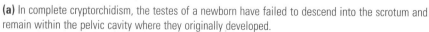

Figure 15.6 :::: **Cryptorchidism.**

(a) In complete cryptorchidism, the testes of a newborn have failed to descend into the scrotum and
remain within the pelvic cavity where they originally developed.
(b) A partial cryptorchidism of the left testis.
Source: Icon Learning Systems.

WORD PARTS (WHEN APPLICABLE)			TERM	DEFINITION
Part	**Type**	**Meaning**		
epididym	r	epididymus	**epididymitis**	inflammation of the epididymus
-itis	s	inflammation	(ep ih did ih MY tiss)	
			erectile dysfunction (ee REK tile diss FUNK shun)	inability to achieve or maintain an erection sufficient to perform sexual intercourse, also called impotency (IM poh ten see); abbreviated **ED**
			genital herpes (JENN ih tal HER peez)	the most common viral STD in North America, it is caused by the herpes simplex virus Type 2 (**HSV-2**) and is characterized by periodic outbreaks of ulcer-like lesions of the genital and anorectal skin and mucous membranes (Figure 15.5)
			gonorrhea (gahn oh REE ah)	an STD infection that is caused by the bacterium *Neisseria gonorrhea,* which produces ulcer-like lesions on the mucous membranes and skin of the genital region and is characterized by urethral discharge (Figure 15.5)
hepat	r	liver	**hepatitis B**	a viral STD, it causes inflammation of the liver and is
-itis	s	inflammation	(hepp ah TYE tiss)	transmitted through any body fluid; abbreviated **HBV**
			human papilloma virus (pap ih LOH ma)	a viral STD that causes wart-like lesions (papillomas, or genital warts) on the skin or mucous membranes of the genitals; lesions on the skin appear like cauliflower-shaped warts, and those on mucous membranes are flattened warts; abbreviated **HPV** (Figure 15.5)
hydr/o	r/cv	water	**hydrocele**	swelling of the scrotum caused by fluid
-cele	s	hernia, swelling	(HIGH droh seel)	accumulation (Figure 15.7 ⠿)

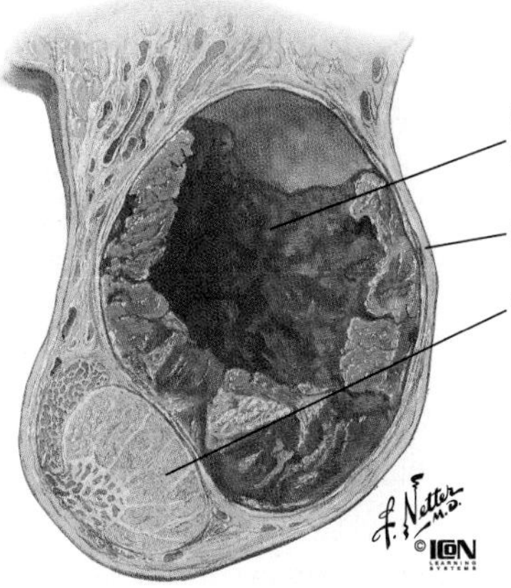

Fluid-filled cavity

Scrotum

Testis

Figure 15.7 ⠿

Hydrocele.
The condition is characterized by the accumulation of fluid within the scrotum.
Source: Icon Learning Systems.

			impotent (IM poh tent)	from the Latin word for *inability,* it refers to a male experiencing erectile dysfunction
orch/i	r/cv	testis	**orchiepididymitis**	inflammation of the testis and epididymis
epididym	r	epididymus	(OR kee EP ih	
-itis	s	inflammation	DID ih MY tiss)	
orch	r	testis	**orchitis**	inflammation of the testis; also known as **orchiditis**
-itis	s	inflammation	(or KYE tiss)	(or kih DYE tiss) or **testitis** (tess TYE tiss)

WORD PARTS (WHEN APPLICABLE)			TERM	DEFINITION
Part	Type	Meaning		
			Peyronie's disease (pay ROHN eez)	induration (hardness) of the erectile tissue within the penis, which can cause erectile dysfunction, and results in a curvature of the penis if the induration is asymmetric
			phimosis (fih MOH siss)	a congenital narrowing of the prepuce opening that prevents it from being drawn back over the glans penis, it can be corrected with circumcision (Figure 15.8::::); when the glans penis becomes strangulated and produces an emergency situation, the condition is often termed paraphimosis (PAR ah fih MOH siss)
			priapism (PRY ah pizm)	an abnormally persistent erection of the penis, often accompanied by pain and tenderness, usually caused by drug overdose
			prostate cancer (PROSS tayt KANN ser)	cancer of the prostate gland, which is often highly invasive and metastatic (Figure 15.9::::)

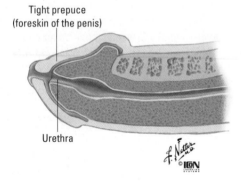

Figure 15.8 ::::

Phimosis. The condition is characterized by an abnormally tight fit of the prepuce over the glans as seen in this illustration of a sectioned penis. It is correctable with circumcision.
Source: Icon Learning Systems

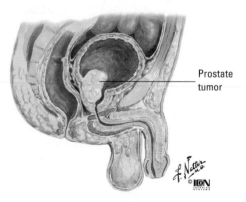

Figure 15.9 ::::

Prostate cancer. In this example, a large mass has grown into the urinary bladder. Prostate cancer is highly metastatic, sending tumor cells to the pelvic area and beyond, where they may form secondary tumor sites.
Source: Icon Learning Systems.

prostat -itis	r s	prostate gland inflammation	**prostatitis** (pross tah TYE tis)	inflammation of the prostate gland
prostat/o cyst -itis	r/cv r s	prostate gland bladder inflammation	**prostatocystitis** (PROSS tah toh siss TYE tiss)	inflammation of the prostate gland and urinary bladder
prostat/o lith	r/cv r	prostate gland stone	**prostatolith** (pross TAH toh lith)	stone in a duct of the prostate gland
prostat/o vesicul -itis	r/cv r s	prostate gland seminal vesicle inflammation	**prostatovesiculitis** (PROSS tah toh vess IK yoo LYE tiss)	inflammation of the prostate gland and seminal vesicles

WORD PARTS (WHEN APPLICABLE)			TERM	DEFINITION
Part	Type	Meaning		
spermat/o lys -is	r/cv r s	seed, sperm dissolution pertaining to	**spermatolysis** (sper mah TALL ih siss)	destruction of sperm by dissolution
			syphilis (SIFF ih liss)	an STD caused by a bacterium called a spirochete (*Treponaema pallidum*), which is transmitted by direct sexual contact and usually first expressed on the skin by red, painless papules that erode to form small ulcers known as **chancres** (Figure 15.5)

[FYI]

Syphilis

The word *syphilis* is derived from the name of a character in a 1530 poem by G. Fracastoro. *Syphilus* was the fictional main character who represented the first sufferer of this sexually transmitted venereal disease.

testicul -ar carcin -oma	r s r s	testis pertaining to cancer tumor	**testicular carcinoma** (tess TIK yoo ler kar sih NOH mah)	cancer originating from a testis, it occurs most often among the 20–29 year-old age group; the most common form is called **seminoma** (sem ih NOH mah), which arises from spermatogenic cells and metastasizes to nearby lymph nodes
testicul -ar	r s	testis pertaining to	**testicular torsion** (tess TIK yoo ler TOR shun)	a condition of a twisted spermatic cord that causes reduced blood flow to the testis; if not corrected immediately, the affected testis can be lost (Figure 15.10::::)
			trichomoniasis (TRIK oh moh NYE ah siss)	an STD caused by the protozoan *Trichomonas,* which infects the urethra and prostate gland to cause urethritis and prostatitis
varic/o -cele	r/cv s	dilated vein hernia, swelling	**varicocele** (VAIR ih koh seel)	abnormal dilation of the veins of the spermatic cord, caused by failure of the valves within the veins (Figure 15.11::::)

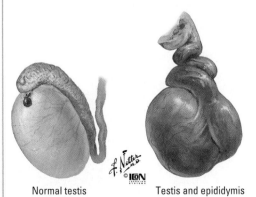

Normal testis and epididymis   Testis and epididymis with torsion

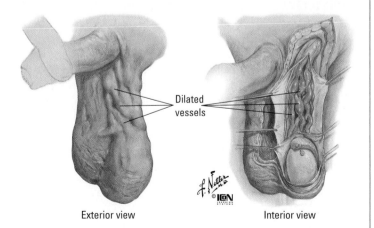

Dilated vessels

Exterior view   Interior view

Figure 15.10 ::::

Testicular torsion.

Source: Icon Learning Systems.

Figure 15.11 ::::

Varicocele. The dilation of veins within the spermatic cord are often visible through the wall of the scrotum.

Source: Icon Learning Systems.

disease focus | Enlarged Prostate

Throughout most of a man's life, the walnut-sized prostate gland produces a milky, alkaline fluid that is an important component of semen. However, usually after age 50, this small structure may become a primary cause of discomfort and, in some cases, can even develop into a life-threatening cancer.

For reasons not well understood, the prostate gland often increases in size as a man ages. In fact, over half of all men in their sixties suffer from an enlarged prostate condition called **benign prostatic hyperplasia** (**BPH**). In this condition, the enlarged gland presses against the urethra, which passes through the center of the prostate. The effects are similar to squeezing a piece of flexible plastic tubing in the center of your fist. Pressure from the prostrate pressing against the urethra leads to problems with urination, including a weakened or hesitant urine stream, leaking of urine, a sensation that the bladder is not completely emptied, and a need to get up several times a night to urinate.

Fortunately, men suffering the discomforts of BPH are not at increased risk for developing cancer, and treatment is usually quite effective. Since about 1980, the most common treatments involve the surgical removal of part of the prostate (**TURP**) or the insertion of small cuts along the neck of the urinary bladder and urethra to widen the urethra (**TUIP**). Both procedures are invasive and involve some risks. According to the American Medical Association, 400,000 such procedures have been performed each year in the United States since 1980. A less invasive technique is the use of microwave-produced heat to destroy unwanted prostate tissue (**TUMT**). However, this procedure may damage surrounding tissue and prostate tissue may grow back.

Recent advances in drug therapy are showing increased promise, particularly in a drug called Proscar, which has demonstrated an ability to stop further growth of the prostate, and in about 24 percent of the cases cause actual shrinkage.

Although the symptoms of BPH can be annoying, it is not life-threatening. However, cancer of the prostate is life-threatening and shares symptoms identical to BPH. Prostate cancer is second only to lung cancer as a deadly form of cancer in men, and in 2002 caused an estimated 39,000 deaths in the United States (American Cancer Society, 2002 published data). In past years, the high incidence of death has been largely due to late diagnosis.

Until recently, the only available technique for diagnosing prostate cancer was a **digital rectal exam** (**DRE**), during which a physician inserts a finger into the rectum and probes for any hard lumps that may indicate the presence of cancer. While this test can identify some malignancies, its accuracy depends on the presence of well-developed lumps that are usually detectable only after metastasis has already begun. During the past 20 years, this physical exam has been assisted by a blood test that detects the presence of a protein called **prostate-specific antigen** (**PSA**). PSA helps to liquefy semen and is normally produced in low levels by cells lining the prostate. Levels greater than four micrograms per liter are considered a possible risk factor that warrants further investigation. High levels of PSA in the blood are a relatively reliable indication of prostate cancer, justifying the need for additional confirmation, usually obtained by biopsy.

SELF QUIZ 15.4

SAY IT—SPELL IT!

Review the terms of the male reproductive system by speaking the phonetic pronunciation out loud, then writing the correct spelling of the term.

1. IM yoo noh dee FISH ehn see SIN drohm _____

2. an OR kizm _____

3. ee REK tile   diss FUNK shun _____

4. kript OR kid izm _____

5. tess TIK yoo ler   kar sih NOH mah _____

6. ep ih did ih MY tiss _____

7. fih MOH siss _____

8. PROSS tah toh siss TYE tiss _____

9. gahn oh REE ah _____

15.6

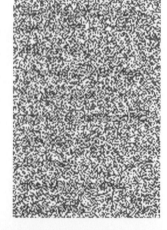

15.7   10. HIGH droh seel   _____

11. bee NINE   pross TAT ik
HIGH per PLAY zee ah   _____

12. PRY ah pizm   _____

13. PROSS tah toh vess IK yoo LYE tiss _____

14. VAIR ih koh seel   _____

15. pay ROHN eez   _____

16. klah MID ee ah   _____

17. OR kee EP ih DID ih MY tiss   _____

18. sper mah TALL ih siss   _____

19. SIFF ih liss   _____

MATCH IT!

Match the term on the left with the correct definition on the right.

_____ 1. andropathy

_____ 2. anorchism

_____ 3. erectile disfunction

_____ 4. balanitis

_____ 5. Peyronie's disease

_____ 6. benign prostatic
hyperplasia

_____ 7. cryptorchidism

_____ 8. epididymitis

_____ 9. hydrocele

_____10. oligospermia

_____11. varicocele

_____12. orchiepididymitis

_____13. testitis

_____14. prostatitis

_____15. testicular torsion

_____16. prostatovesiculitis

a. swelling of the scrotum

b. condition of an undescended testis

c. inflammation of the prostate gland

d. any disease that afflicts only males

e. deficient numbers of sperm

f. a twisted spermatic cord

g. same as orchiditis

h. absence of one or both testes

i. inflammation of a testis and epididymus

j. dilation of the veins of the spermatic cord

k. swollen prostate gland and seminal vesicles

l. inability to achieve and maintain an erection

m. nonmalignant growth of the prostate gland

n. inflammation of the glans penis

o. induration of erectile tissue within the penis

p. inflammation of the epididymus

BREAK IT DOWN!

**Analyze and separate each term into its word parts, labeling each word part
using p = prefix, r = root, cv = combining vowel, and s = suffix.**

1. andropathy   _____

2. anorchism   _____

3. cryptorchidism

4. epididymitis _____

5. orchiepididymitis _____

6. prostatitis _____

7. prostatovesiculitis _____

WORD BUILDING

Construct or recall medical terms from the following meanings.

1. narrowed opening of the prepuce _____

2. abnormally persistent erection _____

3. cancer of the gland surrounding the urethra _____

4. a malignancy arising from a testis _____

5. a condition in which a male cannot achieve an erection _____

6. symptoms include lesions called chancres _____

7. caused by herpes simplex virus Type II _____

8. symptoms include urethral discharge _____

9. caused by a sexually transmitted protozoan _____

FILL IT IN!

Fill in the blanks with the correct terms.

1. An inability to achieve and maintain an erection is known as _____ _____, or impotency. An individual who experiences this condition is recognized as being _____. One cause of this condition is due to the induration of erectile tissue, a disorder known as _____ disease.

2. A condition characterized by a reduced opening of the prepuce is called _____.

3. _____ is an abnormally persistent state of erection, which leads to pain and discomfort.

4. The two most common cancers that are androgenic (arise from male tissues) include _____ _____, which is a malignant form of prostatic hyperplasia, and _____ _____, which has a relatively high occurrence among men in their twenties.

5. A twisted spermatic cord is a condition known as _____ _____, and requires emergency surgery to avoid loss to the affected testis.

6. The virus that causes the syndrome known as _____

   _____ syndrome is HIV.

7. The most common bacterial STD in North America is _____,

   while the most common viral STD is _____

   _____, which is caused by _____

   (abbreviation).

15.10 8. A bacteria-caused STD that forms chancres is _____. Another

   bacteria-caused STD, which causes ulcer-like lesions and urethral discharge, is

   known as _____.

9. An STD that causes inflammation of the liver is the result of infection by the

15.11 _____ virus. An unrelated STD that results in venereal warts is

   caused by _____ (abbreviation).

Treatments, Procedures, and Devices

WORD PARTS (WHEN APPLICABLE)			TERM	DEFINITION
Part	Type	Meaning		
			artificial insemination (ahr tih FISH al in sem ih NAY shun)	a procedure in which semen is introduced into the female reproductive tract using a method other than coitus
balan/o -plasty	r/cv s	glans penis surgical repair	**balanoplasty** (BAL ah noh plass tee)	surgical repair of the glans penis
			circumcision (ser kum SIH zhun)	surgical removal of the prepuce, which involves making a circumscribed incision around the base of the prepuce (Figure 15.12⸬)

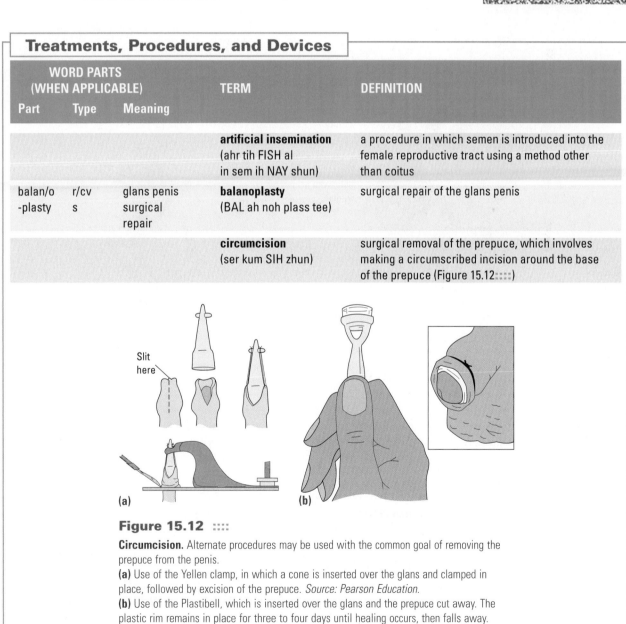

Figure 15.12 ⸬

Circumcision. Alternate procedures may be used with the common goal of removing the prepuce from the penis.
(a) Use of the Yellen clamp, in which a cone is inserted over the glans and clamped in place, followed by excision of the prepuce. *Source: Pearson Education.*
(b) Use of the Plastibell, which is inserted over the glans and the prepuce cut away. The plastic rim remains in place for three to four days until healing occurs, then falls away. *Source: Pearson Education.*

WORD PARTS (WHEN APPLICABLE)			TERM	DEFINITION
Part	Type	Meaning		
			digital rectal examination (DIH jih tal REK tal eks AM ih NAY shun)	a physical examination that involves the insertion of a finger into the rectum to feel the size and shape of the prostate gland through the wall of the rectum; used to screen the patient for BPH and prostate cancer; abbreviated **DRE** (Figure 15.13⁙)
epididym -ectomy	r s	epididymus excision	**epididymectomy** (EP ih did ih MEK toh mee)	excision of the epididymis
hydr/o -cele -ectomy	r/cv s s	water hernia, swelling excision	**hydrocelectomy** (HIGH droh see LEK toh mee)	excision of a hydrocele
orchid -ectomy	r s	testis excision	**orchidectomy** (OR kid EK toh mee)	excision of a testis (Figure 15.14⁙); also called orchiectomy (or kee EK toh mee); a bilateral orchidectomy is commonly called **castration** (kass TRAY shun)

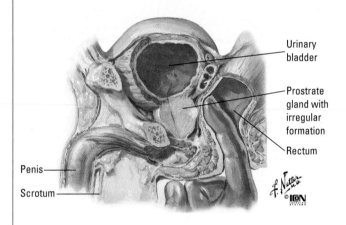

Urinary
bladder

Prostrate
gland with
irregular
formation

Rectum

Penis

Scrotum

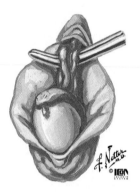

Figure 15.13 ⁙

Digital rectal exam. In this procedure, the index finger is inserted into the rectum to palpate the prostate as a test for signs of BPH or prostate cancer.
Source: Icon Learning Systems.

Figure 15.14 ⁙

Orchidectomy. A testis is removed in this procedure by opening the scrotum and cutting through the spermatic cord.
Source: Icon Learning Systems.

orchid/o -pexy	r/cv s	testis surgical fixation	**orchidopexy** (or KID oh pek see)	surgical fixation of a testis, which draws an undescended testis into the scrotum; also called **orchiopexy** (OR kee oh PEK see)
orchid/o -tomy	r/cv s	testis incision	**orchidotomy** (OR kid OTT toh mee)	incision into a testis; also called **orchiotomy** (OR kee OTT oh mee)
orchi/o -plasty	r/cv s	testis surgical repair	**orchioplasty** (OR kee oh plass tee)	surgical repair of a testis
pen -ile	r s	penis pertaining to	**penile implant** (PEE nile IM plant)	surgical implantation of a penile prosthesis to correct for erectile dysfunction; available options include insertion of semirigid rods and insertion of inflatable balloon-like cylinders (Figure 15.15⁙)

WORD PARTS (WHEN APPLICABLE)			TERM	DEFINITION
Part	Type	Meaning		

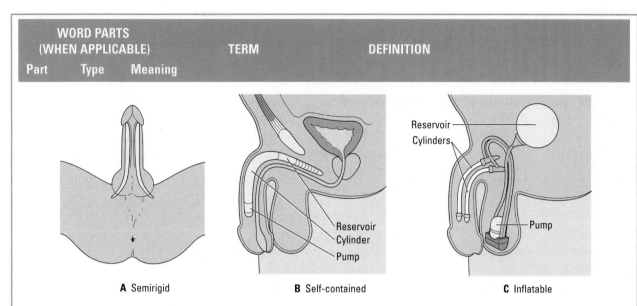

A Semirigid   **B** Self-contained   **C** Inflatable

Figure 15.15 ::::

Penile implants.
(a) Semirigid rods may be surgically implanted into the penis, which provides a partial erection that is persistent. *Source: Pearson Education.*
(b) Inflatable cylinders implanted into the penis may be self-contained, producing an erection when the pump is activated by physical contact. *Source: Pearson Education.*
(c) Inflatable cylinders may alternatively include a pump that requires a more directed hand pumping action to activate. *Source: Pearson Education.*

prostat	r	prostate gland	**prostatectomy** (pross tah TEK toh mee)	excision of a prostate gland to treat prostate cancer and benign prostatic hyperplasia; during a suprapubic prostatectomy, the prostate gland is removed through an incision made above the pubic bone (Figure 15.16::::)
-ectomy	s	excision		

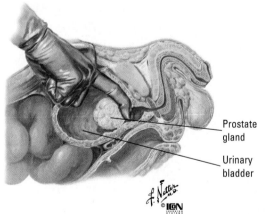

Prostate gland

Urinary bladder

Figure 15.16 ::::

Prostatectomy.
The prostate gland is surgically removed in this procedure. It often involves entry through the anterior abdominal wall, as shown, including a prostatocystotomy.
Source: Icon Learning Systems.

			prostate-specific antigen (PROSS tayt speh SIH fik AN tih jenn)	a clinical test that measures blood levels of the protein prostate-specific antigen; elevated levels suggest the probable presence of prostate cancer, so the test is often used to evaluate cancer treatment progress; abbreviated **PSA**
prostat/o	r/cv	prostate gland	**prostatocystotomy** (pross TAH toh siss TOTT oh mee)	incision into the prostate gland and urinary bladder (Figure 15.16)
cyst/o	r/cv	bladder		
-tomy	s	incision		

WORD PARTS (WHEN APPLICABLE)			TERM	DEFINITION
Part	**Type**	**Meaning**		
prostat/o	r/cv	prostate gland	**prostatolithotomy**	incision into the prostate gland to remove a stone
lith/o	r/cv	stone	(PROSS tah toh lih	that is the source of an obstruction
-tomy	s	incision	THOTT oh mee)	
prostat/o	r/cv	prostate gland	**prostatovesiculectomy**	excision of the prostate gland and seminal vesicles
vesicul	r	seminal vesicle	(pross TAH toh vess ik	
-ectomy	s	excision	yoo LEK toh mee)	
			sterilization	any process that renders an individual unable to
			(ster ih lih ZAY shun)	produce offspring
trans-	p	through, across	**transrectal ultrasound**	placement of an ultrasound probe into the rectum,
			(tranz REK tal)	the sound waves are converted to an image of the
rect	r	rectum		region; the procedure is used to visualize, diagnose,
-al	s	pertaining to		and help treat prostate cancer
trans-	p	through, across	**transurethral incision of the prostate gland**	a surgical procedure that widens the urethra as a treatment for BPH; several small incisions are made
urethr	r	urethra	(tranz yoo REE thral	in the neck of the urinary bladder and the prostate
-al	s	pertaining to	in sih zhun)	gland, allowing the urethra to increase its diameter; abbreviated **TUIP**
trans-	p	through, across	**transurethral microwave thermotherapy**	a therapeutic treatment using microwave heat to destroy excess cells that typify BPH; abbreviated
urethr	r	urethra	(tranz yoo REE thral	**TUMT**
-al	s	pertaining to	MY kroh wayv THER moh THAIR ah pee)	
trans-	p	through, across	**transurethral resection of the prostate gland**	a surgery to treat BPH when the urethra is obstructed; a more complete option than TUIP, it
urethr	r	urethra	(tranz yoo REE thral	involves the resection of prostate tissue using a
-al	s	pertaining to	ree SEK shun)	retroscope inserted through the urethra; the capsule (outer covering) of the prostate and as much tissue as possible is left intact; abbreviated **TURP** (Figure 15.17 ::::)

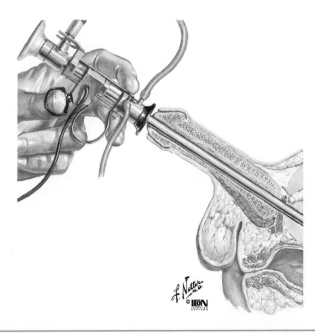

Figure 15.17 ::::

Transurethral resection of the prostate gland.

Source: Icon Learning Systems.

WORD PARTS (WHEN APPLICABLE)			TERM	DEFINITION
Part	Type	Meaning		
vas -ectomy	r s	vessel, duct excision	**vasectomy** (vas EK toh mee)	partial excision of the vas deferens, which causes male sterilization; often shortened to **vas** (Figure 15.18::::)

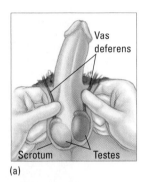 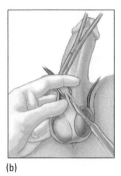 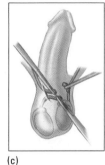 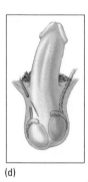

(a) (b) (c) (d)

Figure 15.18 ::::

Vasectomy.

(a) Vas deferens is located within the spermatic cord on both sides.

(b) A small incision is made through the scrotum, and an instrument is inserted that gently separates the vas deferens from other tissues of the spermatic cord. Once separated, the vas is pulled out gently.

(c) The vas deferens is cut and the exposed ends cauterized to close them.

(d) The vas deferens is returned to the spermatic cord, tucked back into the scrotum, and a single suture closes the incision. The vas deferens on the other side is then cut in a duplicate procedure.

WORD PARTS			TERM	DEFINITION
vas/o vas/o -stomy	r/cv r/cv s	vessel, duct vessel, duct surgical creation of an opening	**vasovasostomy** (VAS oh vah SOSS toh mee)	a surgery to restore fertility; it involves creating artificial openings and reconnecting the ends of the vas where they were severed in an earlier vasectomy
vesicul -ectomy	r s	seminal vesicle excision	**vesiculectomy** (veh SIK yoo LEK toh mee)	excision of the seminal vesicles

SELF QUIZ 15.5

SAY IT—SPELL IT!

Review the terms of the male reproductive system by speaking the phonetic pronunciation out loud, then writing the correct spelling of the term.

15.12 1. BAL ah noh plass tee _____

2. EP ih did ih MEK toh mee _____

3. HIGH droh see LEK toh mee _____

4. OR kid EK toh mee _____

15.13 5. or KID oh pek see _____

15.14 6. or kee EK toh mee _____

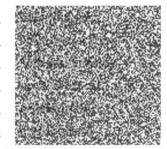

7. pross tah TEK toh mee   _____

8. pross TAH toh siss TOTT oh mee   _____

9. pross TAH toh vess ik yoo
    LEK toh mee   _____

15.15 10. vas EK toh mee   _____

15.16 11. VAS oh vah SOSS toh mee   _____

15.17 12. veh SIK yoo LEK toh mee   _____

MATCH IT!

Match the term on the left with the correct definition on the right.

_____ 1. balanoplasty   a. incision into a testis

_____ 2. epididymectomy   b. excision of the prostate gland and seminal
                                        vesicles

_____ 3. hydrocelectomy   c. surgical repair of a testis

_____ 4. orchioplasty   d. excision of the epididymus

_____ 5. orchidectomy   e. removal of a stone from the prostate gland

_____ 6. orchidopexy   f. excision of the seminal vesicles

_____ 7. orchidotomy   g. incision into the prostate gland and the bladder

_____ 8. prostatectomy   h. removal of a segment of the vas deferens

_____ 9. prostatocystotomy   i. excision of a hydrocele

_____ 10. prostatolithotomy   j. reopening the severed ends of the vas

_____ 11. prostatovesiculectomy k. excision of a testis

_____ 12. vasectomy   l. surgical repair of the glans penis

_____ 13. vasovasostomy   m. removal of the prostate gland

_____ 14. vesiculectomy   n. corrects an undescended testis

BREAK IT DOWN!

**Analyze and separate each term into its word parts by labeling each word
part using p = prefix, r = root, cv = combining vowel, and s = suffix.**

1. balanoplasty   _____

2. epididymectomy   _____

3. hydrocelectomy   _____

4. orchioplasty   _____

5. orchidopexy   _____

6. prostatectomy   _____

7. prostatolithotomy _____

8. vesiculectomy _____

WORD BUILDING

Construct or recall medical terms from the following meanings.

1. compensates for erectile dysfunction _____

2. a surgical cut around the base of the prepuce _____

3. a part of a male physical examination _____

4. a vasectomy achieves this goal _____

5. generates sound waves to visualize the prostate gland _____

6. a blood test to diagnose prostate cancer _____

7. removal of part of the prostate to treat BPH _____

8. widening the urethra to treat BPH _____

9. use of microwave heat to destroy excess cells in BPH _____

FILL IT IN!

Fill in the blanks with the correct terms.

1. A procedure that delivers semen into the female reproductive tract using a method other than coitus is called _____ _____.

2. The surgical procedure that removes the prepuce is known as _____.

3. Benign prostatic hyperplasia may be initially diagnosed during a routine _____ _____ _____, which is part of a complete physical exam for males. If an early diagnosis is made, a blood test for an antigen released by prostate cancer should be given, called a _____ _____ _____, to rule out this disease. Another procedure used to screen for prostate cancer utilizing ultrasound, called _____ _____, involves the insertion of a sound wave probe into the rectum to produce an image.

4. If BPH is diagnosed, several treatment options are available. A surgical procedure that widens the urethra is called _____ _____ of the prostate gland. Another procedure involves the resection of part of the prostate gland in order to open the urethra, called _____ _____ of the prostate gland. A third option involves the use of heat generated by microwave to destroy excess cells, known as transurethal _____ _____.

5. A _____ _____ treats erectile dysfunction by enabling the male to establish an erection.

6. Any process that results in the inability to produce offspring is known as _____.

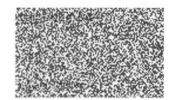

abbreviations of the male reproductive system

The abbreviations that are associated with the male reproductive system are summarized here. Study these abbreviations, and review them in the exercise that follows.

ABBREVIATION	DEFINITION	ABBREVIATION	DEFINITION
AIDS	acquired immunodeficiency syndrome	PSA	prostate-specific antigen
		STD	sexually transmitted disease
BPH	benign prostatic hyperplasia	TUIP	transurethral incision of the
DRE	digital rectal exam		prostate
ED	erectile dysfunction	TUMT	transurethral microwave
HBV	hepatitis B virus		thermotherapy
HIV	human immunodefiency virus	TURP	transurethral resection of the
HPV	human papilloma virus		prostate
HSV-2	herpes simplex virus type 2		

SELF QUIZ 15.6

Fill in the blanks with the abbreviation or the complete medical term.

Abbreviation	Medical Term
1. _____	transurethral microwave thermotherapy
2. PSA	_____
3. _____	sexually transmitted disease
4. HIV	_____
5. _____	transurethral resection of the prostate
6. BPH	_____

15.18 7. _____ acquired immunodeficiency syndrome

8. _____ hepatitis B virus

9. TUIP _____

10. HSV-2 _____

15.19 11. _____ digital rectal exam

12. HPV _____

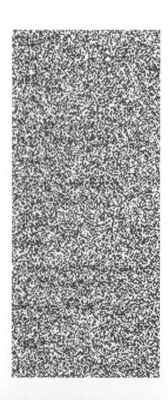

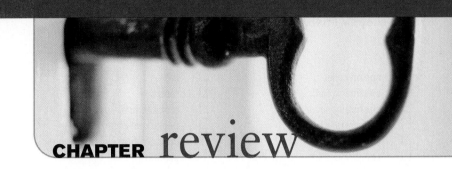

CHAPTER review

In this section, we will review all the word parts and medical terms from this chapter. As in earlier tables, the word roots are shown in **bold**.

Check each word part and medical term to be sure you understand the meaning. If any are not clear, please go back into the chapter and review that term. Then, complete the review exercises that follow.

[word parts **checklist**]

Prefixes

- ❑ im-
- ❑ trans-

Word Roots/Combining Vowels

- ❑ **andr**/o
- ❑ **balan**/o

- ❑ **epididym**/o
- ❑ **orch**/o, **orchid**/o, **orchi**/o
- ❑ **pen**/o
- ❑ **prostat**/o
- ❑ **semin**/o
- ❑ **sperm**/o, **spermat**/o
- ❑ **test**/o, **testicul**/o

- ❑ **vas**/o
- ❑ **vesicul**/o

Suffixes

- ❑ -pexy
- ❑ -rrhea

[medical terminology **checklist**]

- ❑ acquired immunodeficiency syndrome
- ❑ andropathy
- ❑ an**orch**ism
- ❑ artificial in**semin**ation
- ❑ a**sperm**ia
- ❑ azoo**sperm**ia
- ❑ **balan**itis
- ❑ **balan**oplasty
- ❑ **balan**orrhea
- ❑ benign **prostat**ic hyperplasia
- ❑ bulbourethral glands
- ❑ castration
- ❑ chancre
- ❑ chlamydia
- ❑ circumcision
- ❑ coitus
- ❑ Cowper's glands
- ❑ crypt**orchid**ism
- ❑ digital rectal exam
- ❑ ejaculation
- ❑ ejaculatory duct
- ❑ **epididym**ectomy
- ❑ **epididym**is
- ❑ **epididym**itis

- ❑ erectile dysfunction
- ❑ gametes
- ❑ genital herpes
- ❑ genital warts
- ❑ glans **pen**is
- ❑ gonorrhea
- ❑ hepatitis B virus
- ❑ herpes simplex virus Type 2
- ❑ human immunodeficiency virus
- ❑ human papilloma virus
- ❑ hydrocele
- ❑ hydro**cel**ectomy
- ❑ impotency
- ❑ impotent
- ❑ interstitial cells
- ❑ nocturia
- ❑ oligo**sperm**ia
- ❑ **orchid**ectomy
- ❑ **orchid**opexy
- ❑ **orchi**oplasty
- ❑ **orchid**otomy
- ❑ **orch**itis
- ❑ orgasm
- ❑ papillomas
- ❑ **pen**ile implant

- ❑ **pen**is
- ❑ perineum
- ❑ Peyronie's disease
- ❑ phimosis
- ❑ prepuce
- ❑ priapism
- ❑ proctitis
- ❑ **prostat**e cancer
- ❑ **prostat**e gland
- ❑ **prostat**ectomy
- ❑ **prostat**e-specific antigen
- ❑ **prostat**itis
- ❑ **prostat**ocystectomy
- ❑ **prostat**ocystitis
- ❑ **prostat**olith
- ❑ **prostat**olithotomy
- ❑ **prostat**orrhea
- ❑ **prostat**o**vesicul**ectomy
- ❑ **prostat**o**vesicul**itis
- ❑ scrotum
- ❑ semen
- ❑ **semin**al duct
- ❑ **semin**al vesicles
- ❑ **semin**iferous tubules
- ❑ **semin**oma

❑ **sperm** cells	❑ **test**es	❑ trichomoniasis
❑ **sperm**atic cord	❑ **test**is	❑ tubules
❑ **spermat**ogenesis	❑ **test**osterone	❑ **urethr**a
❑ **spermat**olysis	❑ transrectal ultrasound	❑ **urethr**itis
❑ **spermat**ozoa	❑ trans**ureth**ral incision of the	❑ varicocele
❑ sterilization	**prostat**e	❑ **vas** deferens
❑ syphilis	❑ trans**ureth**ral microwave	❑ **vas**ectomy
❑ testicle	thermotherapy	❑ **vas**o**vas**ostomy
❑ **testicul**ar carcinoma	❑ trans**ureth**ral resection of the	❑ venereal disease
❑ **testicul**ar torsion	prostate gland	❑ **vesicul**ectomy

[show what **you know!**]

BREAK IT DOWN!

Analyze and separate each term into its word parts by labeling each word part using p = prefix, r = root, cv = combining vowel, and s = suffix.

		r cv s
Example:	1. andropathy	andr/o/pathy
	2. anorchism	
	3. aspermia	
	4. balanitis	
	5. balanorrhea	
	6. cryptorchidism	
	7. epididymitis	
	8. oligospermia	
	9. orchiepididymitis	
	10. orchitis	
	11. prostatitis	
	12. prostatocystitis	
	13. prostatolith	
	14. prostatorrhea	
	15. prostatovesiculitis	
	16. spermatolysis	
	17. balanoplasty	
	18. epididymectomy	
	19. hydrocelectomy	
	20. orchioplasty	
	21. orchidectomy	
	22. orchidopexy	
	23. prostatocystotomy	

24. prostatolithotomy _____

25. prostatovesiculectomy _____

26. vasectomy _____

27. vasovasostomy _____

28. vesiculectomy _____

WORD BUILDING

Construct or recall medical terms from the following meanings.

Example: 1. absence of one or both testes   _____ anorchism _____

2. inability to achieve or maintain erection   _____

3. a male experiencing erectile dysfunction   _____

4. cancer originating from a testis   _____

5. induration of penile erectile tissue   _____

6. condition of a twisted spermatic cord   _____

7. abnormally persistent erection   _____

8. constriction of the prepuce   _____

9. syndrome caused by HIV   _____

10. ulcer-like lesions caused by HPV   _____

11. implantation of an artificial penis   _____

12. excision of the prepuce   _____

13. blood test that measures PSA   _____

14. process rendering a person unable to produce offspring   _____

15. resection of prostate tissue to treat BPH   _____

16. an STD that causes liver inflammation   _____

17. bacterial STD that causes ulcers called chancres   _____

18. incision into a testis   _____

19. nonmalignant, excessive growth of the prostate   _____

20. swelling of the scrotum due to fluid accumulation   _____

21. virus that causes an STD with wart-like lesions   _____

22. condition of abnormally few sperm   _____

23. inflammation of a testis   _____

24. abnormal dilation of veins in the spermatic cord   _____

CASE STUDIES

Fill in the blanks with the correct terms.

1. A 70-year-old male was admitted as a patient after complaining of the frequent need to void, including throughout the night.

He stated he had no fevers, nausea, or vomiting, although he was experiencing gradually increasing pain in the perineal area.

A physical exam, or (a) _____ _____ _____, revealed an

enlarged prostate without expressed pain or hard nodules. A blood test, or (b) _____

_____ _____, was evaluated to rule out (c) _____

_____ as the possible cause. A low PSA density level of 0.25 provided confidence against this life-

threatening disease. On the basis of the low PSA and DRE results, the diagnosis of benign (d) _____

_____ was recorded. To evaluate the extent of the hypertrophy, sound waves were used in a

(e) _____ _____ procedure. The procedure indicated surgery could successfully

reduce the inflammation of the prostate, or (f) _____. Due to the relatively large hypertrophy, removal

of the inner prostate tissue during a (g) _____ _____

_____ _____ _____, or TURP, is the preferred procedure.

The patient tolerated the procedure well and had minimal bleeding and discomfort during postoperative recovery, and urine

flow returned to near normal levels.

2. A 22-year-old male presented with symptoms that included abnormally few sperm in a semen sample, or

(h) _____, pain in the scrotal and perineal areas, inflammation of the right testis and epididymis,

called (i) _____, and a noticeable lump on his right testis. An evaluation of his medical history

revealed excessive discharge from the glans, called (j) _____, caused by a concurrent infection

resulting in the STD known as (k) _____. The STD was treated with antibiotics and reported as

cleared. A biopsy taken from the right testis was positive for the common form of testicular cancer, known as

(l) _____ _____. The left testis also showed evidence of early metastasis, so

both testes were removed during a (m) _____ _____. Intervention proved effec-

tive, since the patient survived and has made a complete recovery. However, the patient is now

(n) _____, or incapable of producing offspring.

[piece it all **together!**]

CROSSWORD

From the chapter material, fill in the crossword puzzle with answers to the following clues.

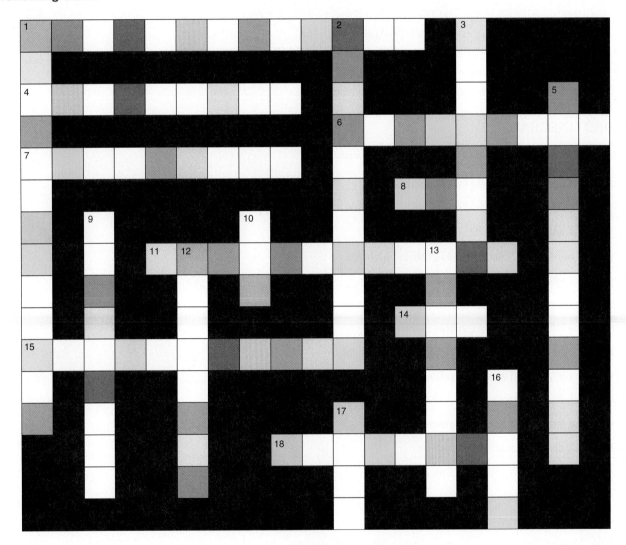

ACROSS

1. Removal of the first pair of male sex glands. (Find puzzle piece 15.17)
4. The cord containing the vas deferens within the scrotum. (Find puzzle piece 15.2)
6. Fluid accumulation within a testis. (Find puzzle piece 15.7)
7. A male sterilization procedure. (Find puzzle piece 15.15)
8. Abbreviation for an exclusively male physical exam. (Find puzzle piece 15.19)
11. Surgical repair of the glans penis. (Find puzzle piece 15.12)
14. Abbreviation for an STD characterized by wart-like lesions. (Find puzzle piece 15.11)
15. Another term for castration when it is doubled. (Find puzzle piece 15.14)
18. An abnormally persistent erection. (Find puzzle piece 15.9)

DOWN

1. Reverses a vasectomy. (Find puzzle piece 15.16)
2. Repairs an undescended testis. (Find puzzle piece 15.13)
3. A man who suffers from erectile dysfunction. (Find puzzle piece 15.8)
5. A condition of few sperm. (Find puzzle piece 15.5)
9. Absence of one or both testes. (Find puzzle piece 15.6)
10. Shortened version of the tube exiting the scrotum. (Find puzzle piece 15.1)
12. The goal of any male sterilization procedure. (Find puzzle piece 15.4)
13. An STD that produces sores known as chancres. (Find puzzle piece 15.10)
16. Normally composed of glandular secretions and sperm. (Find puzzle piece 15.3)
17. The syndrome resulting from HIV infection. (Find puzzle piece 15.18)

WORD UNSCRAMBLE

From the completed crossword puzzle, unscramble:

1. All of the letters that appear in **red** squares __ __ ☐ __ __ __ __ __

   Clue: Also known as testitis

2. All of the letters that appear in **purple** squares __ __ __ __ __ __ ☐ __ __

   Clue: A bacterial STD characterized by urethral discharge

3. All of the letters that appear in **peach** squares __ __ ☐ __ __ __ __ __ __

   Clue: Inflammation of the glans penis

4. All of the letters that appear in **blue** squares __ __ ☐

   Clue: A blood test to detect prostate cancer (abbreviation)

5. All of the letters that appear in **yellow** squares __ __ __ __ __ __ __ __ __ ☐ __

   Clue: Incision into a testis

6. All of the letters that appear in **green** squares __ __ __ __ __ __ __ __ __ ☐

   Clue: Any disease that afflicts only males

7. All of the letters that appear in **pink** squares __ __ ☐ __ __ __ __ __ __ __ __ __ __ __

   Clue: Excision of a hydrocele

8. All of the letters that appear in **gray** squares __ __ ☐ __

   Clue: A surgical treatment to relieve symptoms of BPH (abbreviation)

9. All of the letters that appear in **orange** squares __ ☐ __

   Clue: A short version of the common male sterilization procedure

Now write down each of the letters that are boxed and unscramble them to find the hidden medical term of the male reproductive system: __ __ __ __ __ __ __ __ __.

MEDmedia wrap-up

www.prenhall.com/wingerd

Before you go on to the next chapter, take advantage of the free CD-ROM and study guide website that accompany this book. Simply load the CD-ROM for additional activities, games, animations, videos, and quizzes linked to this chapter. Then visit www.prenhall.com/wingerd for even more!

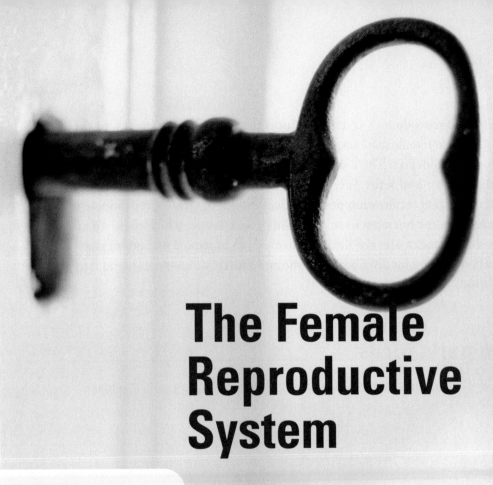

The Female Reproductive System

LEARNING OBJECTIVES

After completing this chapter, you will be able to:

- Define and spell the word parts used to create terms for the female reproductive system

- Identify the major organs of the female reproductive system and describe their structure and function

- Break down and define common medical terms used for symptoms, diseases, disorders, procedures, treatments, and devices associated with the female reproductive system

- Build medical terms from the word parts associated with the female reproductive system

- Pronounce and spell common medical terms associated with the female reproductive system

MEDmedia

www.prenhall.com/wingerd

Enhance your study with the power of multimedia! Each chapter of this book links to activities, games, animations, videos, and quizzes that you'll find on your CD-ROM. Plus, you can click on www.prenhall.com/wingerd, to find a free chapter-specific companion website that's loaded with additional practice and resources.

CD-ROM

- Audio Glossary
- Exercises & Activities
- Flashcard Generator
- Animations
- Videos

 Companion Website

- Exercises & Activities
- Audio Glossary
- Drug Updates
- Current News Update

A secure distance learning course is available at www.prenhall.com/onekey.

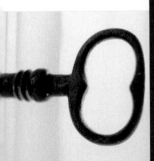

The female reproductive system produces the sex cells, or gametes, of the female. The female gametes are the egg cells, called ova (ovum is the singular form), or oocytes. The female system also provides support for the developing embryo and fetus once fertilization has occurred and makes the process of internal fertilization possible. In addition, the female reproductive system secretes the hormones estrogen and progesterone, which regulate female cycles. Estrogen also regulates the expression of female secondary characteristics including fat distribution, bone and muscle development, and hair distribution.

word parts focus

Let's look at word parts. The following table contains a list of word parts that when combined build many of the terms of the female reproductive system.

PREFIX	DEFINITION	PREFIX	DEFINITION
endo-	within, inner	pre-	before
peri-	around, surrounding		

WORD ROOT	DEFINITION	WORD ROOT	DEFINITION
cervic	neck, cervix	oophor, ovari	ovary
colp	vagina	ov	egg
culd	cul-de-sac	perine	perineum
episi	vulva	py	pus
gynec, gyn	woman	salping	trumpet, fallopian tube
hydr	water		(also eustachian tube)
hyster	uterus	trachel	neck, cervix
mamm, mast	breast	uter	womb, uterus
men, menstru	month, menstruation, menses	vagin	sheath, vagina
metr	uterus	vulv	vulva

[FYI]

Uterus

Hysteria is a Greek word that means *a condition of the uterus.* Some ancient Greeks believed that the uterus was the source of nervous disorders, while Plato argued that the uterus was an animal with an independent mind and emotion, lodged inside a woman and determined to produce children. If the *beast uterus* remained without children, it became ill-tempered and caused a body-wide disturbance, which ended with pregnancy. Thus, a prescription for a *hysterical* female was marriage and pregnancy. This misconceived notion persisted for thousands of years!

SUFFIX	DEFINITION	SUFFIX	DEFINITION
-atresia	closure; absence of a normal body opening	-ial	pertaining to
		-salpinx	trumpet, fallopian tube

SELF QUIZ 16.1

Review the word parts of female reproductive system terminology by working carefully through the exercises that follow. Soon, we will apply this new information to build medical terms.

Success Hint: Once you get to the crossword puzzle at the end of the chapter, remember to check back here for clues! Your clues are indicated by the puzzle icon.

A. Provide the definition of the following prefixes and suffixes.

1. endo-   _____

2. peri-   _____

3. -atresia   _____

4. -ial   _____

B. Provide the word root for each of the following terms.

1. cervix   _____

16.1 2. vagina   _____

3. cul-de-sac   _____

4. vulva   _____

5. woman   _____

6. water   _____

7. uterus   _____

8. breast   _____

9. menstruation   _____

10. ovary   _____

16.2 11. egg   _____

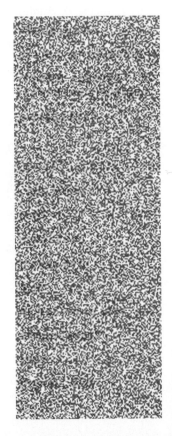

12. pus   _____

13. perineum   _____

14. fallopian tube   _____

15. neck   _____

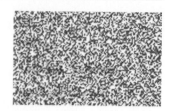

[anatomy and physiology OVeRVIEW]

The primary organs of the female reproductive system are the ovaries. Other female organs support embryonic and fetal development and the internal process of fertilization. They include the fallopian tubes, uterus, vagina, external genitalia, and mammary glands.

The Ovaries

The **ovaries** are the female gonads, and they produce the female gametes (ova) and the female sex hormones. The ovarian hormones are a class of compounds called **estrogens** and **progesterone.** The ovaries are paired, almond-shaped organs located opposite one another against the walls of the pelvic cavity (Figure 16.1⸬).

Each ovary is covered by a layer of cells and is internally divided into a cortex and medulla (Figure 16.2⸬). The cortex contains numerous sac-like ovarian **follicles,** which are in various stages of development (Figure 16.3⸬). Each ovarian follicle contains a single ovum.

In males, sperm development is continuous, but the total number of ova that are produced in a female's lifetime are present in the ovaries at birth, in an immature state. Ova mature and are released on a monthly cycle called the **ovarian cycle;** the release event is called **ovulation.** During this event, the ovum bursts out of a mature ovarian follicle, or **graafian follicle,** through the ovarian wall and into the **peritoneal cavity.** From there, the ovum is usually drawn into a fallopian tube. The ovarian cycle begins at the onset of puberty, and ends about 40 years later at **menopause.**

> **[thinking critically!]**
>
> If a woman lost both her ovaries before the age of 12 years, would she be capable of becoming fertile at puberty?

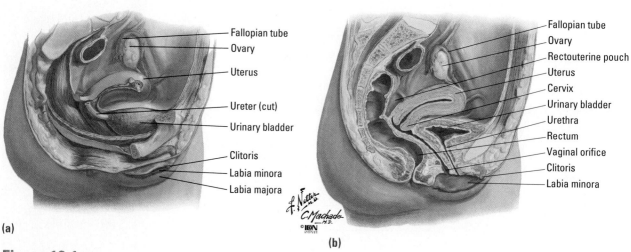

(a)

(b)

Figure 16.1 ⸬

Female reproductive organs.

(a) This side view shows a partial section through the pelvic cavity.

(b) Complete section through the pelvic cavity.

Source: Icon Learning Systems.

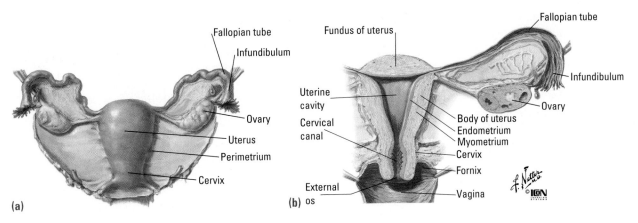

Figure 16.2 ::::

The uterus and nearby structures.
(a) Anterior view of the unsectioned organs.
(b) Sectioned organs, anterior view.
Source: Icon Learning Systems.

The Fallopian Tubes

The **fallopian tubes** are a pair of narrow tubes located along each side of the pelvic cavity wall (Figure 16.2); they are also called **uterine tubes** or **oviducts.** Each tube extends about 10 cm (4 inches) between an ovary and the centrally located uterus and is lined with a ciliated mucous membrane. Beating of the cilia creates a current of mucus, which draws an ovulated ovum inside the tube. If fertilization occurs, it usually happens within the upper one-third of a fallopian tube. At the end of a fallopian tube near the ovary, the tube widens to form a funnel-shaped part that opens into the peritoneal cavity, called the **infundibulum.**

The Uterus

The **uterus** is a pear-shaped organ about the size of a woman's clenched fist. It is suspended just above the floor of the pelvic cavity by ligaments, located between the urinary bladder and the rectum (Figure 16.1). It is separated from the rectum by a narrow space, called the **rectouterine pouch.** The uterus consists of an upper, dome-shaped **fundus,** a central **body** (or **corpus**) that receives the two fallopian tubes, and a lower, narrow **cervix** (Figure 16.2). Internally, the space within the body is the **uterine cavity,** and that within the cervix is the **cervical canal.** The cervical canal opens into the vagina by way of the **external os.**

The wall of the uterus includes an outer layer called the **perimetrium,** a thick layer of muscle known as the **myometrium,** and an inner layer rich in blood vessels known as the **endometrium.** The endometrium provides an implantation site for

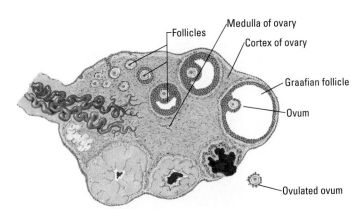

Figure 16.3 ::::

Ovary.
A single ovary is shown sectioned to reveal its internal features. The maturing of the ova and follicles is a gradual process, concluding every 28 days from one of either ovary with the event of ovulation.

the embryo. If implantation occurs, the inner lining of the endometrium will thicken to establish the nourishing **placenta,** which supports the developing child.

The endometrium changes on a monthly cycle by increasing and decreasing in thickness. This cycle is called the **menstrual cycle** because it occurs approximately every 28 days (the term *menstrual* is derived from the Latin word for *month*). **Menses** or menstruation begins when the outer layer of the endometrium breaks away, causing bleeding from the uterus. The cycle begins at the onset of puberty (the first menses of a woman's life is called **menarche**), and ends about 40 years later. A woman who no longer experiences menstrual and ovarian cycles is said to be in **menopause.**

The Vagina

The **vagina** is a thin-walled, tube-shaped organ about 8 to 10 cm (4 to 5 inches) long that functions as a passage between the cervix of the uterus and the outside of the body. (Figure 16.1). The uterus sheds blood during menstruation through the vagina and semen travels to the uterus from the vagina. Because a baby passes through the vagina during (vaginal) childbirth, it is often called the birth canal. At the end that receives the cervix, its wall curves around to form a shallow pocket called the **fornix** (Figure 16.2).

The vagina's opening to the outside is called the **vaginal orifice** (Figure 16.4:::). In young females the mucous membrane may extend across the opening, forming a thin barrier called the **hymen.** The hymen contains blood vessels and tends to bleed when it is first penetrated or ruptured.

> [**FYI**]
>
> **Hymen**
> The ancient Greek god of marriage is named Hymen. Because the ancient Greeks usually married very young (early teens), the brides often started their married life with the hymen intact. According to early Greek customs, it was said that the god Hymen blessed the marriage if, during the first sexual penetration following the wedding ceremony, the thin membrane that partly or completely occludes the vagina was torn. From this early belief, the hymen obtained its name.

[**thinking critically!**]

What layer of the uterus undergoes change during menses every 28 days?

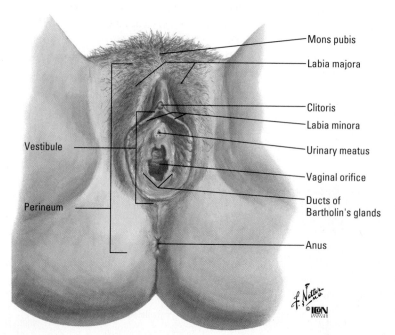

Figure 16.4 ::::

The female external genitalia.
The hymen is not present in this illustration.
Source: Icon Learning Systems.

(Labels in figure: Mons pubis, Labia majora, Clitoris, Labia minora, Urinary meatus, Vaginal orifice, Ducts of Bartholin's glands, Anus, Vestibule, Perineum)

Fornix

The term fornix is the Latin word for *arch* or *vault*. It is an anatomical term that is used to describe an arch-shaped structure. In the case of the fornix of the vagina, the arch is formed by the cervix, which pushes down to rest slightly within the distal end of the vagina. The vagina gives a little, creating the arch-shaped fornix. Because the fornix encircles the cervix, it serves as a good location for the contraceptive diaphragm, which contains an elastic band that snaps into place within the fornix to cover the external os and prevent sperm from penetrating into the uterus.

Female External Genitalia

The structures located outside the vagina are the female external genitalia (Figure 16.4). Collectively, they are known as the **vulva.** The outer part of the vulva includes an elevated, rounded area called the **mons pubis;** two narrow, outer folds of skin called the **labia majora;** and two inner, hair-free folds of skin called the **labia minora.**

The labia minora form the outer margins of an area called the **vestibule,** which represents the inner part of the vulva. From anterior to posterior it contains a small projection called the **clitoris** where the two labia minora meet anteriorly, the urinary meatus, and the vaginal orifice. Near the vaginal orifice is a pair of glands, known as **Bartholin's glands,** which provide lubrication to the vagina. The region between the upper border of the vestibule and the anus is the **perineum,** which sometimes tears during the stress of childbirth.

The Mammary Glands

The mammary glands are the organs that produce milk for infant nourishment. Located in the breasts, they consist of tissue that is modified from sweat glands (Figure 16.5::::)

The breasts of both males and females contain an external, heavily pigmented **areola** that surrounds a centrally located **nipple.** Both structures are very sensitive to touch and contain smooth muscles that cause them to become erect when stimulated by touch, cold, or sexual arousal. Internally, an adult female mammary gland undergoes enlargement during puberty when estrogens increase in production, directing fat tissue to accumulate between the skin and muscle layers. Each adult gland consists of 15 to 20 lobes that radiate around the nipple. Each lobe contains small chambers, which house **alveolar glands.** The alveolar glands produce milk when a woman is lactating, which is under hormonal control.

FYI

Labia

The term labia is the plural form of the Latin word for *lip*. The inner, thin margin of the vulva is the labia minora, which means *small lips* in Latin, and the outer, thick margin is the *labia majora,* which means *large lips* in Latin.

Clitoris

The term clitoris is from the Greek word that means *small hill*. In the female, the clitoris is the homologue of the penis in the male; that is, they originate from similar tissues during embryonic development. Like the penis, the clitoris includes a glans, prepuce, and erectile tissue, but does not contain the urethra.

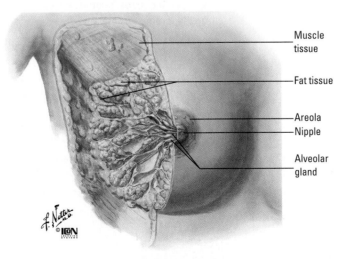

Muscle tissue

Fat tissue

Areola
Nipple

Alveolar gland

Figure 16.5 ::::

The mammary glands.
The alveolar glands communicate with the nipple by way of a system of ducts.
Source: Icon Learning Systems.

getting to the root of it | anatomy and physiology terms

Many of the anatomy and physiology terms are formed from roots that are used to construct the more complex medical terms of the female reproductive system, including symptoms, diseases, and treatments. In this section, we will review the terms that describe the structure and function of the female reproductive system *in relation to their word roots,* which are shown in **bold.**

Study the word roots and terms in this list and complete the review exercises that follow.

Word Root (Meaning)	Terms Formed from the Word Root (Pronunciation)	Definition
cervic (neck, cervix)	**cervix** (SER viks)	the lower, narrow part of the uterus
	cervical canal (SER vih kal)	the interior of the cervix
mamm (breast)	**mamm**ary glands (MAM ah ree)	the organs that secrete milk; they are composed of secretory alveolar glands embedded within the female breasts, which include an areola and a nipple in the center of each
men (month, menstruation, menses)	**men**arche (men AHR kee)	the first menses
	menopause (MEN oh pawz)	the permanent cessation of menses
	menses (MEN seez)	the hemorrhage of the outer endometrial layers that occurs about every 28 days, also called menstruation (MEN stroo AY shun)
metr (uterus)	endo**metr**ium (EHN doh MEE tree um)	the inner, vascular layer of the uterus, which is the site of embryo implantation and menses
	myo**metr**ium (MY oh MEE tree um)	the muscular wall of the uterus
	peri**metr**ium (pair ee MEE tree um)	the outermost layer of the uterus, which is composed of connective tissue
ov (egg)	**ov**a (OH vah)	oocytes (egg cells) that mature within the ovarian follicles of the ovaries; the singular form is ovum
	ovary (OH vah ree)	paired female gonads located in the pelvic cavity which produce estrogens, progesterone and ova
	ovulation (OV yoo LAY shun)	release of an ovum, which occurs every 28 days, on average, from one of the two ovaries
perine (perineum)	**perine**um (pair ih NEE um)	the area between the vulva and the anus in the female
uter (womb, uterus)	**uter**us (YOO ter uss)	a hollow organ located in the pelvic cavity that is the site of embryo implantation, support of the fetus, and menses
vagin (sheath, vagina)	**vagin**a (vah JYE nah)	the tube-shaped organ between the uterus and the vulva, also known as the birth canal, which opens to the uterus at the external os and to the exterior at the vaginal orifice

OTHER IMPORTANT TERMS

The terms in this table are related to the structure and function of the female reproductive system, but are not built from multiple word roots.

alveolar glands (al vee OH lar)	milk-secreting glands within the mammary glands
Bartholin's gland (BAR toh linz)	mucus-secreting glands located outside the vaginal orifice
clitoris (KLIT oh riss)	a small structure located at the anterior end of the vestibule where the labia minora meet, it includes a glans and internal erectile tissue, similar to the male penis
estrogens (ESS troh jenz)	hormones secreted by ovarian tissue that produces female sexual characteristics and prepares the uterus for implantation of an embryo
fallopian tubes (fah LOH pee an)	the paired, narrow tubes that extend between each ovary and the uterus, they are also known as uterine (YOO ter in) tubes and oviducts (OH vih ducts); named after the 16th century anatomist Gabriello Fallopio
fornix (FOR niks)	the shallow pocket at the internal end of the vagina that surrounds the external os of the cervix
follicles (FALL ih klz)	sac-like, hollow balls of supportive cells within the cortex of each ovary, each of which enclose an ovum
Graafian follicle (GRAH fee an)	a mature follicle that participates in ovulation
hymen (HI men)	a thin membrane that partially or completely covers the vaginal orifice prior to penetration into the vagina
infundibulum (IN fun DIB yoo lum)	the expanded, funnel-shaped end of the fallopian tube that opens to the peritoneal cavity
labia majora (LAY bee ah mah JOR ah)	the external ridge of the vulva
labia minora (LAY bee ah mih NOR ah)	the internal, hairless ridge of the vulva
mons pubis (monz PYOO biss)	the anterior-most, elevated part of the vulva in which the prominence is caused by a pad of fat over the symphysis pubis (SIM fih siss PYOO biss)
rectouterine pouch (rek toh YOO ter in POWCH)	a narrow space between the uterus and rectum, also known as Douglas' cul-de-sac
vestibule (VESS tih byool)	the part of the vulva located within the border formed by the labia minora
vulva (VUL vah)	the external female genitalia

SELF QUIZ 16.2

SAY IT—SPELL IT!

Review the terms of the female reproductive system by speaking the phonetic pronunciations out loud, then writing the correct spelling of the term.

Success Hint: Use the audio glossary on the CD and CW for additional help with pronunciation of these terms.

1. al vee OH lar   _____

2. BAR toh linz   _____

3. SER viks   _____

4. KLIT oh riss   _____

5. EHN doh MEE tree um   _____

6. FOR niks   _____

7. HIGH men   _____

8. IN fun DIB yoo lum   _____

9. LAY bee ah   mah JOR ah   _____

10. LAY bee ah   mih NOR ah   _____

11. MAM ah ree   _____

12. monz   PYOO biss   _____

13. MY oh MEE tree um   _____

14. men AHR kee   _____

15. MEN oh pawz   _____

16. MEN seez   _____

17. OV yoo LAY shun   _____

18. rek toh YOO ter in   POWCH   _____

19. YOO ter uss   _____

20. VESS tih byool   _____

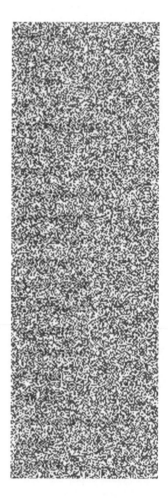

MATCH IT!

Match the term on the left with the correct definition on the right.

_____ 1. ovary

_____ 2. ovum

_____ 3. ovulation

_____ 4. menses

_____ 5. uterus

_____ 6. vagina

_____ 7. endometrium

_____ 8. myometrium

_____ 9. cervix

_____10. graafian follicle

_____11. fallopian tube

_____12. external os

_____13. vulva

_____14. labia minora

_____15. clitoris

_____16. estrogens

_____17. Bartholin's glands

_____18. menopause

a. muscular wall of the uterus

b. a mature ovarian follicle

c. the inner skin-covered ridge of the vulva

d. permanent cessation of menses

e. contains follicles and ova, and produces estrogens

f. the female sex hormones

g. mucous glands near the vaginal orifice

h. an egg cell, or oocyte

i. a small projection that contains erectile tissue

j. the _womb_

k. the _birth canal_

l. the monthly process of ovum release from an ovary

m. the monthly process of endometrial hemorrhage

n. narrow part of the uterus that contains the cervical canal

o. opening between the uterus and vagina

p. female external genitalia

q. inner layer of the uterine wall

r. usual location of ovum fertilization

BREAK IT DOWN!

Analyze and separate each term into its word parts by labeling each word part using p = prefix, r = root, cv = combining vowel, and s = suffix.

1. endometrium   _____

2. cervical   _____

3. perimetrium   _____

4. myometrium   _____

FILL IT IN!

Fill in the blanks with the correct terms.

1. The female gonads are the paired _____, which are located within the pelvic cavity. They contain about two thousand ovarian _____, each of which encloses an _____. Every 28 days, one mature follicle called a _____ follicle releases its ovum during an event known as _____. The female gonads also secrete the female sex hormones known as _____ and progesterone.

2. Each 28-day cycle includes the hemorrhage of the inner lining of the _____, which is known as menstruation or _____. The first such event of a woman's life is called _____. The permanent cessation of these events occurs about 40 years later and is known as _____.

3. The hollow muscular organ that means womb in Latin is the _____. Its muscular layer is called the _____, and the outermost layer of the organ is the _____. The space within the body is called the _____ _____. The narrowed part of the organ is known as the _____, and its interior is a narrow space that is known as the _____ _____, which opens to the vagina by way of a small opening called the _____ _____.

4. If fertilization of an ovum occurs, it normally takes place within the upper one-third of the _____ _____. The expanded end of each tube is called the _____, and the opposite end opens into the uterine cavity.

5. The _____ is a tube-like organ that means *sheath*. It opens to the exterior at the _____ _____, which is at least partly covered by a membrane until it is ruptured, known as the _____.

6. The female external genitalia is also called the _____. It includes an elevated pad, or _____ _____, an outer ridge of skin, called the _____ _____, an inner ridge of hairless skin known as the _____ _____, and an inner area that is called the _____. The inner area includes a small structure that is composed of erectile tissue, called the _____, the urinary meatus, and the vaginal orifice. The _____ is the region between the urinary meatus and the anus.

7. The female adult breasts, or _____ _____, are the milk-producing organs. Each includes a pigmented area in the center, called the _____, which includes a central _____.

16.5 The glands that secrete milk are called _____

_____.

medical terms of the
[female reproductive
system]

Earlier in the chapter, we saw that the vaginal orifice lies between the urinary meatus and the anus, which mark the borders of the perineum. Since the three openings are within the same region, microorganisms may sometimes pass from one opening to another and produce infections. For example, the intestinal bacterium *E. coli* can be spread from the anus to the vaginal orifice and urinary meatus, often due to poor personal hygiene. In a sexually active woman, sexually transmitted diseases (STDs) are the most common infections. Pathogens enter the vagina during sexual intercourse with infected partners. As you may recall, STDs and the pathogens that cause them were described in Chapter 15. Besides infections, other sources of disease may afflict the female reproductive system, including hormonal imbalances, tumors, and inherited disorders.

Diseases of the female reproductive system are often diagnosed during a physical examination. For example, most congenital and sexually transmitted diseases receive an initial diagnosis during an office exam. The disorders that require confirmation or an internal evaluation may be assessed by the noninvasive procedures of MRI, CAT scan, or ultrasound imaging. Diseases of the female reproductive system are usually treated by a physician specializing within the field of **gynecology.** The term is derived from the Greek word for woman, *gynaikos.* It can be written as a constructed term:

gynec/o/logy

in which the root word *gynec* means *woman* and the suffix -logy means *study of.* A physician specializing in gynecology is called a **gynecologist.** This field of medicine is identified in clinics by the abbreviation **GYN.**

[**thinking
critically!**]

In a sexually active woman, what is the most common cause of infection?

let's construct terms!

In this section, we will assemble all of the word parts to construct medical terminology related to the female reproductive system. Abbreviations are used to indicate each word part: **p** = prefix, **r** = root, **cv** = combining vowel, and **s** = suffix. Recall from chapter one that the addition of a combining vowel to the word root creates the combining form for the term. Note that some terms are not constructed from word parts, but they are included here to expand your vocabulary.

The medical terms of the female reproductive system are listed in the following three sections:

- Symptoms and Signs
- Diseases and Disorders
- Treatments, Procedures, and Devices

Each section is followed by review exercises. Study the lists in these tables and complete the review exercises that follow.

Symptoms and Signs

WORD PARTS (WHEN APPLICABLE)			TERM	DEFINITION
Part	Type	Meaning		
a-	p	without, absence of	**amenorrhea** (ah MEN oh REE ah)	absence of menstrual discharge; also called **menostasis** (men oh STAY siss)
men/o	r/cv	month, menstruation		
-rrhea	s	excessive discharge		
dys-	p	bad, abnormal	**dysmenorrhea** (DISS men oh REE ah)	pain during menstruation
men/o	r/cv	month, menstruation		
-rrhea	s	excessive discharge		
hemat/o	r/cv	blood	**hematosalpinx** (HEE mah toh SAL pinks)	blood in a fallopian tube
-salpinx	s	trumpet, fallopian tube		
hydr/o	r/cv	water	**hydrosalpinx** (HIGH droh SAL pinks)	water accumulation in a fallopian tube (Figure 16.6::::)
-salpinx	s	trumpet, fallopian tube		

Uterus

Ovary

Enlarged fallopian tubes

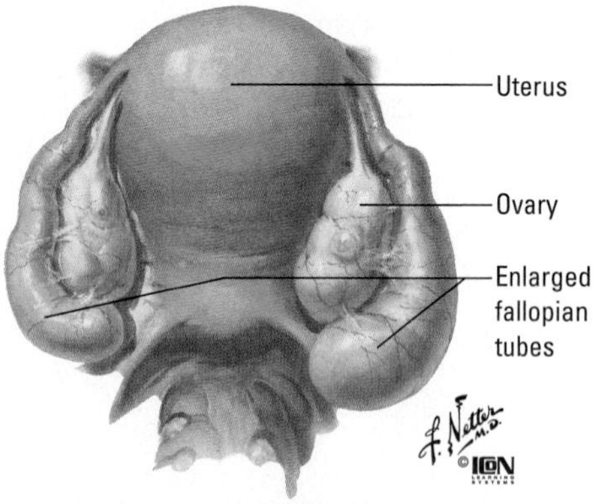

Figure 16.6 ::::

Hydrosalpinx.
The accumulation of fluids within the fallopian tube (hydrosalpinx) is usually caused by an occlusion, causing the tube to enlarge. The common result is the inflammatory condition, salpingitis.
Source: Icon Learning Systems.

leuk/o	r/cv	white	**leukorrhea** (LOO koh REE ah)	white or yellow discharge from the uterus
-rrhea	s	excessive discharge		
mast	r	breast	**mastalgia** (mass TAL jee ah)	pain in the breast
-algia	s	pain		
men/o	r/cv	month, menstruation	**menometrorrhagia** (MEN oh METT roh RAY jee ah)	irregular or excessive bleeding other than during menstruation
metr/o	r/cv	uterus		
-rrhagia	s	bleeding		

WORD PARTS (WHEN APPLICABLE)			TERM	DEFINITION
Part	**Type**	**Meaning**		
men/o	r/cv	month, menstruation	**menorrhagia** (men oh RAY jee ah)	excessive bleeding during menstruation
-rrhagia	s	bleeding		
metr/o	r/cv	uterus	**metrorrhagia** (METT roh RAY jee ah)	bleeding from the uterus at any time other than during normal menstruation
-rrhagia	s	bleeding		
metr/o	r/cv	uterus	**metrorrhea** (meh troh REE ah)	discharge of mucus or pus from the uterus
-rrhea	s	excessive discharge		
olig/o	r/cv	few in number	**oligomenorrhea** (ALL ih goh men oh REE ah)	abnormally reduced discharge during menstruation
men/o	r/cv	month, menstruation		
-rrhea	s	excessive discharge		
py/o	r/cv	pus	**pyosalpinx** (pye oh SAL pinks)	pus within a fallopian tube
-salpinx	s	trumpet, fallopian tube		

SELF QUIZ 16.3

SAY IT—SPELL IT!

Review the terms of the female reproductive system by speaking the phonetic pronunciations out loud, then writing the correct spelling of the term.

1. ah MEN oh REE ah   _____
2. DISS men oh REE ah   _____
3. HEE mah toh SAL pinks   _____
4. HIGH droh SAL pinks   _____
5. LOO koh REE ah   _____
6. mass TAL jee ah   _____
7. MEN oh METT roh RAY jee ah _____
8. meh troh REE ah   _____
9. ALL ih goh men oh REE ah   _____
10. pye oh SAL pinks   _____

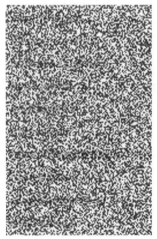

MATCH IT!

Match the term on the left with the correct definition on the right.

_____1. dysmenorrhea

_____2. amenorrhea

_____3. hematosalpinx

_____4. mastalgia

_____5. pyosalpinx

_____6. menometrorrhagia

_____7. hydrosalpinx

_____8. leukorrhea

_____9. oligomenorrhea

16.6 _____10. metrorrhea

_____11. menorrhagia

a. pain in the breast

b. white or yellow uterine discharge

c. abnormally reduced menstrual bleeding

d. pain during menstruation

e. blood in a fallopian tube

f. absence of menstruation

g. water accumulation in a fallopian tube

h. pus within a fallopian tube

i. excessive bleeding during menstruation

j   irregular bleeding during and between menses

k. discharge of mucus or pus from the uterus

BREAK IT DOWN!

Analyze and separate each term into its word parts by labeling each word part using p = prefix, r = root, cv = combining vowel, and s = suffix.

1. amenorrhea   _____

2. dysmenorrhea   _____

3. hematosalpinx   _____

4. mastalgia   _____

5. menometrorrhagia   _____

6. metrorrhea   _____

WORD BUILDING

Construct or recall medical terms from the following meanings.

1. presence of blood in a fallopian tube   _____

2. painful menstruation   _____

3. pain within a breast   _____

4. pus discharge from the uterus   _____

5. nonmenstrual bleeding from the uterus   _____

6. an abnormally reduced menstrual discharge   _____

FILL IT IN!

Fill in the blanks with the correct terms.

1. Changes in menstruation can be signs or symptoms of disease. They include an abnormal reduction of menstrual discharge, or _____, abnormal menstrual pain, or _____, irregular or excessive blood discharge during menstruation, called _____, and the absence of menstrual discharge, called _____.

2. The presence of fluids where they don't belong is a frequent sign of disease. For example, the accumulation of water within a fallopian tube, called a _____, suggests a blockage has occurred. Also, the presence of pus within a fallopian tube, or _____, suggests an infection.

3. An infection may also be signaled by the abnormal discharge of mucus or pus from the uterus, known as _____, or the discharge of yellow-colored material from the uterus, called _____.

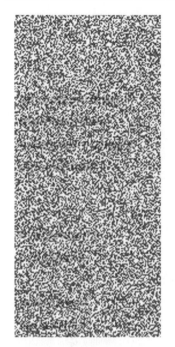

Diseases and Disorders

WORD PARTS (WHEN APPLICABLE)			TERM	DEFINITION
Part	**Type**	**Meaning**		
aden/o	r/cv	gland	**adenomyosis**	an abnormal condition of glandular tissue growth
my	r	muscle	(ADD eh noh my OH siss)	within muscle; in the female, it refers to growth of
-osis	s	condition of		the endometrium into the muscular layer of the uterus
a-	p	without, absence of	**amastia** (ay MASS tee ah)	absence of a breast
mast	r	breast		
-ia	s	condition of		
aden	r	gland	**Bartholin's adenitis**	inflammation of Bartholin's gland; also known as
-itis	s	inflammation	(BAR toh linz add eh NYE tiss)	bartholinitis (BAR toh lin EYE tiss)
			breast cancer (BREST KAN ser)	a malignant tumor arising from breast tissue; the most common form is called an infiltrating ductal carcinoma, abbreviated **IDC** (Figure 16.7::::)
carcin	r	cancer	**carcinoma in situ**	the precancerous form of cervical cancer (Figure
-oma	s	tumor	**(CIS) of the cervix**	16.8::::)

in situ

The term *in situ* is a Latin phrase that literally means *in site*. Its use in modern medicine refers to confinement to a site of origin. Carcinoma in situ describes a tumor that is confined to its organ of origin, rather than a tumor in a secondary site.

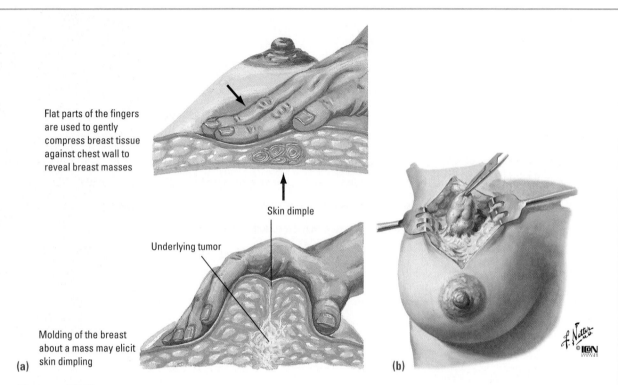

Figure 16.7 ::::

Breast cancer.

(a) The most common form of breast cancer is infiltrating ductal carcinoma, shown here. It can be initially diagnosed by applying pressure (upper figure) and squeezing gently to observe for skin dimpling (lower).
(b) Surgical removal of the primary tumor.
Source: Icon Learning Systems.

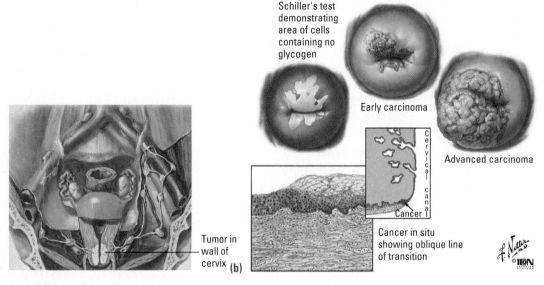

Figure 16.8 ::::

Cervical cancer.

(a) Malignant cells often develop around the external os of the cervix, as shown in this illustration.
(b) Three stages of cervical cancer, as seen through the vaginal orifice during a gynecological exam.
Schiller's test uses vinegar to highlight the area of mutated cells during the early stage of cervical cancer.
In later stages, the carcinoma becomes clearly visible. The lower sections show the transitional zone at
the opening of the external os, where mutations are most likely to occur.
Source: Icon Learning Systems.

WORD PARTS (WHEN APPLICABLE)			TERM	DEFINITION
Part	Type	Meaning		
cervic	r	neck, cervix	**cervical cancer** (SER vih kal KANN ser)	a malignant tumor arising from the cervix; the most common form is squamous cell carcinoma (Figure 16.8)
-al	s	pertaining to		
cervic	r	neck, cervix	**cervical intraepithelial neoplasia** (SER vih kal in trah ep ih THEE lee al nee oh PLAY zee ah)	abnormal development of cells within the cervix resulting in tumor formation, which has the potential of becoming cancerous; abbreviated **CIN**
-al	s	pertaining to		
intra-	p	within		
epi-	p	upon		
thel/i	r/cv	nipple		
-al	s	pertaining to		
neo-	p	new		
-plasia	s	shape, formation		
cervic	r	neck, cervix	**cervicitis** (SER vih SIGH tiss)	inflammation of the cervix
-itis	s	inflammation		
derm	r	skin	**dermoid cyst** (DER moyd sist)	benign tumor arising from ovarian tissue composed of abnormal embryonic tissue (including bone, teeth, hair, and skin)
-oid	s	resemblance to		
			dyspareunia (DISS pah ROO nee ah)	difficult or painful sexual intercourse
endo-	p	within	**endocervicitis** (EHN doh ser vih SIGH tiss)	inflammation of the inner lining of the cervix
cervic	r	neck, cervix		
-itis	s	inflammation		
endo-	p	within	**endometrial cancer** (ehn doh MEE tree al KANN ser)	a malignant tumor arising from endometrial tissue of the uterus, it is one form of uterine cancer (Figure 16.9 ░░░)
metr/i	r/cv	uterus		
-al	s	pertaining to		
endo-	p	within	**endometriosis** (EHN doh mee tree OH siss)	an abnormal condition of the endometrium (of the uterus), in which endometrial tissue grows in various locations in the pelvic cavity, including on the fallopian tubes, uterus, and ovaries (Figure 16.10 ░░░)
metr/i	r/cv	uterus		
-osis	s	condition of		
endo-	p	within	**endometritis** (EHN doh meh TRY tiss)	inflammation of the endometrium (of the uterus)
metr	r	uterus		
-itis	s	inflammation		
fibr/o	r/cv	fiber	**fibrocystic breast disease** (figh broh SISS tik)	formation of one or more benign cysts in the breast (Figure 16.11 ░░░); abbreviated **FBD**
cyst	r	bladder, sac		
-ic	s	pertaining to		
fibr	r	fiber	**fibroid tumor** (FIGH broyd TOO mor)	benign tumor containing fibrous tissue that arises from the myometrium of the uterus; commonly referred to as **fibroids,** the condition is also called myoma of the uterus, fibromyoma, and leiomyoma (Figure 16.12 ░░░)
-oid	s	resemblance to		
			fistula (FISS tyoo lah)	an abnormal passage from one hollow organ to another; a **rectovaginal** (rek toh VAJ ih nal) **fistula** occurs between the vagina and rectum, and a **vesicovaginal** (vess ih koh VAJ ih nal) **fistula** occurs between the bladder and vagina (Figure 16.13 ░░░)
gyn/o	r/cv	woman	**gynopathic** (GYE noh PATH ik)	pertaining to a disease of women
-path	r	disease		
-ic	s	pertaining to		

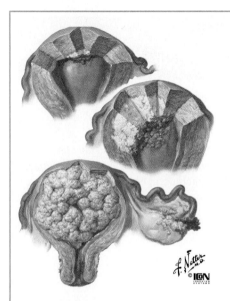

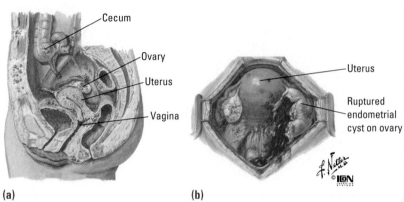

(a)   (b)

Figure 16.9 ::::

Endometrial cancer.

Three stages of endometrial cancer are shown. Note that the mutation arises from the endometrium (top figure), and enters the myometrium later (middle figure). In the bottom figure, the tumor has filled the uterine wall and cavity and has spread to adjacent structures.

Source: Icon Learning Systems

Figure 16.10 ::::

Endometriosis.

(a) Endometrial tissue (red color) has spread throughout the pelvic cavity, attaching to organs and other structures. The tissue behaves like the endometrium, resulting in minor blood loss during menstruation.

(b) Advanced endometriosis can produce blood-filled cysts that are in danger of rupturing, which can result in a life-threatening hemorrhage.

Source: Icon Learning Systems

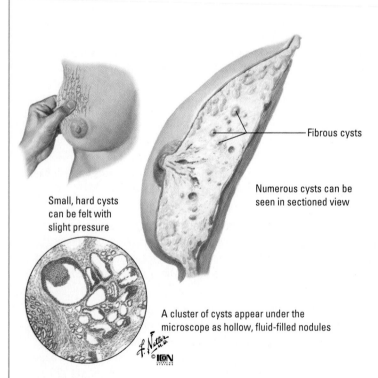

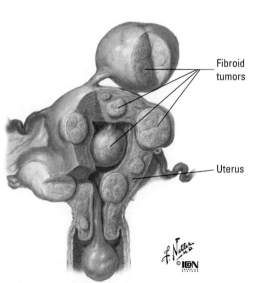

Figure 16.11 ::::

Fibrocystic breast disease.

The condition is characterized by the presence of numerous cysts, which are small, fibrous nodules that are often filled with fluid.

Source: Icon Learning Systems

Figure 16.12 ::::

Fibroid tumors.

Fibroids develop from the uterus to form a variety of hard, round benign structures.

Source: Icon Learning Systems

WORD PARTS (WHEN APPLICABLE)			TERM	DEFINITION
Part	**Type**	**Meaning**		

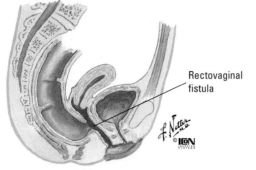

Rectovaginal fistula

Figure 16.13 ::::

Fistula.
The illustration shows a rectovaginal fistula, which is an abnormal passageway between the rectum and vagina.
Source: Icon Learning Systems

Part	Type	Meaning	TERM	DEFINITION
hyster -atresia	r s	uterus closure	**hysteratresia** (hiss ter ah TREE zee ah)	closure of the uterus, resulting in an abnormal obstruction in the uterine canal
mast -itis	r s	breast inflammation	**mastitis** (mass TYE tiss)	inflammation of the breast
mast/o -ptosis	r/cv s	breast falling downward	**mastoptosis** (mass top TOH siss)	condition of a sagging breast
my/o metr -itis	r/cv r s	muscle uterus inflammation	**myometritis** (MY oh meh TRY tiss)	inflammation of the myometrium (of the uterus)
oophor -itis	r s	ovary inflammation	**oophoritis** (oh off oh RYE tiss)	inflammation of an ovary
ovari -an	r s	ovary pertaining to	**ovarian cancer** (oh VAIR ee an)	a malignant tumor arising from an ovary (Figure 16.14::::)

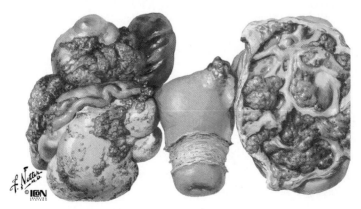

Figure 16.14 ::::

Ovarian cancer.
A carcinoma of the ovary is often an aggressive form of cancer, spreading quickly to other organs of the body. In this illustration, both ovaries have become overcome by the tumors; the right ovary is unsectioned, and the left ovary is sectioned to reveal internal features.
Source: Icon Learning Systems.

Part	Type	Meaning	TERM	DEFINITION
para- ovari -an	p r s	near, alongside ovary pertaining to	**parovarian cyst** (par oh VAIR ee an sist)	a cyst (abnormal fluid-filled sac) of a fallopian tube
			pelvic inflammatory disease	inflammation of the female organs within the pelvic cavity, generally including the ovaries, uterus, and fallopian tubes, usually caused by bacteria; abbreviated **PID**

WORD PARTS (WHEN APPLICABLE)			TERM	DEFINITION
Part	Type	Meaning		
peri- metr -itis	p r s	around, about uterus inflammation	**perimetritis** (PAIR ih meh TRY tiss)	inflammation of the perimetrium (of the uterus) (Figure 16.15::::)
poly- mast -ia	p r s	many breast condition of	**polymastia** (pall ee MAST ee ah)	presence of more than two breasts
pre- menstru -al	p r s	before menstruation pertaining to	**premenstrual syndrome** (pre MEN stroo al SIN drohm)	a collection of symptoms, including tension, irritability, painful breasts (mastalgia), edema, and headache, which usually strike during the ten days preceding menstruation; abbreviated **PMS**
			prolapsed uterus (PRO lapsd)	displacement of the uterus resulting in a downward location, often crowding into the vagina; also called **hysteroptosis** (HISS ter oh TOH siss) (Figure 16.16::::)

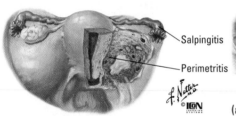

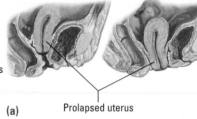

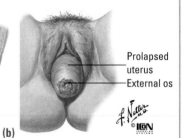

Figure 16.15 ::::

Perimetritis.   The perimetrium of the uterus is inflamed in this condition, usually due to bacterial infection. The infection may quickly spread to nearby structures, such as the fallopian tube, to produce salpingitis. The myometrium may also become inflamed to produce myometritis, as this illustration shows.
Source: Icon Learning Systems

Figure 16.16 ::::

Prolapsed uterus.
(a) A prolapse is the abnormal drop of the uterus into the vagina, representing the most common type of uterine displacement. It is usually caused by weakened uterine ligaments.
(b) A severely prolapsed uterus may extend through the vaginal orifice, as shown.
Source: Icon Learning Systems

salping -itis	r s	trumpet, fallopian tube inflammation	**salpingitis** (sal pin JYE tiss)	inflammation of the fallopian tube (Figure 16.15)
salping/o -cele	r/cv s	tumpet, fallopian tube hernia, swelling	**salpingocele** (sal PING goh seel)	hernia of the fallopian tube
			toxic shock syndrome (TAHK sik SHOK SIN drohm)	an infectious disease characterized by a rapid onset of symptoms including high fever, skin rash, diarrhea, vomiting, and myalgia, followed by hypotension, leading to shock and in severe cases, death; it has been linked to noncotton tampon use and is usually caused by *Staphylococcus aureus;* abbreviated **TSS**

WORD PARTS (WHEN APPLICABLE)			TERM	DEFINITION
Part	**Type**	**Meaning**		
vagin	r	sheath, vagina	**vaginitis** (vaj ih NYE tiss)	inflammation of the vagina, which is also known as **colpitis** (kol PYE tiss); in a common form known as **atrophic vaginitis** (ay TROH fik vaj ih NYE tiss), the usual symptoms of redness and swelling are accompanied by thinning of the vaginal wall and loss of moisture, usually due to a depletion of estrogens (Figure 16.17::::)
-itis	s	inflammation		
vulv/o	r/cv	vulva	**vulvovaginitis** (VUL voh vaj ih NYE tiss)	inflammation of the vulva and vagina
vagin	r	sheath, vagina		
-itis	s	inflammation		

Figure 16.17 ::::

Vaginitis.
(a) Sectioned view of the vagina to show the irritated vaginal lining that is typical of vaginitis.
(b) In the chronic form of vaginitis, fibrous cords develop that may occlude the opening and produce pain during intercourse and menstruation. The view is through a vaginal speculum, an instrument used to open the vagina during a gynecological exam.
Source: Icon Learning Systems

(a)   (b)

disease focus | Cancers of Female Organs

Cancers of female organs collectively form the greatest type of threat to health and life among women. They include cancers of the uterus, breast, and ovaries. According to the American Cancer Society, cancers of the uterus, including cervical cancer and endometrial cancer, are the most common reproductive cancers in women between 15 and 40 years in age. Approximately 14,500 new cases of **cervical cancer** are diagnosed each year in the United States, and about one-third of those cases will result in death. Another 33,500 patients with less aggressive forms of cervical cancer are diagnosed each year.

Uterine cancer is very lethal because most women fail to develop symptoms until later in the disease. Symptoms include vaginal bleeding, pelvic pain, and vaginal discharge. The most effective screening test is the **Pap smear**, although new techniques including **cancer antigen-125 tumor marker** have created additional diagnostic tools.

The primary risk factor for cervical cancer is a history of multiple sex partners, probably due to an association between the cancer and viral infection by one of several human papilloma viruses (HPVs). It is generally believed that early treatment of abnormal but precancerous lesions known as **cervical intraepithelial neoplasia, or CIN,** as detected by Pap smears, may prevent progression to cancer. Without treatment, this precancerous stage often progresses quickly into a severe cervical dysplasia, followed by progression into **carcinoma in situ (CIS) of the cervix** (Figure 16.8). Early treatment of cervical cancer usually includes removal of part of the cervix in a **cervical conization** procedure, while treatment of more advanced cancers involves **hysterectomy,** radiation therapy, and chemotherapy.

Endometrial cancer is slightly less common than cervical cancer (Figure 16.9). About 35,000 new cases are reported each year in the United States, which result in about 6,000 deaths per year. The condition is relatively common among women in the 50 to 70 year age bracket and appears to occur more frequently among women treated with **hormone replacement therapy (HRT),** a treatment to counteract osteoporosis after menopause. Endometrial cancer is aggressive, and there is no satisfactory screening test. Its symptoms include irregular bleeding, and diagnosis usually requires a biopsy. Treatment often involves a **hysterectomy,** followed by radiation therapy.

Breast cancer is the second-most common type of cancer in women, after cancers of the uterus (Figure 16.7). About 80 percent of all breast cancers are a form called **infiltrating ductal carcinoma (IDC),** which arises from cells within the mammary ducts and spreads quickly into adjacent tissues. The most common diagnostic tool for diagnosing breast cancers is **mammography,** often followed by a breast **biopsy** for confirmation. If the cancer remains within the mammary ducts, it is a noninvasive tumor and can be easily treated by a **lumpectomy.** However, if cancerous cells spread to surrounding lymph nodes, the cancer quickly becomes aggressive, requiring more invasive procedures, including **radical mastectomy** or **modified radical mastectomy,** which are followed by radiation therapy and chemotherapy.

The ovaries may also develop cancer (Figure 16.14). In fact, the chance of **ovarian cancer** is 1 in 70 women within the United States; in 1997, 26,800 women were diagnosed and 14,200 deaths were recorded. About 85 percent of ovarian cancers arise from epithelial cells within the ovary. Even though diagnostic procedures like **transvaginal sonography** (TVS) can detect ovarian cancer relatively early, there is a high incidence of false-positive results. In ovarian cancer cases that are detected early, treatment programs are often successful, but many cases are not diagnosed until the disease has progressed. When ovarian cancers are detected later, aggressive treatments like **salpingo-oophorectomy** and **total hysterectomy,** followed with aggressive chemotherapy, become necessary. Unfortunately, these treatments are considered last-ditch efforts to save the patient, and are accompanied by additional risks.

SELF QUIZ 16.4

SAY IT—SPELL IT!

Review the terms of the female reproductive system by speaking the phonetic pronunciations out loud, then writing the correct spelling of the term.

1. ADD eh noh my OH sis _____

16.7 2. DER moyd   sist _____

3. ehn doh MEE tree al   KANN ser _____

4. EHN doh mee tree OH sis _____

5. EHN doh meh TRY tis _____

6. EHN doh ser vih SIGH tis _____

7. fi broh SISS tik _____

8. GYE neh koh MAST ee ah _____

16.8 9. GYE noh PATH ik _____

10. hiss ter ah TREE zee ah _____

11. mass TI tis _____

12. mass top TOH sis _____

13. MY oh meh TRY tis _____

14. oh off oh RYE tis _____

15. par oh VAIR ee an   sist _____

16. PAIR ih meh TRY tis _____

17. sal PING goh seel _____

18. SER vih SIGH tis _____

16.9 19. vaj ih NYE tis _____

20. vess ih koh VAJ ih nal   FISS tyoo lah _____

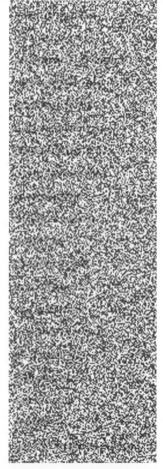

MATCH IT!

Match the term on the left with the correct definition on the right.

_____ 1. breast cancer

   a. benign tumor of the ovary with embryonic tissue

_____ 2. cervical cancer

   b. abnormal fluid-filled sac in a fallopian tube

_____ 3. endometrial cancer

   c. benign tumor arising from the myometrium

_____ 4. toxic shock syndrome

   d. abnormal passage between the bladder and vagina

_____ 5. pelvic inflammatory disease

   e. formation of benign cysts in the breast

_____ 6. cervical intraepithelial neoplasia

   f. also called adenocarcinoma of the breast

_____ 7. parovarian cyst

   g. displacement of the uterus downward

_____ 8. prolapsed uterus

   h. benign form of cervical neoplasia

_____ 9. dermoid cyst

   i. malignant tumor of the cervix

_____10. vesicovaginal fistula

   j. uterine cancer

_____11. fibrocystic breast disease

   k. bacterial infection associated with tampon use

_____12. fibroid tumor

   l. inflammation of pelvic organs

BREAK IT DOWN!

Analyze and separate each term into its word parts, by labeling each word part using p = prefix, r = root, cv = combining vowel, and s = suffix.

1. amastia _____

16.10 2. cervicitis _____

16.11 3. endometriosis _____

4. gynecomastia _____

16.12 5. mastitis _____

6. myometritis _____

16.13 7. perimetritis _____

8. polymastia _____

9. vulvovaginitis _____

WORD BUILDING

Construct or recall medical terms from the following meanings.

1. growth of the endometrium into the myometrium
   _____

2. absence of a breast
   _____

3. inflammation of a Bartholin's gland
   _____

4. any disease of women
   _____

5. inflammation of the vulva and vagina
   _____

6. inflammation of the myometrium
   _____

16.14 7. inflammation of an ovary
   _____

8. hernia of a fallopian tube
   _____

9. inflammation of a breast
   _____

10. inflammation of the cervical inner lining
   _____

11. closure of the uterus
   _____

12. inflammation of the endometrium
   _____

13. endometrial tissue growth in the pelvic area
   _____

FILL IT IN!

Fill in the blanks with the correct terms.

1. A malignant tumor arising from breast tissue is known as breast cancer, or

   _____ of the breast. By contrast, the formation of one or more

   cysts in the breast is a benign condition known as _____ breast

   disease.

2. A cervical neoplasia is an abnormal development of cells within the cervix. The

   precancerous state is called carcinoma _____

   _____ of the cervix, and the early cancerous state is known as

   _____ _____ neoplasia, or more simply,

   _____ _____.

3. A cancer arising from the endometrium is called _____

   _____, or sometimes called _____

   _____. A benign tumor arising from the myometrium of the uterus

16.15 is commonly called _____ _____. In the

   condition known as _____ _____, the uterus is

   displaced in a downward location, often crowding into the vagina.

4. A benign tumor of an ovary that consists of embryonic tissue is known as a

   _____ _____. A tumor of the ovary that is

   malignant results in the disease known as _____

   _____. A cyst that develops within a fallopian tube is called a

   _____ _____.

5. An abnormal passage between the rectum and the vagina is a

_____ _____, and one between the bladder

and vagina is a _____ _____.

6. An inflammatory disease affecting several organs of the female pelvic region

that is often bacterial in origin is known as pelvic _____

_____. A severe bacterial infection that is associated with the

use of certain tampons during menstruation is called _____

_____ _____. A collection of physical and

emotional symptoms that usually strike during the 10 days preceding

menstruation is known as _____ _____.

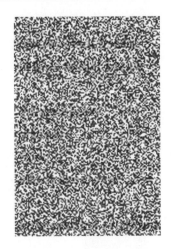

Treatments, Procedures, and Devices

WORD PARTS (WHEN APPLICABLE)			TERM	DEFINITION
Part	Type	Meaning		
colp/o -rraphy	r/cv s	vagina suturing	**anterior and posterior colporrhaphy** (kahl POR ah fee)	surgical repair of a protrusion of the bladder against the anterior vaginal wall and protrusion of the rectum against the posterior vaginal wall; abbreviated **A&P repair**
			biopsy (BYE op see)	removal of a tissue sample for microscopic evaluation, which may be done by aspiration biopsy, endoscopic biopsy, excisional biopsy, or needle biopsy; abbreviated **Bx** (Figure 16.18▦)
			cancer antigen-125 tumor marker (KANN ser AN tih jenn)	a blood test that is used to provide evidence for ovarian cancer, which measures the levels of a protein produced by cancer cells; abbreviated **CA-125**
cervic -al	r s	neck, cervix pertaining to	**cervical conization** (SER vih kal koh nih ZAY shun)	removal of the cone-shaped portion of the cervix
cervic -ectomy	r s	neck, cervix excision	**cervicectomy** (SER vih SEK toh mee)	excision of the cervix; also called **trachelectomy** (TRAY kee LEK toh mee)
colp/o perine/o -rraphy	r/cv r/cv s	vagina perineum suturing	**colpoperineorrhaphy** (KOHLpoh PAIR ih nee OR ah fee)	suture of the vagina and perineum to correct tears
colp/o -plasty	r/cv s	vagina surgical repair	**colpoplasty** (KOHL poh PLASS tee)	surgical repair of the vagina
colp/o -rrhaphy	r/cv s	vagina suturing	**colporrhaphy** (kohl POR ah fee)	suture of the vagina
colp/o -scopy	r/cv s	vagina process of viewing	**colposcopy** (kohl POSS koh pee)	endoscopic examination of the vagina (and cervix) using a modified endoscope called a colposcope (KOHL poh skope)
culd/o -centesis	r/cv s	cul-de-sac surgical puncture	**culdocentesis** (KULL doh sen TEE siss)	surgical puncture into the pelvic cavity to remove fluid from the rectouterine pouch (Douglas' cul-de-sac) (Figure 16.19▦)

WORD PARTS (WHEN APPLICABLE)			TERM	DEFINITION
Part	Type	Meaning		

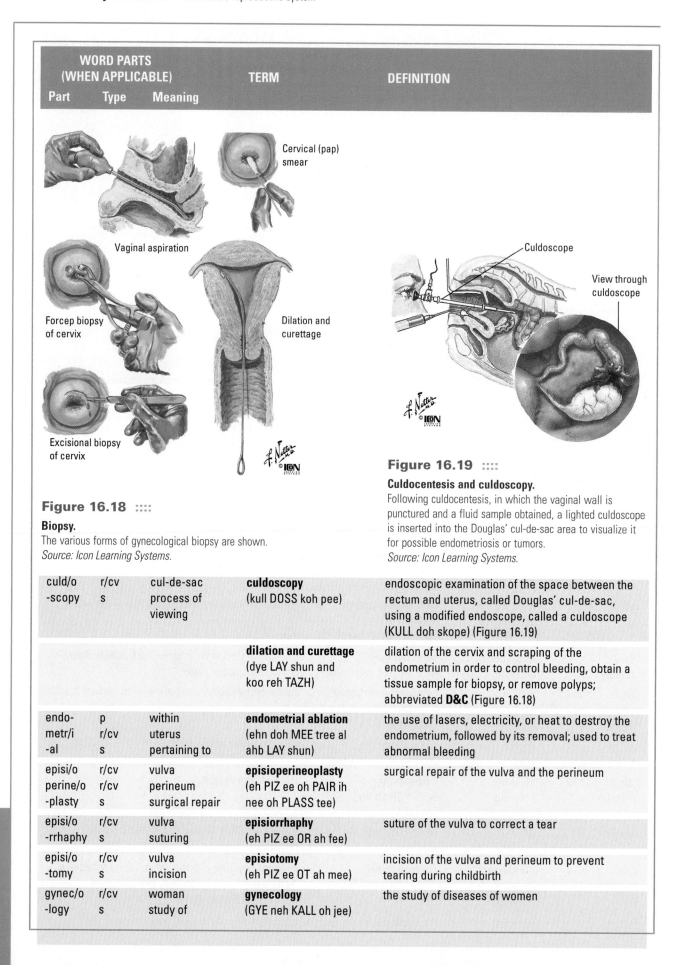

Cervical (pap) smear

Vaginal aspiration

Forcep biopsy of cervix

Dilation and curettage

Excisional biopsy of cervix

Figure 16.18 ::::

Biopsy.
The various forms of gynecological biopsy are shown.
Source: Icon Learning Systems.

Culdoscope

View through culdoscope

Figure 16.19 ::::

Culdocentesis and culdoscopy.
Following culdocentesis, in which the vaginal wall is
punctured and a fluid sample obtained, a lighted culdoscope
is inserted into the Douglas' cul-de-sac area to visualize it
for possible endometriosis or tumors.
Source: Icon Learning Systems.

Part	Type	Meaning	TERM	DEFINITION
culd/o -scopy	r/cv s	cul-de-sac process of viewing	**culdoscopy** (kull DOSS koh pee)	endoscopic examination of the space between the rectum and uterus, called Douglas' cul-de-sac, using a modified endoscope, called a culdoscope (KULL doh skope) (Figure 16.19)
			dilation and curettage (dye LAY shun and koo reh TAZH)	dilation of the cervix and scraping of the endometrium in order to control bleeding, obtain a tissue sample for biopsy, or remove polyps; abbreviated **D&C** (Figure 16.18)
endo- metr/i -al	p r/cv s	within uterus pertaining to	**endometrial ablation** (ehn doh MEE tree al ahb LAY shun)	the use of lasers, electricity, or heat to destroy the endometrium, followed by its removal; used to treat abnormal bleeding
episi/o perine/o -plasty	r/cv r/cv s	vulva perineum surgical repair	**episioperineoplasty** (eh PIZ ee oh PAIR ih nee oh PLASS tee)	surgical repair of the vulva and the perineum
episi/o -rrhaphy	r/cv s	vulva suturing	**episiorrhaphy** (eh PIZ ee OR ah fee)	suture of the vulva to correct a tear
episi/o -tomy	r/cv s	vulva incision	**episiotomy** (eh PIZ ee OT ah mee)	incision of the vulva and perineum to prevent tearing during childbirth
gynec/o -logy	r/cv s	woman study of	**gynecology** (GYE neh KALL oh jee)	the study of diseases of women

WORD PARTS (WHEN APPLICABLE)			TERM	DEFINITION
Part	**Type**	**Meaning**		
gynec/o -logist	r/cv s	woman one who studies	**gynecologist** (GYE neh KALL oh jist)	a physician specializing in women's diseases
			hormone replacement therapy	clinical treatment that includes the replacement of naturally produced hormones with synthetic hormones as a treatment for menopause, abbreviated **HRT**; also called estrogen replacement therapy, abbreviated **ERT**
hymen -ectomy	r s	membrane, hymen excision	**hymenectomy** (HIGH men EK toh mee)	excision of the hymen
hymen/o -tomy	r/cv s	membrane, hymen incision	**hymenotomy** (HIGH men OTT toh mee)	incision into the hymen
hyster -ectomy	r s	uterus excision	**hysterectomy** (HISS teh REK toh mee)	excision of the uterus, which may include surrounding structures; also called **uterectomy** (YOO teh REK toh mee) (Figure 16.20)

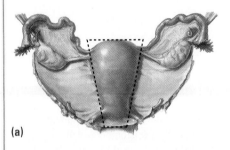

(a)

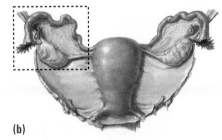

(b)

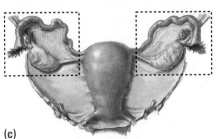

(c)

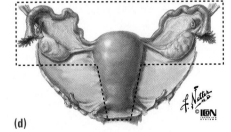

(d)

Figure 16.20

Alternative forms of surgeries involving the uterus, ovaries, and fallopian tubes.
The dotted lines indicate excision.
(a) Hysterectomy.
(b) Right salpingo-oophorectomy.
(c) Bilateral salpingo-oophorectomy.
(d) Bilateral hysterosalpingo-oophorectomy, or panhysterectomy.
Source: Icon Learning Systems

hyster/o -pexy	r/cv s	uterus surgical fixation	**hysteropexy** (HISS ter oh PEK see)	surgical fixation of the uterus
hyster/o salping/o -graphy	r/cv r/cv s	uterus trumpet, fallopian tube recording process	**hysterosalpingography** (HISS ter oh sal pin GOG rah fee)	x-ray procedure that produces an x-ray image of the uterus and fallopian tubes after injection of a radiopaque contrast medium, called a hysterosalpingogram (HISS ter oh sal ping oh gram); abbreviated **HSG** (Figure 16.21)

WORD PARTS (WHEN APPLICABLE)			TERM	DEFINITION
Part	Type	Meaning		

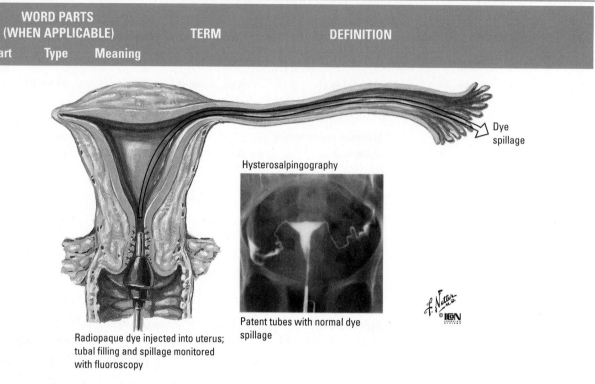

Hysterosalpingography

Dye spillage

Patent tubes with normal dye spillage

Radiopaque dye injected into uterus; tubal filling and spillage monitored with fluoroscopy

Figure 16.21 ⸬

Hysterosalpingogram.   A liquid contrast medium (radiopaque dye) is used to highlight structures by injecting it through the vagina prior to the x-ray. The procedure is usually performed to identify the location of an obstruction within the fallopian tubes or uterus.
Source: Icon Learning Systems

Part	Type	Meaning	TERM	DEFINITION
hyster/o	r/cv	uterus	**hysterosalpingo-oophorectomy** (HISS ter oh sal PING goh oh OFF oh REK toh mee)	excision of the uterus, fallopian tubes, and ovaries (Figure 16.20); when the excision occurs through the abdomen and is bilateral, it is abbreviated **TAH/BSO** (total abdominal hysterectomy/bilateral salpingo-oophorectomy)
salping/o	r/cv	trumpet, fallopian tube		
oophor	r	ovary		
-ectomy	s	excision		
hyster/o	r/cv	uterus	**hysteroscopy** (HISS ter OSS koh pee)	endoscopic examination of the uterine cavity using a modified endoscope called a hysteroscope (HISS ter oh skope)
-scopy	s	viewing instrument		
lapar/o	r/cv	abdomen	**laparoscopy** (lap ahr OSS koh pee)	endoscopic examination of the abdominal or pelvic cavity with a modifed endoscope called a laparoscope (LAP ah roh skope) (Figure 16.22⸬)
-scopy	s	viewing instrument		
mamm/o	r/cv	breast	**mammography** (mam OG rah fee)	x-ray procedure that produces an x-ray image of the breast, called a mammogram (MAM moh gram) (Figure 16.23⸬)
-graphy	s	recording process		
mamm/o	r/cv	breast	**mammoplasty** (MAM moh PLASS tee)	surgical repair of the breasts, resulting in the enlargement or reduction of breast size or removal of a tumor
-plasty	s	surgical repair		

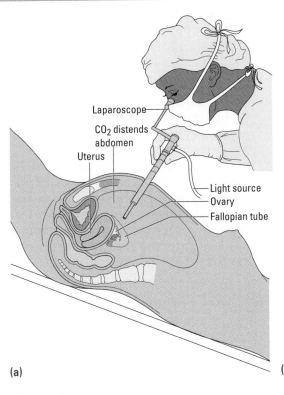

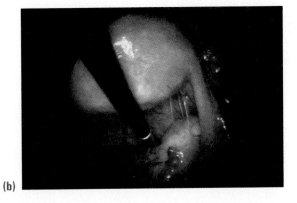

(a)

(b)

Figure 16.22 ::::

Laparoscopy.

(a) A lighted endoscope specialized for insertion into the abdomen, called a laparoscope, is used to view reproductive organs. The laparoscope may also be outfitted with surgical devices for excision of structures.
Source: Pearson Education.

(b) Laparoscopic surgery, as seen from the monitor attached to the laparoscope.
Source: Southern Illinois University/Photo Researchers Inc.

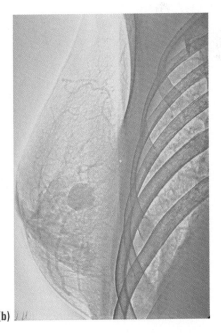

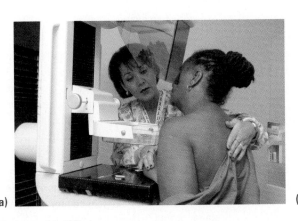

(a)

(b)

Figure 16.23 ::::

Mammography.

(a) A physician assists the patient to assure the breast is placed ideally for the x-ray.

(b) A mammogram. A tumor is visible in this mammogram as the darkened oval structure near the center.

WORD PARTS (WHEN APPLICABLE)			TERM	DEFINITION
Part	**Type**	**Meaning**		
mast	r	breast	**mastectomy**	excision of a breast; in a simple mastectomy, one entire breast is removed, leaving underlying muscles and lymph nodes intact; a **radical mastectomy** (also called Halstead mastectomy) is the removal of the entire affected breast, the underlying chest muscles, and local lymph nodes; a **modified radical mastectomy** is removal of the affected breast and lymph nodes of the underarm, leaving muscle intact; a **lumpectomy** (lump EK toh mee) or tylectomy (tye LEK toh mee) is the removal of the cancerous lesions only, in order to conserve the breast (Figure 16.24▦)
-ectomy	s	excision	(mass TEK toh mee)	

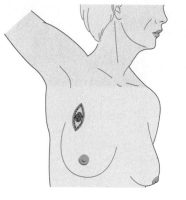

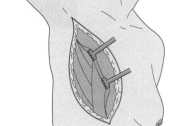

(a) Lumpectomy   **(b)** Modified radical mastectomy

Figure 16.24 ▦

Mastectomy.
(a) A lumpectomy is the removal of the tumor only, with a small margin of surrounding tissue.
Source: Pearson Education.
(b) A modified radical mastectomy involves the removal of all breast tissue and the underarm lymph nodes, but leaves the muscles intact. In a radical mastectomy (not shown), the chest muscles are also removed.
Source: Pearson Education.

WORD PARTS (WHEN APPLICABLE)			TERM	DEFINITION
Part	**Type**	**Meaning**		
mast/o	r/cv	breast	**mastopexy**	surgical fixation of the breast, which is usually performed to elevate pendulous breast tissue
-pexy	s	surgical fixation	(MAST oh pek see)	
my	r	muscle	**myomectomy**	excision of a myoma, or fibroid tumor, from the uterus
-om[a]	s	tumor	(MY oh MEK toh mee)	
-ectomy	s	excision		
oophor	r	ovary	**oophorectomy**	excision of an ovary
-ectomy	s	excision	(oh OFF oh REK toh mee)	
pan-	p	all, entire	**panhysterectomy**	excision of the uterus, ovaries, and fallopian tubes, which are removed through an abdominal incision (Figure 16.20); a radical hysterectomy is a similar procedure, in which the lymph nodes, upper portion of the vagina, and surrounding tissues are also removed
hyster	r	uterus	(PAN HIS teh REK toh mee)	
-ectomy	s	excision		
			Papanicolau smear	a diagnostic procedure in which a sample of cells from the cervix and vagina are removed and examined microscopically for abnormalities; mainly used to screen for cervical cancer; also called **Pap smear** or **Pap test** (Figure 16.25▦)
			(pap an IK oh law)	

WORD PARTS (WHEN APPLICABLE)			TERM	DEFINITION
Part	**Type**	**Meaning**		

> [FYI]
>
> **Papanicolau smear**
> Named after Dr. George Papanicolau, an anatomist and cytologist, the Pap smear is a screening test for ovarian cancer that has made early detection possible. The American Cancer Society recommends annual tests at ages 20 and 21, followed by tests at one-year and three-year intervals.

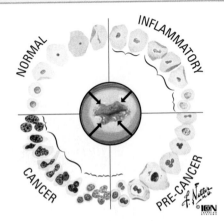

Figure 16.25 ::::

Pap smear.
Cells of the cervix (center) change in appearance as they progress through the various stages of cervical cancer, as shown in this figure. During the pap smear procedure, cells are obtained from the cervix and prepared for microscopic evaluation, then compared to charts. Based on the cells' appearance, a diagnosis and prognosis can be reached.
Source: Icon Learning Systems

Part	Type	Meaning	TERM	DEFINITION
perine/o	r/cv	perineum	**perineorrhaphy**	suture of the perineum to correct a tear
-rrhaphy	s	suturing	(PAIR ih nee OR ah fee)	
salping	r	trumpet, fallopian tube	**salpingectomy** (SAL pin JEK toh mee)	excision of a fallopian tube
-ectomy	s	excision		
salping/o	r/cv	trumpet, fallopian tube	**salpingo-oophorectomy** (sal ping goh oh	excision of a fallopian tube and an ovary, usually from the same side (Figure 16.20)
oophor	r	ovary	OFF oh REK toh mee)	
-ectomy	s	excision		
salping/o	r/cv	trumpet, fallopian tube	**salpingostomy** (SAL ping GOSS toh mee)	surgical creation of an opening through the wall of a fallopian tube, often to treat ectopic tubal pregnancy
-stomy	s	surgical creation of an opening		
son/o	r/cv	sound	**sonohysterography**	ultrasound procedure that records an image of the
hyster/o	r/cv	uterus	(son oh HIST er	uterus with the use of sound waves, called a
-graphy	s	recording process	OG rah fee)	sonohysterogram (son oh HIST er oh gram) and used to evaluate the postoperative status of polyps, myomas, and adhesions of the uterus
trachel/o	r/cv	neck, cervix	**trachelorrhaphy**	suture of the wall of the cervix
-rrhaphy	s	suturing	(tray kee LOR ah fee)	
trans-	p	through, across	**transvaginal sonography**	ultrasound procedure in which a probe is inserted into the vagina to record images of the uterus,
vagin	r	vagina		ovaries, fallopian tubes, and surrounding structures,
-al	s	pertaining to	(trans VAJ ih nal	performed to diagnose ovarian tumors or cysts,
son/o	r/cv	sound	son OG rah fee)	monitor pregnancy, and to monitor ovulation for
-graphy	s	recording process		treating infertility; abbreviated **TVS**

WORD PARTS (WHEN APPLICABLE)			TERM	DEFINITION
Part	**Type**	**Meaning**		
			tubal ligation (TOO bal lye GAY shun)	sterilization procedure by ligating (cutting and tying) the fallopian tubes (Figure 16.26::::)
vagin -al	r s	vaginal pertaining to	**vaginal speculum** (SPEK yoo lum)	instrument for opening the vaginal orifice to permit visual examination of the vagina and beyond (Figure 16.27::::)
vulv -ectomy	r s	vulva excision	**vulvectomy** (vul VEK toh mee)	excision of the vulva

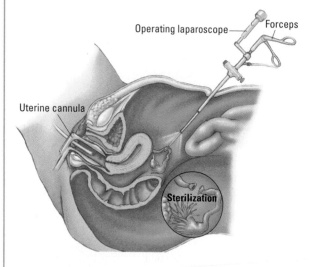

Forceps
Operating laparoscope
Uterine cannula
Sterilization

Figure 16.26 ::::
Tubal ligation.
To minimize the size of the incisions necessary, laparoscopic surgery may be used to enter the abdominal cavity through a small incision, cut the fallopian tubes, and ligate (tie off).

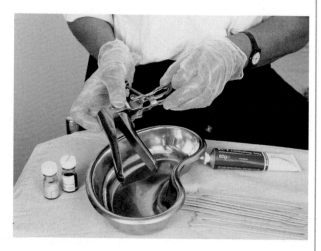

Figure 16.27 ::::
Vaginal speculum.
The instrument is used to increase the diameter of the vaginal canal during a gynecological exam.
Source: Simon Fraser/Science Photo Library/Photo Researchers Inc.

SELF QUIZ 16.5

SAY IT—SPELL IT!

Review the terms of the female reproductive system by speaking the phonetic pronunciations out loud, then writing the correct spelling of the term.

1. HISS ter oh sal pin GOG rah fee _____

2. mam OG rah fee _____

3. son oh HIST er OG rah fee _____

4. kohl POSS koh pee _____

5. HISS ter OSS koh pee _____

6. KULL doh sen TEE siss _____

7. SER vih SEK toh mee _____

8. KOHL poh PAIR ih nee OR ah fee _____

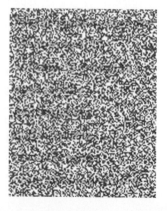

9. KOHL poh PLASS tee   _____

10. eh PIZ ee oh PAIR ih nee oh
    PLASS tee   _____

11. HISS teh REK toh mee   _____

12. HISS ter oh sal PING goh
    oh OFF oh REK toh mee   _____

16.16 13. mass TEK toh mee   _____

14. MY oh MEK toh mee   _____

15. oh OFF oh REK toh mee   _____

16. PAIR ih nee OR ah fee   _____

17. SAL pin JEK toh mee   _____

18. sal ping goh oh OFF oh REK toh mee   _____

19. TRAY kee LEK toh mee   _____

16.17 20. MAM moh PLASS tee   _____

MATCH IT!

Match the term on the left with the correct definition on the right.

_____ 1. cervicectomy

_____ 2. colpoperineorrhaphy

_____ 3. colporrhaphy

_____ 4. radical hysterectomy

_____ 5. hymenotomy

_____ 6. oophorectomy

_____ 7. vulvectomy

_____ 8. episoperineorrhaphy

_____ 9. hysteropexy

_____10. simple mastectomy

_____11. myomectomy

_____12. perineorrhaphy

_____13. salpingostomy

_____14. trachelorrhaphy

_____15. salpingo-oophorectomy

_____16. hormone replacement
        therapy

_____17. dilation & curettage

_____18. cervical conization

_____19. tubal ligation

a. incision into the hymen

b. surgical removal of the vulva

c. surgical fixation of the uterus

d. creation of an opening through the fallopian
   tube

e. excision of the cervix

f. suture of the cervical wall

g. suture of the vagina and perineum

h. suture of the perineum

i. surgical removal of a myoma

j. suture of the vaginal wall

k. excision of a fallopian tube and ovary

l. similar to a panhysterectomy, but more
   extensive

m. surgical repair of the vulva and perineum

n. excision of an ovary

o. removal of one entire breast, leaving other
   tissues intact

p. a sterilization procedure

q. can minimize the effects of postmenopause

r. procedure used to reduce excessive menses

s. removes the cone-shaped part of the cervix

BREAK IT DOWN!

Analyze and separate each term into its word parts by labeling each word part using p = prefix, r = root, cv = combining vowel, and s = suffix.

1. mammography   _____

2. sonohysterography   _____

3. colposcopy   _____

4. hysteroscopy   _____

5. laparoscopy   _____

6. culdocentesis   _____

7. cervicectomy   _____

8. colpoperineorrhaphy   _____

9. episioperineoplasty   _____

10. hymenotomy   _____

11. hysterosalpingo-oophorectomy   _____

WORD BUILDING

Construct or recall medical terms from the following meanings.

1. surgical puncture to remove fluid from Douglas' cul-de-sac   _____

2. endoscope used to view the abdominal or pelvic cavity   _____

3. ultrasound procedure to produce an image of the uterus   _____

4. x-ray procedure to view the uterus and fallopian tubes   _____

5. x-ray procedure to produce an image of the breast   _____

6. endoscope used to view the vagina and cervix   _____

7. views the uterus, ovaries, and fallopian tubes with ultrasound   _____

8. an instrument that widens the vaginal orifice   _____

9. corrects insufficient estrogen levels   _____

10. severs and closes the fallopian tubes   _____

11. removes the inferior part of the cervix _____

12. a blood test for ovarian cancer _____

13. evaluation of cervical or vaginal cells _____

14. removal of a tissue specimen for microscopic study _____

15. opens the vagina and scrapes the endometrium _____

16.18 16. the study of diseases of women _____

FILL IT IN!

Fill in the blanks with the correct terms.

1. A procedure that removes a tissue sample for microscopic evaluation is called a

   _____. A similar test in which cells from the cervix and vagina

   are removed for microscopic evaluation is a _____

   _____. The cervix is first dilated and the endometrium is then

   scraped to obtain a tissue sample, or to remove polyps or control bleeding in a

   _____ _____ _____.

2. A blood test that is used to evaluate for ovarian cancer is called the

   _____ _____ tumor marker.

3. A _____ _____ is an instrument that is used

   to widen the vaginal orifice to permit visual examination or perform a procedure.

   A procedure that requires this instrument is the _____

   _____, in which the cone-shaped portion of the cervix is removed.

4. A _____ _____ is a surgical procedure that

   provides permanent sterilization of the patient.

5. Naturally produced hormones may be replaced in _____

   _____ therapy in postmenopausal women.

abbreviations of the female reproductive system

The abbreviations that are associated with the female reproductive system are summarized here. Study these abbreviations, and review them in the exercise that follows.

ABBREVIATION	DEFINITION	ABBREVIATION	DEFINITION
A&P repair	anterior and posterior colporrhaphy	CIN	cervical intraepithelial neoplasia
		CIS	carcinoma in situ
Bx	biopsy	D&C	dilation and curettage
CA-125	cancer antigen-125 tumor marker	ERT	estrogen replacement therapy
		FBD	fibrocystic breast disease

ABBREVIATION	DEFINITION	ABBREVIATION	DEFINITION
GYN	gynecology	PMS	premenstrual syndrome
HRT	hormone replacement therapy	TAH/BSO	total abdominal hysterectomy/
HSG	hysterosalpingogram		bilateral salpingo-oophorectomy
Pap smear (test)	Papanicolau smear (or test)	TSS	toxic shock syndrome
PID	pelvic inflammatory disease	TVS	transvaginal sonography

SELF QUIZ 16.6

Fill in the blanks with the abbreviation or the complete medical term.

Abbreviation	Medical Term
1. _____	cervical intraepithelial neoplasia
2. D&C	_____
3. _____	carcinoma in situ
16.19 4. HRT	_____
5. _____	cancer antigen-125 tumor marker
6. PMS	_____
7. _____	estrogen replacement therapy
16.20 8. TSS	_____
16.21 9. _____	pelvic inflammatory disease
10. TVS	_____
16.22 11. _____	gynecology
12. Bx	_____
13. _____	Papanicolau smear
14. A&P repair	_____
15. _____	fibrocystic breast disease
16. TAH/BSO	_____

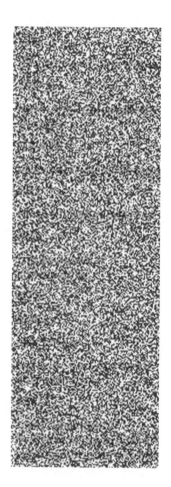

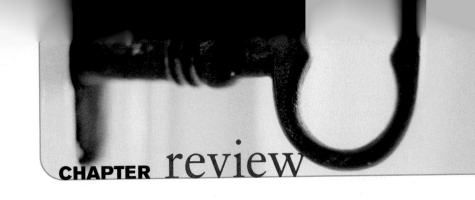

In this section, we will review all the word parts and medical terms from this chapter. As in earlier tables, the word roots are shown in **bold**.

Check each word part and medical term to be sure you understand the meaning. If any are not clear, please go back into the chapter and review that term. Then, complete the review exercises that follow.

[word parts **checklist**]

Prefixes

- ❑ endo-
- ❑ peri-
- ❑ pre-

Word Roots/Combining Vowels

- ❑ **cervic**/o
- ❑ **colp**/o
- ❑ **culd**/o
- ❑ **episi**/o
- ❑ **gyn**/o
- ❑ **gynec**/o
- ❑ **hydr**/o
- ❑ **hyster**/o
- ❑ **mamm**/o
- ❑ **mast**/o
- ❑ **men**/o, **menstru**/o
- ❑ **metr**/o
- ❑ **oophor**/o, **ovari**/o
- ❑ **ov**/i, **ov**/o
- ❑ **perine**/o
- ❑ **py**/o
- ❑ **salping**/o
- ❑ **trachel**/o
- ❑ **uter**/o
- ❑ **vagin**/o
- ❑ **vulv**/o

Suffixes

- ❑ -atresia
- ❑ -ial
- ❑ -salpinx

[medical terminology **checklist**]

- ❑ **aden**o**my**osis
- ❑ adenocarcinoma of the breast
- ❑ alveolar glands
- ❑ a**mast**ia
- ❑ a**men**orrhea
- ❑ Bartholin's adenitis
- ❑ Bartholin's glands
- ❑ biopsy
- ❑ breast cancer
- ❑ Cancer Antigen-125 Tumor Marker
- ❑ **cervic**al canal
- ❑ **cervic**al cancer
- ❑ **cervic**al conization
- ❑ **cervic**al neoplasia
- ❑ **cervic**ectomy
- ❑ **cervic**itis
- ❑ cervix
- ❑ clitoris
- ❑ **colp**ography
- ❑ **colp**o**perine**orrhaphy
- ❑ **colp**orrhaphy
- ❑ **culd**ocentesis
- ❑ **culd**ocentesis
- ❑ **culd**oscopy
- ❑ dermoid cyst
- ❑ dilation and curettage
- ❑ dys**men**orrhea
- ❑ endo**cervic**itis
- ❑ endo**metr**ial cancer
- ❑ endo**metr**iosis
- ❑ endo**metr**itis
- ❑ endo**metr**ium
- ❑ **episi**o**perine**oplasty
- ❑ **episi**orrhaphy
- ❑ estrogen
- ❑ fallopian tube
- ❑ fibrocystic breast disease
- ❑ fibroid tumor
- ❑ fistula
- ❑ follicle
- ❑ fornix
- ❑ graafian follicle
- ❑ **gynec**o**mast**ia
- ❑ **gyn**opathic
- ❑ hematosalpinx
- ❑ hormone replacement therapy
- ❑ **hydr**osalpinx
- ❑ hymen
- ❑ **hymen**ectomy
- ❑ **hymen**otomy
- ❑ **hyster**atresia
- ❑ **hyster**ectomy
- ❑ **hyster**opexy
- ❑ **hyster**o**salping**ography
- ❑ **hyster**o**salping**o-**oophor**ectomy
- ❑ **hyster**oscopy
- ❑ infundibulum
- ❑ labia majora
- ❑ labia minora
- ❑ laparoscopy
- ❑ leukorrhea

- lumpectomy
- **mamm**ary gland
- **mamm**ography
- **mamm**oplasty
- **mast**algia
- **mast**ectomy
- **mast**itis
- **mast**opexy
- **mast**optosis
- **men**arche
- **menometr**orrhagia
- **men**opause
- **men**orrhagia
- **men**ses
- **metr**orrhagia
- **metr**orrhea
- mons pubis
- myomectomy

- myo**metr**itis
- myo**metr**ium
- oligo**men**orrhea
- **oopho**rectomy
- **oopho**ritis
- **ov**a
- **ov**arian cancer
- **ov**ary
- **ov**ulation
- pan**hyster**ectomy
- Papanicolau smear
- par**ovari**an cyst
- pelvic inflammatory disease
- peri**metr**itis
- **perine**orrhaphy
- poly**mast**ia
- pre**menstru**al syndrome
- prolapsed **uter**us

- **py**osalpinx
- **salping**ectomy
- **salping**itis
- **salping**ocele
- **salping**ostomy
- sono**hyster**ography
- toxic shock syndrome
- trachelorrhaphy
- trans**vagin**al sonography
- tubal ligation
- **uter**us
- **vagin**a
- **vagin**al speculum
- **vagin**itis
- vestibule
- **vulv**a
- **vulv**ectomy
- **vulv**o**vagin**itis

[show what **you know!**]

BREAK IT DOWN!

Analyze and separate each term into its word parts by labeling each word part using p = prefix, r = root, cv = combining vowel, and s = suffix.

Example:	1. gynecopathic	<div align="center">r cv r s gynec/o/path/ic</div>
	2. amenorrhea	
	3. dysmenorrhea	
	4. hydrosalpinx	
	5. mastalgia	
	6. metrorrhagia	
	7. endocervicitis	
	8. endometritis	
	9. hysteratresia	
	10. mastitis	
	11. myometritis	
	12. oophoritis	
	13. perimetritis	
	14. vulvovaginitis	
	15. culpoperineorrhaphy	
	16. oophorectomy	
	17. mastectomy	
	18. panhysterectomy	

19. salpingostomy _____

20. trachelorrhaphy _____

21. vulvectomy _____

22. mammography _____

23. culdoscopy _____

24. laparoscopy _____

25. culdocentesis _____

WORD BUILDING

Construct or recall medical terms from the following meanings.

Example: 1. absence of menstrual discharge _____ amenorrhea _____

2. blood in a fallopian tube _____

3. white or yellow discharge from the uterus _____

4. pain in the breast _____

5. excessive bleeding during menstruation _____

6. abnormally reduced bleeding during menstruation _____

7. growth of endometrial tissue into the myometrium _____

8. absence of a breast _____

9. inflammation of the cervix _____

10. closure of the uterus _____

11. condition of a sagging breast _____

12. hernia of a fallopian tube _____

13. inflammation of the vulva and vagina _____

14. malignant tumor arising from a breast _____

15. malignant tumor arising from an ovary _____

16. displacement of the uterus downward _____

17. abnormal passageway between bladder and vagina _____

18. one or more benign cysts in a breast _____

19. excision of a fallopian tube and ovary _____

20. excision of uterus, ovaries, and fallopian tubes _____

21. excision of a fibroid tumor from the uterus _____

22. surgical fixation of the breast _____

23. suture of the perineum to correct a tear _____

24. endoscopic examination of the uterus _____

25. x-ray of the breast _____

26. incision into the hymen _____

CASE STUDIES

Fill in the blanks with the correct terms.

1. A 45-year-old woman was admitted after complaining of excessive pain during menstruation, or

   (a) _____, that was often accompanied by excessive bleeding, or (b)_____. A

   white discharge, or (c)_____, was also mentioned by the patient, usually between periods. A prior

   treatment in which the cervix was dilated and the endometrium scraped, called a (d)_____

   _____ _____, did not eliminate the symptoms. The woman had no prior his-

   tory of reproductive disease, STD, or cancer. A scraping of the vagina and cervix for microscopic evaluation of cells, or

   (e)_____ _____, showed abnormalities of cells. Culturing the cells indicated

   a type of virus that produces vaginal warts, called (f)_____, was present and may have been the

   source of the abnormalities. Further evaluation of the cervix, in which a tissue sample is removed with the aid of endoscopy

   and known as (g)_____, indicated a population of mutated cells that are precancerous, a condition

   called (h)_____ _____ _____

   _____ _____. This finding was confirmed by a negative blood test for ovar-

   ian cancer cells, called (i)_____ _____ _____

   _____. To eliminate the possibility of a neoplasm from developing, the location of the anaplastic cell

   population, at the end of the cervix, was surgically removed in a (j)_____

   _____ procedure.

2. A 75-year-old woman was admitted following her personal observation of a painless, small lump near the nipple of her right

   breast, which had been noticed for just three months. A physical exam revealed the presence of dimpled skin around the nip-

   ple of the right breast, in addition to a small, hard lump. An x-ray of the breast, or (k)_____, indicated

   the presence of a 2 cm tumor, providing further evidence for the condition of (l)_____

   _____. An alternative diagnosis of (m)_____ _____

   was ruled out due to the dimpled skin and x-ray, but a small tissue sample was removed for testing, called a

   (n)_____ to confirm this, which it did. The patient requested a minor surgery to conserve the breast,

   called (o)_____, and refused follow-up treatment of chemotherapy and radiation therapy. Unfortu-

   nately, the patient was readmitted five years later for additional treatment, due to the appearance of additional tumors and

   lymphadenopathy. Extensive removal of breast and surrounding tissues in a (p)_____

   _____ procedure was performed.

[piece it all **together!**]

CROSSWORD

From the chapter material, fill in the crossword puzzle with answers to the following clues.

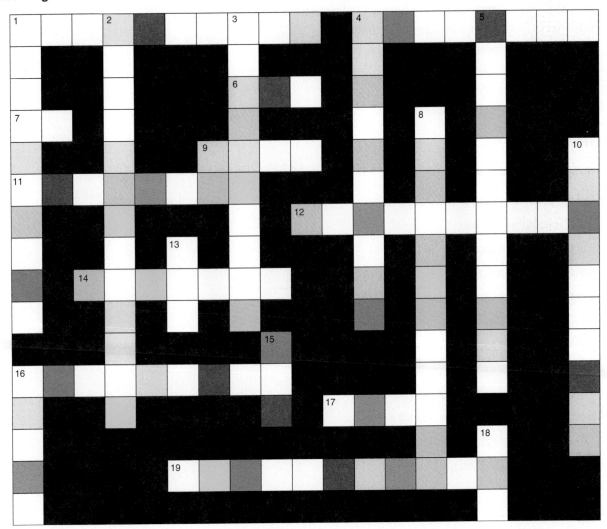

ACROSS

1. The study of women. (Find puzzle piece 16.18)
4. Inflammation of a breast. (Find puzzle piece 16.12)
6. Abbreviation for inflammation of pelvic organs. (Find puzzle piece 16.21)
7. A word root for egg. (Find puzzle piece 16.2)
9. A word root for vagina. (Find puzzle piece 16.1)
11. Milk-secreting glands within the breast. (Find puzzle piece 16.5)
12. Inflammation of the constricted portion of the uterus (Find puzzle piece 16.10)
14. A benign tumor arising from the myometrium. (Find puzzle piece 16.15)
16. Inflammation of the "sheath." (Find puzzle piece 16.9)
17. A benign, often fluid-filled tumor; one type is dermoid. (Find puzzle piece 16.7)
19. Surgical repair of the breasts. (Find puzzle piece 16.17)

DOWN

1. Pertaining to any disease of women. (Find puzzle piece 16.8)
2. Condition of endometrial tissue outside of the uterus. (Find puzzle piece 16.11)
3. Inflammation of an ovary. (Find puzzle piece 16.14)
4. Discharge of mucus or pus from the uterus. (Find puzzle piece 16.6)
5. The expanded end of a fallopian tube. (Find puzzle piece 16.3)
8. Inflammation of the outermost layer of the uterus. (Find puzzle piece 16.13)
10. Surgical removal of a breast. (Find puzzle piece 16.16)
13. Abbreviation for a hormonal therapy after menopause. (Find puzzle piece 16.19)
15. Bacterial infection associated with tampon use (abbreviation). (Find puzzle piece 16.20)
16. Female external genitalia. (Find puzzle piece 16.4)
18. Abbreviation for the study of women. (Find puzzle piece 16.22)

WORD UNSCRAMBLE

From the completed crossword puzzle, unscramble:

1. All of the letters that appear in **red** squares __ __ __ ☐ __ __ __ __

   Clue: Also known as vaginitis

2. All of the letters that appear in **purple** squares __ __ ☐ __ __ __ __

   Clue: Results from a radical mastectomy

3. All of the letters that appear in **peach** squares __ __ __ __ ☐ __ __ __ __

   Clue: Cessation of menses, often occurring around age 50

4. All of the letters that appear in **blue** squares __ __ ☐ __ __ __ __

   Clue: A "pipe" from one hollow organ to another

5. All of the letters that appear in **yellow** squares __ __ __ __ __ __ __ __ ☐ __

   Clue: Surgical removal of small tumors from a breast

6. All of the letters that appear in **green** squares __ __ ☐ __ __ __

   Clue: Also known as mammary gland

7. All of the letters that appear in **pink** squares __ __ ☐ __ __

   Clue: The female organ that produces ova and estrogen

8. All of the letters that appear in **gray** squares __ __ __ __ __ ☐ __ __ __ __ __

   Clue: Surgical removal of uterus

Now write down each of the letters that are boxed and unscramble them to find the hidden medical term of the female reproductive system: __ __ __ __ __ __ __ __ .

MEDmedia wrap up

www.prenhall.com/wingerd

Before you go on to the next chapter, take advantage of the free CD-ROM and study guide website that accompany this book. Simply load the CD-ROM for additional activities, games, animations, videos, and quizzes linked to this chapter. Then visit www.prenhall.com/wingerd for even more!

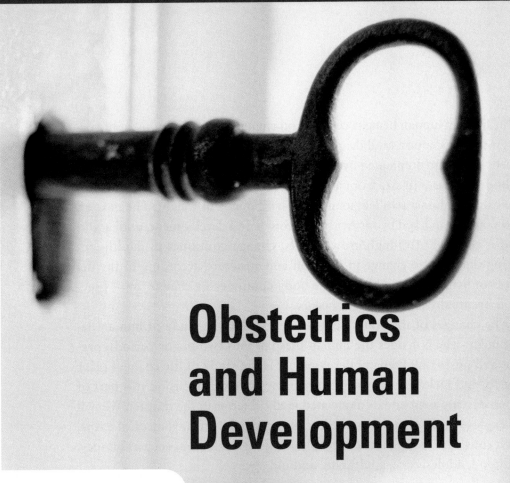

Obstetrics and Human Development

LEARNING OBJECTIVES

After completing this chapter, you will be able to:

- Define and spell the word parts used to create terms for obstetrics and human development

- Identify the major organs of obstetrics and human development and describe their structure and function

- Break down and define common medical terms used for symptoms, diseases, disorders, procedures, treatments, and devices associated with obstetrics and human development

- Build medical terms from the word parts associated with obstetrics and human development

- Pronounce and spell common medical terms associated with obstetrics and human development

MEDmedia

www.prenhall.com/wingerd

Enhance your study with the power of multimedia! Each chapter of this book links to activities, games, animations, videos, and quizzes that you'll find on your CD-ROM. Plus, you can click on www.prenhall.com/wingerd, to find a free chapter-specific companion website that's loaded with additional practice and resources.

CD-ROM
- Audio Glossary
- Exercises & Activities
- Flashcard Generator
- Animations
- Videos

Companion Website
- Exercises & Activities
- Audio Glossary
- Drug Updates
- Current News Update

A secure distance learning course is available at www.prenhall.com/onekey.

The life of a human being is centered on change. From the moment life begins at conception until death, the body changes in many ways. The first months of life are dominated by cell division and body growth, during which the body increases in size from a tiny period dot on this page to a newborn infant that is almost two feet long and 6–10 pounds in weight. The next 18 or so years are marked by further body growth and development, until adulthood is reached. Although growth ends, change continues in adulthood, causing the body to change in function and structure according to the demands of living. Even in old age the body continues its change, until function is eventually lost and death occurs.

The changes of the body are described within the study of human development, which divides the human lifespan into two major periods, prenatal and postnatal. Prenatal development is the study of life changes prior to birth, and includes the issues of pregnancy. We will focus on this part of human development and its associated medical terms in the chapter. We will also explore the field of postnatal development and its related medical terms, which considers the changes of life following the birth event such as infancy, childhood, adolescence, adulthood, and old age.

word parts focus

Let's look at word parts. The following table contains a list of word parts that when combined build many of the terms of obstetrics and human development.

PREFIX	DEFINITION	PREFIX	DEFINITION
ante-	before	nulli-	none
micro-	small	post-	after
multi-	many		

WORD ROOT	DEFINITION	WORD ROOT	DEFINITION
amni, amnion	amnion or amniotic fluid	gravid, gravidar	pregnancy
chori	membrane, chorion	lact	milk
cyes, cyesi	pregnancy	nat	birth
embry	embryo	obstetr	midwife, prenatal development
fet	fetus	omphal	umbilicus (navel)
ger, geront	old age	par, part	parturition or labor

WORD ROOT	DEFINITION	WORD ROOT	DEFINITION
ped, pediatr	child	pseud	false
pelv	pelvis, washbasin	puerper	childbirth
presby	old age	toc	birth, labor
prim	first		

SUFFIX	DEFINITION	SUFFIX	DEFINITION
-lytic	to loosen	-tocia	birth, labor
-rrhexis	rupture		

SELF QUIZ 17.1

Review the word parts of obstetrics and human development terminology by working carefully through the exercises that follow. Soon, we will apply this new information to build medical terms.

Success Hint: Once you get to the crossword puzzle at the end of the chapter, remember to check back here for clues! Your clues are indicated by the puzzle icon.

A. Provide the definition of the following prefixes and suffixes.

1. ante- _____

2. multi- _____

3. -tocia _____

4. nulli- _____

5. post- _____

6. -rrhexis _____

7. micro- _____

B. Provide the word root for each of the following terms.

1. amnion _____

2. chorion _____

3. embryo _____

4. fetus _____

5. pregnancy _____

6. milk _____

7. birth _____

8. umbilicus _____

9. labor _____

10. childbirth _____

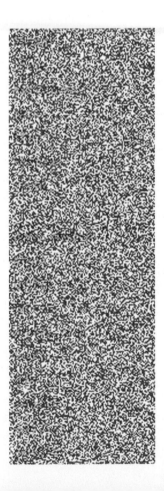

11. old age   _____

17.1 12. child   _____

13. first   _____

17.2 14. birth, labor   _____

[anatomy and physiology overview]

Human development is a continuous process of body change that begins at the moment of fertilization and continues until death. It is divided into two periods: prenatal development and postnatal development. **Prenatal development** refers to the changes that occur during the mother's pregnancy, prior to birth. The clinical field of **obstetrics** is focused on this period of life. Obstetrics also supports the mother throughout pregnancy, during childbirth, and during the first month or so following childbirth. **Postnatal development** refers to the changes that occur to the child after birth, such as body growth, puberty, and later, aging in an adult. Terms associated with prenatal and postnatal human development and the phases of human life appear in Table 17.1:::, while anatomy and physiology terms follow.

Prenatal Development and Pregnancy

A new life begins when a gamete from a male and a gamete from a female unite to form a fertilized egg, or **zygote** (Figure 17.1::::). The process of gamete union is known as **fertilization,** or **conception.** A single sperm cell penetrates the cell membrane of the ovum after it has ovulated. Soon after penetration has occurred, the sperm cell's DNA unites with the ovum's DNA to form a cell with a complete complement of genetic material. Fertilization marks the beginning of **pregnancy,** or **cyesis,** which normally lasts 280 days or 9 calendar months (10 lunar months). Pregnancy is divided into three segments, or **trimesters,** each of which supports the process of prenatal development.

Prenatal development proceeds immediately after fertilization, beginning with the division of the zygote into two cells, then four cells, then sixteen cells, and so on. After about two days of dividing, the structure has formed into a cluster of cells that include an **embryo** (Figure 17.2::::). Associated with the embryo is a group of cells that will form supporting structures. The structures include a thin membrane called the **amnion** that surrounds and protects the embryo, an outer membrane known as the **chorion** that eventually unites with the endometrium to form the **placenta,** and a **yolk sac** that will later help to form the **umbilical cord** (Figure 17.3::::). At about the eighth day after fertilization, the embryo implants within the endometrium of the uterus. For the next seven weeks of development, the embryo increases in size and complexity within the uterine cavity.

By the eighth week of development, the embryo has grown and taken form, at which point it is called a **fetus** (Figure 17.3). The fetus continues growing and developing for approximately 32 more weeks until its weight signals the mother's brain to begin producing the hormone oxytocin, which stimulates contractions of the uterine wall. Once contractions increase in frequency and strength, the process of **labor** begins.

Labor is a four-stage process that involves the gradual dilation of the cervix, accompanied by the increasing strength and duration of uterine contractions (Figure 17.4::::). Labor is the process that terminates pregnancy and brings about the birth, or **parturition,** of the child. The time period from delivery of the child until the

[FYI]

Pregnancy
The Old Latin version of the word pregnancy is *praegnas.* It is composed of the Latin words *prae,* which means *before,* and *gnatus,* meaning *to be born.*

Table 17.1 ::: Terms Related to Prenatal and Postnatal Human Development	
adolescence (add oh LESS ens)	period of life between the start of puberty and attainment of complete height
adulthood (ah DULT hood)	period of life between attainment of complete height and the moment of death
antepartum (AN tee PAR tum)	occurring before childbirth
childhood	period of life between infancy and puberty
gravida (GRAV ih dah)	a pregnant woman
gravidopuerperal (GRAV ih doh pyoo ER per al)	pertaining to pregnancy and puerperium
infancy (IN fan see)	the period of life between birth and the first year or two of life
intrapartum (IN trah PAR tum)	occurring during labor and childbirth
multigravida (MULL tee GRAV ih dah)	a pregnant woman who has been previously pregnant one or more times
multipara (mull TIP ah rah)	a woman who has given birth to an infant (either alive or dead) two or more times; also called a multip
natal (NAY tal)	pertaining to birth
neonate (NEE oh nayt)	the period of life between birth and 28 days; abbreviated **NB** (for newborn)
nulligravida (null ih GRAV ih dah)	a woman who has never been pregnant
nullipara (null IP ah rah)	a woman who has not given birth to an infant, either alive or dead
para (PAIR ah)	a woman who has given birth to an infant, either alive or dead
postnatal development (pohst NAY tal)	period of life between the moment of birth and the moment of death
postpartum (pohst PAR tum)	occurring after childbirth
pregnancy (PREG nahn see)	a woman's state between conception and birth; also known as gestation (jes TAY shun) or cyesia (sigh EE see ah)
premature infant (pree MAH TYOOR)	an infant born before reaching 37 weeks of prenatal development
prenatal development (pree NAY tal)	period of life between conception and birth
primigravida (preem ih GRAV ih dah)	a woman in her first pregnancy
primipara (preem IP ah rah)	a woman who has given birth to one infant, either alive or dead
puerpera (pyoo ER per ah)	a woman who has just given birth
puerperal (pyoo ER per al)	adjective meaning pertaining to the period after puerperium (childbirth)
puerperium (pyoo er PEER ee um)	period of the mother's life from the termination of labor to the return to the state of having a reproductively capable uterus
senescence (seh NESS ens)	the process or state of aging
trimester (TRY mess ter)	a third of the period of pregnancy with a duration of approximately three months, or thirteen and one-third weeks

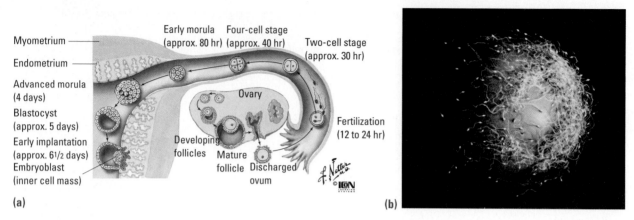

(a)

(b)

Figure 17.1 ::::

Fertilization and implantation.

(a) Fertilization usually occurs in the upper one-third of the fallopian tube. The fertilized egg, or zygote, is slowly moved to the uterus, where implantation normally occurs. The implanted ball of cells includes an embryo and supporting cells. *Source: Icon Learning Systems.*

(b) Photograph of an ovum surrounded by numerous sperm cells. Successful penetration of one sperm into the ovum results in fertilization, or conception. *Source: Custom Medical Stock Photo, Inc.*

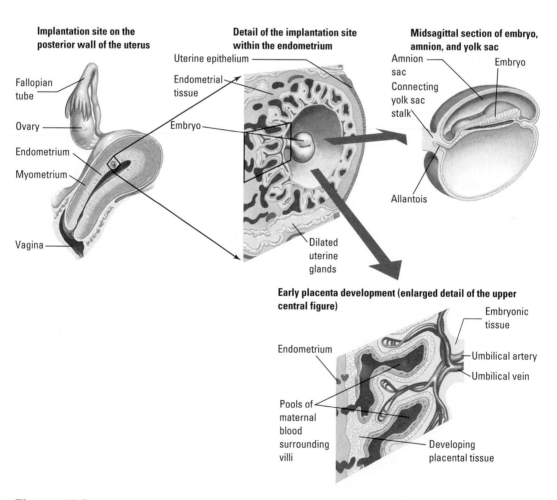

Figure 17.2 ::::

Early prenatal development. During this stage, the embryo becomes implanted within the endometrium of the uterus, giving rise to an early placenta. *Source: Pearson Education.*

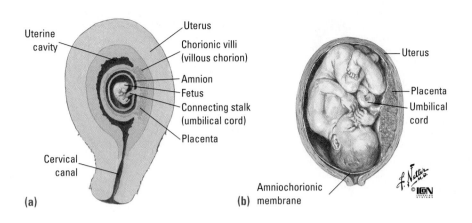

(a)

(b)

Figure 17.3 ⸬⸬

Prenatal growth.

Growth during the prenatal stage is rapid, resulting from the differentiation of tissues and an increase in cell numbers.
(a) Section through the pregnant uterus about eight weeks after fertilization.
(b) Section through the uterus about six months after fertilization. *Source: Icon Learning Systems.*

mother's reproductive organs return to normal, or about six weeks later, is known as **puerperium.**

Postnatal Development

Postnatal development begins immediately after birth and continues until death. It includes the changes that occur during infancy, childhood, adolescence, adulthood, and old age (Figure 17.5⸬⸬).

Infancy is the period of life during which the individual adjusts to the world outside the womb. Human beings experience a transition from a life of total submersion in a regulated fluid (the **amniotic fluid** that envelops the fetus) to a life of independence in a biologically hostile world.

During the first month after birth, the newborn is referred to as a **neonate.** The neonate begins life with its first gasp of air at birth. This event causes fluids in the

[**thinking critically!**]

What two structures, one from the developing embryo and one from the mother, contribute to form the placenta?

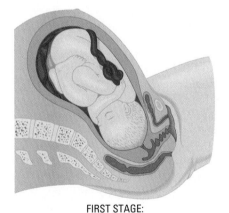

FIRST STAGE:
(a) First uterine contraction to dilation of cervix

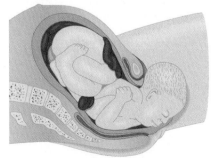

SECOND STAGE:
(b) Birth of baby or expulsion

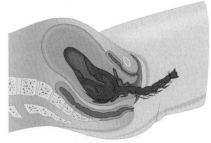

THIRD STAGE:
(c) Delivery of placenta

Figure 17.4 ⸬⸬

Labor.

(a) The first stage of labor occurs when the cervix dilates and the child's head enters the birth canal. *Source: Pearson Education.*
(b) The second stage of labor is the expulsion of the child, caused by uterine contractions that are hormonally induced. *Source: Pearson Education.*
(c) The third stage is the expulsion of the placenta. *Source: Pearson Education.*
The fourth stage (not shown) is the extrusion of afterbirth tissues and fluids.

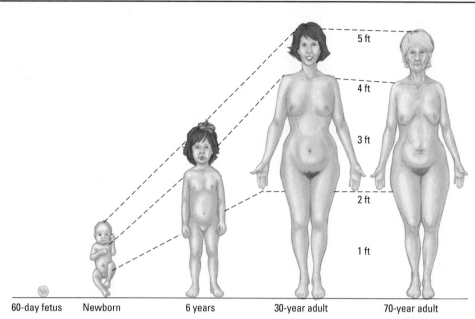

Figure 17.5 ::::

Postnatal development.
The body changes throughout postnatal life, as illustrated in this figure.

60-day fetus   Newborn   6 years   30-year adult   70-year adult

lungs to be expelled, and air rushes in to replace them. As the lungs inflate with air, changes occur in the neonate's circulatory system that result in a redirection of blood flow to the lungs for the first time. In the following weeks and months, the **infant** undergoes rapid brain growth and development, muscle growth and coordination, and growth of most body tissues and organs.

After the first or second year, the infant has become a child capable of responding to the surrounding world. The next ten years or so make up the period of **childhood.** Childhood is marked by a slower growth rate that is accompanied with continued brain, muscle, and bone development.

By the age of 10 to 12 years, **puberty** begins and lasts until the age of 16 to 18 years. This stage in life is known as **adolescence.** It is characterized by the development of secondary sexual characteristics, such as body hair and muscle development in males and fat deposition at the breasts and hips in females. The maximum body height is reached during this stage.

The attainment of full adult height marks the end of adolescence and the beginning of **adulthood.** This period of life lasts the longest, for it extends to old age. It is characterized by a lack of vertical growth, and the slow effects of aging that begin to accumulate as the years go by. The effects of aging include increased fat deposition, gradual muscle loss, a slowing of the metabolic rate, and thinning of the skin.

The last stage in human development is old age, or **senescence.** It usually begins between the ages of 65 and 75 years, and is marked by bone fragility and a resulting loss of posture, muscle atrophy, and slowing of nervous responses. The skin continues to thin and lose its elasticity, producing wrinkles. Old age ultimately ends with death, when all body functions stop as a result of the failure of one or more vital organs.

[**thinking critically!**]

How does adolescence differ from childhood?

getting to the root of it | anatomy and physiology terms

Many of the anatomy and physiology terms are formed from roots that are used to construct the more complex medical terms of obstetrics and human development, including symptoms, diseases, and treatments. In this section, we will review the terms that describe the structure and function of obstetrics and human development *in relation to their word roots,* which are shown in **bold.**

Study the word roots and terms in this list and complete the review exercises that follow.

Word Root (Meaning)	Terms Formed from the Word Root (Pronunciation)	Definition
amni, amnion (amnion or amniotic fluid)	**amnion** (AM nee on)	the embryonic and fetal membrane that encloses the embryo and fetus and is filled with a watery fluid called amniotic fluid; also called an amniotic sac
cyes, cyesi (pregnancy)	**cyes**is (sigh EE siss)	pregnancy
chori (membrane, chorion)	**chori**on (KOR ee on)	the outer embryonic membrane that forms the fetal side of the placenta
embry (embryo)	**embry**o (EM bree oh)	the developing human from the second day after conception until the eighth week
	embryogenic (EM bree oh JENN ik)	adjective meaning producing an embryo
fet (fetus)	**fet**us (FEE tuss)	the developing human from the eighth week after conception to the moment of birth
lact (milk)	**lact**ogenic (LAK toh JENN ik)	adjective meaning producing milk
par, part (parturition or labor)	**part**urition (par too RISH un)	the event of childbirth

[FYI]

Embryo
The term *embryo* is a Greek word composed of two parts: *em,* which means *inside,* and *bryo,* which means *to swell.* Although the modern meaning of the term refers to the first eight weeks of life after conception, the Greeks captured its most amazing feature: rapid growth within!

Fetus
The term *fetus* is the Latin word for *offspring,* and during the days of the Roman Empire was used as a reference to the young while still in the womb. Today, the term refers to the period of human development between the eighth week after conception until birth.

OTHER IMPORTANT TERMS
The terms in this table are related to the structure and function of obstetrics and human development, but are not built from multiple word roots.

conception (kon SEPP shun)	the moment of fertilization, or union of a male and female gamete
labor (LAY ber)	the process of expulsion of the fetus and placenta from the uterus involving the gradual dilation of the cervix, accompanied by the increasing strength and duration of uterine contractions
lochia (LOH kee ah)	vaginal discharge that normally follows childbirth
meconium (meh KOH nee um)	the first stool of a newborn, which is usually a greenish-black semisolid
placenta (plah SEHN tah)	the organ that provides an exchange of materials between the mother and the fetus; it is composed of the inner layer of the endometrium and fetal tissues, including the chorion
placental blood barrier (plah SEHN tal)	composed of the capillary walls, basement membrane, and chorion, it divides the mother's blood from the fetal blood supply
puberty (PYOO ber tee)	the physical, mental, and emotional changes that occur during the period of adolescence
umbilical cord (um BILL ih kal KORD)	the cord-like connection that extends between the fetal side of the placenta and the fetus; it includes an artery and vein that carry materials between the mother and fetus
zygote (ZIGH goht)	the cell resulting from the union of a male sperm with a female ovum

[FYI]

Labor
The term *labor* is a Latin word that means *toil, suffering*. Interestingly, there is no synonym for the difficult, usually painful process that results in the delivery of the neonate.

SELF QUIZ 17.2

Success Hint: Use the audio glossary on the CD and CW for additional help with pronunciation of these terms.

SAY IT—SPELL IT!

Review the terms of obstetrics and human development by speaking the phonetic pronunciations out loud, then writing the correct spelling of the term.

1. LOH kee ah   _____

2. meh KOH nee um   _____

3. EM bree oh JENN ik   _____

4. LAK toh JENN ik   _____

5. GRAV ih dah   _____

6. PAIR ah   _____

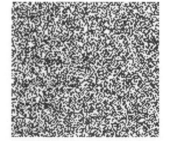

7. pyoo ER per ah _____

8. AN tee PAR tum _____

9. GRAV ih doh pyoo ER per al _____

10. IN trah PAR tum _____

11. MULL tee GRAV ih dah _____

12. mull TIP ah rah _____

13. null ih GRAV ih dah _____

14. null IP ah rah _____

15. preem ih GRAV ih dah _____

16. preem IP ah rah _____

MATCH IT!

Match the term on the left with the correct definition on the right.

_____ 1. adolescence

a. period of life between conception and the eighth week

_____ 2. adulthood

b. period of life between childhood and adulthood

_____ 3. amnion

c. mother's state between conception and childbirth

_____ 4. prenatal development

d. outermost embryonic membrane; contributes to placenta

_____ 5. labor

e. period of life between birth and 28 days

_____ 6. pregnancy

f. longest lasting stage of life before senescence

_____ 7. parturition

g. membrane that encloses the fetus in a watery world

_____ 8. postnatal development

h. begins with the onset of puberty

_____ 9. chorion

i. the four-stage process of childbirth

_____ 10. placenta

j. birth of a child

_____ 11. umbilical cord

k. period of life between conception and parturition

_____ 12. fetus

l. manages exchange of materials between mother and fetus

_____ 13. embryo

m. old age

_____ 14. neonate

n. period of life between the eighth week after conception and birth

_____ 15. adolescence

o. period of life between birth and death

_____ 16. senescence

p. connection between placenta and fetus

_____ 17. natal

q. producing an embryo

_____ 18. lactogenic

r. pertaining to birth

_____ 19. embryogenic

s. production of milk

_____ 20. lochia

t. the first stool of a newborn infant

_____ 21. meconium

u. vaginal discharge that often follows childbirth

BREAK IT DOWN!

Analyze and separate each term into its word parts by labeling each word part using p = prefix, r = root, cv = combining vowel, and s = suffix.

1. antepartum   _____

2. gravidopuerperal   _____

3. intrapartum   _____

4. multigravida   _____

5. multipara   _____

6. nulligravida   _____

7. primipara   _____

8. puerperal   _____

FILL IT IN!

Fill in the blanks with the correct terms.

1. The period of _____, also known as gestation, or

   _____ is the mother's state between fertilization, or

   _____, and the birth of the child.

2. When a woman is pregnant, she may be described as a _____.

   A woman who has given birth to a child, either alive or dead, is known as a

   _____. A newborn who has been born less than 37 weeks after

   conception is called a _____ infant. Regardless of the status of

   the child, a mother who has just given birth is known as _____.

3. During the first 28 days following childbirth, the child is called a

   _____. This period of life is followed by a slowing of growth,

   known as _____.

4. The slow-growth period ends with the onset of _____, during

   which secondary sexual characteristics begin to appear. The appearance of

   secondary sexual changes marks the period of life known as

   _____, which continues until complete height is attained.

5. It is followed by _____, which is the period of life that lasts the

   longest. The last period of life is characterized by changes accompanied with aging,

   and is called _____.

6. The period of life between conception and birth is called _____

   _____. The fertilized egg begins dividing soon after it is fertilized

   to form a cluster of cells that will eventually become a human, called an

   _____.

17.3

17.4

7. After the eighth week, the developing organism becomes known as a

   _____.

8. Other dividing cells form supporting structures, including an inner membrane that encloses the fetus within a water-filled sac. The sac is called the

   _____, and the fluid within it bathes and surrounds the fetus

   and is called _____ _____. Another

   supporting structure is the outermost embryonic membrane, which forms the

   fetal side of the _____ and is known as the

   _____. A supporting structure known as the yolk sac joins

   other tissues to form the _____ _____, which

   carries material between the mother and fetus.

17.5 9. The fetal stage ends with childbirth, or _____. The process of

   birth consists of four stages, and is known as _____.

10. A vaginal discharge that often follows childbirth is called _____.

   The newborn's first stool is a greenish-black semisolid material called

   _____.

medical terms of
obstetrics and human development

At the beginning of this chapter, you learned that obstetrics is the medical discipline concerned with prenatal development, pregnancy, childbirth, and the period following childbirth. The term *obstetrics* is derived from the Latin word *obstetrix*, which means *midwife*. It is often referred to in a clinical setting by its abbreviated form, **OB.** A physician specializing in obstetrics is known as an **obstetrician.** An obstetrician or clinic may combine specialties with **gynecology;** this combination of fields is commonly known as **OB/GYN.**

Soon after birth, the care of the developing child falls into a different field of medical specialty, known as **pediatrics.** This term is derived from the Greek word *paiatrikos,* which means *relating to child healing.* A medical specialist in this field is called a **pediatrician.** A pediatrician usually follows child patients through the adolescent stage of life.

When an individual reaches adulthood, commonly recognized as the age of 18 years in most hospitals, patient care is transferred to a **general practitioner (GP).** The GP maintains primary medical care of a person into his or her old age, usually considered to be around 65 years of age. The period of old age is managed within the field of medicine known as **geriatrics,** and it is studied within the field of **gerontology.** Both terms of old age are derived from the Greek word for old man, *gerontos.* Gerontology can be written as a constructed term:

geront/o/logy

in which the word root geront means *old man* and the suffix -logy means *study of.* A physician specializing in gerontology is called a **gerontologist.**

The diseases of obstetrics and human development often have profound effects on the health and wellbeing of a person's entire life. They include diseases of prenatal development, pregnancy, and postnatal development.

The disorders associated with prenatal development are generally known as **congenital anomalies,** since they are present at birth (the word *congenital* literally means *with development*). Congenital anomalies are usually caused by a genetic mutation, although the movement of a pathogen across the placental barrier may be another cause. For example, the viruses that cause rubella and AIDS can cross the placental barrier to pass from the infected mother to the fetus. In either case, the effect is often a lifelong defect.

Pregnancy may also be plagued by disorders, often arising from infectious diseases but also by anatomical defects or tumors. Diseases of pregnancy carry the added threat of imposing long-lasting harm upon the unborn child.

Diseases that afflict pregnancy and prenatal development are often diagnosed during regular checkups that are routine for tracking a pregnancy. The most cost-effective technique for examining a developing fetus and mother includes sonography, or ultrasound. When combined with computer graphics that can improve resolution, detail, and add color to enhance certain features, the resulting images provide the obstetrician with a valuable diagnostic tool that does not increase the stress of the mother or fetus. If the ultrasound image suggests clinical problems, other imaging techniques can be employed to provide additional evidence, including x-ray imaging and endoscopy.

As you have learned in other chapters of this book, postnatal development may be affected by nearly all forms of disease, including congenital diseases, infectious diseases, metabolic disorders that alter hormonal production, and tumors. In addition, the aging process, or senescence, plays a major part in the progression of disease later in life, mainly by reducing the effectiveness of the immune response.

> **[thinking critically!]**
>
> What is the medical specialization that would most likely treat an infectious disease that has crossed the placental barrier?

let's construct terms!

In this section, we will assemble all of the word parts to construct medical terminology related to obstetrics and human development. Abbreviations are used to indicate each word part: **p** = prefix, **r** = root, **cv** = combining vowel, and **s** = suffix. Recall from Chapter 1 that the addition of a combining vowel to the word root creates the combining form for the term. Note that some terms are not constructed from word parts, but they are included here to expand your vocabulary.

The medical terms of obstetrics and human development are listed in the following three sections:

- Symptoms and Signs
- Diseases and Disorders
- Treatments, Procedures, and Devices

Each section is followed by review exercises. Study the lists in these tables and complete the review exercises that follow.

Symptoms and Signs

WORD PARTS (WHEN APPLICABLE)			TERM	DEFINITION
Part	Type	Meaning		
amni/o	r/cv	amnion, amniotic fluid	**amniorrhea** (AM nee oh REE ah)	abnormal discharge of amniotic fluid
-rrhea	s	excessive discharge		
dys-	p	bad, abnormal	**dystocia**	difficult labor
-tocia	s	birth, labor	(diss TOH see ah)	
hyper-	p	excessive	**hyperemesis**	severe nausea and emesis (vomiting) during
-emesis	s	vomiting	**gravidara**	pregnancy that can cause severe dehydration in the
gravidar	r	pregnancy	(HIGH per EM eh siss	mother and fetus
-a	s	singular	grav ih DAR ah)	
lact/o	r/cv	milk	**lactorrhea**	an abnormal, spontaneous discharge of milk
-rrhea	s	excessive discharge	(LAK toh REE ah)	
poly-	p	many	**polyhydramnios**	excessive amniotic fluid
hydr	r	water	(PALL ee high	
amni/o	r/cv	amnion, amniotic fluid	DRAM nee ohs)	
-s	s	plural		
pseud/o	r/cv	false	**pseudocyesis**	a false pregnancy
cyes	r	pregnancy	(SOO doh sigh EE siss)	
-is	s	pertaining to		

SELF QUIZ 17.3

SAY IT—SPELL IT!

Review the terms of obstetrics and human development by speaking the phonetic pronunciations out loud, then writing the correct spelling of the term.

1. AM nee oh REE ah _____

17.6 2. diss TOH see ah _____

3. HIGH per EM eh siss   grav ih DAR ah _____

4. LAK toh REE ah _____

5. PALL ee high DRAM nee ohs _____

6. SOO doh sigh EE siss _____

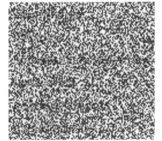

MATCH IT!

Match the term on the left with the correct definition on the right.

_____1. pseudocyesis

a. excessive amniotic fluid

_____2. polyhydramnios

b. difficult labor

_____3. dystocia

c. severe nausea and vomiting during pregnancy

_____4. lactorrhea

d. false pregnancy

_____5. amniorrhea

e. abnormal, spontaneous milk discharge

_____6. hyperemesis gravidara

f. abnormal discharge of amniotic fluid

BREAK IT DOWN!

Analyze and separate each term into its word parts by labeling each word part using p = prefix, r = root, cv = combining vowel, and s = suffix.

1. dystocia   _____

2. hyperemeis gravidara   _____

3. lactorrhea   _____

4. polyhydramnios   _____

5. pseudocyesis   _____

WORD BUILDING

Construct or recall medical terms from the following meanings.

1. spontaneous milk discharge   _____

2. a false pregnancy   _____

3. severe nausea and vomiting while pregnant   _____

4. excessive amniotic fluid   _____

5. abnormal discharge of amniotic fluid   _____

6. a difficult labor   _____

FILL IT IN!

Fill in the blanks with the correct terms.

1. A symptom of a difficult, often painful labor is known as _____. It may be preceded by an uncomfortable and potentially hazardous pregnancy that includes severe nausea and vomiting, a symptom called _____ _____.

2. The abnormal discharge of amniotic fluid during pregnancy, which is a symptom called _____, can threaten normal development of the fetus.

3. A false pregnancy is known as _____.

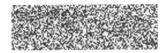

4. The spontaneous discharge of milk, called _____, can be an embarrassment in public places, although it does not threaten fetal health.

Diseases and Disorders

WORD PARTS (WHEN APPLICABLE)			TERM	DEFINITION
Part	**Type**	**Meaning**		
			abortion (ah BOR shun)	termination of pregnancy by expulsion of the embryo or fetus from the uterus; a natural expulsion is also called a **miscarriage** or **spontaneous abortion (SAB)**, and an abortion induced by surgery or drugs is called a **therapeutic abortion (TAB)**
			abruptio placentae (ah BRUP shee oh plah SEN tee)	premature separation of the placenta from the uterine wall, resulting in either premature birth or fetal death (Figure 17.6::::)

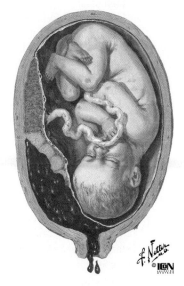

Figure 17.6 ::::

Abruptio placentae.
The placenta becomes prematurely detached from the uterine wall.
Source: Icon Learning Systems.

WORD PARTS			TERM	DEFINITION
amnion	r	amnion or amniotic fluid	**amnionitis** (AM nee oh NYE tiss)	inflammation of the amnion
-itis	s	inflammation		
amni/o	r/cv	amnion or amniotic fluid	**amniorrhexis** (AM nee oh REK siss)	rupture of the amnion
-rrhexis	s	rupture		
			breech birth	abnormal childbirth in which the buttocks, feet, or knees emerge first
			cervical effacement (SER vih kal ee FAYS ment)	progressive obliteration of the cervical canal during labor
chori/o	r/cv	membrane, chorion	**chorioamnionitis** (KOR ee oh AM nee oh NYE tiss)	inflammation of the chorion and amnion
amnion	r	amnion or amniotic fluid		
-itis	s	inflammation		

WORD PARTS (WHEN APPLICABLE)			TERM	DEFINITION
Part	Type	Meaning		
chori/o	r/cv	membrane, chorion	**choriocarcinoma** (KOR ee oh KAR sih NOH mah)	cancer of the chorion
carcin	r	cancer		
-oma	s	tumor		
			cleft palate (PAHL aht)	congenital abnormality in which the roof of the mouth fails to close during prenatal development, leaving a fissure (Figure 17.7▦)

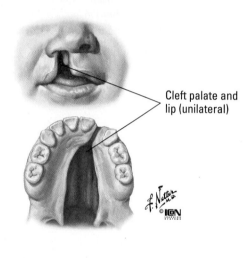

Cleft palate and lip (unilateral)

Figure 17.7 ▦
Cleft palate.
A congenital defect in which the bones of the upper palate fail to grow to the center and fuse, leaving a space between the mouth and the nasal cavity. A cleft palate is usually accompanied by deformity of the lip, called cleft lip.
Source: Icon Learning Systems.

WORD PARTS			TERM	DEFINITION
			congenital anomaly (kon JENN ih tal ah NOM ah lee)	an abnormality present at birth
			Down syndrome (SIN drohm)	congenital disorder caused by a genetic defect in chromosome 21, resulting in degrees of mental retardation and other physical defects; also called trisomy 21 and formerly known as "mongolism"
			eclampsia (eh KLAMP see ah)	a condition characterized by convulsions and possibly coma, during pregnancy, which may follow preeclampsia

[FYI]

Eclampsia

The term *eclampsia* is derived from the Greek word *eclampsis,* which means to *shine forth rapidly or flash.* It refers to a sudden development, and was chosen to be used for this condition in modern times because of the sudden onset of convulsions that often marks the disease.

WORD PARTS			TERM	DEFINITION
			ectopic pregnancy (ek TOP ik PREG nan see)	a pregnancy occurring outside of the uterus (Figure 17.8▦)
embry/o	r/cv	embryo	**embryotocia** (EM bree oh TOH see ah)	expulsion, or abortion, of the embryo
-tocia	s	birth, labor		

WORD PARTS (WHEN APPLICABLE)			TERM	DEFINITION
Part	**Type**	**Meaning**		

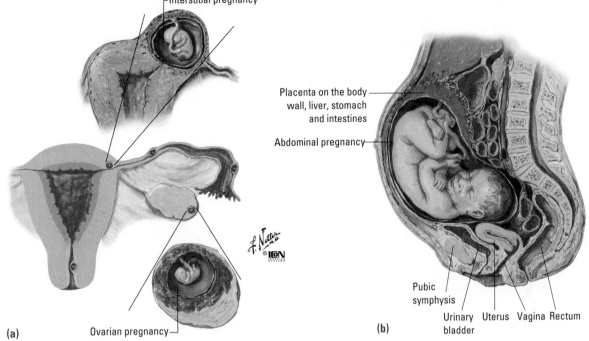

(a)

Interstitial pregnancy

Ovarian pregnancy

Placenta on the body wall, liver, stomach and intestines

Abdominal pregnancy

(b)

Pubic symphysis

Urinary bladder — Uterus — Vagina — Rectum

Figure 17.8 ::::

Ectopic pregnancies.

(a) An ectopic pregnancy may occur in any of the locations shown. Interstitial pregnancy is the most common, with implantation occurring near the union of a fallopian tube and uterus. An ovarian pregnancy has the unfortunate result of destroying the ovary.
(b) An abdominal pregnancy is shown at full term. Note that the fetus is surrounded by the amnion, but outside of the uterus.
Source: Icon Learning Systems.

erythr/o	r/cv	red	**erythroblastosis**	a condition of newborns in which red blood cells are
blast/o	r/cv	germ, bud	**fetalis**	destroyed (by hemolysis) due to an incompatibility
-sis	s	state of	(eh RITH roh blass	between the mother's blood and baby's blood
fet	r	fetus	TOH siss	occurring when the mother is Rh negative and has
-al	s	pertaining to	fee TAL iss)	previously had an Rh positive child, and making
-is	s	pertaining to		subsequent Rh positive children susceptible (Figure 17.9::::)
esophag/e	r/cv	esophagus	**esophageal atresia**	congenital absence of part of the esophagus,
-al	s	pertaining to	(eh soff ah JEE al	resulting in the inability of food to pass between the
atresia		closure, absence of a normal body opening	ah TREE zee ah)	child's mouth and stomach (Figure 17.10::::)
			fetal alcohol syndrome (FEE tal AL koh hall SIN drohm)	a condition caused by alcohol ingestion during pregnancy, it can cause brain dysfunction and growth abnormalities in the newborn; abbreviated **FAS**

WORD PARTS (WHEN APPLICABLE)			TERM	DEFINITION
Part	Type	Meaning		

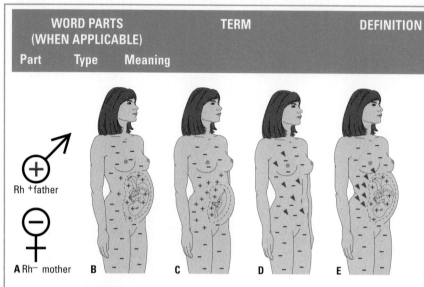

Figure 17.9 ::::

Erythroblastosis fetalis.
(a) The condition occurs with an Rh-positive father and Rh-negative mother.
(b) First pregnancy with an Rh-positive fetus stimulates the mother's blood to form antibodies against the fetal blood.
(c) As the placenta separates during birth, the mother is further exposed to the Rh-positive blood, increasing her blood's reaction against it.
(d) The mother carries antibodies against the Rh-positive blood.
(e) In a subsequent pregnancy with an Rh-positive fetus, the mother's antibodies attack the Rh-positive blood of the fetus, causing hemolysis of the fetal red blood cells.
Source: Pearson Education.

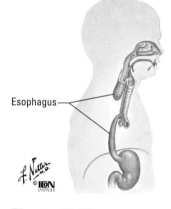

Figure 17.10 ::::

Esophageal atresia.
This congenital anomaly results in the inability to swallow or digest food, and requires surgical correction.
Source: Icon Learning Systems.

Part	Type	Meaning	TERM	DEFINITION
			hyaline membrane disease (HIGH ah linn)	disease of newborns, and particularly of premature infants, in which certain cells of the lungs fail to mature by birth, leading to a tendency for lung collapse that may be followed by death; abbreviated **HMD,** it is also called respiratory distress syndrome of the newborn, or **RDS**
hyster/o -rrhexis	r/cv s	uterus rupture	**hysterorrhexis** (HISS ter oh REK siss)	rupture of the uterus
micro- cephal -y	p r s	small head process of	**microcephaly** (MY kroh SEFF ah lee)	congenital abnormality of a small head
omphal -itis	r s	umbilicus inflammation	**omphalitis** (OM fah LYE tiss)	inflammation of the umbilicus (navel)
omphal/o -cele	r/cv s	umbilicus hernia, swelliing	**omphalocele** (OM fall oh seel)	congenital herniation at the umbilicus, in which a segment of the small intestine pushes through the abdominal wall (Figure 17.11::::)
			placenta previa (plah SEN tah PREH vee ah)	abnormal attachment of the placenta, in which it implants in the lower segment of the uterus near, or obstructing, the external os (Figure 17.12::::)
			preeclampsia (pree eh KLAMP see ah)	an abnormal development of high blood pressure that may be accompanied with proteinuria and edema, all due to toxemia during pregnancy; also known as pregnancy-induced hypertension, or **PIH**

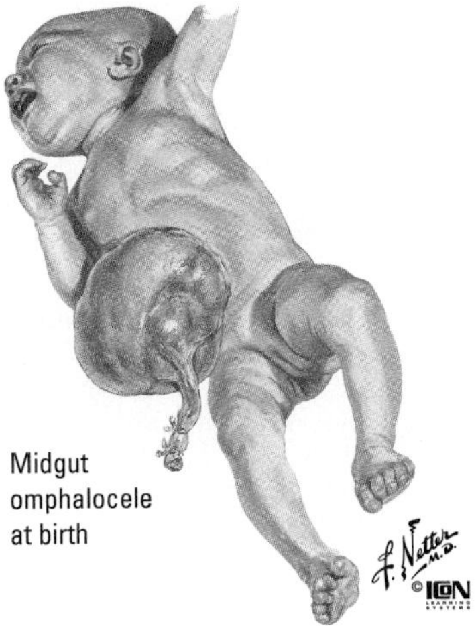

WORD PARTS (WHEN APPLICABLE)			TERM	DEFINITION
Part	Type	Meaning		

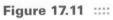

Figure 17.11 ::::

Omphalocele.
In this example, an omphalocele has formed near the entry of the umbilical cord into the newborn.
Source: Icon Learning Systems.

Midgut omphalocele at birth

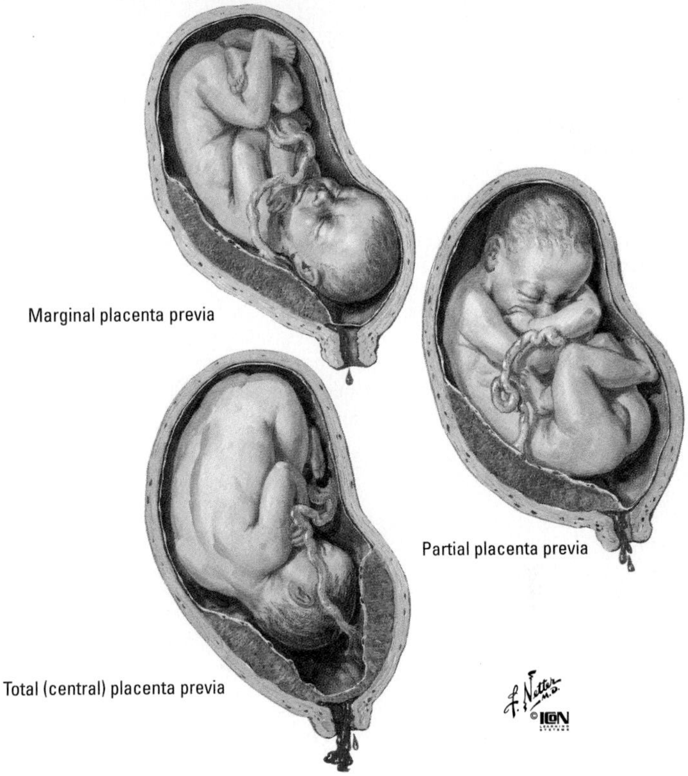

Figure 17.12 ::::

Placenta previa.
The condition is caused by the development of the placenta over the cervical canal, creating an occlusion. Three types of placenta previa are illustrated.
Source: Icon Learning Systems.

Marginal placenta previa

Partial placenta previa

Total (central) placenta previa

			rubella (roo BELL ah)	an acute disease caused by the rubella virus (*Rubivirus*), which is capable of crossing the placental barrier to infect a fetus, producing abnormalities in prenatal development; also called German measles and epidemic roseola
salping/o cyes -is	r/cv r s	fallopian tube pregnancy pertaining to	**salpingocyesis** (sal PING goh sigh EE siss)	an abnormal pregnancy in which the embryo has implanted within the fallopian tube; it is a form of ectopic pregnancy (Figure 17.13::::)
			spina bifida (SPY nah BIFF ih dah)	a congenital defect of the vertebral column resulting from an absence of the vertebral arches and often leading to a severe inflammation of the spinal meninges, called a hydrocele spinalis (Figure 17.14::::)
toxoplasm -osis	r s	a bacterium condition of	**toxoplasmosis** (TAHK soh plaz MOH siss)	caused by the bacterium *Toxoplasma gondii*, which may be contracted by exposure to animal feces (most commonly from household pets such as cats), this disease can cross the placental blood barrier to infect the fetus, causing birth defects or miscarriage

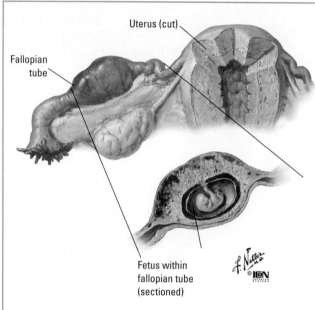

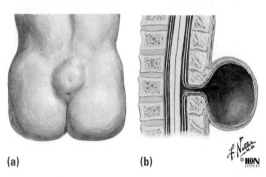

Figure 17.13 ::::

Salpingocyesis.

In this type of ectopic pregnancy, implantation has occurred within a fallopian tube, as shown.

Source: Icon Learning Systems.

Figure 17.14 ::::

Spina bifida.

(a) This congenital anomaly is characterized by the lack of vertebral arches in one or more vertebrae. The lack of a vertebral arch often causes the spinal cord or meninges to bend outward, due to lack of support.

(b) The bending of the meninges leads to inflammation, which is often manifested by a fluid-filled sac called a hydrocele spinalis, shown in this cross section.

Source: Icon Learning Systems.

disease focus | Crossing the Placental Blood Barrier

The placenta is the life-supporting organ of the fetus. It is composed of two parts, one from the mother and one from the fetus. The mother's contribution is a portion of the inner lining of the uterus, while the contribution of the fetus is a membrane that has originated from the embryo, called the chorion. In between the mother's and fetus' parts is a thin membrane, composed of two thin layers of cells and protein fibers. This membrane is the placental blood barrier, which divides the mother's blood from the fetal blood supply. It forms a barrier that prevents the mixing of maternal blood cells and fetal blood cells, while permitting the passage of tiny molecules of nutrients, gases, and waste materials.

In a normal placenta, the movement of most potentially harmful substances, such as wandering white blood cells, red blood cells that might be incompatible, bacteria, fungi, and viruses, from the mother's blood supply to the fetus is prevented. However, some disease-causing substances are known to be transmitted from mother to fetus, often resulting in birth defects or premature death. In most cases, these substances are transmitted only when the placental blood barrier becomes torn.

Tearing may occur if the mother receives a traumatic injury during pregnancy, but it frequently occurs during the birth process. The result of a torn placenta is the mixing of blood between the mother and child. If the mother is carrying pathogens or toxins, such as the virus that causes herpes or the bacteria that causes syphilis, in her bloodstream at the time the placenta tears, the child is at risk of contracting the disease through blood-to-blood contact. The child may also be in danger if the mother's and child's blood types are not compatible, and the amount of blood mixed is significant.

A torn placental blood barrier is not the only way infections or toxic substances spread from mother to child. Certain microorganisms and drugs may cross the intact barrier. For example:

- The virus that causes **rubella** (German measles) is capable of crossing the placental barrier. If the mother is infected during the first trimester of her pregnancy, there is great danger that the virus will infect the developing embryo and cause severe birth defects or miscarriage.

- The bacterium *Toxoplasma gondii* is the microorganism that causes the infectious disease **toxoplasmosis**. This disease may be contracted by exposure to animal feces, most commonly from house pets like cats. Although *Toxoplasma* normally has little effect on adults, it can quickly cross the placental barrier and infect the fetus, causing birth defects or miscarriage.

- For a brief period during the 1950s, a drug called **thalidomide** was administered to pregnant women experiencing distress. This drug has been shown to cause dramatic birth defects in infants, including the underdevelopment of arms and legs.

- If ingested during pregnancy, alcohol can cross the placental blood barrier and has been shown to cause brain dysfunction and growth abnormalities in newborns, producing a condition known as **fetal alcohol syndrome,** or **FAS.** To prevent this potential disaster, pregnant women are advised to abstain from all sources of alcohol.

- Research has shown that HIV, the virus that causes AIDS, will infect the child if the barrier is torn in any way, but HIV is capable of crossing the placental blood barrier from the mother's bloodstream to the child's even without a tear.

Although the placental blood barrier provides protection for the developing embryo and fetus, protection is not complete. In addition to the consequences of tearing as a result of trauma, the barrier can be crossed by certain chemicals and pathogens to cause harm to the developing child. Therefore, obstetricians and expecting mothers must be on their guard to minimize the hazards of life before birth.

SELF QUIZ 17.4

SAY IT—SPELL IT!

Review the terms of obstetrics and human development by speaking the phonetic pronunciations out loud, then writing the correct spelling of the term.

1. AM nee oh NYE tiss _____
2. AM nee oh REK siss _____
- 17.7   3. KOR ee oh AM nee oh NYE tiss _____
- 17.8   4. KOR ee oh KAR sih NOH mah _____
5. EM bree oh TOH see ah _____
6. eh RITH roh blass TOH siss   fee TAL iss _____
7. HISS ter oh REK siss _____
8. MY kroh SEFF ah lee _____
- 17.9   9. OM fah LYE tiss _____
10. OM fall oh seel _____
- 17.10   11. sal PING goh sigh EE siss _____
- 17.11   12. ah BOR shun _____
13. ah BRUP shee oh plah SEN tee _____
14. SER vih kal   ee FAYS ment _____
15. kon JENN ih tal   ah NOM ah lee _____
16. eh soff ah JEE al   ah TREE zee ah _____
17. plah SEN tah   PREH vee ah _____
18. pree eh KLAMP see ah _____
19. SPY nah   BIFF ih dah _____

MATCH IT!

Match the term on the left with the correct definition on the right.

_____ 1. amnionitis

_____ 2. hysterorrhexis

_____ 3. erythroblastosis fetalis

_____ 4. salpingocyesis

_____ 5. omphalitis

_____ 6. microcephaly

_____ 7. chorioamnionitis

_____ 8. abruptio placentae

_____ 9. miscarriage

_____ 10. abortion

_____ 11. preeclampsia

_____ 12. rubella

_____ 13. Down syndrome

_____ 14. esophageal atresia

_____ 15. spina bifida

_____ 16. hyaline membrane disease

_____ 17. cleft palate

_____ 18. eclampsia

_____ 19. cervical effacement

_____ 20. breech birth

_____ 21. placenta previa

a. inflammation of the chorion and amnion

b. congenital anomaly of an abnormally small head

c. inflammation of the amnion

d. ectopic pregnancy in the fallopian tube

e. rupture of the uterus

f. inflammation of the navel

g. fetal hemolysis due to blood incompatibility

h. end of pregnancy by expulsion of the fetus

i. viral disease that can cause congenital anomalies

j. natural expulsion of the fetus

k. caused by incomplete lung development in premature infants

l. birth involving presentation of the feet or buttocks first

m. premature separation of the placenta from the uterus

n. failure of vertebral arches to develop

o. a congenital disorder caused by genetic defects in chromosome #21

p. obliteration of the cervical canal during labor

q. incomplete development of the esophagus

r. pregnancy with an abnormally high blood pressure

s. a disorder in which the palate fails to close during development

t. abnormal attachment of the placenta

u. a disorder characterized by convulsions during pregnancy

BREAK IT DOWN!

Analyze and separate each term into its word parts by labeling each word part using p = prefix, r = root, cv = combining vowel, and s = suffix.

1. amnionitis   _____

2. amniorrhexis   _____

3. choriocarcinoma   _____

4. embryotocia _____

5. hysterorrhexis _____

6. microcephaly _____

7. salpingocyesis _____

WORD BUILDING

Construct or recall medical terms from the following meanings.

1. inflammation of the navel _____

2. rupture of the uterus _____

3. inflammation of the chorion and amnion _____

4. cancer of the chorion _____

5. rupture of the chorion _____

6. ectopic pregnancy in a fallopian tube _____

7. congenital herniation of the umbilicus _____

8. inflammation of the amnion _____

FILL IT IN!

Fill in the blanks with the correct terms.

17.12 1. In the condition known as _____ _____, the placenta separates from the uterine wall prematurely, often causing the natural expulsion of the fetus, or _____. Any expulsion of a fetus, whether natural or artificially induced, is known as _____.

2. An abnormal birth in which the child is delivered with the feet or buttocks first is called a _____ birth.

3. In some cases, labor may cause an obliteration of the cervical canal, a condition known as _____ _____.

4. Any abnormality that is present at birth is called a _____ _____. An example of a genetically caused anomaly is an incomplete palate, or _____ _____, which results in disfigurement of the face. It can be corrected with surgery. Another genetic anomaly that can be surgically corrected is _____ _____, in which the esophagus is incomplete at birth.

In the genetic anomaly known as _____ _____, the newborn lacks vertebral arches of the spine.

5. A severe anomaly that includes numerous symptoms and is caused by a genetic mutation in chromosome #21 is called _____

_____.

6. A virus may also cause congenital anomalies. An example is

17.13   _____, or German measles, which is passed from the mother to the child during pregnancy. Yet another type of genetic anomaly is the result of incomplete development in the lungs, making it difficult for the infant's premature lungs to inflate after an exhalation. This condition is known as

_____ _____ disease.

7. A pregnancy that is experienced outside of the uterus is called

17.14   _____ _____. In these cases, the benefit of a placenta is not realized, so it usually leads to a miscarriage. In the condition

17.15   _____ _____, a placenta is present, but it is abnormally attached, usually blocking the external os.

8. A pregnancy may be accompanied by an abnormally high blood pressure, which includes proteinuria and edema. This condition is known as

_____. In some cases, it may be followed by a more severe condition characterized by convulsions and possible coma and death, called

_____.

Treatments, Procedures, and Devices

WORD PARTS (WHEN APPLICABLE)			TERM	DEFINITION
Part	Type	Meaning		
			abortifacient (a BOR tih FAY shent)	a drug that induces abortion
amni/o -centesis	r/cv s	amnion, amniotic fluid surgical puncture	**amniocentesis** (AM nee oh sehn TEE siss)	surgical puncture through the amnion and aspiration of a small amount of amniotic fluid for the purpose of analyzing the fluid for possible fetal abnormalities (Figure 17.15::::)
amni/o -graphy	r/cv s	amnion, amniotic fluid recording process	**amniography** (AM nee OG rah fee)	x-ray imaging of the amnion after the injection of a contrast medium, which provides an image of the amnion and fetus known as an amniogram (AM nee oh gram)
amni/o -scopy	r/cv s	amnion, amniotic fluid process of viewing	**amnioscopy** (AM nee OSS koh pee)	examination of amniotic fluid and the fetus with an endoscope, called an amnioscope, which is introduced into the cervical canal
amni/o -tomy	r/cv s	amnion, amniotic fluid incision	**amniotomy** (AM nee OTT oh mee)	incision through the amnion, which ruptures the membrane as an inducement to labor
			cesarean section (seh ZAIR ee an SEK shun)	surgical delivery by making an incision through the abdomen and uterus; abbreviated **C-section**

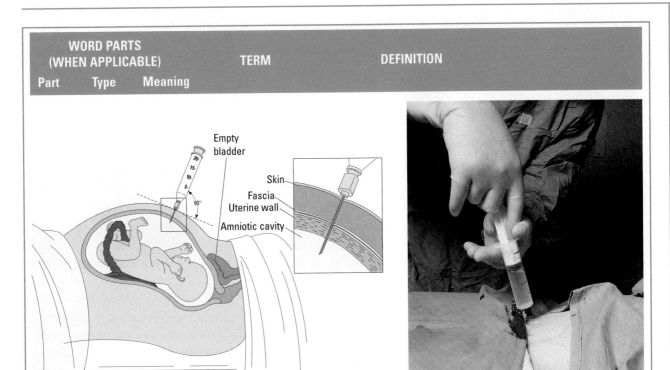

WORD PARTS (WHEN APPLICABLE)			TERM	DEFINITION
Part	**Type**	**Meaning**		

Figure 17.15 ::::

Amniocentesis.
(a) In this examination procedure, amniotic fluid is aspirated with a syringe that is inserted through the abdominal wall, uterine wall, and amnion.
(b) Photograph of the procedure. Amniotic fluid is a slightly yellowish color, which can be seen within the syringe.
Source: Pearson Education.

> ### [FYI]
>
> **Cesarean section**
> The term *cesarean section* was first used to describe this surgical alternative to vaginal birth during Roman times, because it was thought that Julius Caesar was born in this way. However, his family name, Caesar, had its origin from such a birth, which literally means *to cut*, centuries before the birth of Julius.

Part	Type	Meaning	Term	Definition
embry/o	r/cv	embryo	**embryology**	study of embryonic development
-logy	s	study of	(EM bree ALL oh jee)	
episi/o	r/cv	vulva	**episiotomy**	incision through the perineum, often during labor to
-tomy	s	incision	(eh peez ee OTT oh mee)	prevent its tearing (Figure 17.16::::)
fet/o	r/cv	fetus	**fetometry**	measurement of the size of the fetus
-metry	s	measurement	(fee TOM eh tree)	(Figure 17.17::::)
geriatr	r	old age	**geriatrics**	the medical discipline concerned with old age
-ic	s	pertaining to	(jair ee AT riks)	
-s	s	plural		
geront/o	r/cv	old age	**gerontologist**	a physician practicing in the field of gerontology
-logist	s	one who studies	(jair on TALL oh jist)	
geront/o	r/cv	old age	**gerontology**	the medical discipline concerned with the effects of
-logy	s	study of	(jair on TALL oh jee)	aging; abbreviated **GER**

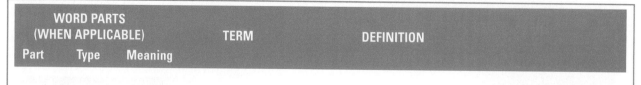

Part	Type	Meaning		

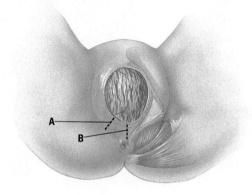

Figure 17.16 ::::

Episiotomy.
Two alternate surgeries (A and B) are indicated by the dotted lines, both of which are intended to reduce the risk of tearing during parturition. *Source: Pearson Education.*

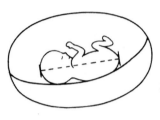
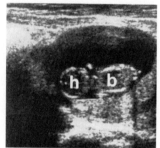

Figure 17.17 ::::

Fetometry.
(a) A sketch of the ultrasound image shown in (b), which is performed in order to create a measurement of the fetus. In this example, the measurement is from the crown of the head to the buttocks.
(b) Ultrasound image of the fetus.
Source: Callen, P.W. Ultrasonography on obstetrics and gynecology (2nd ed., p. 50). Copyright 1998, with permission from Elsevier Science.

Part	Type	Meaning	TERM	DEFINITION
obstetr	r	midwife, prenatal development	**obstetrical sonography** (ob STET rih kal son OG rah fee)	ultrasound imaging of the pregnant uterus to observe fetal development (Figure 17.18::::)
-ic	s	pertaining to		
-al	s	pertaining to		
son/o	r/cv	sound		
-graphy	s	recording process		
obstetr	r	midwife, prenatal development	**obstetrician** (OB steh TRISH an)	a physician practicing in the field of obstetrics
-ic	s	pertaining to		
-ian	s	pertaining to		
obstetr	r	midwife, prenatal development	**obstetrics** (ob STET riks)	the medical discipline concerned with prenatal development, pregnancy, childbirth, and the 42-day period following childbirth; abbreviated **OB.**
-ic	s	pertaining to		
-s	s	plural		
pediatr	r	child	**pediatrician** (pee dee ah TRISH an)	a physician practicing in the field of pediatrics
-ic	s	pertaining to		
-ian	s	pertaining to		
pediatr	r	child	**pediatrics** (pee dee AT riks)	the medical discipline concerned with infancy, childhood, and adolescence; abbreviated **PED**
-ic	s	pertaining to		
-s	s	plural		
pelv/i	r/cv	bowl, pelvis	**pelvimetry** (pell VIHM eh tree)	measurement of a mother's pelvis to determine the potential size of the birth canal
-metry	s	measurement		

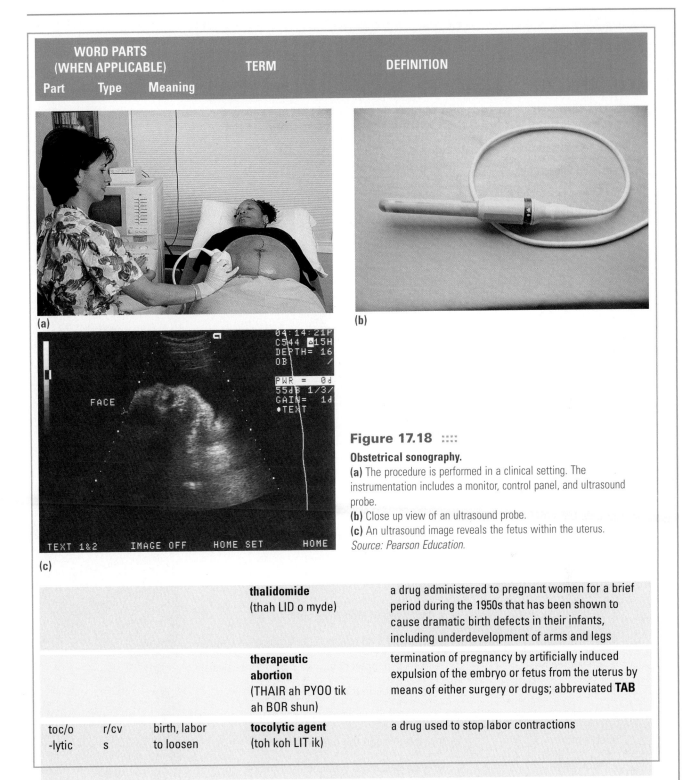

WORD PARTS (WHEN APPLICABLE)			TERM	DEFINITION
Part	**Type**	**Meaning**		

Figure 17.18 ⠿

Obstetrical sonography.
(a) The procedure is performed in a clinical setting. The instrumentation includes a monitor, control panel, and ultrasound probe.
(b) Close up view of an ultrasound probe.
(c) An ultrasound image reveals the fetus within the uterus.
Source: Pearson Education.

Part	Type	Meaning	Term	Definition
			thalidomide (thah LID o myde)	a drug administered to pregnant women for a brief period during the 1950s that has been shown to cause dramatic birth defects in their infants, including underdevelopment of arms and legs
			therapeutic abortion (THAIR ah PYOO tik ah BOR shun)	termination of pregnancy by artificially induced expulsion of the embryo or fetus from the uterus by means of either surgery or drugs; abbreviated **TAB**
toc/o -lytic	r/cv s	birth, labor to loosen	**tocolytic agent** (toh koh LIT ik)	a drug used to stop labor contractions

SELF QUIZ 17.5

SAY IT—SPELL IT!

Review the terms of obstetrics and human development by speaking the phonetic pronunciations out loud, then writing the correct spelling of the term.

1. AM nee oh sehn TEE siss _____

2. AM nee OG rah fee _____

3. AM nee OSS koh pee _____

17.16 4. AM nee OTT oh mee _____

5. seh ZAIR ee an   SEK shun _____

17.17 6. eh peez ee OTT oh mee _____

7. fee TOM eh tree _____

8. ob STET rih kal   son OG rah fee _____

9. pell VIHM eh tree _____

10. toh koh LIT ik _____

11. ob STET riks _____

12. pee dee AT riks _____

17.18 13. jair on TALL oh jee _____

MATCH IT!

Match the term on the left with the correct definition on the right.

_____ 1. amniocentesis   a. measures the size of a fetus

_____ 2. tocolytic agent   b. birth by an incision through the abdomen and uterus

_____ 3. amniotomy   c. ultrasound of a pregnant uterus and the fetus within

_____ 4. cesarean section   d. a drug used to stop labor contractions

_____ 5. pelvimetry   e. endoscopic evaluation of the amnion and fetus

_____ 6. amniography   f. surgical aspiration of amniotic fluid for analysis

_____ 7. amnioscopy   g. incision through the amnion

_____ 8. obstetrical sonography h. measurement of a female pelvis

_____ 9. episiotomy   i. incision through the perineum

_____10. fetometry   j. x-ray procedure to evaluate the amnion (and fetus)

BREAK IT DOWN!

Analyze and separate each term into its word parts by labeling each word part using p = prefix, r = root, cv = combining vowel, and s = suffix.

1. tocolytic _____

2. fetometry _____

3. amniotomy   _____

4. pelvimetry   _____

5. amniography   _____

6. amniocentesis   _____

WORD BUILDING

Construct or recall medical terms from the following meanings.

1. puncture of the amnion and
   withdrawal of amniotic fluid   _____

2. incision through the amnion   _____

3. study of embryonic development   _____

4. a physician specializing in the care
   of children   _____

5. medical field specializing in prenatal
   development   _____

6. ultrasound imaging of the pregnant
   uterus   _____

7. incision through the perineum to
   prevent tearing   _____

FILL IT IN!

Fill in the blanks with the correct terms.

1. A physician who treats people in their senior years is a _____

2. A physician who treats pregnant women, follows prenatal development, and
   assists at childbirth is known as an _____.

3. A physician who treats infant, childhood, and adolescent patients works within
   the medical field of _____.

4. The surgical aspiration of amniotic fluid is called an _____. It
   may be accompanied by an ultrasound imaging procedure, known as
   _____ _____, in an effort to evaluate the fetus.

5. In a vaginal delivery, an _____ is often recommended to avoid
   tearing of the vulva. A nonvaginal delivery involves surgery to extract the newborn
   in a procedure called a _____ _____.

abbreviations of obstetrics and human development

The abbreviations that are associated with obstetrics and human development are summarized here. Study these abbreviations, and review them in the exercise that follows.

ABBREVIATION	DEFINITION	ABBREVIATION	DEFINITION
C-section	cesarean section	OB/GYN	obstetrics/gynecology
EDD	expected date of delivery	PED	pediatrics
DOB	date of birth	PIH	pregnancy-induced hypertension
GER	gerontology	RDS	respiratory distress syndrome
HMD	hyaline membrane disease		(of the newborn)
LMP	last menstrual period	SAB	spontaneous abortion
NB	newborn	TAB	therapeutic abortion
OB	obstetrics		

SELF QUIZ 17.6

Fill in the blanks with the abbreviation or the complete medical term.

Abbreviation	Medical Term
17.19 1. DOB	_____
2. _____	hyaline membrane disease
17.20 3. OB	_____
17.21 4. _____	respiratory distress syndrome
17.22 5. TAB	_____
6. _____	last menstrual period
7. C-section	_____
8. _____	expected date of delivery
9. PED	_____
10. _____	gerontology
11. NB	_____
12. _____	obstetrics/gynecology
13. SAB	_____
14. _____	pregnancy-induced hypertension

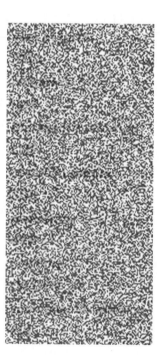

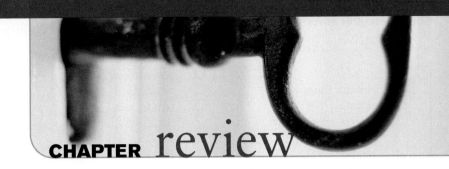

In this section, we will review all the word parts and medical terms from this chapter. As in earlier tables, the word roots are shown in **bold.**

Check each word part and medical term to be sure you understand the meaning. If any are not clear, please go back into the chapter and review that term. Then, complete the review exercises that follow.

[word parts **checklist**]

Prefixes

- ☐ ante-
- ☐ micro-
- ☐ multi-
- ☐ nulli-
- ☐ post-

Word Roots/Combining Vowels

- ☐ **amni**/o, **amnion**/o
- ☐ **chori**/o
- ☐ **cyes**i/o

- ☐ **cyes**/o
- ☐ **embry**/o
- ☐ **fet**/o, **fet**/i
- ☐ **ger**/o, **geront**/o
- ☐ **gravid**/o, **gravidar**/o
- ☐ **lact**/o
- ☐ **nat**/o
- ☐ **obstetr**/o
- ☐ **omphal**/o
- ☐ **par**/o, **part**/o
- ☐ **ped**/o, **pediatr**/o

- ☐ **pelv**/o
- ☐ **presby**/o
- ☐ **prim**/i
- ☐ **pseud**/o
- ☐ **puerper**/o
- ☐ **toc**/o

Suffixes

- ☐ -lytic
- ☐ -rrhexis
- ☐ -tocía

[medical terminology **checklist**]

- ☐ abortifacient
- ☐ abortion
- ☐ abruptio placentae
- ☐ adolescence
- ☐ adulthood
- ☐ **amni**ocentesis
- ☐ **amni**ography
- ☐ **amni**on
- ☐ **amni**onitis
- ☐ **amni**orrhea
- ☐ **amni**orrhexis
- ☐ **amni**oscopy
- ☐ **amni**otomy
- ☐ antepartum
- ☐ breech birth
- ☐ cesarean section (C-section)
- ☐ **cerv**ical effacement
- ☐ childhood
- ☐ **chori**o**amnion**itis
- ☐ **chori**o**carcin**oma
- ☐ **chori**on

- ☐ cleft palate
- ☐ conception
- ☐ con**gen**ital anomaly
- ☐ **cyes**is
- ☐ date of birth (DOB)
- ☐ Down syndrome
- ☐ dys**toc**ia
- ☐ eclampsia
- ☐ ectopic pregnancy
- ☐ **embryo**
- ☐ **embryo**gen**ics
- ☐ **embryo**logy
- ☐ **embryo**tocia
- ☐ episiotomy
- ☐ erythro**blast**osis **feta**lis
- ☐ **esophage**al atresia
- ☐ expected date of delivery (EDD)
- ☐ **fet**ometry
- ☐ **fet**us
- ☐ **geront**ology (GER)
- ☐ **gravid**a

- ☐ **gravid**o**puerper**al
- ☐ hyaline membrane disease (HMD)
- ☐ hyperemesis **gravid**arum
- ☐ **hyster**orrhexis
- ☐ infancy
- ☐ intra**part**um
- ☐ labor
- ☐ **lact**ogenic
- ☐ **lact**orrhea
- ☐ last **menstru**al period (LMP)
- ☐ lochia
- ☐ meconium
- ☐ micro**ceph**aly
- ☐ miscarriage
- ☐ multi**gravid**a
- ☐ multi**para**
- ☐ **nat**al
- ☐ neo**nat**e
- ☐ newborn (NB)
- ☐ nulli**gravid**a

- ☐ nulli**para**
- ☐ **obstetri**cal **son**ography
- ☐ **obstetri**cs (OB)
- ☐ **obstetri**cs/**gynec**ology (OB/GYN)
- ☐ **omphal**itis
- ☐ **omphal**ocele
- ☐ **par**a
- ☐ parturition
- ☐ **pediatri**cs (PED)
- ☐ **pelv**imetry
- ☐ placenta
- ☐ placenta previa
- ☐ post**nat**al development
- ☐ post**part**um
- ☐ preeclampsia
- ☐ pregnancy
- ☐ pregnancy-induced hypertension (PIH)
- ☐ premature infant
- ☐ pre**nat**al development
- ☐ primi**gravid**a
- ☐ primi**par**a
- ☐ **pseud**ocyesis
- ☐ **puerper**a
- ☐ **puerper**al
- ☐ **puerper**ium
- ☐ respiratory distress syndrome (RDS)
- ☐ rubella
- ☐ **salping**ocyesis
- ☐ senescence
- ☐ spina bifida
- ☐ spontaneous abortion (SAB)
- ☐ therapeutic abortion (TAB)
- ☐ **toc**olytic agent
- ☐ **umbilic**al cord
- ☐ zygote

[show what **you know!**]

BREAK IT DOWN!

Analyze these medical terms by separating each term into its word parts, labeling each word part using p = prefix, r = root, cv = combining vowel, and s = suffix.

Example:	1. multipara	<div align="center">p r multi/para</div>
	2. multipartum	_____
	3. postpartum	_____
	4. embryogenic	_____
	5. gerontology	_____
	6. pseudocyesis	_____
	7. gravidopuerperal	_____
	8. lactogenic	_____
	9. amnionitis	_____
	10. amniocentesis	_____
	11. omphalitis	_____
	12. microcephaly	_____
	13. chorioamnionitis	_____
	14. embryotocia	_____

WORD BUILDING

Construct or recall medical terms from the following meanings.

Example:	1. a woman previously pregnant one or more times	<div align="center">multigravida</div>
	2. term for a child less than 28 days after birth	_____

3. occurring after childbirth   _____

4. study of embryonic development   _____

5. pertaining to birth   _____

6. a woman who has never been pregnant   _____

7. a woman in her first pregnancy   _____

8. a false pregnancy   _____

9. pertaining to the period after childbirth   _____

10. termination of pregnancy by expulsion
    of the fetus   _____

11. separation of the placenta from the
    uterine wall   _____

12. severe nausea and vomiting during pregnancy   _____

13. rupture of the uterus   _____

14. abnormal discharge of amniotic fluid   _____

15. congenital absence of vertebral arches   _____

16. x-ray imaging of the amnion   _____

17. delivery of a child through an incision into
    the abdomen and uterus   _____

18. a drug used to stop labor contractions   _____

19. termination of pregnancy by medical
    intervention   _____

CASE STUDIES

Fill in the blanks with the correct terms.

1. A 42-year-old patient who had not had children, or was (a)_____, was evaluated after complaining of

    cessation of menstruation and pain in the abdomen. A pregnancy test confirmed the cause was pregnancy, with an EDD of

    175 days. She was scheduled for (b) _____ care, a measurement of her pelvic birth canal, or

    (c) _____, and surgical aspiration of a sample of amniotic fluid, or (d) _____,

    to check for possible birth defects of the (e) _____. She was assigned a physician specializing in the

    treatment of pregnancy and prenatal development, or an (f) _____, to follow her progress and

    prepare her for (g) _____, or childbirth. Since all evaluations indicated a normal pregnancy, she was

    scheduled for routine weekly checkups. At the start of the third trimester, her pelvic region and fetus were evaluated with

    (h) _____ _____, which provided ultrasound imaging of the fetus. The proce-

    dure indicated the fetus was turned to exit from the birth canal in a feet-first position, or (i) _____

    _____. A subsequent ultrasound confirmed the position, so the patient was scheduled for surgical de-

    livery, or (j) _____ _____ in which the child was birthed through an abdominal

    and uterine incision. Nine weeks later, as a result of the procedure, a normal female was born. For the next 28 days, the

    newborn, or (k) _____, and the (l) _____ mother were evaluated weekly. After

28 days, the infant was transferred to a physician specializing in the care of children, or a (m) _____,

and the mother returned to her (n) _____ _____.

2. A 22-year-old pregnant female was admitted to the OB ward after complaining of severe headache, nausea, and weight loss.

Her medical history indicated she was (o) _____, having given birth once; her blood type is Rh– while

that of her husband is Rh+, and she had become pregnant with this child 45 days previously. Her obstetrician scheduled her

for blood tests and amniocentesis. The results of the blood test indicated acute hypertension during pregnancy, or

(p) _____. Evidence further indicated a likelihood that this condition would worsen into

(q) _____, which is life-threatening. The amniocentesis indicated a breakage in fetal

chromosome #21, or (r) _____ _____. The parents were consulted about

the genetic evidence, and elected for an induced expulsion of the fetus, or (s) _____

_____.

 piece it all **together!**

CROSSWORD

**From the chapter material, fill in the crossword puzzle with answers to the
following clues.**

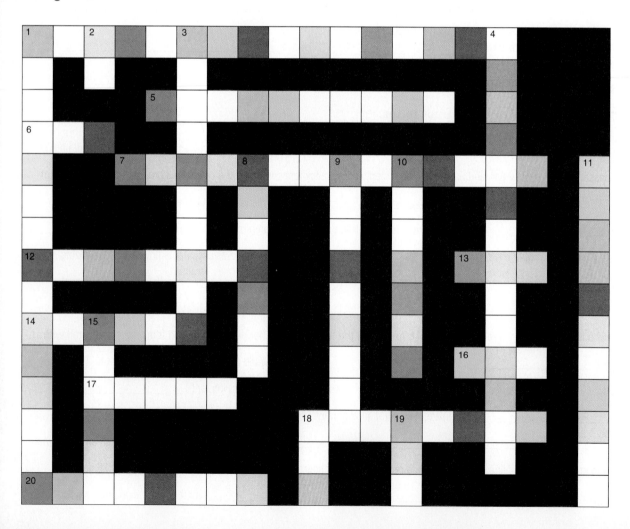

ACROSS

1. Inflammation of the chorion and amnion. (Find puzzle piece 17.7)
5. Incision through the perineum to prevent tearing during birth. (Find puzzle piece 17.17)
6. Abbreviation for an alternate term of HMD. (Find puzzle piece 17.21)
7. An abnormal attachment of the placenta. (Find puzzle piece 17.15)
12. A common cause of miscarriage (first word only). (Find puzzle piece 17.12)
13. A word root for *birth, labor.* (Find puzzle piece 17.2)
14. A synonym for *pregnancy.* (Find puzzle piece 17.3)
16. A word root for *child.* (Find puzzle piece 17.1)
17. A common word for *parturition.* (Find puzzle piece 17.5)
18. Difficult labor. (Find puzzle piece 17.6)
20. Expulsion of the embryo or fetus from the uterus. (Find puzzle piece 17.11)

DOWN

1. Cancer of the chorion. (Find puzzle piece 17.8)
2. Abbreviation for *obstetrics.* (Find puzzle piece 17.20)
3. Inflammation of the navel. (Find puzzle piece 17.9)
4. Implantation of the embryo in a fallopian tube (Find puzzle piece 17.10)
8. Implantation outside of the uterus. (Find puzzle piece 17.14)
9. A surgical procedure that induces labor. (Find puzzle piece 17.16)
10. A viral disease that can cross the placental blood barrier. (Find puzzle piece 17.13)
11. The field of medicine that treats old age diseases. (Find puzzle piece 17.18)
15. The first eight weeks of development. (Find puzzle piece 17.4)
18. Abbreviation for a date entered into the birth certificate (Find puzzle piece 17.19)
19. Abbreviation for an induced abortion. (Find puzzle piece 17.22)

WORD UNSCRAMBLE

From the completed crossword puzzle, unscramble:

1. All of the letters that appear in **red** squares __ ☐ __ __ __ __ __ __ __ __ __ __ __ __

   Clue: Aspiration of amniotic fluid to evaluate it for birth defects

2. All of the letters that appear in **purple** squares __ ☐ __ __ __ __ __ __

   Clue: A woman who has just given birth

3. All of the letters that appear in **peach** squares __ __ __ __ ☐ __ __ __ __

   Clue: A drug that is used to stop labor contractions

4. All of the letters that appear in **blue** squares __ __ __ ☐ __ __ __ __ __ __

   Clue: The field of medicine that treats pregnancy and childbirth

5. All of the letters that appear in **yellow** squares __ __ __ __ __ __ ☐ __ __ __

   Clue: An anomaly (disease or disorder) that is present at birth

6. All of the letters that appear in **green** squares __ __ __ __ __ ☐ __ __ __

   Clue: A severe condition of PIH

7. All of the letters that appear in **pink** squares __ ☐ __ __ __

   Clue: Pertaining to birth

8. All of the letters that appear in **gray** squares __ __ __ __ ☐

   Clue: From the Latin word for *toil, suffering*

9. All of the letters that appear in **brown** squares __ ☐ __ __

   Clue: A woman who has experienced childbirth

Now write down each of the letters that are boxed and unscramble them to find the hidden medical term of obstetrics and human development: __ __ __ __ __ __ __ __ __.

MEDmedia wrap-up

www.prenhall.com/wingerd

Before you go on to the next chapter, take advantage of the free CD-ROM and study guide website that accompany this book. Simply load the CD-ROM for additional activities, games, animations, videos, and quizzes linked to this chapter. Then visit www.prenhall.com/wingerd for even more!

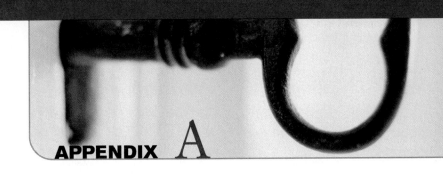

[word parts arranged alphabetically and defined]

The word parts that have been presented in this textbook are summarized with their definitions for quick reference. The chapter numbers correspond to the first chapter in which the word part is described. Prefixes are listed first, followed by combining forms and suffixes.

PREFIX	DEFINITION	CHAPTER	PREFIX	DEFINITION	CHAPTER
a-	without, absence of	4	macro-	large	11
ad-	toward	9	meta-	after, change	3
an-	without, absence of	4	micro-	small	11
ana-	up, toward, apart	2	mono-	single	6
ante-	before	15	multi-	many	17
anti-	against, opposing	9	my-	muscle	5
bi-	two	2	myo-	muscle	5
bin-	two	7	neo-	new	3
brady-	slow	10	nulli-	none	17
di-	two	6	ortho-	straight, normal	5
dia-	around, passing through	5, 14	pan-	all, entire	6
dys-	bad, abnormal	3	para-	near, alongside; departure	5
e-	to remove	7		from normal	
en-	within, upon, on, over	14	per-	through	4
endo-	within, inner, absorbing	1	peri-	around, about, surrounding	10
ep-	upon, on, over	4	poly-	many	5
epi-	upon	2	post-	after	17
eu-	normal, good	11	pre-	before	1
ex-	outside, away from	9	pro-	forward, preceding	11
exo-	outside, away from	9	quad-	four	5
hemi-	one-half	6	re-	back	13
homo-	same	11	sub-	beneath	4
hydro-	water	6	sym-	together, joined	5
hyper-	excessive	3	syn-	together, joined	5
hypo-	under, below normal	2	tachy-	rapid, fast	10
im-	not	14	tetra-	four	6
inter-	between	10	trans-	through, across, beyond	14
intra-	within	1	uni-	one	2

COMBINING FORM	DEFINITION	CHAPTER	COMBINING FORM	DEFINITION	CHAPTER
abdomin/o	abdomen, abdominal cavity	2	card/o	heart	2
acou/o	hearing	8	cardi/o	heart	10
acoust/o	hearing	8	carp/o	wrist	5
acr/o	extremity, extreme	9	cartil/o	gristle, cartilage	5
aden/o	gland	3	caud/o	tail	2
adren/o	adrenal gland	9	cec/o	blind intestine, cecum	13
aer/o	air or gas	8	cel/o	hernia, protrusion	5
albumin/o	albumin	14	celi/o	abdomen, abdominal cavity	13
alveol/o	alveolus (air sac)	12	cephal/o	head	2
amni/o	amnion, amniotic fluid	17	cerebell/o	cerebellum (little brain)	6
amnion/o	amnion, amniotic fluid	17	cerebr/o	cerebrum (brain)	6
an/o	anus	13	cerumin/o	wax	7
andr/o	male	9	cervic/o	cervix, neck	16
angi/o	blood vessel	10	cheil/o	lip	13
ankyl/o	crooked	5	chir/o	hand	5
anter/o	front	2	chol/e	bile, gall	13
aort/o	aorta	10	choledoch/o	common bile duct	13
appendic/o	to hang onto, appendix	13	chondr/o	cartilage	3
aque/o	water	8	chori/o	membrane, chorion	17
arche/o	first, beginning	16	chromat/o	color	11
arter/o	artery	10	clon/o	spasm	5
arteri/o	artery	10	col/o	colon	13
arthr/o	joint	5	colp/o	vagina	16
astheni/o	weakness	6	conjunctiv/o	to bind together, conjunctiva	7
atel/o	imperfect, incomplete	12			
ather/o	fat	10	cor/o	pupil	7
atri/o	atrium	10	core/o	pupil	7
aud/o	hearing	8	corne/o	horny, cornea	7
audi/o	hearing	8	coron/o	crown, circle	10
aur/i	ear	8	cortic/o	tree bark, outer covering, cortex	9
aut/o	self	4			
azot/o	urea, nitrogen	14	cost/o	rib	5
bacter/o	bacteria	11	cran/o	skull, cranium	2
balan/o	glans penis	15	crani/o	skull, cranium	2
bi/o	life	4	crin/o	to secrete	9
bil/i	bile	13	crypt/o	hidden	4
blast/o	germ, bud	11	culd/o	cul-de-sac	16
blephar/o	eyelid	7	cutane/o	skin	4
bronch/i	bronchus (airway)	12	cyan/o	blue	10
bronch/o	bronchus (airway)	12	cyes/i	pregnancy	17
burs/o	purse or sac; bursa	5	cyes/o	pregnancy	17
calc/i	calcium	9	cyst/o	bladder, sac	14
cancer/o	cancer	3	cyt/o	cell	3
carcin/o	cancer	3	dacry/o	tear	7

COMBINING FORM	DEFINITION	CHAPTER	COMBINING FORM	DEFINITION	CHAPTER
dent/i	teeth	13	gloss/o	tongue	13
derm/o	skin	4	gluc/o	glucose, sugar	9
dermat/o	skin	4	glut/o	buttock	2
diaphragmat/o	diaphragm	2	glyc/o	glycogen, sugar	9
dipl/o	double	7	glycos/o	sugar	14
dips/o	thirst	9	gravid/o	pregnancy	17
dist/o	away	2	gravidar/o	pregnancy	17
diverticul/o	small blind pouch, diverticulum	13	gyn/o	woman	16
			gynec/o	woman	16
dors/o	back	2	halat/o	breath	13
duct/o	lead, move	5	hem/o	blood	11
duoden/o	twelve, duodenum	13	hemat/o	blood	11
dur/o	hard	6	hepat/o	liver	13
ech/o	sound	10	hern/o	protrusion, hernia	13
electr/o	electricity	10	herni/o	protrusion, hernia	13
embol/o	a throwing in	6	heter/o	other	4
embry/o	embryo	17	hidr/o	sweat	4
encephal/o	brain	6	hist/o	tissue	3
endocrin/o	endocrine	9	hom/o	sameness, unchanging	2
enter/o	small intestine	13	hormon/o	to set in motion	9
epididym/o	epididymis	15	hydr/o	water	14
epiglott/o	epiglottis	12	hymen/o	hymen	16
episi/o	vulva	16	hyster/o	uterus	16
eryth/o	red	4	iatr/o	to heal	2
erythr/o	red	10	idi/o	person, self	2
esophag/o	gullet, esophagus	13	ile/o	ileum of small intestine, to roll	13
esthesi/o	sensation	6			
eti/o	cause (of disease)	2	ili/o	flank, groin, ilium of the pelvis	5
fasci/o	fascia	5			
femor/o	thigh	2	immun/o	exempt; immunity	11
fet/i	fetus	17	infect/o	to enter, invade	2
fet/o	fetus	17	infer/o	below	2
fibr/o	fiber	3	inguin/o	groin	2
fibul/o	clasp of buckle, fibula	5	ir/o	rainbow, iris	7
fovea/o	small pit	7	irid/o	rainbow, iris	7
gangli/o	ganglion	6	isch/o	to hold back, deficiency, blockagestomach	10
gastr/o	stomach	13			
gen/o	formation, cause, produce	3	ischi/o	haunch, hip joint, ischium	5
			jejun/o	empty, jejunum	13
ger/o	old age	17	kal/i	potassium	9
geront/o	old age	17	kerat/o	hard, horny; cornea	4
gingiv/o	gums	13	ket/o	ketone bodies	9
gli/o	glue, neuroglia	6	keton/o	ketone bodies	14
glomerul/o	little ball, glomerulus	14	kinesi/o	motion	5

COMBINING FORM	DEFINITION	CHAPTER	COMBINING FORM	DEFINITION	CHAPTER
kyph/o	hump	5	nas/o	nose	12
labyrinth/o	labyrinth, internal ear	8	nat/o	birth	17
lacrim/o	tear	7	natr/o	sodium	9
lact/o	milk	17	necr/o	death	4
lamin/o	thin, lamina	5	nephr/o	kidney	14
lapar/o	abdomen, abdominal cavity	13	neur/o	sinew or cord, nerve, fascia	3
laryng/o	larynx	12	noct/i	night	14
later/o	side	2	nucl/o	kennel, nucleus	3
lei/o	smooth	3	nyct/o	night, nocturnal	7
leuk/o	white	4	nyctal/o	night, nocturnal	7
lingu/o	tongue	13	obstetr/o	midwife, prenatal development	17
lip/o	fat, lipid	3	ocul/o	eye	7
lith/o	stone	13	olig/o	few in number	14
lob/o	lobe	12	omphal/o	umbilicus (navel)	17
lord/o	bent forward	5	onc/o	tumor	3
lumb/o	loin, lower back	2	onych/o	nail	4
lymph/o	clear water or fluid	11	oophor/o	ovary	16
lys/o	dissolution	6	opt/o	eye, vision	7
mal/o	bad	3	opthalm/o	eye	7
mamm/o	breast	16	or/o	mouth	13
mast/o	breast	16	orch/o	testis or testicle	15
meat/o	opening	14	orchi/o	testis or testicle	15
medi/o	middle	2	orchid/o	testis or testicle	15
megal/o	abnormally large	9	organ/o	tool	3
melan/o	dark, black	3	orth/o	straight	5
men/o	month, menstruation	16	oste/o	bone	3
menstru/o	month, menstruation	16	ot/o	ear	8
mening/o	meninges, membrane	6	ov/i	egg	16
menisc/o	cresent-shaped moon, meniscus membrane	5	ov/o	egg	16
ment/o	mind	6	ovari/o	ovary	16
metr/o	uterus	16	ox/o	oxygen	12
mon/o	one	11	pachy/o	thick	4
muc/o	mucus	12	palat/o	roof of mouth, palate	13
my/o	muscle	3	pancreat/o	sweetbread, pancreas	9, 13
myc/o	fungus	4	par/o	parturition or labor	17
myel/o	bone marrow; spinal cord; medulla; myelin	5	parathyroid/o	parathyroid	9
			pariet/o	wall	5
myelon/o	bone marrow; spinal cord; medulla; myelin	5	part/o	parturition or labor	17
			patell/o	small pan, patella	5
myos/o	muscle	5	path/o	disease	3
myring/o	membrane; eardrum	8	pector/o	chest	2
myx/o	mucus	9	ped/o	child	5

COMBINING FORM	DEFINITION	CHAPTER	COMBINING FORM	DEFINITION	CHAPTER
pediatr/o	child	17	radicul/o	nerve root	6
pelv/i	basin, pelvis	2	rect/o	straight, erect, rectum	13
pen/o	penis	15	ren/o	kidney	14
peps/o	digestion	13	retin/o	net, retina	7
perine/o	perineum	16	rhabd/o	rod	3
peritone/o	to stretch over, peritoneum	13	rhin/o	nose	12
			rhytid/o	wrinkles	4
petr/o	stone	5	sacr/o	sacred, sacrum	5
phac/o	lens	7	salping/o	tube: eustachian tube; fallopian tube	7; 16
phag/o	eat, swallow	13			
phak/o	lens	7	sarc/o	flesh, muscle	3
phalang/o	row of soldiers	5	scler/o	thick, hard; sclera	4; 7
pharyng/o	pharynx (throat)	12	scoli/o	curved	5
phas/o	speech	6	seb/o	sebum, oil	4
phleb/o	vein	10	semin/o	seed	15
phot/o	light	7	sept/o	wall, partition	12
physi/o	nature	2	sial/o	saliva, salivary gland	13
physis/o	growth	5	sigm/o	the letter "s," sigmoid colon	13
plegi/o	paralysis	6			
pleur/o	pleura	12	sinus/o	cavity	12
pneum/o	lung or air	12	somat/o	body	6
pneumat/o	lung or air	12	somn/o	sleep	12
pod/o	foot	5	son/o	sound	8
poikil/o	irregular	11	sperm/o	seed	15
polyp/o	polyp	13	spermat/o	seed	15
poster/o	back	2	sphygm/o	pulse	10
presby/o	old age	7	spin/o	spine or thorn	2
prim/i	first	17	spir/o	breathe	12
proct/o	anus	13	splen/o	spleen	11
prostat/o	prostate gland	15	spondyl/o	vertebra	5
proxim/o	near	2	staped/o	stapes	8
pseud/o	false	17	staphyl/o	grape-like clusters (bacterium)	11
psych/o	mind	6			
pub/o	grown up	5	stasis/o	standing still	2
puerper/o	childbirth	17	steat/o	fat	13
pulmon/o	lung	12	sten/o	narrowness, constriction	10
py/o	pus	12	stern/o	chest, sternum	5
pyel/o	pelvis (renal)	14	steth/o	chest	10
pylor/o	pylorus	13	stigmat/o	point	7
quad/o	four gate keeper	6	stomat/o	mouth	13
quadr/i	four	6	strept/o	twisted or gnarled (bacterium)	11
rachi/o	spine	5			
radi/o	spoke of a wheel, radius	5	super/o	above	2
radic/o	nerve root	6	synov/o	binding eggs; synovial	5

COMBINING FORM	DEFINITION	CHAPTER	COMBINING FORM	DEFINITION	CHAPTER
synovi/o	binding eggs; synovial	5	umbilic/o	navel	2
syndesm/o	binding together	5	ur/o	urine	14
tars/o	flat surface	5	ureter/o	ureter	14
taxi/o	reaction to a stimulus	5	urethr/o	urethra	14
ten/o	to stretch out; tendon	5	urin/o	urine	14
tend/o	to stretch out; tendon	5	uter/o	womb, uterus	16
tendin/o	to stretch out; tendon	5	uvul/o	grape, uvula	13
test/o	testis, testicle	15	vagin/o	sheath, vagina	16
testicul/o	small testis, testicle	15	valvul/o	little valve	10
thalam/o	thalamus	6	varic/o	dilated vein	10
thel/o	nipple	3	vas/o	blood vessel; duct	10; 15
therm/o	heat	11	vascul/o	little blood vessel	10
thorac/o	thorax (chest)	2	ven/o	vein	10
thromb/o	clot	10	ventr/o	front, belly	2
thym/o	wart-like, thymus gland	11	ventricul/o	little belly or cavity, ventricle	10
thyr/o	shield, thyroid	9			
toc/o	birth, labor	17	vers/o	turn	5
tom/o	cut, section	2	vertebr/o	joint, vertebra	5
ton/o	tone, tension, pressure	7	vesic/o	bladder, sac	14
toxic/o	poison	7	vesicul/o	vesicle (seminal vesicle)	15
trache/o	trachea	12	vitr/o	glassy	7
trachel/o	neck, cervix	16	vitre/o	glassy	7
trich/o	hair	4	vulv/o	vulva	16
tubercul/o	little mass of swelling	12	xanth/o	yellow	4
tympan/o	eardrum	8	xer/o	dry	4

SUFFIX	DEFINITION	CHAPTER	SUFFIX	DEFINITION	CHAPTER
-a	singular	5	-cele	hernia, swelling, protrusion	6
-ac	pertaining to	10			
-acusis	hearing condition	8	-centesis	surgical puncture	5
-ad	toward	2	-clasia	break apart	5
-al	pertaining to	1	-clasis	break apart	5
-algesia	pain	6	-clast	break apart	5
-algia	pain	5	-crit	separate	11
-apheresis	removal	10	-cusis	hearing condition	8
-ar	pertaining to	12	-cyte	cell	11
-ary	pertaining to	12	-desis	surgical fixation, fusion	5
-asthenia	weakness	5	-drome	run, running	9
-atresia	closure; absence of a normal body opening	16	-dynia	pain	5
			-eal	pertaining to	12
			-ectasis	expansion, dilation	12
-capnia	carbon dioxide	12	-ectomy	excision	4

SUFFIX	DEFINITION	CHAPTER	SUFFIX	DEFINITION	CHAPTER
-elle	small	3	-paresis	paralysis (minor)	6
-emesis	vomiting	13	-pathy	disease	5
-emetic	vomiting	13	-penia	abnormal reduction in number, deficiency	11
-emia	blood (condition of)	9			
-gen	formation, cause, produce	3	-pepsia	digestion	13
			-pexy	surgical fixation, suspension	12
-genesis	origin, cause	3			
-genic	pertaining to formation, causing, producing	3	-phagia	eating or swallowing	4
			-phasia	speaking	6
-gram	recording	6	-phil	loving, affinity for	11
-graph	instrument for recording	10	-philia	loving, affinity for	11
			-phobia	fear	7
-graphy	recording process	10	-phonia	sound or voice	12
-hemia	blood (condition of)	11	-phylaxis	protection	11
-ia	diseased state (condition of)	4	-physis	growth	5
			-plasia	shape, formation	3
-ial	pertaining to	16	-plasm	something shaped	3
-iasis	condition of	13	-plasty	surgical repair	4
-iatry	treatment, specialty	5	-plegia	paralysis (major)	5
-ic	pertaining to	2	-pnea	breathing	12
-ion	pertaining to	4	-poiesis	formation	11
-ior	pertaining to	2	-practic	one who practices	5
-is	pertaining to	4	-ptosis	falling downward (condition of)	5
-ism	condition or disease	9			
-ist	one who practices	5	-ptysis	spit out a fluid	12
-itis	inflammation	4	-rrhagia	bleeding, hemorrhage	7
-lepsy	seizure	6	-rrhaphy	suturing	13
-logist	one who studies	3	-rrhea	excessive discharge	4
-logy	study of	3	-rrhexis	rupture	10
-lytic, -lysis	to loosen, dissolve	11, 17	-salpinx	trumpet, fallopian tube	16
-malacia	softening	4	-sarcoma	malignant tumor	3
-meter	measuring instrument	12	-schisis	split, fissure	5
-metry	measurement	11	-sclerosis	hardening	10
-oid	resemblance to	6	-scope	viewing instrument	3
-oma	abnormal swelling, tumor	3	-scopy	process of viewing	3
			-sis	state of	3
-opia	vision	7	-some	body	3
-opsy	view of	4	-spasm	sudden, involuntary muscle contraction	12
-osis	process or condition that is usually abnormal	3			
			-stasis	standing still	3
-otomy	cutting into, excision	5	-stenosis	narrowing, constriction	10
-ous	pertaining to	4	-stomy	surgical creation of an opening	11
-oxia	oxygen	12			

SUFFIX	DEFINITION	CHAPTER	SUFFIX	DEFINITION	CHAPTER
-tic	pertaining to	5	-trophy	nourishment, development	14
-tocia	birth, labor	17			
-tome	cutting instrument	4	-um	pertaining to	3
-tomy	incision	11	-uria	urine, urination	14
-tripsy	surgical crushing	14	-y	process of	2

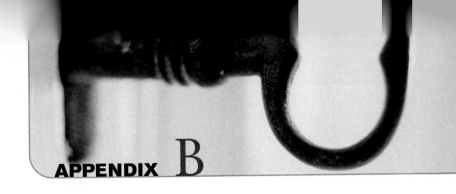

APPENDIX B

[abbreviations]

The abbreviations from Chapters 1–17 are presented in alphabetical order.
Additional abbreviations are also included to establish a complete listing of medical
abbreviations. In each case, the abbreviations are presented in the form in which
they are most common within the health care environment.

ABBREVIATION	DEFINITION	ABBREVIATION	DEFINITION
AA	Alcoholics Anonymous	AMA	American Medical Association
A	anterior	amb	ambulatory
A&P	auscultation and percussion	AMBS	American Medical Board of Specialists
A&P repair	anterior and posterior colporrhaphy		
A&P resection	abdominoperineal resection	AMI	acute myocardial infarction
A&W	alive and well	AML	acute myelocytic leukemia
ab	abortion	amt	amount
abd	abdomen	ant	anterior
ABE	acute bacterial endocarditis	AODM	adult-onset (Type II) diabetes mellitus
ABGs	arterial blood gases	AP	anterioposterior
ac	before meals	AP	angina pectoris
ACL	anterior cruciate ligament	ARDS	adult (acute) respiratory distress syndrome
ACTH	adrenocorticotrophic hormone		
AD	right ear (in Latin, *auris dexter*)	ARM	artificial rupture of membranes
AD	Alzheimer's disease	ARMD	age-related macular degeneration
ADL	activities of daily living	AS	left ear (in Latin, *auris sinister*)
ad lib	as desired	ASA	aspirin (aspirinic salicylic acid)
Adeno-Ca	adenocarcinoma	ASCVD	arteriosclerotic cardiovascular disease
ADH	antidiuretic hormone		
AFB	acid-fast bacilli	ASD	atrial septal defect
Afib	atrial fibrillation	ASHD	arteriosclerotic heart disease
AIDS	acquired immune deficiency syndrome	Ast	astigmatism
AKA	above-knee amputation	as tol	as tolerated
alb	albumin	AU	both ears (in Latin, *aures unitas*)
ALL	acute lymphocytic leukemia	AUL	acute undifferentiated leukemia
ALS	amyotrophic lateral sclerosis	AV	atrioventricular
alt dieb	alternate days	AVR	aortic valve replacement
alt hor	alternate hours	ax	axillary (armpit region)
alt noct	alternate nights	BA	bronchial asthma
AMA	against medical advice	BBB	bundle branch block

ABBREVIATION	DEFINITION	ABBREVIATION	DEFINITION
BC	Bowman's capsule	CI	coronary insufficiency
BCC	basal cell carcinoma	CIN	cervical intraepithelial neoplasia
BE	barium enema	circ	circumcision
bid	twice a day	cl	clinic
BK	below knee	Cl	chloride
BKA	below-knee amputation	CLD	chronic liver disease
BM	bowel movement	CLL	chronic lymphocytic leukemia
BOM	bilateral otitis media	cl liq	clear liquid
BP	blood pressure	cm	centimeter
BPH	benign prostatic hyperplasia	CML	chronic myelogenous leukemia
BR	bed rest	CNS	central nervous system
BRP	bathroom privileges	c/o	complains of
BS	blood sugar	CO	carbon monoxide
BSO	bilateral salpingo-oophorectomy	CO_2	carbon dioxide
BUN	blood urea nitrogen	CIS	carcinoma in situ
Bx	biopsy	COLD	chronic obstructive lung disease
bx	biopsy	cond	condition
C	Celsius	COPD	chronic obstructive pulmonary
Ca	calcium		disease
CA	cancer	CP	cerebral palsy
CA-125	Cancer Antigen-125 Tumor Marker	CPK	creatine phosphokinase
CABG	coronary artery bypass graft	CPN	chronic pyelonephritis
CAD	coronary artery disease	CPR	cardiopulmonary resuscitation
cal	calorie	CRD	chronic respiratory disease
cap	capsule	creat	creatinine
CAPD	continuous ambulatory peritoneal	CRF	chronic renal failure
	dialysis	CRNA	certified registered nurse-anesthetist
cath	catheter, catheterization	C-section	cesarean section
CBC	complete blood count	CS	cesarean section
CBR	complete bed rest	CT (CAT) scan	computed (axial) tomography scan
CBS	chronic brain syndrome	CT	calcitonin
cc	cubic centimeter	CTS	carpal tunnel syndrome
CC	colony count	Cu	copper
CCU	coronary care unit	CVA	cerebrovascular accident (stroke)
CDH	congenital dislocation of the hip	CVP	central venous pressure
CEA	carcinoma embryonic antigen	CXR	chest x-ray
CF	cystic fibrosis	D&C	dilation and curettage
CHB	complete heart block	DAT	diet as tolerated
CHD	coronary heart disease	DC	discontinued
chemo	chemotherapy	del	delivery
CHF	congestive heart failure	DI	diabetes insipidus
CHO	carbohydrate	DIC	diffuse intravascular coagulation
chol	cholesterol	diff	differential (blood count)

ABBREVIATION	DEFINITION	ABBREVIATION	DEFINITION
DLE	discoid lupus erythmatosus	FACP	Fellow of the American College of Physicians
DM	diabetes mellitus		
DNA	deoxyribonucleic acid	FACS	Fellow of the American College of Surgeons
DOA	dead on arrival		
DOB	date of birth	FBD	fibrocystic breast disease
Dr	dram	FBS	fasting blood sugar
DRG	diagnosis-related group	Fe	iron
DRE	digital rectal exam	FHT	fetal heart tones
D/S	dextrose in saline	flu	influenza
DT	delirium tremens	FOB	fetal occult blood
DTR	deep tendon reflexes	FSH	follicle-stimulating hormone
DVT	deep vein thrombosis	FTT	failure to thrive
D/W	dextrose in water	FUO	fever of undetermined origin
Dx	diagnosis	Fx	fracture
E	enema	g	gram
EBL	estimated blood loss	GB series	gallbladder series
ECHO	echocardiogram	GC	gonorrhea
ECG	electrocardiogram	GER	gerontology
EchoEG	echoencephalography	GERD	gastroesophageal reflux disease
ECT	electroconvulsive therapy	GH	growth hormone
ED	erectile dysfunction	GI	gastrointestinal
EDD	expected date of delivery	GSW	gunshot wound
EEG	electroencephalogram	GTT	glucose tolerance test
EENT	eye, ear, nose, and throat	GU	genitourinary
EGD	esophagogastroduodenoscopy	GYN	gynecology
EKG	electrocardiogram	h	hour
EM	emmetropia	H	hypodermic
EMG	electromyogram	HB	heart block
ENT	ear, nose, and throat	HBV	hepatitis B virus
EP	ectopic pregnancy	HCl	hydrochloric acid
EP	evoked potential	HCO_3	bicarbonate
ERCP	endoscopic retrograde cholangiopancreatography	HCT, Hct	hematocrit
		HCVD	hypertensive cardiovascular disease
ERT	estrogen replacement therapy	HD	hemodialysis
ESR	erythrocyte sedimentation rate	Hg	mercury
ESRD	end-stage renal disease	HGB, Hgb	hemoglobin
ESLW	extracorporeal shockwave lithotripsy	HHD	hypertensive heart disease
		H&H	hemoglobin and hematocrit
etio	etiology	HHD	hypertensive heart disease
ETOH	ethanol	HIV	human immunodeficiency virus
EUS	endoscopic ultrasound	HMD	hyaline membrane disease
ex	external	HNP	herniated nucleus pulposus
F	Fahrenheit	H_2O	water

ABBREVIATION	DEFINITION	ABBREVIATION	DEFINITION
H$_2$O$_2$	hydrogen peroxide	LH	luteinizing hormone
HOB	head of bed	LLL	left lower lobe (of lung)
H&P	history and physical examination	LLQ	left lower quadrant
HPV	human papilloma virus	LMP	last menstrual period
HRT	hormone replacement therapy	LOC	loss of consciousness
hs	hour of sleep	LP	lumbar puncture
ht	height	LPN	licensed practical nurse
HSG	hysterosalpingogram	LR	lactated Ringer's
HSV-2	herpes simplex virus Type 2	LTB	laryngotracheobronchitis
HTN	hypertension	LUL	left upper lobe
Hx	history	LUQ	left upper quadrant
hypo	hypodermic	LVN	licensed vocational nurse
IBD	inflammatory bowel disease	mcg	microgram
IBS	irritable bowel syndrome	MCH	mean corpuscular hemoglobin
ICU	intensive care unit	MCV	mean corpuscular volume
IDDM	insulin-dependent diabetes mellitus	MD	muscular dystrophy
I&D	incision and drainage	MD	medical doctor
IHD	ischemic heart disease	mEq	milliequivalent
IM	intramuscular	Mets	metastasis
inf	inferior	MG	myasthenia gravis
I&O	intake and output	mg	milligram
INR	international normalized ratio	MI	myocardial infarction
IPPR	intermittent positive pressure	mL	milliliter
	breathing	mm	millimeter
irrig	irrigation	MM	multiple myeloma
isol	isolation	MOM	milk of magnesia
IUD	intrauterine device	MR	may repeat
IV	intravenous	MRA	magnetic resonance angiography
IVC	intravenous cholangiogram	MRCP	magnetic resonance
IVP	intravenous pyelogram		cholangiopancreatography
K	potassium	MRI	magnetic resonance imaging
KCl	potassium chloride	MRSA	methicillin-resistant staphylococcus
kg	kilogram		aureus
KUB	kidney, ureter, and bladder x-ray	MS	multiple sclerosis
KVO	keep vein open	MSH	melanocyte-stimulating hormone
L	liter	MVP	mitral valve prolapse
lac	laceration	N&V	nausea and vomiting
LAP	laparotomy	Na	sodium
LAS	lymphadenopathy syndrome	NA	nursing assistant
LASIK	laser-assisted in situ keratomileusis	NaCl	sodium chloride (salt)
lat	lateral	NB	newborn
L&D	labor and delivery	neuro	neurology
LE	lupus erythematosus	NG	nasogastric

ABBREVIATION	DEFINITION	ABBREVIATION	DEFINITION
NICU	neonatal intensive care unit	PDR	*Physician's Desk Reference*
NICU	neurology intensive care unit	PE	pulmonary embolism
NIVA	noninvasive vascular assessment	PE	physical examination
NIDDM	noninsulin-dependent diabetes mellitus	PED	pediatrics
		PEG	percutaneous endoscopic gastrostomy
noc	night		
noct	night	per	by
NPO	nothing by mouth	PERRLA	pupils equal, round, reactive to light and accommodation
NRDS	neonatal respiratory distress syndrome		
		PET	positron emission tomography
NS	normal saline	PFT	pulmonary function test
NSR	normal sinus rhythm	PICC	peripherally inserted central catheter
NVS	neurovital signs	PICU	pediatric intensive care unit
O	objective	PID	pelvic inflammatory disease
O_2	oxygen	PIH	pregnancy-induced hypertension
OA	osteoarthritis	PKU	phenylketonuria
OB	obstetrics	PLT	platelet count
OB/GYN	obstetrics/gynecology	PMS	premenstrual syndrome
OD	right eye (in Latin, *oculus dexter*)	PNS	peripheral nervous system
OM	otitis media	po	postoperation
OP	outpatient	po	orally
Ophth	ophthalmic	post-op	postoperatively
OR	operating room	PP	postpartum
ortho	orthopedics	PPBS	postprandial blood sugar
OS	left eye (in Latin, *oculus sinister*)	PPD	purified protein derivative
OSA	obstructive sleep apnea	pr	per rectum
OT	occupational therapy	PRBC	packed red blood cells
OT	oxytocin	pre-op	preoperation
Oto	otology	PRK	photorefractive keratotomy
OU	each eye (in Latin, *oculus uterque*)	PRL	prolactin
oz	ounce	prn	as needed
P	phosphorus	PSA	prostate-specific antigen
PA	physician's assistant	pt	patient
PA	posteroanterior	PT	prothrombin time
PAC	premature atrial contractions	PT	physical therapy
Pap smear (test)	Papanicolau smear (or test)	PTCA	percutaneous transluminal coronary angioplasty
PAT	paroxysmal atrial tachycardia		
pc	after meals	PTH	parathyroid hormone
PCP	*Pneumocystis carinii* pneumonia	PTT	partial thromboplastin time
PCU	progressive care unit	PUL	percutaneous ultrasound lithotripsy
PCV	packed cell volume	PVC	premature ventricular contractions
PD	Parkinson's disease	PVD	peripheral vascular disease
PDA	patent ductus arteriosus	Px	prognosis

ABBREVIATION	DEFINITION	ABBREVIATION	DEFINITION
Px	physical examination	SO	salpingo-oophorectomy
q	every	SPECT	single-photon emission computed tomography
qd	every day		
qid	four times a day	SqCCa	squamous cell carcinoma
qn	every night	ss	one-half
qod	every other day	SSE	soapsuds enema
qt	quart	St	stage (of cancer development)
R	rectal	staph	staphylococcus
R	right	stat	immediately
RA	rheumatoid arthritis	STD	sexually transmitted disease
RAIU	radioactive iodine uptake	strep	streptococcus
RBC	red blood cell or red blood count	subq	subcutaneous
RDS	respiratory distress syndrome	sup	superior
reg	regular	supp	suppository
REM	rapid eye movement	surg	surgery
resp	respiration	SVD	spontaneous vaginal delivery
RHD	rheumatic heart disease	T_3	triiodothyronine
RK	radial keratotomy	T_4	thyroxine
RLL	right lower lobe	T&A	tonsillectomy and adenoidectomy
RLQ	right lower quadrant	tab	tablet
RN	registered nurse	TAB	therapeutic abortion
ROM	range of motion	TAH	total abdominal hysterectomy
RP	retrograde pyelogram	TAH/BSO	total abdominal hysterectomy/ bilateral salpingo-oophorectomy
RR	recovery room		
rt	right	TAT	tetanus antitoxin
rt	routine	TB	tuberculosis
RT	respiratory therapy	TCDB	turn, cough, deep breathe
RUL	right upper lobe	TCT	thrombin clotting time
Rx	prescription	TEE	transesophageal echocardiogram
SA	sinoatrial	temp	temperature
SAB	spontaneous abortion	THA	total hip arthroplasty
SBE	subacute bacterial endocarditis	THR	total hip replacement
SBE	self breast examination	TIA	transient ischemic attack
sc	subcutaneous	tid	three times a day
SCI	spinal cord injury	TKA	total knee arthroplasty
SG	specific gravity	TKR	total knee replacement
SHG	sonohistogram	TM	tympanic membrane
SICU	surgical intensive care unit	TNM	tumor, node, metastasis
SIDS	sudden infant death syndrome	TPN	total parenteral nutrition
SL	semilunar (pertaining to the heart valve)	tr	tincture
		trach	tracheostomy
SLE	systemic lupus erythematosus	TSH	thyroid-stimulating hormone
SMR	submucous resection	TSS	toxic shock syndrome

ABBREVIATION	DEFINITION	ABBREVIATION	DEFINITION
TUIP	transurethral incision of the prostate	UVR	ultraviolet radiation
TULIP	transurethal laser incision of the prostate	VA	visual acuity
		vag	vaginal
TUMT	transurethral microwave thermotherapy	VBAC	vaginal birth after cesarean section
TURP	transurethral resection of the prostate	VC	vital capacity
		VCUG	voiding cystourethrogram
TV	tidal volume	VD	venereal disease
TVH	total vaginal hysterectomy	Vertebrae	
TVS	transvaginal sonography	T1 through T12	the twelve thoracic vertebrae
TWE	tapwater enema	C1 through C7	the seven cervical vertebrae
Tx	treatment	L1 through L5	the five lumbar vertebrae
U	unit	VLAP	visual ablation of the prostate
UA	urinalysis	VPS	ventilation-perfusion scanning
UGI	upper gastrointestinal	VS	vital signs
UNG	ointment	WA	while awake
UPPP	uvulopalatopharyngoplasty	WBC	white blood cell
URI	upper respiratory infection	W/C	wheelchair
US	ultrasound	wt	weight
UTI	urinary tract infection	XRT	radiation therapy
UV	ultraviolet		

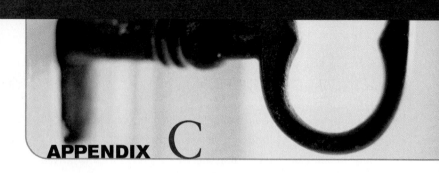

[endings in medical terminology]

1. **Plural endings.** The following list provides a summary of plural endings that are in common use with medical terms. Examples are provided to demonstrate how these endings are applied.

ENDINGS SINGULAR	PLURAL	EXAMPLES SINGULAR	PLURAL
-a	-ae	fistula	fistulae
-ax	-aces	hemothorax	hemothoraces
-ex	-ices	cortex	cortices
-is	-es	mastoiditis	mastoidites
-ix	-ices	cicatrix	cicatrices
-ma	-mata	fibroma	fibromata
-on	-a	contusion	contusia
-um	-a	bacterium	bacteria
-us	-i	fungus	fungi
-y	-ies	episiotomy	episiotomies

2. **Adjective endings.** The list below provides a summary of suffixes that mean "pertaining to" and form an adjective (a description of a noun) when combined with a root.

ENDING	EXAMPLE	DEFINITION
-ac	cardiac	pertaining to the heart
-al	endotracheal	pertaining to within the trachea
-ar	submandibular	pertaining to below the mandible
-ary	pulmonary	pertaining to a lung
-eal	esophageal	pertaining to the esophagus
-ic	leukemic	pertaining to leukemia
-ous	fibrous	pertaining to fiber
-tic	cyanotic	pertaining to cyanotic (blue)

3. **Diminutive endings.** The endings listed below provide the meaning of "small" to the word of origin.

ENDING	EXAMPLE	DEFINITION
-icle	ossicle	small bone
-ole	bronchiole	small bronchus (airway)
-ula	macula	small macule (spot)
-ule	pustule	small pimple

4. **Diagnostic endings.** The endings in this list summarize the suffixes that are in common use to indicate measurements, treatments, and procedures.

ENDING	MEANING	EXAMPLE	DEFINITION
-gram	record	bronchogram	recording of bronchus image
-graph	recording instrument	sonograph	ultrasound instrument
-graphy	process of recording	echocardiography	procedure of heart recording
-iatrics	treatment	pediatrics	treatment of children
-iatry	treatment	psychiatry	treatment of the mind
-logy	study of	oncology	study of cancer
-logist	one who studies	audiologist	one who studies hearing
-ist	one who specializes	optometrist	specialist in eye measurement
-meter	instrument of measure	spirometer	instrument measuring breathing
-metry	process of measuring	spirometry	process of measuring breathing
-scope	instrument for exam	endoscope	instrument for examination within
-scopy	examination	endoscopy	examination within

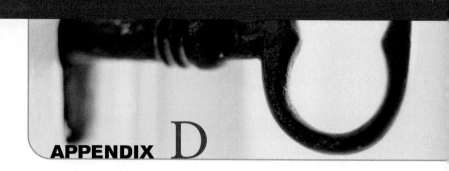

[pharmacology terms]

The major terms that are in common use in the field of pharmacology (preparation and dispensation of medicines) are provided. The pronunciation guide and definition of each term is included.

absorption (ab SORP shun): the process of taking in, in which a drug moves into the body toward the target organ or tissue.

ACE inhibitor (AYSS in HIB ih tor): angiotensin-converting enzyme inhibitor, a category of antihypertensive drugs that suppress the renin pathway to reduce blood pressure.

administration (ad min ih STRA shun): providing a drug treatment to a patient.

adverse reaction (ad VERS re AK shun): a harmful reaction to a drug that was administered at the proper dosage.

ampule (AM puhl): a sealed container containing a sterile solution to be used for injection.

analgesic (an al JEE zik): a compound that produces a reduced response to painful stimuli.

anesthetic (an ess THET ik): a compound that depresses neuronal function, resulting in a loss of the ability to perceive pain and other sensations.

antacid (ant ASS id): a substance that neutralizes or buffers an acid, usually taken orally to reduce hydrochloric acid in the stomach.

antianemic (an tee a NEE mik) **agent:** a drug that is used to treat or prevent anemia.

antianxiety (an tee ang ZI eh tee) **agent:** a drug that is used to treat anxiety such as fear, worry, or apprehension; usually a sedative or minor tranquilizer.

antiarrhythmic (an tee a RITH mik): a drug that is used to treat cardiac arrhythmia.

antibiotic (AN tee BYE ott ik): a chemical substance derived from a biological source (a mold or bacteria) that inhibits the growth of other microorganisms.

anticoagulant (AN tye koh AG yoo LANT): a drug that prevents or delays blood coagulation.

anticonvulsant (an tee kon VUL sant): a drug that reduces or prevents convulsive disorders, such as epilepsy.

antidepressant (an tee dee PRESS ant): a drug that counteracts depression.

antidiabetic (an tee DYE ah bet ik): a drug that reduces the amount of glucose in the blood; also called **hypoglycemic.**

antidiarrheal (an tee dye ah REE al): a drug that relieves the symptoms of diarrhea, usually by absorbing water from the large intestine and altering intestinal motility.

antidiuretic (an tee dye yoor EH tik): a drug that reduces the formation and excretion of urine.

antiemetic (an tee ee MET ik): a drug that is used to prevent or reduce nausea and vomiting.

antihistamine (an tih HISS tah meen): a class of drugs that suppress the action of histamines in order to counter the effects of inflammation.

antihormones (an te HOR mohnz): substances that inhibit or otherwise prevent the normal effects of certain hormones.

antihypertensive (an tee high per TEN sihv): a drug or treatment that reduces high blood pressure.

anti-inflammatory (an tee in FLAM a tor ee): a drug or treatment that reduces inflammation by acting on body function.

antimutagenic (an tee myoo tah JEN ik): a drug or treatment that reduces a substance's ability to form mutations in cells.

antineoplastic (an tee nee oh PLASS tik): a drug that is used to destroy or inhibit cancer cells, usually by inhibiting the synthesis of DNA.

antipsychotic (an tee sigh KOH tik): a drug that counteracts the symptoms of psychosis, such as schizophrenia and major behavioral disorders.

antiseptic (an tih SEP tik): a substance that prevents infection by inhibiting the growth of microorganisms.

antispasmodic (an tee spaz MOD ik): a drug or treatment that inhibits muscle contractions to relieve convulsions or spasms.

antitoxin (an tee TAHKS inn): an antibody that forms in response to antigenic poisonous substances. The antibody is often collected from its biological origin and concentrated for use in treatment against the antigenic toxin.

antitussive (an tee TUSS iv): a drug or treatment that relieves coughing.

bactericidal (bak teer ee SIGH dal): a drug or treatment that destroys bacteria.

barbiturate (barr BIHCH yoor aht): a derivative of barbituric acid, which acts as a depressant on the central nervous system. They are usually used as tranquilizers and hypnotics.

beta blocker (BAY ta block er): an agent that suppresses the rate and force of heart contractions by inhibition of beta adrenergic receptors.

bioavailability (bye oh ah vayl ah BILL ih tee): the percentage of a drug that is available to the target organ or tissue.

biotoxin (bye oh TAHKS inn): any toxic substance formed in a living organism.

biotransformation (bye oh trans for MAY shun): the changes that occur to a chemical due to biological action within the body.

calcium channel blockers: a class of drugs that inhibit the movement of calcium ions into muscle cells, which thereby inhibits muscle contraction. They are useful in the treatment of heart disease that involve coronary spasms.

capsule (KAP suhl): a small container that is soluble in water, which is used for the oral administration of a dose of medication. It is abbreviated **cap.**

carcinogen (kar SIN oh jenn): any substance that causes cancer.

cardiotonic (kar dee oh TOHN ik): a substance that exerts a favorable effect upon the action of the heart by increasing the force and efficiency of its contractions.

catabolic (kat ah BOHL ik): relating to catabolism, which is the metabolic breakdown of chemicals to produce energy in the form of ATP.

chemotherapy (KEE moh THAIR ah pee): treatment of disease by the use of chemical agents. The term is usually used to describe agents used in the treatment of cancer.

contraindication (kon trah in dih KAY shun): a symptom or circumstance that renders the administration of a drug to be inadvisable.

detoxify (dee TAHK sih fye): to diminish or remove the poisonous quality of a substance or pathogen.

disinfectant (diss in FEK tant): a chemical that destroys microorganisms, and is thereby often used to sanitize objects and surfaces.

distribution (diss trih BYOO shun): the pattern of absorption of drug molecules by the body once the drug has been administered.

diuretic (dye yoor EH tik): a drug that increases the production of urine by increasing water reabsorption within the kidneys. It is often prescribed to reduce water retention by the body, which reduces blood pressure, edema, and congestive heart failure.

dose: the quantity of a drug that is to be administered at one time.

drug: a therapeutic agent; any substance (other than food) that is used in the diagnosis, prevention, or treatment of a disease.

drug fast: microorganisms that become tolerant or resistant to an antimicrobial drug treatment.

drug clearance: the elimination of a drug from the body, usually through excretion by the kidneys, lungs, liver, or intestinal tract.

drug interactions: the modification of a drug that results from the drug interacting with itself or with other drugs, components of the diet, or other chemicals that are administered. The modification can be either desirable or undesirable.

effect: the biological effect of the administration of a particular drug. The effect may be **local** if it is confined to the site of administration, or **systemic** if the effect is more widespread.

enteral (ENT er ahl): administration of a drug by the oral route (by way of the intestines), as distinguished from parenteral. Enteral administration is the most common route.

Food and Drug Administration (FDA): the federal agency responsible for evaluation and regulation of pharmaceuticals in the U.S. The FDA also enforces regulations dealing with the manufacture and distribution of food and cosmetics. The mission of the FDA is the protection of American citizens from the sale of impure or unhealthy substances.

formula (FOR myoo lah): a prescription that includes directions for the compounding of a medical preparation.

formulary (FOR myoo lahr ree): a compilation of drugs and other relevant information that is used as a reference library by health professionals to prescribe treatment.

genotoxic (jee noh TAHK sik): a substance that is capable of damaging DNA and therefore may cause mutation or cancer.

grain: a minute hard particle of any substance or a unit of weight equivalent to 1/60 of a dram (1/437.5 ounce).

gram: a unit of mass in the metric system, equivalent to 15.432 grains.

granule (GRAHN yool): a very small pill that is usually gelatin coated or sugar coated.

hormone (HOR mohn): a chemical substance, usually a protein or steroid, that is secreted by an endocrine gland and transported by the circulatory system throughout the body. Upon making physical contact with a target cell, the hormone enters the cell and induces changes in metabolism, growth rate, protein synthesis, or synthesis of other compounds. The changes the hormone induces can have profound effects on body function.

homeopathy (hoh mee OPP ah thee): a system of medical treatment centered on the theory that large doses of a certain drug given to a healthy person will produce conditions that are relieved by the same drug in small doses during a diseased state.

hypnotics (hip NOTT iks): drugs that depress central nervous system function, resulting in drowsiness. They are used as sedatives and to produce sleep.

immunodeficiency (IM yoo noh dee FISH ehn see): a condition resulting from defective immune mechanisms, characterized by a frequent and rapid onset of infectious diseases.

infusion (inn FYOO zhun): the introduction of a fluid (other than blood) directly into a vein.

inhalation (inn hah LAY shun): a treatment that involves breathing in of a spray or vapor. The medication, known as the inhalant, is absorbed through capillaries in the mucous membranes of the upper respiratory tract.

injection (inn JEHK shun): introduction of a substance into the body with the use of a hollow needle. The injection may be beneath the skin (**subcutaneous** or **hypodermic**), into muscular tissue (**intramuscular,** or **IM**), into a vein (**intravenous,** or **IV**), or into the rectum (**rectal**).

laxative (LAHKS ah tihv): a substance that promotes bowel movement without pain or violent action. Laxatives work by softening the stool (decreasing water reabsorption), increasing the bulk of the feces, or lubricating the intestinal wall.

muscle relaxant: a drug that reduces muscle contraction.

nonprescription drugs: drugs that are not required (by the FDA) to be sold with a medical prescription. They are also called **over the counter** (**OTC**) drugs.

non-steroidal anti-inflammatory drugs: abbreviated **NSAIDs,** they are a class of drugs that reduce the symptoms of inflammation (swelling, redness, and pain) and are not steroidal compounds. The most common NSAID is aspirin (salicylic acid).

ointment (OYNT ment): a semisolid, medicated mixture that is topically (externally) applied.

oral (OR ahl): the mouth, the most common route of drug administration.

parenteral (pah RENT er ahl): introduction of medication through a route other than the oral (intestinal) or inhalation (lungs) routes. It involves injection that may be subcutaneous, intravenous, intramuscular, or rectal.

pharmacist (FARM ah sist): a health professional formally trained to formulate and dispense prescription drugs and other medications.

pharmacodynamic (farm ah koh dye NAM ik): relating to drug action.

pharmacology (farm ah KALL oh jee): the science of drugs and their sources, chemistry, action within the body, and uses.

pharmacotherapy (farm ah koh THAIR ah pee): the treatment of disease by means of drugs.

pharmacy (FARM ah see): the practice of preparing and dispensing drugs; also, a place where drugs are prepared and dispensed.

placebo (plah SEs boh): a neutral, ineffective substance that is identical to a known drug, which is administered to a patient for the suggestive effect or during blind testing.

potency (POH ten see): the pharmacological activity of a drug. It is used to determine the amount of a drug to be administered in order to cause the desired effect.

prescription (pree SKRIP shun): a written order for pharmacotherapy, provided by an authorized health professional.

routes of administration: the various ways in which a drug may be administered; the options include subcutaneous injection, intravenous injection, intramuscular injection, rectal injection, oral, vaginal, rectal, or topical.

sedative (SED ah tiv): an agent that reduces central nervous system activity, producing a calming, quieting effect that is usually used to treat anxiety.

side effects: a reaction by the body resulting from a treatment program that is a diversion from the desired effects. The reaction can be beyond the desired effect, and is usually undesirable.

solution (suh LYOO shun): a chemical mixture that includes a dissolved substance (solute) in a liquid medium (solvent).

stimulant (STIHM yool ant): an agent that increases the rate of activity of a body function.

superscription (SOO per skrip shun): the beginning of a prescription, consisting of the command recipe "take."

suppository (suh POZ ih tor ee): a medication that is introduced into one of the body orifices (other than the mouth), such as rectum, vagina, or urethra. It is usually a solid mass that melts at body temperature.

suspension (suh SPEN shun): a mixture of solid particles in a liquid medium that do not dissolve. The solid particles are usually dispersed through the liquid by blending.

tablet (TAB let): a small solid that contains medication for oral administration. Tablets may be designed to be swallowed whole, chewed, or dissolved prior to administration.

topical (TAHP ih kuhl): administration of a drug onto the surface of the skin.

toxicity (tahk SISS ih tee): the state of being poisonous. It is the level at which a drug's concentration in the body produces serious adverse effects.

toxicology (TAHK sih KALL oh jee): the science of poisons, in which the source, chemical properties, and body responses to poisonous substances are studied.

trade name: the name provided to a drug by its manufacturer, and commonly used by the health community to identify the drug.

tranquilizer (TRAN kwill eye zer): a drug that brings tranquility, or a calming effect, to the mind without depression. It is abbreviated **trank.**

transdermal (trans DERM al): administration of a drug topically to unbroken skin for its absorption into deeper tissues.

United States Pharmacopeia (FARM ah KOP ee ah): abbreviated **USP,** it is a reference text approved by the Federal Food, Drug, and Cosmetic Act containing specifications for drugs, such as chemical properties, uses, recommended dosage levels, contraindications, adverse side effects, etc.

vasoconstrictor (vaz oh kon STRIK tor): a chemical that causes blood vessels to constrict, which reduces blood flow and elevates blood pressure. Also called **vaso-pressors.**

vasodilator (vaz oh DYE lay tor): a chemical that causes blood vessels to relax, resulting in dilation that increases blood flow and lowers blood pressure. Due to their effect, they are in common use for acute heart failure.

vitamin (VYE tah min): an organic compound that is required for normal function of cells. Most vitamins are produced by the body, but those that are not are known as **essential vitamins** and must be included in the diet.

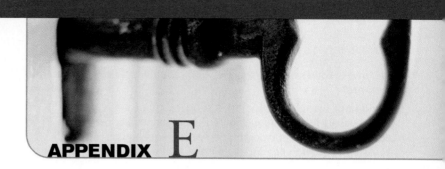

[alternative medicine: therapies and treatments]

The growing field of alternative medicine includes disciplines from the Far East, India, the Arab world, and lessons learned from the ancients. The list that follows provides definitions and pronunciation guides for the primary terms associated with alternative medicine.

acupressure (ACK yoo preh shur): the physical stimulation of pressure points on the body surface, usually to divert or suppress pain.

acupuncture (ACK yoo punk shur): the piercing with fine needles on the body surface along peripheral nerve routes to produce surgical anesthesia, relieve pain, and promote healing.

Alexander technique (al ecks AN der tech NEEK): the improvement of posture, body movement, breathing, and physiological functions by the use of exercises.

apiotherapy (a pee oh THAIR ah pee): the use of honey bee products, such as venom and royal jelly, to treat inflammatory and degenerative diseases.

applied kinesiology (kih nee zee AHL oh jee): the use of manipulative, hands-on treatments to stimulate or relax muscles in an attempt to resolve health challenges.

aromatherapy (a roh mah THAIR ah pee): the topical use of aromatic oils obtained from plants in an effort to treat stress, minor infections, and immune disorders.

Ayurvedic (a yur VAY dik) **medicine:** an ancient practice that includes the use of herbs, music, oils, massage, and yoga. It places equal emphasis on the mind, body, and spirit in an effort to achieve and maintain health.

balneotherapy (bal nee oh THAIR ah pee): the treatment of disease by the use of bathing in oil scented baths.

biofeedback (bye oh FEED bak): a method of training and self healing that involves the playback of data recording the physiological activities of the body.

chelation (kee LAY shun) **therapy:** the use of chemicals that chelate, or form a complex with metal ions, within the body by their oral or intravenous administration. It is used in the treatment of arterial disease.

clay therapy: the therapeutic use of very fine mineral particles suspended in water that form a thick paste. The clay is usually administered topically as a poultice, but may also be taken orally as an elixir to treat intestinal problems.

colon cleansing: the use of water or mixtures that are introduced into the colon by the anal route in an effort to cleanse the colon. The therapy removes waste matter that may interfere with healthy function.

craniosacral (kray nee oh SAHK ral) **therapy:** the manipulation of the bones of the cranium to treat conditions associated with the brain and spinal cord.

energy medicine: the use of electromagnetic diagnostic devices to identify electrical fields generated by the body in an effort to detect imbalances that cause disease.

environmental medicine: the study of environmental influences on the development of disease, such as electromagnetic radiation (EMR), pesticide exposure, allergens, and solar radiation.

enzyme therapy: the oral administration of plant and animal enzymes to improve digestion and absorption of nutrients.

fasting: abstinence from eating foods for a controlled period of time in an effort to allow the body to eliminate toxins and promote health.

Feldenkrais (FEHL dehn kris) **method:** the application of slow, gentle body movements to increase range of motion, improve flexibility, and increase muscle coordination.

glandular (GLAN dyoo lar) **therapy:** the use of natural and synthetic hormones in the treatment of disease.

herbal (ER bahl) **medicine:** the use of herbs (certain plant materials) by oral or topical administration to restore or maintain health.

holistic (hoh LISS tik) **medicine:** a medical practice that entertains all aspects of healing, including the physical, mental, and spiritual components of an individual.

homeopathy (hoh mee OPP ah thee): a system of medical treatment centered on the theory that large doses of a certain drug given to a healthy person will produce conditions that are relieved by the same drug in small doses during a diseased state.

hydrotherapy (high droh THAIR ah pee): the use of various forms of water (steam, hot water, cold water, or ice), either internally or externally, to combat disease and maintain health.

hypnotherapy (hip noh THAIR ah pee): the use of hypnosis (the power of mental suggestion) to encourage the patient to make adjustments in lifestyles in order to improve health.

juice therapy: the oral administration of various nutritious juices to combat disease and maintain health.

light therapy: the use of light in various forms (ultraviolet, visible with color filters, or laser light) to combat pain, mental states of depression or anxiety, and other conditions.

manipulation (mah nip yoo LAY shun): movement of parts of the body by another person to reduce pain, improve mobility, and improve physiological function.

magnetic field therapy: the use of magnets to reduce the symptoms of inflammation (pain, swelling, redness), joint injury, and anxiety.

massage (mah SAHJ): **therapy:** gentle pushing and kneading of the surface of the body to increase blood flow, relieve nervous tension, and relax muscles.

meditation (med ih TAY shun): a discipline of the mind based on focusing, usually upon a single word or thought, that produces clarity of thinking and reduces anxiety.

moxibustion (mahks ih BUS chun): the use of an herb that is ignited and burned on or near a point on the skin to achieve a reduction of pain or stress.

naturopathic (NATCH yoor oh path ik) **medicine:** a combination of healing remedies that is based on the patient's individual needs and exploits the body's natural ability to heal. It treats the underlying causes of the disease with the use of nontoxic remedies, with the idea of providing maximum support to the body's natural defense mechanisms.

osteopathy (OSS tee OPP ah thee): a form of medicine that combines manipulation of the musculoskeletal system, physical therapy, herbal medicine, and physical medicine to help restore health. An osteopathic doctor (OD) practices in a way similar to a medical doctor (MD), and is often included within a conventional medical staff.

oxygen therapy: the use of oxygen in various forms to promote healing, with the underlying concept that the oxygen will destroy pathogens in the body.

phytotherapeutics (fye toh thair ah PYOO tiks): the generalized use of plant materials in the treatment of disease and maintenance of health.

prayer therapy: the use of prayer to a higher power to help combat disease and restore health.

Qigong (KYE gong): a combination of activities, including exercise, meditation, and breathing, that are intended to increase the flow of energy through the body, improve blood flow, and enhance immunity.

reflexology (ree fleks ALL oh jee): a pressure technique in which nerve tracts that carry reflex information are pressed, presumably activating electrochemical currents along nerves for the purpose of improving function of internal body organs.

rolfing (ROHL fing): manipulation of the areas of the body containing loose connective tissue (mainly beneath the skin surface) to improve mobility of muscles and joints.

rotation diet: a diet plan that is based on the rotation of foods throughout the week, with an emphasis on avoiding a repetition of foods.

self hypnosis (hip NOH siss): a mental discipline that involves concentration to promote behaviors that are desired and resist behaviors that are not desired.

shiatsu (she AHT soo): a manipulation therapy involving the gentle touch of fingers, hands, and feet in order to reduce tension. It also includes passive exercises to achieve tension reduction.

vibrational massage (vye BRAY shun al mah SAHJ): the use of mechanical vibrations to provide massage to body surfaces in an effort to reduce tension and relieve stress.

watsu (waht SOO): immersion into warm water to the chest that combines aquatic exercise with manipulation by a practitioner.

yoga (YOH gah): an exercise discipline that emphasizes balance (posture and equilibrium), controlled breathing, slow movements, and meditation to reduce tension and relieve stress. The exercise routines also improve joint mobility and muscle conditioning.

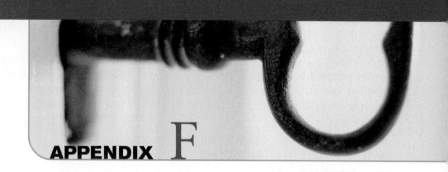

APPENDIX F

[answers to chapter review exercises]

Chapter 1

Show What You Know!

Break It Down!

       r s
1. ven/ous

      p   r s
2. hypo/tens/ion

       r   s
3. arthr/itis

       r cv s
4. gastr/o/logy

      p   r   s
5. pre/hepat/itis

       r cv r cv s
6. hepat/o/gastr/o/pathy

       r cv r s
7. oste/o/path/ic

Word Building
1. osteopathy
2. arthritis
3. hepatic
4. pregastric
5. subcardiac
6. arthrology
7. venous
8. hepatopathic
9. osteoarthropathology
10. gastritis

Fill It In!
1. (a) THRY (b) OSS (c) short
2. (d) long
3. (e) vowel (f) third

Piece It All Together!

Across
1. arteri
3. hyper
5. tens
6. pathy
7. hepat
9. itis
10. osteitis

Down
1. arthro
2. ic
3. hypo
4. pathic
8. di
10. o

Word Unscramble
1. cardio
2. post
3. hypertension
4. hepatic
Hidden term: osteopathy

Chapter 2

Show What You Know!

Break It Down!

      p   r s
1. ana/tom/y

       r cv s
2. physi/o/logy

       r cv s
3. cran/i/al

      p   r   s s
4. uni/lat/er/al

       r cv r cv s
5. anter/o/med/i/al

       r   cv r s s
6. poster/o/lat/er/al

       r   s
7. cephal/ic

       r   cv r s
8. abdomin/o/pelv/ic

      p   r   s
9. epi/gastr/ic

      p   r cv s
10. hypo/chondr/i/ac

       r cv s
11. home/o/stasis

Word Building

1. anatomy
2. cranial
3. distal
4. bilateral
5. medial
6. transverse
7. midsagittal
8. cranial cavity
9. thoracic cavity
10. abdominopelvic cavity
11. brachium
12. abdominal region
13. umbilical
14. anteroposterior

Case Study

1. a. symptoms; b. disease; c. cranial; d. sign; e. abdominal; f. right lumbar region; g. idiopathic; h. homeostasis; i. posterior; j. cranial cavity; k. spinal cord; l. pathology

Piece It All Together!

Across

1. anatomy
4. dist
6. hypo
7. pelvic
8. spinal
9. epi
10. front
12. equal
13. lumbar
14. umbilical

Down

2. anterior
3. mediolateral
5. superior
6. homeo
11. ili

Word Unscramble

1. idiopathic
2. symptom
3. dorsal
4. ventral
5. femoral
6. belly

Hidden terms: spleen, liver

Chapter 3

Show What You Know!

Break It Down!

    r cv s
1. cyt/o/logy

    r cv s
2. cyt/o/logist

    r cv s
3. cyt/o/plasm

    r cv s
4. chrom/o/some

    r   s
5. organ/elle

    r cv s
6. hist/o/logy

    p   r cv s
7. epi/thel/i/um

    r cvs
8. card/i/ac

    r cv r s
9. neur/o/gli/al

    p   s
10. ana/plasia

    r   s
11. carcin/oma

    r cv s
12. carcin/o/gen

    p   s
13. dys/plasia

    p   r cv s
14. epi/thel/i/oma

    r cv r s
15. fibr/o/sarc/oma

    p   s
16. hyper/plasia

    r cv r cv r   s
17. lei/o/my/o/sarc/oma

    p   s
18. meta/stasis

    r   s
19. melan/oma

    p   s
20. neo/plasm

    r cv r s
21. onc/o/gen/ic

    r cv s
22. onc/o/logist

    r cv r cv r   s
23. rhabd/o/my/o/sarc/oma

Word Building

1. cell
2. tissue
3. organelle
4. nucleus
5. epithelial tissue
6. glandular epithelium
7. connective tissue
8. muscle tissue
9. cardiac muscle tissue
10. skeletal muscle tissue
11. nervous tissue
12. benign tumor
13. malignant tumor

14. cancer
15. oncologist
16. remission
17. fibroma
18. leiomyoma
19. lipoma
20. metastasis
21. melanoma
22. neoplasm
23. tumorogenic

Case Study

1. a. oncology; b. tissues; c. histology; d. mutations; e. mutated;
   f. anaplasia; g. skeletal; h. nervous; i. epithelial; j. connective;
   k. tumors (neoplasms); l. organs; m. oncologist; n. myosarcoma;
   o. spread; p. metastatic; q. chemotherapy; r. radiotherapy;
   s. prognosis

Piece It All Together!

Across

1. cells
3. cytology
6. stasis
8. onco
9. AP
12. skeletal
16. membrane

Down

1. chromosome
2. lipo
3. cytoplasm
4. tissue
5. gland
7. sarc
10. nerve
11. neuro
13. fibr
14. DNA
15. neo

Word Unscramble

1. oncology
2. muscle
3. lip/o
4. dysplasia
5. melanoma
6. cancer
7. tissue
8. my/o

Hidden term: neoplasm

Chapter 4

Show What You Know!

Break It Down!

     p r s
1. epi/derm/is

     r   s
2. dermat/itis

     r   s
3. ecchym/osis

     r cv s
4. onych/o/malacia

     r cv r s
5. lei/o/derm/a

     r   r s
6. hidr/aden/itis

     r cv r s
7. scler/o/derm/a

     r cv r s
8. dermat/o/fibr/oma

     r cv r s
9. trich/o/myc/osis

     p r s
10. per/cutane/ous

     r cv s
11. derm/a/tome

     r cv r s
12. onych/o/krypt/osis

     p r s
13. par/onych/ia

     r cv s
14. rhytid/o/plasty

     r cv r s
15. kerat/o/gen/ic

     r cv r s
16. leuk/o/derm/a

     r cv s
17. dermat/o/plasty

     p r s
18. hypo/derm/ic

     r cv r s
19. erythr/o/derm/a

     r   r s
20. pachy/derm/a

     r cv s
21. onych/o/phagia

     r cv r s
22. lei/o/derm/a

     r cv r s
23. onych/o/myc/osis

Word Building

1. biopsy
2. abscess
3. cellulitis
4. erythroderma
5. onychomycosis
6. carbuncle
7. xeroderma
8. necrosis

9. epithelium
10. abrasion
11. furuncle
12. impetigo
13. nevus
14. macule
15. emollient
16. dermatologist
17. keloid
18. onychokryptosis
19. onychophagia
20. actinic keratosis
21. xanthoderma
22. leiodermia
23. hyperhidrosis
24. pachyderma
25. seborrhea
26. leukoderma

Case Study

1. a. dermatology; b. dermatitis; c. erythroderma; d. keratogenic; e. actinic keratosis; f. pustules; g. pruritis; h. ulcers; i. cicatrices; j. keloids; k. biopsy; l. dermatome; m. percutaneous; n. debridement; o. dermabrasion; p. dermatoautoplasty

Piece It All Together!

Across

1. gland
3. protection
6. seborrhea
8. epi
9. bio
10. acne
11. nevus
12. onychectomy
14. keratogenic
16. decubitus
17. SLE
18. erythroderma

Down

2. dermatologist
4. connective
5. necr
6. sebum
7. bio
13. macule
15. cut

Word Unscramble

1. verruca
2. herpes
3. cyst
4. dermatitis
5. onych/o
6. leukoderma
7. sebaceous

Hidden term: vesicle

Chapter 5

Show What You Know!

Word Building

1. osteomalacia
2. osteoporosis
3. paraplegia
4. scoliosis
5. tendonitis
6. arthrogram
7. meniscitis
8. arthrotomy
9. myasthenia
10. myocoele
11. carpal tunnel syndrome
12. compression fracture
13. Paget's disease
14. herniated disk
15. arthroplasty
16. tenodynia
17. bursolith
18. ankylosis
19. bradykinesia
20. synoviosarcoma
21. arthrodesis
22. maxillitis
23. myoclonus
24. osteopetrosis
25. cranioschisis
26. atrophy

Case Studies

1. a. compound; b. tendonitis; c. myalgia; d. myositis; e. polymyositis; f. Pott's; g. tendonitis; h. osteonecrosis; i. osteomyelitis; j. osteochondritis; k. arthrocentesis; l. femur; m. osteitis; n. arthroscopy; o. podiatrist; p. orthotist; q. prosthetic

2. r. dyskinesia; s. orthopedics; t. kyphosis; u. osteoporosis; v. osteoarthritis; w. osteosarcoma; x. osteocarcinoma

Piece It All Together!

Across

1. achondroplasia
5. tendo
6. lamina
8. rachiotomy
11. ACL
12. gout
13. hard
15. pain
16. costectomy
19. ribs
20. TKR
21. fascia
22. syn
23. strain

Down

1. arthrochondritis
2. polymyositis

3. spiral
4. ataxia
7. myalgia
9. chiro
10. osteoclasis
14. ortho
17. myo
18. sprain
21. fun

Word Unscramble
1. osteitis
2. dyskinesia
3. atrophy
4. arthroscopy
5. osteoporosis
6. tenodynia
7. bursitis
8. Colles'
9. scoliosis
Hidden term: orthotics

Chapter 6

Show What You Know!

Break It Down!

        r   cv s
1. psych/i/atry

        p   s
2. dys/phasia

        p   r   s
3. hypo/thalam/us

        r   s
4. cerebell/itis

        r   cv r   s
5. cerebr/o/vascul/ar

        r   s
6. encephal/itis

        p   r   s
7. hydro/cephal/y

        r   cv r   cv s
8. mening/o/myel/o/cele

        p   r   s
9. hyper/esthesi/a

        r   s
10. myel/itis

        r   s
11. neur/asthenia

        r   s
12. neur/oma

        p   s
13. para/plegia

        p   r   s
14. poly/neur/itis

        r   cv r   s
15. psych/o/somat/ic

        r   s
16. crani/ectomy

        r   cv s
17. crani/o/tomy

        r   cv s
18. neur/o/lysis

        r   cv s
19. radic/o/tomy

        r   cv s
20. psych/o/pathy

        r   cv s
21. neur/o/rraphy

Word Building
1. aphasia
2. cephalalgia
3. cerebellitis
4. cerebrovascular disease
5. glioma
6. encephalomalacia
7. duritis
8. hyperesthesia
9. encephalitis
10. meningocele
11. multiple sclerosis
12. myelitis
13. neurasthenia
14. neuroma
15. neuralgia
16. paresthesia
17. hemiplegia
18. polyneuritis
19. psychopathy
20. quadriplegia
21. radiculitis
22. craniectomy
23. craniotomy
24. neurorraphy
25. neurolysis
26. neurotomy

Case Studies
1. a. cephalalgia; b. neuralgia; c. dysphasia; d. deep tendon reflexes; e. polyneuritis; f. analgesics; g. syncope; h. hemiplegia; i. computed tomography; j. magnetic resonance imaging; k. subdural; l. intracranial; m. craniotomy
2. n. senile; o. epilepsy; p. dysphasia; q. agnosia; r. Alzheimer's disease; s. cerebral thrombosis; t. cerebral angiogram; u. cerebrovascular accident; v. hemiplegia; w. dementia; x. psychosis; y. encephalomalacia

Piece It All Together!

Across
1. neurologist
5. myelin
6. meninges
8. polio
9. glia

10. ganglion
12. stroke
13. pia
14. coma
15. dementia
16. yellow
18. parasthesia
19. axons

Down

2. radicotomy
3. gangliitis
4. tomography
5. meningocele
7. glioma
11. neuritis
15. dura
17. CT

Word Unscramble

1. myelitis
2. psycho
3. agnosia
4. glioma
5. neurosis
6. encephalitis
7. duritis
8. gray

Hidden term: epilepsy

Chapter 7

Show What You Know!

Break It Down!

      r   cv s
1. ophthalm/o/logy

      r   r s
2. presby/op/ia

     r cv r   s
3. scler/o/keratin/itis

     r cv r   s
4. retin/o/blast/oma

     r   cv s
5. blephar/o/ptosis

      p   r s
6. hyper/op/ia

     r cv s
7. irid/o/plegia

       r   s
8. conjunctiv/itis

       r   s
9. ophthalm/algia

     r cv r s
10. phot/o/retin/itis

     r cv r s
11. ocul/o/myc/osis

       r s
12. dipl/opia

       r cv r s
13. dacry/o/cyst/itis

       r cv r s
14. corne/o/ir/itis

       r   s
15. kerat/itis

       r   s
16. irid/ectomy

Word Building

1. astigmatism
2. blepharitis
3. glaucoma
4. hordeolum
5. nystagmus
6. asthenopia
7. blepharoptosis
8. emmetropia
9. diplopia
10. ophthalmoplegia
11. myopia
12. ophthalmorrhagia
13. oculomycosis
14. pterygium
15. strabismus
16. blepharoplasty
17. vitrectomy

Case Study

1. a. ophthalmalgia; b. conjunctivitis; c. esotropia; d. iridoplegia; e. ophthalmologist; f. opthalmoscope; g. tonometry; h. tonometer; i. detached retina; j. emmetropia; k. fluorescein angiography; l. scleral buckling

Piece It All Together!

Across

1. ophthalmologist
7. cornea
8. myopia
9. cataract
12. kerato
13. diplopia

Down

2. asthenopia
3. lens
4. glaucoma
5. scleromalacia
6. presbyopia
10. pupils
11. RK

Word Unscramble

1. lens
2. mydriatic
3. strabismus
4. retina
5. keratitis

Hidden term: LASER

Chapter 8

Show What You Know!

Break It Down!

       r   a
1. ot/algia

       r   cv s
2. mastoid/o/tomy

     p s
3. an/acusis

       r   s
4. labyrinth/itis

     r cv r s
5. ot/o/scler/osis

     r cv s
6. ot/o/pathy

Word Building

1. tympanoplasty
2. anacusis
3. labyrinthitis
4. otalgia
5. otitis media
6. otorrhea
7. otopathy
8. paracusis
9. cerumen impaction
10. stapedectomy

Case Study

1. a. paracusis; b. otalgia; c. otorrhea; d. otorrhagia; e. tinnitis; f. vertigo; g. audiogram; h. otitis media; i. labyrinthitis; j. eustachian; k. mastoidectomy; l. labyrinthectomy; m. anacusis

Piece It All Together!

Across

1. otosclerosis
6. paracusis
7. OM
9. eardrum
10. neuroma

Down

1. otopathy
2. otorrhea
3. otoscopy
4. stapedectomy
5. AU
8. cochlea

Word Unscramble

1. incus
2. TM
3. ear
4. otopathy
5. ear
6. otoscope

Hidden term: stapes

Chapter 9

Show What You Know!

Break It Down!

       p   r cv s
1. endo/crin/o/logy

       r   s   s
2. adren/al/itis

       p   r s s
3. hyper/thyr/oid/ism

       r   s
4. pancreat/itis

       p   r s
5. hypo/glyc/emia

     r cv r cv p   s
6. adren/o/cortic/o/hyper/plasia

       r cv s
7. adren/o/megaly

       p   r cv s
8. endo/crin/o/pathy

       p   r   cvs
9. ex/ophthalm/o/s

       p   r   s
10. hyper/insulin/ism

       p   r r s s
11. hyper/para/thyr/oid/ism

       p   r s
12. hypo/calc/emia

       p   r   s
13. hypo/natr/emia

       p   r s s
14. para/thyr/oid/oma

       p   r   s
15. hypo/phys/ectomy

       p   r s s
16. para/thyr/oid/ectomy

       r s cv s
17. thyr/oid/o/tomy

       r cv r   r s   s
18. thyr/o/para/thyr/oid/ectomy

Word Building

1. endocrinopathy
2. hyperthyroidism
3. hypophysectomy
4. adrenalitis
5. hyponatremia
6. hypercalcemia
7. parathyroidoma
8. pituitary gigantism
9. adrenalopathy
10. hirsutism
11. hypoparathyroidism
12. hyperinsulinism

13. pancreatitis
14. hyperglycemia

Case Studies

1. a. endocrinology; b. polydipsia; c. ketosis; d. acidosis; e. fasting blood sugar; f. glucose; g. hyperglycemia; h. insulin; i. type II diabetes
2. j. hirsutism; k. adrenopathy; l. hyperadrenalism; m. adrenomegaly; n. Cushing's; o. hyperglycemia; p. adrenocortico-hyperplasia; q. testosterone; r. virilism; s. cortex

Piece It All Together!

Across

1. endocrinopathy
7. pancreatitis
9. hormone
11. hyperglycemia
15. GTT
16. Addison's
17. polydipsia

Down

1. exophthalmos
2. DM
3. crino
4. adrenomegaly
5. ketosis
6. insulin
8. thal
10. nicotyxo
12. pineal
13. goiter
14. FBS

Word Unscramble

1. cretinism
2. hirsutism
3. diabetes
4. thyroid
5. acidosis
6. iodine
7. hypoglycemia
8. syndrome

Hidden answer: Cushing's

Chapter 10

Show What You Know!

Break It Down!

1.   r cv r s
   cardi/o/vascul/ar

2.   r cv r   s
   atri/o/ventricul/ar

3.   p r s
   peri/cardi/um

4.   r cv r s
   angi/o/card/itis

5.   r   s
   angi/oma

6.   r cv   s
   arteri/o/sclerosis

7.   r cv r cv r
   angi/o/sten/o/sis

8.   p   r   s
   a/rrhythm/ia

9.   p   r   s
   brady/cardi/a

10.   r cv s
   cardi/o/dynia

11.   r cv r cv s
   cardi/o/my/o/pathy

12.   r cv r   s
   cardi/o/valvul/itis

13.   p   r   s
   endo/card/itis

14.   p   r   s
   hyper/tens/ion

15.   p   r   s
   hypo/phys/ectomy

16.   r cv r   s
   my/o/card/itis

17.   p   r   s
   poly/arter/itis

18.   r   s
   aneurysm/ectomy

19.   r cv s
   angi/o/gram

20.   r cv s
   angi/o/rrhaphy

21.   r cv r cv s
   electr/o/cardi/o/graphy

Word Building

1. cardiomyopathy
2. angiocarditis
3. angiostenosis
4. angioma
5. arteriosclerosis
6. bradycardia
7. cardiodynia
8. angiogenesis
9. cardiomegaly
10. endocarditis
11. dysrhythmia
12. hypertension
13. myocardial infarction
14. myocarditis
15. epicarditis
16. phlebitis
17. angiogram
18. angioplasty
19. angioscopy
20. arteriotomy

21. auscultation
22. echocardiography
23. electrocardiography
24. endarterectomy
25. pericardiostomy

Case Studies

1. a. angina pectoris; b. cardiology; c. cardiologist; d. perfusion deficit; e. electrocardiography; f. stress echogradiography; g. block; h. myocardial infarction; i. angiostenosis; j. atherosclerosis; k. pericarditis; l. endocarditis; m. pericardostomy
2. n. hypertension; o. arteriogram; p. angiospasm; q. aneurysm; r. arteriorrhexis; s. aneurysmectomy; t. angiorrhaphy
3. u. myocardial infarction; v. coronary artery disease; w. ischemia; x. coronary occlusion; y. atherosclerosis; z. arteriosclerosis; aa. balloon angioplasty; bb. coronary artery bypass graft

Piece It All Together!

Across

1. cardiology
3. angioma
5. venogram
7. ischemia
9. myocardial
11. venule
12. artery
13. angiogram
14. His
15. embolism
17. thrombus

Down

1. cardiomyopathy
2. dys
3. angio
4. atherosclerosis
6. MI
8. aneurysm
10. cardiac
11. vein
15. EKG
16. BP

Word Unscramble

1. aorta
2. sinoatrial
3. endocarditis
4. embolus
5. atherectomy
6. coronary
7. varicose
8. angiospasm

Hidden term: aneurysm

Chapter 11

Show What You Know!

Break It Down!

    r cv s
1. erythr/o/cyte

    r cv s
2. hemat/o/poiesis

    r cv s
3. leuk/o/cyte

    r cv s
4. hemat/o/logist

    p p r s
5. an/iso/cyt/osis

    p r
6. dys/crasia

    r cv r s
7. erythr/o/blast/osis

    r cv s
8. erythr/o/penia

    r cv r s
9. hem/o/chromat/osis

    r cv s
10. hem/o/lysis

    r cv s
11. hem/o/philia

    r s
12. leuk/emia

    p r s
13. macro/cyt/osis

    r cv p s
14. myel/o/dys/plasia

    p r s
15. poly/cyt/hemia

    r cv r s
16. poikil/o/cyt/osis

    r s
17. septic/emia

    r cv s
18. hemat/o/crit

    r cv s
19. hem/o/stasis

    r s
20. plasma/pheresis

    r cv s
21. thromb/o/lysis

    r r s
22. lymph/aden/itis

    r r cv s
23. lymph/aden/o/pathy

    r cv s
24. splen/o/megaly

    r r s
25. lymph/aden/ectomy

    r r cv s
26. lymph/angi/o/graphy

    r s
27. splen/ectomy

    r s
28. thym/ectomy

       r   cv s
29. immun/o/logy

       r   cv s
30. lymph/o/cyte

       p   r
31. macro/phage

       r   cv s
32. neutr/o/phil

       r   s
33. bacter/emia

       r   cv   s
34. immun/o/suppression

       r   cv r   s
35. staphyl/o/cocc/emia

       r   s
36. tox/emia

Word Building
1. anemia
2. anisocytosis
3. dyscrasia
4. erythroblastosis fetalis
5. erythropenia
6. hemochromatosis
7. hemophilia
8. leukemia
9. macrocytosis
10. microcytosis
11. myelodysplasia
12. polycythemia
13. poikilocytosis
14. septicemia
15. anticoagulant
16. homologous transfusion
17. hematocrit
18. hemostasis
19. platelet count
20. Hodgkin's disease
21. lymphadenitis
22. lymphadenopathy
23. lymphoma
24. splenomegaly
25. thymoma
26. lymph node dissection
27. splenopexy
28. acquired immune deficiency syndrome
29. allergy
30. anaphylaxis
31. autoimmune disorder
32. bacteremia
33. diphtheria
34. fungemia
35. immunodeficiency
36. influenza
37. malaria
38. plague
39. staphylococcemia

40. vaccine
41. immunization

Case Studies
1. a. dyscrasia; b. blood chemistry; c. hematocrit; d. erythrocyte sedimentation rate; e. anemia; f. pernicious; g. iron deficiency; h. differential count; i. anisocytosis; j. poikilocytosis; k. myelodysplasia; l. leukemia
2. m. lymphadenitis; n. lymphadenopathy; o. lymphoma; p. Hodgkin's disease; q. lymphadenography; r. lymph node dissection; s. splenomegaly; t. differential count; u. infection; v. septicemia; w. staphylococcemia; x. antibiotic; y. immunodeficiency; z. immunotherapy

Piece It All Together!

Across
1. hematology
4. immune
7. anemia
8. hematocrit
11. polycythemia
12. blood
13. septicemia
14. node
15. staph
17. hemophilia
19. splenomegaly
21. tonsil
22. basophil

Down
1. hematopoiesis
2. toxin
3. greek
5. mono
6. erythropenia
9. plasma
10. thick
16. lymph
18. iron
20. LAS

Word Unscramble
1. antibody
2. hemoglobin
3. anaphylaxis
4. tetanus
5. macrophage
6. malaria
7. anemia
Hidden term: toxemia

Chapter 12

Show What You Know!

Break It Down!

       r   s
1. laryng/itis

       r   s
2. trache/itis

r cv s
3. bronch/o/scope

p s
4. hypo/pnea

p s
5. hyper/capnia

r cv r
6. hem/o/thorax

p s
7. a/pnea

p s
8. dys/pnea

r cv s
9. rhin/o/rrhagia

p s
10. dys/phonia

r s
11. thorac/algia

p r
12. hyper/ventilation

r s
13. bronch/itis

p s
14. hyp/oxia

r cv s
15. bronch/i/ectasis

r cv r s
16. coccidioid/o/myc/osis

r cv r s
17. rhin/o/myc/osis

r cv r s
18. nas/o/pharyng/itis

r s
19. sinus/itis

r cv s
20. sept/o/plasty

r cv s
21. thorac/o/centesis

r cv r cv s
22. laryng/o/trache/o/tomy

r cv s
23. ox/i/metry

r cv s
24. spir/o/metry

r cv s
25. trache/o/tomy

r s
26. laryng/ectomy

Word Building
1. laryngitis
2. anoxia
3. chronic obstructive pulmonary disease
4. eupnea

5. apnea
6. hypoxemia
7. dyspnea
8. hypercapnia
9. bronchiectasis
10. pneumatocele
11. pneumoconiosis
12. hyperventilation
13. bronchitis
14. cystic fibrosis
15. tracheitis
16. upper respiratory infection
17. asphyxia
18. bronchogram
19. pleurocentesis
20. respiratory distress syndrome
21. rhinoplasty
22. oximetry
23. tracheoplasty
24. pulmonary neoplasm
25. auscultation
26. respiratory distress syndrome

Case Studies
1. a. auscultation; b. pulse oximeter; c. pulmonary function tests;
d. spirometer; e. hypoxemia; f. pneumonia; g. acid fast;
h. *Pneumocystis cariini;* i. AIDS; j. pulmonary angiography
2. k. coryza; l. rhinitis; m. laryngotracheobronchitis; n. bronchodi-
lating; o. TB (tuberculosis); p. acid fast; q. tuberculosis; r. pulmonary angiography
3. s. apnea; t. hemoptysis; u. pulmonary carcinoma; v. bronchoscope; w. bronchitis; x. emphysema; y. bronchitis; z. chronic
obstructive pulmonary disease

Piece It All Together!

Across
1. atelectasis
4. CPR
6. pneumonia
7. PCP
8. pyo
9. legionellosis
11. epistaxis
13. tracheotomy
14. coryza
15. mucus
16. ARDS
18. auscultation

Down
1. alveoli
2. lung
3. tracheostenosis
4. croup
5. rhinomycosis
10. asthma
12. bronch
17. OSA

Word Unscramble
1. emphysema
2. empyema
3. rhinitis
4. TB
5. pleurisy
6. spirometer
7. NRDS
8. asphyxia
9. VPS

Hidden term: pertussis

Chapter 13

Show What You Know!

Break It Down!

    p   r   s
1. a/phag/ia

    p   r   s
2. dys/peps/ia

    p   r   s
3. hyper/bilirubin/emia

     r   s
4. appendic/itis

    r   cv r   s
5. choledoch/o/lith/iasis

   r s
6. col/itis

      r   s
7. diverticul/osis

    r   s
8. enter/itis

    r cv s
9. gastr/o/malacia

    r cv s
10. gloss/o/pathy

    r   s
11. hepat/oma

    r   s
12. periton/itis

    r cv s
13. bronch/i/ectasis

    r   s
14. polyp/osis

     r cv s
15. abdomin/o/centesis

    r cv s
16. an/o/plasty

    p   r   s
17. anti/emet/ic

    r cv s
18. cheil/o/rrhaphy

    r cv r cv s
19. chol/e/cyst/o/gram

    r cv r cv s
20. laryng/o/trache/o/tomy

    r   s
21. gastr/ectomy

    r cv r cv r cv s
22. esophag/o/gastr/o/duoden/o/scopy

    r   s
23. gingiv/ectomy

     r   s
24. hemorrhoid/ectomy

    r cv r cv r cv s
25. uvul/o/palat/o/pharyng/o/plasty

    p   r   s
26. dys/peps/ia

    r cv s
27. hepat/o/megaly

Word Building
1. dyspepsia
2. hepatomegaly
3. dysphagia
4. cheilitis
5. cholangioma
6. cholecystitis
7. cholelithiasis
8. colitis
9. colorectal cancer
10. enteritis
11. gastromalacia
12. ileitis
13. hepatoma
14. sialoadenitis
15. stomatitis
16. abdominoplasty
17. appendectomy
18. cholangiogram
19. colostomy
20. gastrectomy
21. proctoscopy
22. laparoscopy
23. glossorrhaphy
24. polypectomy
25. uvulopalatopharyngoplasty

Case Studies
1. a. nausea; b. diarrhea; c. flatus; d. ulcer; e. antacids; f. cholelithiasis; g. proctoscopy; h. sigmoidoscopy; i. gastroscopy; j. enema; k. upper GI; l. fecal occult; m. peptic ulcer; n. gastrectomy; o. *Helicobacter pylori*
2. p. diarrhea; q. flatus; r. constipation; s. lactose intolerance; t. irritable bowel syndrome; u. Crohn's disease; v. inflammatory bowel; w. barium enema; x. laparoscopy; y. diverticulitis; z. intussesception; aa. ileus; bb. colectomy

Piece It All Together!

Across
1. gastroenterocolitis
5. ulcer

10. cirrhosis
11. dyspepsia
12. stool
13. polyp
15. cathartic
16. rrhaphy
17. steatorrhea
18. ilieitis
19. hepatoma

Down

1. gastromalacia
2. sialoadenitis
3. cancer
4. laparotomy
6. cholecystitis
7. ascites
8. dysentery
9. EUS
14. pepsia

Word Unscramble

1. hernia
2. diarrhea
3. ileus
4. colitis
5. cheilitis
6. giardiasis
Hidden term: nausea

Chapter 14

Show What You Know!

Break It Down!

    r cv s
1. ur/o/logy
    r cv s
2. nephr/o/logist
    r   s
3. albumin/aria
    p s
4. an/uria
    r s
5. azot/emia
    p s
6. dys/uria
    p r s
7. en/ur/esis
    r   s
8. hemat/uria
    r s
9. cyst/itis
    r cv r s
10. glomerul/o/nephr/itis
    r cv r s
11. nephr/o/lith/iasis

    r cv s
12. ureter/o/stenosis
    r cv r s
13. urethr/o/cyst/itis
    r s
14. cyst/ectomy
    r cv s
15. meat/o/tomy
    r cv s
16. nephr/o/plexy
    r cv s
17. pyel/o/stomy
    r cv s
18. ureter/o/tomy
    r cv s
19. urethr/o/plasty
    r cv s
20. urethr/o/tomy
    r cv r s
21. vesic/o/urethr/al
    r cv r cv s
22. cyst/o/pyel/o/graphy
    r cv r cv s
23. cyst/o/ureter/o/gram
    r cv s
24. hem/o/dialysis
    r cv s
25. nephr/o/graphy
    r cv s
26. pyel/o/gram
    r cv s
27. ren/o/graphy
    r cv s
28. meat/o/scope

Word Building

1. anuresis
2. anuria
3. bacteriuria
4. cystolith
5. nephritis
6. hematuria
7. ureterocele
8. enuresis
9. nephrolithiasis
10. urinary tract infection
11. nephropexy
12. pyelostomy
13. urethroplasty
14. ureterostomy
15. cystogram
16. nephrography
17. nephrosonography
18. intravenous pyelogram
19. meatoscopy

20. nephroscope
21. blood urea nitrogen
22. urinometer
23. urinalysis
24. urinary catheterization

Case Studies

1.a. dysuria; b. nocturia; c. urinalysis; d. renal calculi; e. ureterolithiasis; f. urology; g. urologist; h. bloodstream; i. intravenous pyelogram; j. nephroscopy; k. renal calculi; l. lithotripsy

2.m. urinalysis; n. albuminuria; o. hematuria; p. cystopyelography; q. nephrotomography; r. nephroscopy; s. nephromegaly; t. polycystic disease; u. pyelonephritis; v. hemodialysis; w. renal transplant

Piece It All Together!

Across

1. glomerulonephritis
7. cystopyelography
8. UTI
11. enuresis
14. pyelithotomy
15. pyelo
16. uremia
19. renal
20. azotemia

Down

2. lithotripsy
3. ureter
4. pyelogram
5. UA
6. hypo
9. ketonuria
10. polyuria
12. IVP
13. polycystic
17. meato
18. void
19. RP

Word Unscramble

1. urine
2. renogram
3. cystogram
4. hemodialysis
5. nephroma
6. oliguria
7. cystolith

Hidden term: urology

Chapter 15

Show What You Know!

Break It Down!

     r cv s
1. andr/o/pathy

     p r s
2. an/orch/ism

     p r s
3. a/sperm/ia

     r   s
4. balan/itis

     r cv s
5. balan/o/rrhea

     r   r s
6. crypt/orchid/ism

     r   s
7. epididym/itis

     p r s
8. oligo/sperm/ia

     r   r   s
9. orchi/epididym/itis

     r s
10. orch/itis

     r   s
11. prostat/itis

     r cv r s
12. prostat/o/cyst/itis

     r cv s
13. prostat/o/lith

     r cv s
14. prostat/o/rrhea

     r cv r s
15. prostat/o/vesicul/itis

     r cv s
16. spermat/o/lysis

     r cv s
17. balan/o/plasty

     r s
18. epididym/ectomy

     p r s
19. hydro/cel/ectomy

     r cv s
20. orchi/o/plasty

     r s
21. orchid/ectomy

     r cv s
22. orchid/o/pexy

     r cv r   s
23. prostat/o/cyst/ectomy

     r cv r cv s
24. prostat/o/lith/o/tomy

     r cv   r   s
25. prostat/o/vesicul/ectomy

     r s
26. vas/ectomy

     r cv r cv s
27. vas/o/vas/o/stomy

     r   s
28. vesicul/ectomy

Word Building

1. anorchism
2. erectile dysfunction

3. impotent
4. testicular carcinoma
5. Peyronie's disease
6. testicular torsion
7. priapism
8. phimosis
9. AIDS
10. papillomas
11. penile implant
12. circumcision
13. prostate-specific antigen
14. sterilization
15. transurethral resection of the prostate gland
16. hepatitis B
17. syphilis
18. orchidotomy
19. benign prostatic hyperplasia
20. hydrocele
21. human papilloma virus
22. oligospermia
23. orchitis
24. varicocele

Case Studies

1.a. digital rectal exam; b. prostate specific antigen; c. prostate cancer; d. prostatic hyperplasia; e. transrectal ultrasound; f. prostatitis; g. transurethral resection of the prostate
2.h. oligospermia; i. orchiepididymitis; j. balanorrhea; k. gonorrhea; l. testicular carcinoma; m. bilateral orchidectomy; n. sterile

Piece It All Together!

Across

1. vesiculectomy
4. spermatic
6. hydrocele
7. vasectomy
8. DRE
11. balanoplasty
14. HPV
15. orchiectomy
18. priapism

Down

1. vasovasostomy
2. orchidopexy
3. impotent
5. oligospermia
9. anorchism
10. vas
12. aspermia
13. syphilis
16. semen
17. AIDS

Word Unscramble

1. orchitis
2. gonorrhea
3. balanitis
4. PSA
5. orchidotomy

6. andropathy
7. hydrocelectomy
8. TUIP
9. vas
Hidden term: chlamydia

Chapter 16

Show What You Know!

Break It Down!

1.   r cv r s
   gynec/o/path/ic

2.   p r cv s
   a/men/o/rrhea

3.   p   r cv s
   dys/men/o/rrhea

4.   r cv s
   hydr/o/salpinx

5.   r   s
   mast/algia

6.   r cv s
   metr/o/rrhagia

7.   p   r   s
   endo/cervic/itis

8.   p   r cv s
   endo/metr/i/osis

9.   r   s
   hyster/atresia

10.   r   s
   mast/itis

11.   r cv r s
   my/o/metr/itis

12.   r   s
   oophor/itis

13.   p   r   s
   peri/metr/itis

14.   r cv r s
   vulv/o/vagin/itis

15.   r cv p p s
   colp/o/peri/neo/rrhapy

16.   r   s
   oophor/ectomy

17.   r   s
   mast/ectomy

18.   p   r   s
   pan/hyster/ectomy

19.   r   s
   salping/ostomy

20.   r cv s
   trachel/o/rrhaphy

21.   r   s
   vulv/ectomy

22.   r cv s
   mamm/o/graphy

r cv s
23. culd/o/scopy

r cv s
24. lapar/o/scopy

r cv s
25. culd/o/centesis

Word Building

1. amenorrhea
2. hematosalpinx
3. leukorrhea
4. mastalgia
5. menorrhagia
6. oligomenorrhea
7. endometriosis
8. amastia
9. cervicitis
10. hysteratresia
11. mastoptosis
12. salpingocele
13. vulvovaginitis
14. breast cancer
15. ovarian cancer
16. prolapsed uterus
17. vesicovaginal fistula
18. fibrocystic breast disease
19. salpingo-oophorectomy
20. hysterosalpingo-oophorectomy
21. fibroidectomy
22. mastopexy
23. episiotomy
24. hysteroscopy
25. mammography
26. hymenotomy

Case Studies

1.a. dysmenorrhea; b. menorrhagia; c. leukorrhea; d. dilation and curettage; e. Papanicolau (Pap) smear; f. HPV (human papillomavirus); g. colposcopy; h. carcinoma in situ of the cervix; i. Cancer Antigen-125 Tumor Marker; j. cervical conization

2.k. mammography; l. breast cancer; m. dermoid cyst; n. biopsy; o. lumpectomy; p. radical mastectomy

Piece It All Together!

Across

1. gynecology
4. mastitis
6. PID
7. ov
9. colp
11. alveolar
12. cervicitis
14. fibroid
16. vaginitis
17. cyst
19. mammoplasty

Down

1. gynecopathic
2. endometriosis

3. oophoritis
4. metrorrhea
5. infundibulum
8. perimetritis
10. mastectomy
13. HRT
15. TSS
16. vulva
18. GYN

Word Unscramble

1. colpitis
2. amastia
3. menopause
4. fistula
5. lumpectomy
6. breast
7. ovary
8. hysterectomy

Hidden term: Pap smear

Chapter 17

Show What You Know!

Break It Down!

p r s
1. multi/par/a

p r s
2. multi/part/um

p r s
3. post/part/um

r cv r s
4. embry/o/gen/ic

r cv s
5. geront/o/logy

p r
6. pseudo/cyesis

r cv r s
7. gravid/o/puerper/al

r cvr s
8. lact/o/gen/ic

r s
9. amnion/itis

r cv s
10. amni/o/centesis

r s
11. omphal/itis

p r s
12. micro/cephal/y

r cv r s
13. chori/o/amnion/itis

r cv s
14. embry/o/tocia

Word Building

1. multigravida
2. puerpera

3. postpartum
4. embryology
5. natal
6. nulligravida
7. primigravida
8. pseudocyesis
9. puerperal
10. abortion
11. abruptio placentae
12. hyperemesis gravidarum
13. hysterorrhexis
14. amniorrhea
15. spina bifida
16. amniography
17. cesarean section
18. tocolytic agent
19. therapeutic abortion

Case Studies

1.a. nulligravida; b. prenatal; c. pelvimetry; d. amniocentesis;
e. fetus; f. obstetrician; g. parturition; h. obstetrical sonography;
i. breech birth; j. cesarean section; k. neonate; l. puerperal;
m. pediatrician; n. general practitioner

2.o. multigravida; p. preeclampsia; q. eclampsia; r. Down syndrome; s. therapeutic abortion

Piece It All Together!

Across

1. chorioamnionitis
5. episiotomy
6. RDS
7. placenta previa

12. abruptio
13. toc
14. cyesia
16. ped
17. birth
18. dystocia
20. abortion

Down

1. choriocarcinoma
2. OB
3. omphalitis
4. salpingocyesis
8. ectopic
9. amniotomy
10. rubella
11. gerontology
15. embryo
18. DOB
19. TAB

Word Unscramble

1. amniocentesis
2. puerpera
3. tocolytic
4. obstetrics
5. congenital
6. eclampsia
7. natal
8. labor
9. para

Hidden term: multipara

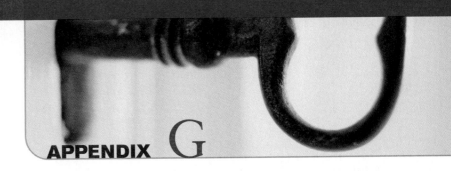

[answers to self quiz exercises]

Chapter 1

Self Quiz 1.1

Definition
1. side
2. liver
3. common state
4. heart
5. vein
6. joint
7. artery
8. stomach
9. bone
10. to stretch
11. disease

Word Root
1. norm
2. later
3. tens
4. arthr
5. hepat
6. oste
7. cardi
8. ven
9. gastr
10. arteri
11. path

Self Quiz 1.2

Definition
1. within
2. above, beyond, excessive
3. away from
4. within
5. to come before
6. under
7. to follow after
8. below, under, deficient
9. two

Prefix
1. ab-
2. hyper-
3. intra-
4. bi-
5. hypo-
6. endo-
7. post-
8. pre-
9. sub

Self Quiz 1.3

Definition
1. use of an instrument for viewing
2. inflammation
3. disease
4. pertaining to
5. study of
6. pertaining to
7. measure
8. an instrument used for viewing
9. pertaining to

Suffix
1. -al
2. -itis
3. -pathy
4. -ic
5. -logy
6. -ous
7. -meter
8. -scope
9. -scopy

Self Quiz 1.4

Definition
1. heart
2. liver
3. vein
4. joint
5. artery
6. stomach
7. bone
8. disease

Combining Form
1. arthr/o
2. hepat/o
3. oste/o
4. cardi/o
5. ven/o
6. gastr/o
7. arteri/o
8. path/o

Self Quiz 1.5

Define It!
1. study of arteries
2. pertaining to above the stomach
3. study of bone
4. disease of bone and joint
5. pertaining to disease of heart
6. pertaining to after a vein

Match It!
1. d
2. f
3. g
4. c
5. h
6. b
7. a
8. e

Self Quiz 1.6

Word Building
1. arthropathy
2. osteitis
3. cardiology
4. gastric
5. hypohepatic
6. gastrohepatic

Break It Down!

    r cv s
1. arthr/o/pathy
    r   s
2. oste/itis
     r cv s
3. cardi/o/logy
    r   s
4. gastr/ic
     p   r s
5. hypo/hepat/ic
     r cv r   s
6. gastr/o/hepat/ic

Self Quiz 1.7

Say It—Spell It!
1. cardiology
2. carditis
3. arteriocarditis

4. myocardium
5. osteopathic

Fill It In!
1. ALL
2. DYE
3. long
4. en doh kar DYE tiss

End It!
1. carditides
2. papilla
3. ova
4. gastrolysis
5. osteitides
6. axilla

Chapter 2

Self Quiz 2.1

Definition
1. two
2. pertaining to
3. pertaining to
4. pertaining to
5. up, toward, apart
6. one
7. beneath

Word Root
1. anter
2. dors
3. poster
4. cephal
5. card
6. abdomin
7. physi
8. path
9. medi
10. stasis
11. thorac
12. ventr
13. tom
14. super
15. ili
16. infect
17. eti
18. iatr

Self Quiz 2.2

Say It—Spell It!
1. anatomy
2. anterior
3. posterior
4. caudal
5. cephalic
6. distal
7. proximal
8. dorsal
9. ventral
10. inferior
11. superior
12. lateral
13. medial

Match It!
1. d
2. a
3. f
4. b
5. c
6. e
7. j
8. m
9. l
10. k
11. g
12. h
13. i
14. o
15. n
16. r
17. p
18. q

Break It Down!
1. anter/ior (r s)
2. poster/ior (r s)
3. caud/al (r s)
4. cephal/ic (r s)
5. dist/al (r s)
6. proxim/al (r s)
7. dors/al (r s)
8. ventr/al (r s)
9. infer/ior (r s)
10. super/ior (r s)
11. later/al (r s)
12. medi/al (r s)
13. poster/o/anter/ior (r cv r s)
14. uni/later/al (p r s)
15. medi/o/later/al (r cv r s)
16. epi/gastr/ic (p r s)
17. hypo/gastr/ic (p r s)
18. hypo/chondr/iac (p r s)
19. ili/ac (r s)
20. lumb/ar (r s)
21. umbilic/al (r s)

Word Building
1. bilateral
2. cephalic
3. ventral
4. posteroanterior
5. distal
6. superolateral
7. medial
8. mediolateral
9. posterolateral
10. inferior
11. medial

Fill It In!
1. anatomical plane
2. frontal/coronal
3. vertical/equal
4. transverse
5. ventral cavity
6. dorsal/ventral
7. cranial cavity
8. viscera
9. back
10. thoracic
11. abdominal
12. cranial cavity/spinal cavity
13. thoracic/diaphragm
14. pelvic/abdominopelvic
15. spinal
16. endocrine
17. urinary system
18. heart
19. cephalic/cervical
20. inguinal
21. lumbar/abdominal
22. chest
23. femoral
24. hypo-/beneath/gastr/pertaining to
25. epigastric/umbilical
26. iliac/umbilical
27. ili/pertaining to
28. home/o

Self Quiz 2.3

Match It!
1. c
2. d
3. e
4. a
5. b

Word Building
1. fever
2. pain
3. sensation
4. sign
5. symptom

Fill It In!
1. symptom/sign
2. fever
3. pain
4. sensation

Self Quiz 2.4

Say It—Spell It!
1. iatrogenic
2. idiopathic
3. inflammation
4. sequelae
5. acute
6. chronic
7. disease
8. infection
9. trauma

Match It!
1. c
2. d
3. b
4. a
5. h
6. g
7. e
8. i
9. f

Break It Down!
```
      r  cv  r  s
```
1. iatr/o/gen/ic
```
      r  cv  r  s
```
2. idi/o/path/ic
```
         r  s
```
3. infect/ion
```
         r  s
```
4. chron/ic

Word Building
1. acute
2. chronic
3. disease
4. iatrogenic
5. idiopathic
6. infection
7. inflammation
8. sequelae
9. trauma

Fill It In!
1. pathology
2. idiopathic
3. infections/inflammation
4. disease
5. trauma

Self Quiz 2.5

Say It—Spell It!
1. prognosis
2. diagnosis
3. etiology
4. ultrasound
5. pathology
6. endoscopy

Match It!
1. d
2. f
3. i

4. b
5. g
6. a
7. e
8. h
9. c

Break It Down!
```
         p     r   s
```
1. endo/scop/y
```
         r  cv  s
```
2. eti/o/logy
```
         r  cv  s
```
3. path/o/logy
```
         r  cv  s
```
4. path/o/logist

Word Building
1. prognosis
2. diagnosis
3. CAT
4. pathology
5. ultrasound
6. PET scan
7. etiology

Fill It In!
1. etiology/study of
2. diagnosis
3. prognosis
4. MRI
5. CAT scan

Self Quiz 2.6
1. positron emission tomography scan
2. CAT scan
3. magnetic resonance imaging
4. ant
5. posterior
6. inf
7. superior
8. med
9. lateral
10. AP
11. posteroanterior

Chapter 3

Self Quiz 3.1

Prefix/Suffix
1. neo-
2. epi-
3. -osis
4. -sis
5. dys- or mal-
6. -genesis
7. -stasis
8. -plasia
9. -oma
10. -some
11. -al, -um, -ic

Word Root
1. lip
2. carcin

3. sarc
4. fibr
5. melan
6. neur
7. lei
8. onc
9. rhabd
10. my
11. thel
12. hist

Self Quiz 3.2

Say It—Spell It!
1. chromosome
2. cytoplasm
3. epithelial
4. tissue
5. epithelium
6. organ
7. organelle
8. organism
9. neuroglial
10. neuron
11. nucleus

Match It!
1. d
2. a
3. c
4. b
5. j
6. k
7. h
8. g
9. l
10. e
11. f
12. i

Break It Down!
```
         r  cv  s
```
1. cyt/o/plasm
```
         r   s
```
2. organ/elle
```
         r  cv  s
```
3. chrom/o/some
```
         p    r  cv s
```
4. epi/thel/i/um
```
         r   s
```
5. organ/ism

Word Building
1. cell membrane
2. nucleus
3. DNA
4. genes
5. tissue
6. connective tissue
7. skeletal muscle
8. nervous tissue
9. neuron
10. epithelium

11. heart muscle
12. neuroglial cells

Fill It In!
1. atoms/molecules
2. cell/tissue
3. cell
4. cytoplasm
5. plasma
6. boundary/ regulate
7. small tool
8. organelles
9. nucleus
10. DNA
11. color/body
12. tissue/ histologist
13. epithelium/secretions/glands
14. connective/support
15. muscle/contracting
16. muscle/skeletal/smooth/cardiac
17. nervous tissue/neurons/neuroglial

Self Quiz 3.3

Say It—Spell It!
1. anaplasia
2. dysplasia
3. hyperplasia
4. metastasis
5. remission

Match It!
1. c
2. d
3. a
4. e
5. b

Break It Down!
    p   r
1. dys/plasia
    p   r
2. ana/plasia
     p   r
3. hyper/plasia
     p   r
4. meta/stasis

Word Building
1. remission
2. metastasis
3. dysplasia
4. anaplasia
5. hyperplasia

Fill It In!
1. mutation/dysplasia/anaplasia
2. metastasis
3. remission

Self Quiz 3.4

Say It—Spell It!
1. adenocarcinoma
2. adenoma
3. carcinoma
4. carcinogen

5. epithelioma
6. fibroma
7. fibrosarcoma
8. leiomyoma
9. leiomyosarcoma
10. lipoma
11. lymphoma
12. melanoma
13. myoma
14. neoplasm
15. neuroma
16. oncogenic
17. osteosarcoma
18. rhabdomyoma
19. rhabdomyosarcoma
20. sarcoma
21. benign
22. cancer
23. cancer in situ
24. malignant

Match It!
1. d
2. c
3. b
4. a
5. j
6. l
7. m
8. e
9. g
10. k
11. f
12. i
13. h

Break It Down!
    r   s
1. fibr/oma
    r   s
2. carcin/oma
    r cv s
3. carcin/o/gen
   p r cv s
4. epi/thel/i/oma
    r cv r s
5. fibr/o/sarc/oma
    r cv r s
6. lei/o/my/oma
    r s
7. lip/oma
    r   s
8. melan/oma
   r cv r cv r   s
9. lei/o/my/o/sarc/oma
    r s
10. my/oma
    p   r
11. neo/plasm
    r   s
12. neur/oma
    r cv s
13. onc/o/genic

    r cv r s
14. rhabd/o/my/oma
    r cv r cv r   s
15. rhabd/o/my/o/sarc/oma
    r   s
16. sarc/oma

Word Building
1. neuroma
2. sarcoma
3. liposarcoma
4. rhabdomyoma
5. benign tumor
6. cancer in situ
7. fibrosarcoma
8. carcinogen
9. epithelioma

Fill It In!
1. benign/malignant
2. sarcoma/epithelioma
3. skeletal muscle
4. neuroma
5. fat/lipoma

Self Quiz 3.5

Say It—Spell It!
1. chemotherapy
2. cytology
3. histologist
4. oncology
5. radiotherapy
6. cytologist
7. histology

Break It Down!
    r cv s
1. onc/o/logy
    r cv s
2. onc/o/logist
    r cv s
3. cyt/o/logy
    r cv s
4. cyt/o/logist

Word Building
1. chemotherapy
2. oncology
3. histology
4. cytologist
5. radiotherapy

Fill It In!
1. oncology/oncologist
2. cytology/cytologist
3. histology/histologist
4. chemotherapy/radiotherapy

Self Quiz 3.6
1. chemo
2. adenocarcinoma
3. St
4. cancer
5. TNM
6. metastasis

Chapter 4

Self Quiz 4.1

Definition
1. upon, on, over
2. within
3. through
4. beneath
5. surgical removal
6. diseased condition
7. pertaining to
8. inflammation
9. softening
10. view of
11. excessive discharge
12. condition of
13. pertaining to
14. eating or swallowing
15. surgical repair
16. instrument used to cut material

Word Root
1. aden
2. auto
3. bi
4. cutane, derm, derma, dermat
5. crypt
6. eryth, erythr
7. hidr
8. heter
9. kerat
10. leuk
11. myc
12. necr
13. onych
14. pachy, scler
15. rhytid
16. seb
17. trich

Self Quiz 4.2

Say It—Spell It!
1. integumentary
2. epidermis
3. dermis
4. keratin
5. melanin
6. collagen
7. elastin
8. follicle
9. lunula
10. eponychium
11. cuticle
12. sebaceous
13. sebum

Fill It In!
1. to cover/protection
2. epidermis/epithelial/connective/keratin
3. melanin
4. collagen/elastin
5. root/follicle/keratin
6. sebum/receptors

Match It!
1. e
2. j
3. h
4. b
5. f
6. c
7. i
8. a
9. g
10. k
11. d

Self Quiz 4.3

Say It—Spell It!
1. verruca
2. urticaria
3. edema
4. induration
5. nevus
6. cyst
7. alopecia
8. papule
9. contusion
10. diaphoresis

Match It!
1. j
2. d
3. b
4. f
5. o
6. a
7. c
8. i
9. l
10. n
11. m
12. p
13. h
14. k
15. g
16. e

Word Building
1. abrasion
2. nevus
3. alopecia
4. comedo
5. contusion
6. furuncle
7. diaphoresis
8. induration
9. fissure
10. laceration
11. pallor
12. pustule
13. petechiae
14. vesicle

Fill It In!
1. abrasion
2. abscess

3. alopecia
4. cicatrix
5. comedo
6. diaphoresis
7. induration
8. contusion
9. cyst
10. erythema/edema
11. laceration
12. pruritus/pallor/petechiae
13. vesicles/pustules

Self Quiz 4.4

Say It—Spell It!
1. scleroderma
2. onychophagia
3. necrosis
4. impetigo
5. decubitus ulcer
6. trichomycosis

Fill It In!
1. decubitus ulcers
2. carbuncle
3. eczema
4. basal cell carcinoma
5. acne
6. gangrene
7. tinea/scabies/pediculosis

Match It!
1. h
2. f
3. d
4. g
5. b
6. e
7. c
8. a

Break It Down!
```
         r    s
1. dermat/itis
          r   cv r   s
2. dermat/o/fibr/oma
         r   cv   r
3. erythr/o/derma
         r   cv  s
4. seb/o/rrhea
          r    cv   s
5. onych/o/malacia
            r     r
6. pachy/derma
          r   cv r    s
7. onych/o/krypt/osis
```

Word Building
1. cellulitis
2. carbuncle
3. impetigo
4. scabies
5. dermatitis
6. erythroderma

7. hyperhidrosis
8. necrosis
9. onychomalacia
10. onychophagia
11. trichomycosis
12. xeroderma

Self Quiz 4.5

Say It—Spell It!
1. biopsy
2. debridement
3. dermabrasion
4. dermatoautoplasty
5. dermatoheteroplasty
6. dermatome
7. dermatoplasty
8. emollient
9. onychectomy
10. percutaneous
11. rhytidectomy
12. rhytidoplasty

Match It!
1. e
2. a
3. g
4. c
5. h
6. d
7. k
8. i
9. l
10. b
11. j
12. f

Break It Down!
```
        r   cv  s
```
1. dermat/o/plasty
```
        r    s
```
2. derma/tome
```
        r   cv  s
```
3. rhytid/o/plasty
```
        r   cv  r    s
```
4. dermat/o/auto/plasty
```
        r    s
```
5. onych/ectomy

Word Building
1. dermatologist
2. biopsy
3. dermatoplasty
4. rhytidectomy
5. rhytidoplasty

Self Quiz 4.6
1. bx
2. basal cell carcinoma
3. sc
4. systemic lupus erythematosus
5. SqCCa

Chapter 5

Self Quiz 5.1

Definition
1. without
2. bad, difficult
3. straight, normal
4. alongside, near
5. many
6. four
7. together, joined
8. pain
9. weakness
10. a puncture
11. to break apart
12. surgical fixation
13. pain
14. disease
15. cutting, incision
16. paralysis
17. growth
18. falling downward
19. split, fissure

Word Root
1. ankyl
2. arthr
3. chir
4. clon
5. cost
6. crani
7. kinesi
8. kyph
9. lord
10. scoli
11. myel, myelon
12. my, myos
13. oste
14. ped
15. petr
16. pod
17. rachi
18. spondyl, vertebr
19. synovi
20. taxi
21. ten, tend, tendin

Self Quiz 5.2
1. diaphysis
2. epiphysis
3. periosteum
4. endosteum
5. cranium
6. sphenoid
7. zygomatic
8. appendicular
9. clavicles
10. scapula
11. phalanges
12. ischium
13. synovial

Match It!
1. e

2. j
3. g
4. k
5. m
6. c
7. b
8. f
9. a
10. d
11. h
12. i
13. n
14. l

Break It Down!
```
        p   r   s
```
1. end/oste/um
```
        p    r    s
```
2. peri/oste/um
```
        p    r
```
3. dia/physis
```
        p    r
```
4. epi/physis
```
        r  cv  s
```
5. oste/o/cyte

Word Building
1. articular cartilage
2. bursa
3. tarsals
4. carpals
5. cartilaginous joint
6. circumduction
7. facial bones
8. fibrous joint
9. fibula
10. dorsiflexion
11. plantar flexion
12. lacrimal bones
13. mandible
14. meniscus
15. occipital bone
16. pectoral girdle
17. pelvic girdle
18. pubis
19. radius
20. thoracic vertebrae
21. vertebral column
22. coccyx
23. compact bone
24. frontal bone
25. nasal bones

Fill It In!
1. musculoskeletal
2. support/storage
3. supination
4. patella
5. spongy
6. collagen/osteocytes/osteoclasts
7. Red
8. muscle/ligament
9. movement/heat
10. fasciae/tendon

11. hard
12. abduction
13. depression/elevation

Self Quiz 5.3

Say It—Spell It!
1. myalgia
2. bradykinesia
3. dyskinesia
4. arthralgia
5. hypertrophy
6. atrophy
7. ataxia
8. tenodynia

Break It Down!

    r   s
1. arthr/algia
    p r s
2. a/taxi/a
    p s
3. a/trophy
      p   r s
4. brady/kinesi/a
     p   r   s
5. dys/kinesi/a
    p   s
6. dys/trophy
    p   s
7. hyper/trophy
    r   s
8. my/algia
    r cv s
9. ten/o/dynia

Fill It In!
1. ataxia
2. arthralgia
3. bradykinesia
4. dyskinesia
5. dystrophy
6. tenodynia
7. myalgia

Self Quiz 5.4

Say It—Spell It!
1. achondroplasia
2. arthrochondritis
3. carpoptosis
4. cranioschisis
5. epichondylitis
6. kyphosis
7. meniscitis
8. myococele
9. osteoarthritis
10. osteochondritis
11. osteomalacia
12. polymyositis
13. quadriplegia
14. scoliosis
15. synoviosarcoma
16. Paget's disease

Break It Down!

    r cv s
1. arthr/o/tomy
     r cv   s
2. crani/o/schisis
     r   s
3. my/asthenia
    r cv r s
4. oste/o/fibr/oma
     p   r   s
5. poly/myos/itis
      r   s
6. lord/osis

Fill It In!
1. bursolith
2. chondromalacia
3. cranioschisis
4. diskitis/kyphosis
5. epichondylitis/dyskinesia
6. myositis/myalgia
7. osteitis/maxillitis
8. Osteoarthritis
9. bunion
10. Colles'/Pott's
11. simple/compound
12. comminuted
13. spiral
14. epiphyseal
15. Duchenne's
16. herniated
17. Marfan's
18. Paget's/osteoblasts
19. strain/sprain
20. gout/pain

Self Quiz 5.5

1. arthrocentesis
2. arthroclasia
3. arthrodesis
4. arthroplasty
5. arthroscopy
6. bursectomy
7. chiropractic
8. chondrectomy
9. costectomy
10. cranioplasty
11. craniotomy
12. electromyography
13. fasciotomy
14. laminectomy
15. meniscectomy
16. myorrhaphy
17. osteoclasis
18. osteopathy
19. rachiotomy
20. spondylosyndesis
21. synovectomy
22. tenomyoplasty
23. tenorrhaphy
24. podiatry

Match It!
1. d

2. f
3. i
4. l
5. b
6. m
7. c
8. n
9. p
10. o
11. s
12. j
13. g
14. q
15. h
16. a
17. r
18. k
19. e

Fill It In!
1. chiropractor/podiatrist/orthopedics/
   bursotomy/bursectomy
2. arthroscopy/meniscectomy
3. craniotomy/cranioplasty
4. myasthenia/electromyography
5. arthrodesis/arthroclasia
6. costectomy
7. laminectomy/herniated/lamina
8. syn-
9. prostheses
10. osteology/arthrology

Self Quiz 5.6

1. SCI
2. total knee arthroplasty
3. RA
4. myasthenia gravis
5. HNP
6. electromyogram
7. ACL
8. total hip replacement
9. L1–L5
10. carpal tunnel syndrome
11. ROM
12. osteoarthritis
13. TKR
14. the 12 thoracic vertebrae

Chapter 6

Self Quiz 6.1

Definition
1. without
2. two
3. bad, abnormal
4. one-half
5. water
6. single
7. all, entire
8. four
9. pain
10. hernia or swelling
11. treatment, specialty
12. inflammation

13. resemblance to
14. slight paralysis
15. speaking
16. paralysis
17. seizure

Word Root
1. astheni
2. cephal
3. cerebell
4. cerebr
5. dur
6. esthesi
7. gangli/ganglion
8. lys
9. mening
10. ment or psych
11. myel
12. neur
13. phas
14. plegi
15. quad
16. radic, radicul
17. somat
18. thalam
19. cran, crani
20. encephal
21. gli

Self Quiz 6.2

Say It—Spell It!
1. neuron
2. neuroglia
3. dendrites
4. axons
5. myelin
6. neurotransmitter
7. meninges
8. dura mater
9. pia mater
10. cerebrum
11. cerebral hemispheres
12. corpus callosum
13. cerebral cortex
14. cerebellum
15. diencephalon
16. thalamus
17. hypothalamus
18. medulla
19. cerebrospinal
20. afferent
21. efferent
22. ganglia

Fill It In!
1. central/peripheral
2. autonomic
3. cerebrum/hemispheres/cortex
4. cerebellum
5. arachnoid/dura
6. medulla
7. hypothalamus
8. yellow/ventricles

9. 31/roots
10. motor/ganglion

Match It!
1. j
2. l
3. o
4. k
5. c
6. n
7. m
8. i
9. h
10. b
11. d
12. e
13. f
14. g
15. a

Self Quiz 6.3

Say It—Spell It!
1. cephalalgia
2. hyperesthesia
3. aphasia
4. dysphasia
5. neuralgia
6. neurasthenia
7. paresthesia

Match It!
1. e
2. d
3. g
4. f
5. c
6. b
7. a

Break It Down
1. cephal/algia
    r   s
2. hyper/esthes/ia
    p   r   s
3. a/phas/ia
    p r s
4. neur/algia
    r   s
5. neur/astheni/a
    r   r   s

Word Building
1. cephalalgia
2. hyperesthesia
3. neuralgia
4. neurasthenia
5. dysphasia
6. paresthesia

Self Quiz 6.4

Say It—Spell It!
1. cerebral aneurysm
2. encephalitis
3. gangliitis
4. glioma

5. cerebellitis
6. meningocele
7. multiple sclerosis
8. myelitis
9. neuritis
10. hemiplegia
11. poliomyelitis
12. polyneuritis
13. radiculitis

Match It!
1. l
2. c
3. g
4. i
5. a
6. n
7. m
8. b
9. d
10. e
11. h
12. f
13. k
14. j

Break It Down!
    r   s   r cv r   s
1. cerebr/al arteri/o/scler/osis
    r   s
2. encephal/itis
    r   cv   s
3. encephal/o/malacia
    r   s
4. gangli/itis
    p   r   s
5. hydro/cephal/y
    r   s
6. mening/itis
    r cv r cv s
7. mening/o/myel/o/cele
    r cv r cv s
8. neur/o/arthr/o/pathy
    r   r
9. quadri/plegia
    p   r   s
10. poly/neur/itis
    r cv   r   s
11. psych/o/somat/ic

Word Building
1. cerebral aneurysm
2. cerebrovascular accident
3. duritis
4. encephalitis
5. glioma
6. meningitis
7. meningomyelocele
8. shingles
9. narcolepsy
10. cerebral palsy
11. coma
12. AD
13. epilepsy

Fill It In!
1. agnosia
2. Alzheimer's/dementia
3. epilepsy
4. palsy
5. Parkinson's
6. sciatica
7. Shingles
8. narcolepsy
9. transient/syncope
10. cerebral palsy
11. stroke

Self Quiz 6.5

Say It—Spell It!
1. craniectomy
2. ganglionectomy
3. neurectomy
4. neurolysis
5. neurorrhaphy
6. neurotomy
7. radicotomy
8. echoencephalography

Match It!
1. e
2. c
3. d
4. b
5. a

Break It Down!
1. crani/ectomy
2. crani/otomy
3. ganglion/ectomy
4. neur/o/lysis
5. neur/o/plasty
6. radic/otomy

Word Building
1. craniectomy
2. craniotomy
3. neurolysis
4. neurorrhaphy
5. paresthesia
6. ganglionectomy
7. radicotomy, rhizotomy
8. anesthetic
9. echoencephalography
10. evoked potential studies
11. cerebral angiography
12. computed tomography
13. sedative
14. neurologist

Fill It In!
1. tomography/MRI/evoked/PET
2. EEG

3. angiography
4. sedatives
5. CT
6. Anesthesia

Self Quiz 6.6
1. EP
2. positron emission tomography
3. TIA
4. electroencephalogram
5. CAT scan
6. magnetic resonance imaging
7. PD
8. cerebral palsy
9. EchoEG
10. deep tendon reflexes
11. MS
12. cerebrovascular accident
13. AD
14. amyotrophic lateral sclerosis

Chapter 7
Self Quiz 7.1

Definition
1. two
2. within
3. pain
4. vision
5. fear
6. paralysis
7. drooping
8. partial or near
9. drainage of fluid
10. hemorrhage

Word Root
1. blephar
2. conjunctiv
3. corne
4. dacry, lacrim
5. ir, irid
6. kerat
7. nyct, nyctal
8. ocul, ophthalm, opt
9. phac, phak
10. phot
11. presby
12. scler
13. stigmat
14. vitre
15. humor
16. retina
17. fovea
18. cor, core

Self Quiz 7.2

Say It—Spell It!
1. aqueous humor
2. choroid
3. iris
4. pupil
5. conjunctiva

6. cornea
7. sclera
8. lacrimal
9. meibomian
10. retina
11. vitreous humor

Match It!
1. j
2. e
3. i
4. a
5. b
6. g
7. d
8. c
9. h
10. m
11. f
12. o
13. k
14. l
15. n

Fill It In!
1. conjunctiva/lacrimal
2. sclera/cornea
3. iris/lens/choroid
4. pupil
5. anterior/aqueous humor/posterior/ vitreous humor
6. retina/photoreceptors/rods/cones/ fovea centralis/optic disc

Self Quiz 7.3

Say It—Spell It!
1. asthenopia
2. blepharoptosis
3. emmetropia
4. leukocoria
5. ophthalmalgia
6. ophthalmorrhagia

Match It!
1. d
2. f
3. a
4. e
5. c
6. b

Break It Down!
1. asthen/opia
2. blephar/o/ptosis
3. emmetr/opia
4. leuk/o/cor/ia
5. ophthalm/algia
6. ophthalm/o/rrhagia

Word Building
1. emmetropia
2. ophthalmorrhagia
3. ophthalmalgia
4. asthenopia
5. leukocoria
6. blepharoptosis

Self Quiz 7.4

Say It—Spell It!
1. astigmatism
2. chalazion
3. conjunctivitis
4. corneoiritis
5. dacryocystitis
6. diplopia
7. endophthalmitis
8. glaucoma
9. hyperopia
10. iridoplegia
11. myopia
12. nyctalopia
13. nystagmus
14. photoretinitis
15. presbyopia
16. pterygium
17. retinoblastoma
18. retinopathy
19. sclerokeratitis
20. scleromalacia
21. strabismus

Match It!
1. d
2. f
3. j
4. a
5. h
6. b
7. e
8. c
9. g
10. i

Break It Down!
    p r   s
1. a/stigmat/ism
      r cv r s
2. corne/o/ir/itis
       r cv r s
3. dacry/o/cyst/itis
      p   s
4. hyper/opia
     r cv s
5. irid/o/plegia
       r   cv s
6. ocul/o/myc/osis
       r   cv s
7. ophthalm/o/plegia
     r cv s
8. phot/o/retin/itis
     r cv s
9. retin/o/pathy

     r cv r   s
10. scler/o/kerat/itis
     r cv s
11. scler/o/malacia

Word Building
1. cataract
2. chalazion
3. detached retina
4. photophobia
5. pterygium
6. retinitis pigmentosa
7. scotoma

Fill It In!
1. asthenopia/diplopia
2. blepharoptosis/blepharitis
3. conjunctivitis/dacryocystitis/ keratitis/iritis/corneoiritis
4. iridoplegia
5. glaucoma/ophthalmopathy
6. strabismus/esotropia/diplopia
7. presbyopia/retinopathy/detached retina/cataract

Self Quiz 7.5

Say It—Spell It!
1. ophthalmology
2. blepharoplasty
3. keratometry
4. ophthalmoscopy
5. ophthalmologist

Break It Down!
     r cv s
1. opt/o/metry
       r cv s
2. blephar/o/plasty
      r cv s
3. kerat/o/plasty
      r   s
4. kerat/ectomy
      r   s
5. irid/ectomy
     r cv s
6. ton/o/metry

Match It!
1. h
2. e
3. k
4. a
5. i
6. b
7. c
8. d
9. l
10. g
11. f
12. k

Fill It In!
1. iridectomy
2. radial keratotomy/photorefractive keratectomy/keratoplasty

3. tonometer/vitrectomy
4. strabotomy

Self Quiz 7.6
1. OS
2. emmetropia
3. OU
4. right eye
5. EENT
6. visual acuity
7. PRK
8. radial keratotomy
9. Ast

Chapter 8
Self Quiz 8.1

Definition
1. pain
2. without
3. partial or near
4. hearing condition
5. excessive discharge
6. hemorrhage
7. without
8. inflammation

Word Root
1. aur/ot
2. mast
3. myring
4. salping
5. staped
6. tympan
7. labyrinth

Self Quiz 8.2

Say It—Spell It!
1. stapes
2. Eustachian
3. vestibule
4. incus
5. cochlea
6. malleus
7. tympanic
8. auricle
9. labyrinth

Match It!
1. d
2. f
3. a
4. h
5. g
6. b
7. i
8. e
9. c

Word Building
1. external auditory canal
2. mastoid process
3. tympanic membrane
4. tympanic cavity
5. cerumen

Fill It In!
1. audation/tympanic/mastoid
2. auricle/auditory/cerumen
3. tympanic/Eustachian/ossicles/malleus/incus/stapes
4. labyrinth/cochlea/semicircular/vestibule/organ of Corti

Self Quiz 8.3

Say It—Spell It!
1. tinnitus
2. vertigo
3. otalgia
4. anacusis
5. hyperacusis
6. paracusis
7. otorrhagia
8. otorrhea

Match It!
1. c
2. a
3. b
4. e
5. f
6. d
7. h
8. g

Break It Down!
1. para/cusis (p s)
2. ot/algia (r s)
3. an/acusis (p s)
4. hyper/acusis (p s)
5. ot/o/rrhea (r cv s)

Word Building
1. anacusis
2. hyperacusis
3. otalgia
4. paracusis
5. tinnitus
6. vertigo
7. otorrhea
8. otorrhagia

Fill It In!
1. vertigo/tinnitus
2. anacusis/paracusis
3. hyperacusis/otalgia
4. otorrhea/otorrhagia

Self Quiz 8.4

Say It—Spell It!
1. mastoiditis
2. myrigitis
3. otitis media
4. otosclerosis
5. presbyacusis
6. Menière's

Match It!
1. f
2. c
3. h
4. i
5. g
6. d
7. e
8. b
9. a

Break It Down!
1. acoust/ic neur/oma (r s r s)
2. labyrinth/itis (r s)
3. mast/oid/itis (r s s)
4. ot/algia (r s)
5. myring/itis (r s)
6. presby/acusis (r s)

Word Building
1. acoustic neuroma
2. myringitis
3. otitis externa
4. otopathy
5. Menière's disease
6. labyrinthitis
7. mastoiditis
8. otitis media
9. cerumen impaction
10. presbyacusis
11. otosclerosis

Fill It In!
1. otitis media/Eustacian/mastoiditis/paracusis
2. myringitis/otitis media
3. otopathy/paracusis/anacusis/presbyacusis

Self Quiz 8.5

Say It—Spell It!
1. otorhinolaryngology
2. acoumetry
3. labyrinthectomy
4. mastoidectomy
5. myringoplasty
6. otoscopy
7. tympanometry

Match It!
1. f
2. e
3. d
4. a
5. c
6. b

Break It Down!
1. acou/metry (r s)
2. audi/o/metry (r cv s)
3. mast/oid/ectomy (r s s)
4. myring/o/tomy (r cv s)
5. ot/o/scopy (r cv s)
6. tympan/o/plasty (r cv s)

Word Building
1. acoumetry
2. audiometry
3. labyrinthectomy
4. mastoidectomy
5. mastoidotomy
6. myringoplasty
7. myringotomy
8. otoscopy
9. stapedectomy
10. tympanometry
11. tympanoplasty

Fill It In!
1. acoumetry/audiometry/audiogram
2. stapedectomy
3. mastoidectomy/mastoidotomy
4. tympanoplasty
5. myringotomy
6. otoscopy/otologist

Self Quiz 8.6
1. right ear
2. AS
3. otology
4. tympanic membrane
5. AU
6. ear, nose, throat
7. OM

Chapter 9

Self Quiz 9.1

Definition
1. against, opposing
2. within, absorbing
3. outside, away from
4. together
5. running
6. blood
7. resembling
8. shape, formation

Word Root
1. acr
2. aden
3. ren
4. andr
5. calc
6. cortic
7. crin
8. dips
9. gluc
10. kal

11. megal
12. natr
13. thyr
14. tox

Self Quiz 9.2

Say It—Spell It!
1. pituitary
2. pineal
3. thyroid
4. parathyroid
5. adrenal
6. pancreas
7. islets of Langerhans

Match It!
1. d
2. g
3. f
4. i
5. b
6. a
7. h
8. c
9. e

Fill It In!
1. hormones/pituitary/adenohypophysis/oxytocin
2. pineal
3. thyroid/glucose
4. parathyroid/calcium
5. adrenal/cortex
6. pancreas/insulin/glucagon

Self Quiz 9.3

Say It—Spell It!
1. acidosis
2. ketosis
3. polydipsia
4. polyuria
5. exophthalmos
6. goiter
7. hypersecretion
8. hyposecretion

Match It!
1. d
2. e
3. b
4. a
5. f
6. c

Break It Down!
```
          r   s
1. acid/osis
          r   s
2. ket/osis
        p   r   s
3. poly/dips/ia
        p   r   s
4. poly/ur/ia
        p    r   cv s
5. ex/ophthalm/o/s
```

Word Building
1. polydipsia
2. polyuria
3. ketosis
4. acidosis
5. exophthalmos
6. goiter

Fill It In!
1. acidosis/ketosis
2. polyuria/polydipsia
3. exophthalmos
4. goiter

Self Quiz 9.4

Say It—Spell It!
1. syndrome
2. acromegaly
3. adrenalitis
4. adrenomegaly
5. calcipenia
6. hypercalcemia
7. hyperinsulinism
8. hyperkalemia
9. hyperthyroidism
10. hypoglycemia
11. hyponatremia
12. hypoparathyroidism
13. parathyroidoma
14. myxedema

Match It!
1. i
2. h
3. f
4. g
5. a
6. k
7. b
8. c
9. l
10. n
11. d
12. e
13. j
14. w
15. r
16. p
17. u
18. o
19. m
20. s
21. v
22. q
23. t

Break It Down!
```
        p    r  cv  s
1. endo/crin/o/logy
        r  cv    r   s
2. acr/o/megal/y
      p   r  cv   r   cv  p    s
3. ad/ren/o/cortic/o/hyper/plasia
```

```
       r  cv  s
4. adren/o/pathy
       p     r  cv  s
5. endo/crin/o/pathy
       p    r   s
6. hyper/glyc/emia
       p    r   s
7. hyper/insulin/ism
       p   r   s
8. hyper/kal/emia
       p     p   r  s   s
9. hyper/para/thyr/oid/ism
       p    r   s
10. hypo/glyc/emia
        p   r   s   s
11. hypo/thyr/oid/ism
        p   r   s   s
12. para/thyr/oid/ism
```

Fill It In!
1. acromegaly/gigantism/dwarfism/endocrinopathy
2. adrenalitis/adrenomegaly/adrenopathy
3. parathyroidoma/hyperparathyroidism/hypercalcemia/hypoparathyroidism/hypocalcemia
4. pancreatitis/hyperinsulinism/hyperglycemia
5. diabetes mellitus/ketosis/II/insulin
6. Addison's/hirsutism/virilism/Cushing's
7. goiter/thyroid/cretinism
8. gigantism/dwarfism
9. tetany

Self Quiz 9.5

Say It—Spell It!
1. adrenalectomy
2. hypophysectomy
3. parathyroidectomy
4. thyroidotomy
5. radioiodine
6. thyroidectomy

Match It!
1. d
2. e
3. g
4. b
5. k
6. a
7. i
8. c
9. j
10. f
11. h

Break It Down!
```
        p    r  cv  s
1. endo/crin/o/logist
        r   s    s
2. thyr/oid/otomy
       r  cv  p   r  s     s
3. thyr/o/para/thyr/oid/ectomy
```

```
        p   r  cv  s
```
4. endo/crin/o/pathy

Word Building
1. fasting blood sugar
2. glucose tolerance test
3. radioactive iodine uptake
4. postprandial blood sugar
5. thyroxine test
6. hormone replacement therapy
7. thyroid scan
8. parathyroidectomy
9. radioiodine therapy
10. thyroidotomy

Fill It In!
1. adrenalectomy/thyroidectomy/
   parathyroidectomy/
   thyroparathyroidectomy
2. hyperthyroidism/exophthalmos/
   radioiodine/iodine/thyroid scan/HRT
3. fasting blood sugar/glucose tolerance/
   postprandial blood

Self Quiz 9.6
1. glucose tolerance test
2. RAIU
3. postprandial blood sugar
4. DI
5. fasting blood sugar
6. HRT
7. diabetes mellitus

Chapter 10

Self Quiz 10.1

Definition
1. slow
2. within, inner
3. between
4. around
5. fast
6. pertaining to
7. removal
8. pain
9. hardening

Word Root
1. angi, angin
2. aort
3. arter, arteri
4. ather
5. atri
6. card, cardi
7. coron
8. isch
9. pector, steth
10. phleb
11. sphygm
12. sten
13. thromb
14. varic
15. vas
16. ven
17. ech
18. electr

Self Quiz 10.2

Say It—Spell It!
1. cardiovascular
2. aorta
3. arteriole
4. atrioventricular
5. atrium
6. bicuspid
7. capillaries
8. diastole
9. endocardium
10. endothelium
11. myocardium
12. semilunar
13. sinoatrial
14. systole
15. vasoconstriction
16. vasodilation
17. ventricle
18. venule

Match It!
1. o
2. n
3. h
4. m
5. c
6. i
7. a
8. j
9. d
10. b
11. e
12. f
13. l
14. k
15. g

Fill It In!
1. heart/blood
2. pericardial/pericardial sac/
   pericardium/epicardium
3. myocardium/endocardium/atria/
   ventricles
4. tricuspid/pulmonary/pulmonary
5. left atrium/mitral/aortic/aorta
6. conduction/sinoatrial/atrioventricular/ His
7. arteries/veins/interstitial/capillaries/
   muscle/vasoconstriction/arterioles/
   venules

Label It!
1. right atrium
2. left ventricle
3. mitral valve
4. pericardial sac
5. right ventricle
6. aortic valve
7. aorta
8. pulmonary trunk

Self Quiz 10.3

Say It—Spell It!
1. angiospasm

2. arrhythmia
3. angiostenosis
4. bradycardia
5. cardiodynia
6. cardiogenic
7. dysrhythmia
8. tachycardia

Break It Down!
```
        r  cv  r   s
```
1. angi/o/sten/osis
```
        p   r    s
```
2. a/rrythm/ia
```
        p    r   s
```
3. brady/card/ia
```
        r  cv  s
```
4. cardi/o/dynia
```
        p    r   s
```
5. dys/rhythm/ia

Fill It In!
1. Dysrhythmia
2. angiostenosis
3. cardiogenic/cardiodynia
4. tachycardia/bradycardia

Self Quiz 10.4

Say It—Spell It!
1. angiocarditis
2. angioma
3. arteriorrhexis
4. arteriosclerosis
5. atherosclerosis
6. cardiomyopathy
7. cardiovalvulitis
8. endocarditis
9. hypertension
10. myocardial infarction
11. myocarditis
12. pericarditis
13. phlebitis
14. polyarteritis
15. thromboangiitis obliterans

Break It Down!
```
        r  cv  r   s
```
1. angi/o/card/itis
```
        r  cv  r   s
```
2. cardi/o/vascul/ar
```
        r   s
```
3. angi/oma
```
        r  cv  r    s
```
4. arteri/o/scler/osis
```
        r  cv r  cv  s
```
5. cardi/o/my/o/pathy
```
        r  cv  r   s
```
6. cardi/o/valvul/itis
```
        p    r    s
```
7. endo/card/itis
```
        p    r    s
```
8. peri/card/itis
```
        p     r     s
```
9. poly/arter/itis
```
        r   cv  r   s
```
10. thromb/o/angi/itis
```
```

Match It!
1. e
2. k
3. l
4. p
5. g
6. a
7. n
8. b
9. m
10. f
11. h
12. o
13. c
14. i
15. d
16. j

Fill It In!
1. cardiology
2. angiocarditis
3. polyarteritis/myocarditis/endocarditis/cardiovalvulitis/pericarditis
4. phlebitis/thromboangiitis/angioma/arteriosclerosis
5. atherosclerosis/myocardial infarction/MI
6. cardiomyopathy
7. Hypertension/hypotension
8. aneurysm
9. angina pectoris/ischemia/arrest/heart attack
10. occlusion/coronary artery disease/embolism/thrombus/thrombosis
11. cor pulmonale/congestive/fibrillation/flutter
12. congenital/atrial septal/coarctation/aorta/septal/Fallot

Word Building
1. embolism
2. heart murmur
3. flutter
4. heart block
5. coronary occlusion
6. cardiac arrest
7. blood pressure
8. palpitation
9. ischemia
10. congestive heart failure
11. atrial septal defect
12. claudication
13. coartaction of the aorta

Self Quiz 10.5

Say It—Spell It!
1. aneurysmectomy
2. angiogram
3. arteriogram
4. aortogram
5. venogram
6. angioplasty
7. angiorrhaphy
8. angioscopy
9. arteriotomy

10. atherectomy
11. auscultation
12. catheterization
13. defibrillation
14. echocardiography
15. electrocardiogram
16. embolectomy
17. endarterectomy
18. hemorrhoidectomy
19. pericardiostomy
20. phlebectomy
21. phlebotomy
22. valvuloplasty

Break It Down!
```
         r  cv  r    s
```
1. angi/o/sten/osis
```
        r         s
```
2. aneurysm/ectomy
```
      r  cv  s
```
3. angi/o/gram
```
       r  cv  s
```
4. arteri/o/gram
```
      r  cv   s
```
5. angi/o/plasty
```
      r  cv  s
```
6. angi/o/rrhaphy
```
       r    s
```
7. arteri/o/tomy
```
      r       s
```
8. ather/ectomy
```
     r  cv   r   cv  s
```
9. ech/o/cardi/o/graphy
```
      r  cv   r   cv s
```
10. electr/o/cardi/o/gram
```
       r      s
```
11. embol/ectomy
```
      p    r      s
```
12. end/arter/ectomy
```
       p    r  cv  s
```
13. peri/cardi/o/stomy
```
      r   cv  s
```
14. valvul/o/plasty

Match It!
1. h
2. j
3. l
4. k
5. o
6. n
7. a
8. g
9. d
10. b
11. e
12. m
13. c
14. f
15. i

Fill It In!
1. aneurysmectomy/angiogram/aortogram/coronary angiogram

2. angioscopy/atherectomy/endarterectomy/angioplasty/stent/bypass graft
3. auscultation/stethoscope
4. electrocardiography/ECG or EKG/echocardiography/stress ECHO/Doppler
5. pacemaker/Holter

Self Quiz 10.6
1. atrial septal defect
2. HHD
3. myocardial infarction
4. MRA
5. electrocardiogram
6. CHF
7. coronary artery disease
8. CPR
9. coronary artery bypass graft
10. AV
11. blood pressure
12. SA
13. deep vein thrombosis

Chapter 11
Self Quiz 11.1

Definition
1. large
2. small
3. to separate
4. condition of blood
5. abnormal decrease
6. loving, affinity for
7. formation
8. up, toward
9. forward, preceding
10. protection
11. to dissolve
12. equal
13. same
14. cell
15. condition of
16. surgical fixation, suspension

Word Root
1. blast
2. erythr
3. hem, hemat
4. leuk
5. poikil
6. therm
7. thromb
8. aden
9. immun
10. lymph
11. staphyl
12. path
13. strept
14. splen
15. thym
16. bacteria
17. mon

Self Quiz 11.2

Say It—Spell It!
1. hemoglobin
2. leukocytes
3. hematopoiesis
4. fibrinogen
5. coagulation
6. erythrocytes
7. antibody
8. antigen
9. immunity
10. lymph
11. lymphocyte
12. thoracic
13. neutrophil

Match It!
1. f
2. h
3. a
4. c
5. i
6. e
7. j
8. b
9. g
10. d
11. m
12. p
13. o
14. k
15. r
16. l
17. n
18. q
19. s

Break It Down!
    r cv s
1. erythr/o/cyte
    r cv s
2. leuk/o/cyte
     r cv s
3. hemat/o/poiesis
     r cv s
4. lymph/o/cyte

Fill It In!
1. erythrocytes/leukocytes/platelets
2. plasma/fibrinogen/serum
3. coagulation
4. lymph/lymphatic capillaries/lymph nodes
5. thoracic duct
6. spleen/thymus gland/lymphatic nodules/tonsils
7. infection/phagocytes/monocytes/lymphocytes/immune
8. T cells/B cells/antigens/antibodies
9. basophils

Self Quiz 11.3

Say It—Spell It!
1. bacteremia
2. anisocytosis
3. erythropenia
4. splenomegaly
5. toxemia
6. macrocytosis
7. poikilocytosis

Match It!
1. d
2. a
3. h
4. g
5. b
6. c
7. f
8. e

Break It Down!
    r cv s
1. erythr/o/penia
    r s
2. tox/emia
    r cv r s
3. poikil/o/cyt/osis
    r cv r s
4. splen/o/megal/y
    p   r r s
5. poly/cyt/hem/ia

Word Building
1. bacteremia
2. splenomegaly
3. macrocytosis
4. toxemia
5. polycythemia
6. hemorrhage
7. hemolysis
8. erythropenia

Fill It In!
1. anisocytosis/erythropenia/hemorrhage
2. Toxemia/toxins
3. hemolysis/bacteremia
4. macrocytosis/polycythemia

Self Quiz 11.4

Say It—Spell It!
1. allergy
2. anaphylaxis
3. aplastic anemia
4. diphtheria
5. erythroblastosis fetalis
6. fungemia
7. hemophilia
8. hemochromatosis
9. immunodeficiency
10. lymphadenitis
11. lymphadenopathy
12. lymphoma
13. leukemia
14. myelodysplasia
15. mononucleosis
16. autoimmune
17. septicemia
18. staphylococcemia
19. thymoma

Match It!
1. b
2. g
3. i
4. f
5. k
6. c
7. a
8. e
9. j
10. q
11. m
12. o
13. l
14. h
15. p
16. n
17. t
18. s
19. r
20. w
21. v
22. u

Break It Down!
    r s
1. leuk/emia
    r cv s
2. hem/o/philia
    r s
3. fung/emia
    r cv r s
4. erythr/o/blast/osis
    r cv r s
5. mon/o/nucle/osis
    r cv r s
6. hem/o/chromat/osis
    r cv p r s
7. myel/o/dys/plas/ia
    r s
8. thym/oma

Fill It In!
1. anemia/aplastic/iron deficiency/pernicious/folic acid/sickle cell
2. polycythemia
3. dyscrasia/hemochromatosis/hemophilia/septicemia
4. anaphylaxis/allergy
5. autoimmune
6. staphylococcemia/staph/gas gangrene
7. Hodgkin's disease/thymoma/lymphoma
8. mononucleosis
9. rabies/tetanus/botulism/diphtheria
10. AIDS

Self Quiz 11.5

Say It—Spell It!
1. coagulation
2. anticoagulant
3. hematocrit

4. hemostasis
5. plasmapheresis
6. lymphadenectomy
7. thymectomy
8. lymphadenography
9. vaccine
10. lymphangiography
11. lymphadenotomy
12. splenectomy
13. vaccination
14. lymphangiogram
15. splenopexy

Match It!
1. c
2. f
3. g
4. b
5. a
6. e
7. d
8. i
9. n
10. j
11. k
12. m
13. o
14. h
15. l

Break It Down!

    r cv s
1. hemat/o/crit
    r cv s
2. hem/o/stasis
     r   r cv s
3. lymph/angi/o/graphy
    p   s
4. pro/phylaxis
    r   s
5. splen/ectomy

Fill It In!
1. splenomegaly/splenopexy/splenectomy
2. blood chemistry/blood culture/complete blood count
3. hematocrit/hemoglobin/red blood count/white blood count
4. thrombolysis/PLT/coagulation time
5. lymphadenopathy/lymphadenitis
6. lymph node dissection/lymphadenography/lymphadenectomy
7. immunization/vaccinations/attenuation
8. hematology

Self Quiz 11.6
1. complete blood count
2. AIDS
3. red blood cell (or count)
4. ESR
5. prothrombin time
6. INR
7. lymphadenopathy syndrome
8. PTT
9. white blood cell (or count)

10. HGB, Hgb
11. hematocrit

Chapter 12
Self Quiz 12.1

Definition
1. without
2. normal, good
3. many
4. all, total
5. pain
6. carbon dioxide
7. dilation
8. sound, voice
9. breathing
10. condition
11. protrusion
12. surgical opening

Word Root
1. laryng
2. trache
3. glottis
4. nas, rhin
5. pleur
6. sinus
7. thorac
8. pulmon, pneum
9. alveol
10. muc
11. ox
12. pneum
13. py
14. somn
15. sept
16. pharyng
17. spir
18. narrowing, constriction

Self Quiz 12.2

Say It—Spell It!
1. alveoli
2. bronchi
3. bronchioles
4. diaphragm
5. expiration
6. inspiration
7. larynx
8. pharynx
9. respiration
10. trachea
11. ventilation

Match It!
1. f
2. e
3. j
4. h
5. l
6. g
7. b
8. k
9. i

10. a
11. c
12. d

Fill It In!
1. respiration/oxygen
2. nasal cavity/mucous
3. pharynx
4. larynx/glottis/epiglottis
5. trachea
6. bronchi/bronchial tree
7. bronchioles/alveoli
8. respiratory/alveolar
9. lung/pleurae
10. inspiration/ventilation

Self Quiz 12.3

Say It—Spell It!
1. apnea
2. bradypnea
3. bronchospasm
4. dysphonia
5. dyspnea
6. epistaxis
7. hemothorax
8. hemoptysis
9. hypercapnia
10. hyperpnea
11. hyperventilation
12. hypoxia
13. hypoxemia
14. hypopnea
15. laryngospasm
16. orthopnea
17. rhinorrhagia
18. thoracalgia
19. eupnea

Match It!
1. c
2. g
3. a
4. e
5. f
6. b
7. h
8. d
9. l
10. m
11. n
12. o
13. p
14. k
15. q
16. r
17. i
18. j

Break It Down!

    p s
1. brady/pnea
    p   s
2. dys/phonia

p   s
3. dys/pnea
   p   s
4. epi/staxis
   r   cv   s
5. hem/o/ptysis
   r   cv   r
6. hem/o/thorax
   p   s
7. hyper/capnia
   p   s
8. hyper/pnea
   p   s
9. hypo/capnea
   p   s
10. hypo/pnea
    p   r   s
11. hyp/ox/emia
    p   r   s
12. hyp/ox/ia
    r   cv   s
13. laryng/o/spasm
    r   cv   s
14. orth/o/pnea
    r   cv   s
15. rhin/o/rrhagia
    r   s
16. thorac/algia

Self Quiz 12.4

Say It—Spell It!
1. atelectasis
2. asthma
3. bronchiectasis
4. bronchitis
5. diaphragmatocele
6. emphysema
7. epiglottitis
8. cor pulmonale
9. coryza
10. croup
11. laryngotracheobronchitis
12. laryngitis
13. legionellosis
14. nasopharyngitis
15. pneumatocele
16. pneumoconiosis
17. pneumonia
18. pneumonitis
19. pansinusitis
20. pertussis
21. pyothorax
22. pleuritis
23. rhinitis
24. rhinomycosis
25. sinusitis
26. cystic fibrosis
27. tonsillitis
28. tracheostenosis

Match It!
1. h
2. i

3. g
4. a
5. e
6. d
7. c
8. b
9. f
10. m
11. b
12. n
13. k
14. o
15. l

Break It Down!
   p   s
1. atel/ectasis
   p   r   cv   s
2. dia/phragmat/o/cele
   p   r   s
3. epi/glott/itis
   r   s
4. trache/itis
   r   cv   s
5. pneumat/o/cele
   r   cv   r   s
6. nas/o/pharyng/itis
   r   cv   r   s
7. rhin/o/myc/osis
   r   cv   s
8. bronch/i/ectasis
   p   r   s
9. pan/sinus/itis
   r   cv   r   s
10. trache/o/sten/osis
    r   cv   r
11. py/o/thorax
    r   s
12. tubercul/osis

Fill It In!
1. ARDS
2. asphyxia
3. asthma
4. apnea
5. obstructive pulmonary/smoking
6. emphysema/cor pulmonale
7. coryza
8. croup
9. Cystic fibrosis
10. pneumonia/pulmonary edema
11. Legionellosis/*Pneumocystis carinii*/pleural effusion
12. pertussis
13. upper respiratory

Self Quiz 12.5

Say It—Spell It!
1. antihistamine
2. bronchdilation
3. bronchogram
4. bronchography
5. bronchoplasty
6. endoscopy

7. laryngoscopy
8. endotracheal intubation
9. laryngectomy
10. laryngocentesis
11. laryngoplasty
12. laryngotracheotomy
13. lobectomy
14. oximetry
15. pleurocentesis
16. pneumobronchotomy
17. pneumonectomy
18. rhinoplasty
19. septoplasty
20. septotomy
21. sinusotomy
22. spirometry
23. thoracocentesis
24. tracheoplasty
25. tracheostomy
26. tracheotomy

Match It!
1. k
2. f
3. g
4. a
5. j
6. b
7. i
8. e
9. h
10. d
11. n
12. o
13. c
14. l
15. m

Break It Down!
   p   r
1. anti/histamine
   r   cv   s
2. bronch/o/gram
   p   r   s
3. endo/trache/al
   r   cv   s
4. spir/o/metry
   r   s
5. laryng/ectomy
   r   s
6. lob/ectomy
   r   cv   s
7. ox/i/metry
   r   cv   s
8. pleur/o/centesis
   r   cv   r   cv   s
9. pneum/o/bronch/o/tomy
   r   cv   s
10. sept/o/tomy
    r   cv   s
11. thorac/o/centesis
    r   cv   s
12. trache/o/plasty

Word Building

1. TB skin test
2. resuscitation
3. auscultation
4. arterial blood gases
5. chest CT scan
6. mechanical ventilation
7. acid-fast bacilli smear
8. chest x-ray
9. pulmonary function tests

Fill It In!

1. acid-fast bacilli
2. auscultation
3. spirometer/pulmonary function
4. arterial blood gas
5. chest CT scan
6. chest x-ray
7. mechanical ventilation
8. ventilation-perfusion
9. TB skin test
10. resuscitation

Self Quiz 12.6

1. vital capacity
2. LTB
3. hyaline membrane disease
4. TB
5. tidal volume
6. ARDS
7. cardiopulmonary resuscitation
8. PPD
9. chest x-ray
10. CF
11. respiratory distress syndrome
12. COPD
13. arterial blood gases
14. OSA
15. pulmonary embolism
16. PCP
17. upper respiratory infection

Chapter 13

Self Quiz 13.1

Definition

1. puncture
2. vomiting
3. digestion
4. toward
5. bad, abnormal
6. all, entire
7. around
8. back

Word Root

1. abdomin
2. an
3. append
4. bil
5. col
6. choledoch
7. diverticul
8. duoden
9. gingiv
10. hern
11. ile
12. jejun
13. cheil
14. hepat
15. or, stomat
16. palat
17. pancreat
18. periton
19. polyp
20. pylor
21. rect
22. sial
23. sigm
24. enter
25. gastr
26. dent
27. phag
28. gloss, lingu
29. uvul
30. emesis

Self Quiz 13.2

Say It—Spell It!

1. esophagus
2. gallbladder
3. gastrointestinal
4. cecum
5. colon
6. tongue
7. uvula
8. pancreas
9. duodenum
10. jejunum
11. pylorus

Match It!

1. g
2. f
3. q
4. r
5. k
6. d
7. c
8. e
9. m
10. l
11. p
12. b
13. o
14. h
15. i
16. a
17. n
18. j

Fill It In!

1. oral cavity/soft palate/uvula
2. pharynx/esophagus/peristalsis/abdominal/peritoneum
3. gastric/pepsin/mucus/pylorus
4. digestion/absorption/villi/duodenum/pyloric valve/jejunum/cecum
5. colon/rectum/defecation/anus
6. bile/fats/gallbladder/saliva/pancreatic juice

Self Quiz 13.3

Say It—Spell It!

1. aphagia
2. dyspepsia
3. hematemesis
4. hyperbilirubinemia
5. gastrodynia
6. steatorrhea
7. hepatomegaly
8. dysphagia
9. nausea

Match It!

1. c
2. e
3. f
4. b
5. a
6. d
7. m
8. l
9. j
10. k
11. i
12. h
13. g

Break It Down!

1. a/phag/ia (p r s)
2. dys/peps/ia (p r s)
3. gastr/o/dynia (r cv s)
4. hyper/bil/i/rubin/emia (p rcv r s)
5. hemat/emesis (r s)

Self Quiz 13.4

Say It—Spell It!

1. adhesion
2. anorexia nervosa
3. bulimia
4. dysentery
5. diverticulosis
6. gastroenterocolitis
7. gastromalacia
8. glossitis
9. hepatitis
10. hernia
11. ileitis
12. intussusception
13. gingivitis
14. cheilitis
15. cholangioma
16. choledokolithiasis
17. cholecystitis
18. colitis
19. colorectal cancer

20. pancreatitis
21. peritonitis
22. polyp
23. proctoptosis
24. rectocele
25. cirrhosis
26. sialoadenitis
27. sialolith
28. stomatitis
29. volvulus
30. uvulitis

Match It!
1. i
2. j
3. d
4. c
5. k
6. l
7. e
8. a
9. h
10. b
11. g
12. f
13. p
14. r
15. t
16. m
17. s
18. q
19. o
20. n

Break It Down!
    r s s
1. append/ic/itis
    r s
2. cheil/itis
    r cv r   s
3. chol/e/lith/iasis
    r s
4. col/itis
    r   s
5. diverticul/itis
    r   s
6. enter/itis
    r   s
7. esophag/itis
    r cv r   s
8. gastr/o/enter/itis
    r   s
9. gingiv/itis
    r   s
10. gloss/itis
    r   s
11. hepat/oma
    r   s
12. ile/itis
    r   s
13. pancreat/itis
    r   s
14. polyp/osis

    r   s
15. proct/itis

Fill It In!
1. adhesion
2. anorexia nervosa/bulimia
3. ascites/jaundice/cirrhosis
4. Crohn's/ileitis
5. diarrhea/flatus/bowel syndrome
6. ileus/intussusception/volvulus
7. vomit/nausea
8. hiatal hernia/direct inguinal
9. duodenal ulcer/gastric ulcer
10. colorectal cancer/hepatoma

Self Quiz 13.5

Say It—Spell It!
1. abdominoperineal
2. abdominoplasty
3. abdominocentesis
4. anoplasty
5. antiemetic
6. antispasmodic
7. esophagogastroduodenoscopy
8. hemorrhoidectomy
9. herniorrhaphy
10. gingivectomy
11. cheilorrhaphy
12. cholangiopancreatography
13. choledocholithotomy
14. cholecystectomy
15. colonoscopy
16. colostomy
17. laparoscopy
18. laparotomy
19. polypectomy
20. proctoscopy
21. celiotomy
22. sigmoidoscopy
23. vagotomy
24. uvulopalatopharyngoplasty

Match It!
1. f
2. l
3. i
4. n
5. c
6. p
7. q
8. s
9. b
10. g
11. e
12. r
13. o
14. a
15. d
16. m
17. t
18. h
19. k
20. j

Break It Down!
    r   cv s
1. abdomin/o/centesis
    r cv   s
2. an/o/plasty
    p   s
3. anti/emetic
    r   s
4. append/ectomy
    r cv   s
5. cheil/o/rrhaphy
    r   r cv s
6. chol/angi/o/gram
    r   cv r cv s
7. choledoch/o/lith/o/tomy
    r   r cv   r   cv s
8. chol/angi/o/pancreat/o/graphy
    r cv s
9. colon/o/scopy
    r   cv r   cv   r   cv s
10. esophag/o/gastr/o/duoden/o/scopy
    r   cv s
11. gloss/o/rrhaphy
    r   cv s
12. lapar/o/scopy
    r   cv s
13. sigmoid/o/scopy
    r   s   s
14. hemorrh/oid/ectomy
    r   cv s
15. herni/o/rrhaphy

Word Building
1. cathartic
2. fecal occult blood test
3. upper GI series
4. gastric lavage
5. stool culture and sensitivity
6. gavage
7. barium enema

Fill It In!
1. enema/lower GI/upper GI
2. cathartic
3. nasogastric/gavage
4. gastric lavage
5. fecal occult
6. stool culture

Self Quiz 13.6
1. EGD
2. barium enema
3. IBD
4. upper GI series
5. UPPP
6. nausea and vomiting
7. ERCP
8. irritable bowel syndrome
9. EUS
10. abdominoperineal resection
11. GERD

Chapter 14

Self Quiz 14.1

Definition
1. without
2. on top of
3. surgical crushing
4. nourishment
5. urine or urination
6. under

Word Root
1. azot
2. albumin
3. blast
4. cyst, vesic
5. glomerul
6. glyc, glycos, gluc
7. hydr
8. lith
9. meat
10. nephr
11. olig
12. pyel
13. py
14. ren
15. ur, urin
16. urethr

Self Quiz 14.2

Say It—Spell It!
1. glomerulus
2. urinary meatus
3. nephron
4. renal corpuscle
5. ureters
6. urethra
7. internal urethral sphincter
8. external urethral sphincter
9. urine
10. urinary bladder
11. hilum
12. micturition

Match It!
1. c
2. k
3. o
4. g
5. b
6. l
7. i
8. a
9. e
10. m
11. d
12. n
13. j
14. h
15. f

Fill It In!
1. kidneys/renal cortex/renal medulla/ renal pelvis

2. nephrons/renal corpuscle/Bowman's capsule/glomerulus
3. ureter/urinary bladder/urethra/ urethral/urinary meatus/external urethral sphincter

Self Quiz 14.3

Say It—Spell It!
1. albuminuria
2. anuresis
3. anuria
4. azotemia
5. bacteriuria
6. diuresis
7. dysuria
8. enuresis
9. glycosuria
10. hematuria
11. nocturia
12. oliguria
13. polyuria
14. proteinuria
15. pyuria
16. ketonuria

Match It!
1. k
2. d
3. i
4. h
5. e
6. p
7. o
8. b
9. j
10. c
11. g
12. a
13. m
14. f
15. n
16. l

Break It Down!
      r   s
1. albumin/uria
      p s
2. an/uresis
      r   s
3. azot/emia
     r cv s
4. bacter/i/uria
      p s
5. dys/uria
      p s
6. en/uresis
      r   s
7. glycos/uria
      r   s
8. keton/uria

Word Building
1. nocturia
2. bacteriuria

3. glycosuria
4. anuria
5. dysuria
6. enuresis
7. azotemia
8. diuresis

Self Quiz 14.4

Say It—Spell It!
1. epispadias
2. glomerulonephritis
3. hydronephrosis
4. hypospadias
5. incontinence
6. nephritis
7. nephroblastoma
8. nephrohypertrophy
9. nephrolithiasis
10. nephroma
11. nephromegaly
12. nephroptosis
13. pyelitis
14. pyelonephritis
15. polycystic kidney
16. renal calculi
17. renal hypertension
18. cystitis
19. cystolith
20. cystocele
21. uremia
22. ureteritis
23. ureterolithiasis
24. ureterocele
25. ureterostenosis
26. urethrocystitis
27. urinary retention
28. urinary suppression

Match It!
1. e
2. g
3. m
4. j
5. r
6. s
7. l
8. q
9. f
10. a
11. p
12. d
13. k
14. h
15. c
16. b
17. i
18. o
19. n
20. w
21. t
22. y
23. u

24. x
25. z
26. v

Break It Down!

1. cyst/itis
   r   s
2. cyst/o/cele
   r cv s
3. cyst/o/lith
   r cv s
4. glomerul/o/nephr/itis
   r   cv r   s
5. hydr/o/nephr/itis
   r cv r   s
6. nephr/o/blast/oma
   r cv r   s
7. nephr/o/megaly
   r cv s
8. pyel/o/nephr/itis
   r cv r   s
9. hypo/spadias
   p   r

Fill It In!

1. epispadias/hypospadias
2. incontinence
3. polycystic kidney
4. renal calculi
5. renal hypertension/urinary suppression
6. urinary tract infection/voiding/urinary retention

Self Quiz 14.5

Say It—Spell It!

1. cystography
2. cystorrhaphy
3. cystoureterogram
4. cystoureterography
5. cystourethrogram
6. cystourethrography
7. hemodialysis
8. lithotripsy
9. nephrectomy
10. nephrogram
11. nephrography
12. nephrolysis
13. nephropexy
14. nephrosonography
15. nephrostomy
16. nephrotomogram
17. pyelithotomy
18. ureterostomy
19. ureterogram
20. pyelogram
21. urethropexy
22. urethroplasty
23. urethroscopy
24. urethrostomy
25. urinometer
26. ureterectomy
27. vesicourethral

Match It!

1. p
2. e
3. h
4. b
5. n
6. q
7. d
8. l
9. k
10. g
11. c
12. m
13. j
14. o
15. a
16. i
17. f
18. t
19. x
20. w
21. u
22. z
23. r
24. s
25. v
26. y

Break It Down!

1. cyst/o/lith/o/tomy
   r cv r cv s
2. cyst/o/pyel/o/graphy
   r cv r cv s
3. cyst/o/ureter/o/gram
   r cv r cv s
4. meat/o/tomy
   r cv s
5. nephr/o/son/o/graphy
   r cv r cv s
6. nephr/o/lys/is
   r cv r s
7. nephr/o/tom/o/gram
   r cv r cv s
8. ren/o/graphy
   r cv s
9. ureter/o/gram
   r cv s
10. urethr/o/stomy
    r cv s
11. urethr/o/scope
    r cv s
12. ureter/o/stomy
    r cv s
13. urethr/o/tomy
    r cv s
14. vesic/o/urethr/al
    r cv r   s

Word Building

1. urinary catheter
2. specific gravity
3. renal transplant
4. fulguration

5. urinalysis
6. kidney, ureter, and bladder x-ray
7. peritoneal dialysis
8. nephroscope
9. hemodialysis
10. cystourethrography
11. nephrotomography
12. intravenous pyelogram
13. cystopyelogram
14. meatoscope
15. cystoscopy

Fill It In!

1. creatinine/specific gravity/urinalysis
2. blood urea nitrogen
3. peritoneal dialysis/renal transplant
4. kidney/ureter/urinary catheter/fulguration

Self Quiz 14.6

1. urinalysis
2. RP
3. Bowman's capsule
4. VCUG
5. intravenous pyelogram
6. KUB
7. hemodialysis
8. UTI
9. catheter, catheterization

Chapter 15

Self Quiz 15.1

Definition

1. not
2. through, across, beyond
3. surgical fixation
4. excessive discharge

Word Root

1. epididym
2. test, orch, orchid, orchi
3. balan
4. prostat
5. andr
6. sperm, spermat
7. vas
8. vesicul
9. pen

Self Quiz 15.2

Say It—Spell It!

1. bulbourethral
2. ejaculation
3. epididymus
4. penis
5. perineum
6. prostate
7. scrotum
8. semen
9. seminal vesicles
10. seminiferous tubules
11. spermatic cord
12. testis

13. testosterone
14. vas deferens

Match It!
1. m
2. l
3. i
4. j
5. b
6. d
7. a
8. c
9. h
10. n
11. f
12. k
13. e
14. g

Fill It In!
1. testes/scrotum/sperm cells/
   seminiferous tubules/testosterone
2. epididymus/vas deferens/spermatic
   cord/ejaculatory duct/urethra
3. semen/seminal vesicles/prostate
   gland/bulbourethral glands
4. penis/glans penis/prepuce

Self Quiz 15.3

Say It—Spell It!
1. azoospermia
2. balanorrhea
3. prostatorrhea
4. chancres
5. aspermia
6. oligospermia
7. urethritis
8. proctitis
9. papillomas

Match It!
1. b
2. c
3. a
4. e
5. f
6. d

Break It Down!
        p r cv r   s
1. a/zo/o/sperm/ia
        r   cv s
2. balan/o/rrhea
        r   cv s
3. prostat/o/rrhea
        r   cv r   s
4. olig/o/sperm/ia
        r   s
5. proct/itis

Word Building
1. azoospermia
2. balanorrhea
3. prostatorrhea
4. papilloma

5. oligospermia
6. aspermia
7. chancres

Self Quiz 15.4

Say It—Spell It!
1. immunodeficiency syndrome
2. anorchism
3. erectile dysfunction
4. cryptorchidism
5. testicular carcinoma
6. epididymitis
7. phimosis
8. prostaocytosis
9. gonorrhea
10. hydrocele
11. benign prostatic hyperplasia
12. priapism
13. prostatovesiculitis
14. varicocele
15. Peyronie's
16. chlamydia
17. orchiepididymitis
18. spermatolysis
19. syphilis

Match It!
1. d
2. h
3. l
4. n
5. o
6. m
7. b
8. p
9. a
10. e
11. j
12. i
13. g
14. c
15. f
16. k

Break It Down!
        r   cv s
1. andr/o/pathy
        p   r   s
2. an/orch/ism
        r   r   s
3. crypt/orchid/ism
        r   s
4. epididym/itis
        r   cv   r   s
5. orch/i/epididym/itis
        r   s
6. prostat/itis
        r   cv r   s
7. prostat/o/vesicul/itis

Word Building
1. phimosis
2. priapism

3. prostate cancer
4. testicular cancer
5. impotent
6. syphilis
7. genital herpes
8. gonorrhea
9. trichomoniasis

Fill It In!
1. erectile dysfunction/impotent/Peyronie's
2. phimosis
3. Priapism
4. prostate cancer/testicular carcinoma
5. testicular torsion
6. acquired immunodeficiency
7. chlamydia/genital herpes/HSV-2
8. syphilis/gonorrhea
9. hepatitis B/HPV

Self Quiz 15.5

Say It—Spell It!
1. balanoplasty
2. epididymectomy
3. hydrocelectomy
4. orchidectomy
5. orchidopexy
6. orchiectomy
7. prostatectomy
8. prostatocystotomy
9. prostatovesiculectomy
10. vasectomy
11. vasovasostomy
12. vesiculectomy

Match It!
1. l
2. d
3. i
4. c
5. k
6. n
7. a
8. m
9. g
10. e
11. b
12. h
13. j
14. f

Break It Down!
        r   cv s
1. balan/o/plasty
        r   s
2. epididym/ectomy
        r   cv r   s
3. hydr/o/cel/ectomy
        r   cv s
4. orchi/o/plasty
        r   cv s
5. orchid/o/pexy
        r   s
6. prostat/ectomy

r   cv r cv s
7. prostat/o/lith/o/tomy
r   s
8. vesicul/ectomy

Word Building
1. penile implant
2. circumcision
3. digital rectal exam
4. sterilization
5. transrectal ultrasound
6. prostate-specific antigen
7. transurethral resection of the prostate
8. transurethral incision of the prostate
9. transurethral microwave thermotherapy

Fill It In!
1. artificial insemination
2. circumcision
3. digital rectal exam/prostate specific antigen/transrectal ultrasound
4. transurethral incision/transurethral resection/microwave thermotherapy
5. penile implant
6. sterilization

Self Quiz 15.6
1. TUMT
2. prostate specific antigen
3. STD
4. human immunodeficiency virus
5. TURP
6. benign prostatic hypertrophy (or hyperplasia)
7. AIDS
8. HBV
9. transurethral incision of the prostate
10. herpes simplex virus type 2
11. DRE
12. human papilloma virus

Chapter 16

Self Quiz 16.1

Definition
1. within, inner
2. around, surrounding
3. closure; absence of a normal body opening
4. pertaining to

Word Root
1. cervic
2. colp, vagin
3. culd
4. episi, vulv
5. gynec, gyn
6. hydr
7. hyster, metr, uter
8. mamm, mast
9. men
10. oophor, ovari
11. ov
12. py
13. perine
14. salping, salpinx
15. trachel, cervic

Self Quiz 16.2

Say It—Spell It!
1. alveolar
2. Bartholin's
3. cervix
4. clitoris
5. endometrium
6. fornix
7. hymen
8. infundibulum
9. labia majora
10. labia minora
11. mammary
12. mons pubis
13. myometrium
14. menarche
15. menopause
16. menses
17. ovulation
18. rectouterine pouch
19. uterus
20. vestibule

Match It!
1. e
2. h
3. l
4. m
5. j
6. k
7. q
8. a
9. n
10. b
11. r
12. o
13. p
14. c
15. i
16. f
17. g
18. d

Break It Down!
p   r cv s
1. endo/metr/i/um
r   s
2. cervic/al
p   r cv s
3. peri/metr/i/um
r cv r cv s
4. my/o/metr/i/um

Fill It In!
1. ovaries/follicles/ovum/graafian/ovulation/estrogens
2. endometrium/menses/menarche/menopause
3. uterus/myometrium/perimetrium/uterine cavity/cervix/cervical canal/external os
4. fallopian tube/infundibulum
5. vagina/vaginal orifice/hymen
6. vulva/mons pubis/labia majora/labia minora/vestibule/clitoris/perineum
7. mammary glands/areola/nipple/alveolar glands

Self Quiz 16.3

Say It—Spell It!
1. amenorrhea
2. dysmenorrhea
3. hematosalpinx
4. hydrosalpinx
5. leukorrhea
6. mastalgia
7. menometrorrhagia
8. metrorrhea
9. oligomenorrhea
10. pyosalpinx

Match It!
1. d
2. f
3. e
4. a
5. h
6. j
7. g
8. b
9. c
10. k
11. i

Break It Down!
p   r cv s
1. a/men/o/rrhea
p   r cv s
2. dys/men/o/rrhea
r   cv s
3. hemat/o/salpinx
r   s
4. mast/algia
r cv r cv s
5. men/o/metr/o/rrhagia
r   cv s
6. metr/o/rrhea

Word Building
1. hematosalpinx
2. dysmenorrhea
3. mastalgia
4. metrorrhea
5. metrorrhagia
6. oligomenorrhea

Fill It In!
1. oligomenorrhea/dysmenorrhea/menometrorrhagia/amenorrhea
2. hydrosalpinx/pyosalpinx
3. metrorrhea/leukorrhea

Self Quiz 16.4

Say It—Spell It!
1. adenomyosis
2. dermoid cyst
3. endometrial cancer
4. endometriosis
5. endometritis
6. endocervicitis

7. fibrocystic
8. gynecomastia
9. gynopathic
10. hysteratresia
11. mastitis
12. mastoptosis
13. myometritis
14. oophoritis
15. parovarian cyst
16. perimetritis
17. salpingocele
18. cervicitis
19. vaginitis
20. vesicovaginal fistula

Match It!
1. f
2. i
3. j
4. k
5. l
6. h
7. b
8. g
9. a
10. d
11. e
12. c

Break It Down!

    p   r   s
1. a/mast/ia
    r   s
2. cervic/itis
    p   r cv s
3. endo/metr/i/osis
    r cv r   s
4. gynec/o/mast/ia
    r   s
5. mast/itis
    r cv r   s
6. my/o/metr/itis
    p   r   s
7. peri/metr/itis
    p   r   s
8. poly/mast/ia
    r cv r   s
9. vulv/o/vagin/itis

Word Building
1. adenomyosis
2. amastia
3. Bartholin's adenitis
4. gynopathic
5. vulvovaginitis
6. myometritis
7. oophoritis
8. salpingocele
9. mastitis
10. endocervicitis
11. hysteratresia
12. endometritis
13. endometriosis

Fill It In!
1. adenocarcinoma/fibrocystic
2. in situ/cervical intraepithelial/cervical cancer
3. endometrial cancer/uterine cancer/fibroid tumor/prolapsed uterus
4. dermoid cyst/ovarian cancer/parovarian cyst
5. rectovaginal fistula/vesicovaginal fistula
6. inflammatory disease/toxic shock syndrome/premenstrual syndrome

Self Quiz 16.5

Say It—Spell It!
1. hysterosalpingography
2. mammography
3. sonohysterography
4. colposcopy
5. hysteroscopy
6. culdocentesis
7. cervicectomy
8. colpoperineorrhaphy
9. colpoplasty
10. episioperinoplasty
11. hysterectomy
12. hysterosalpingo-oopherectomy
13. mastectomy
14. myomectomy
15. oophorectomy
16. perineorrhaphy
17. salpingectomy
18. salpingo-oophorectomy
19. trachelectomy
20. mammoplasty

Match It!
1. e
2. g
3. j
4. i
5. a
6. n
7. b
8. m
9. c
10. o
11. i
12. h
13. d
14. f
15. k
16. q
17. r
18. s
19. p

Break It Down!

    r cv s
1. mamm/o/graphy
    r cv r cv s
2. son/o/hyster/o/graphy
    r cv s
3. colp/o/scopy
    r cv s
4. hyster/o/scopy

    r cv s
5. lapar/o/scopy
    r cv s
6. culd/o/centesis
    r   s
7. cervic/ectomy
    r cv r cv s
8. colp/o/perine/o/rrhaphy
    r cv r cv s
9. episi/o/perine/o/plasty
    r   s
10. hymen/otomy
    r cv r cv r   s
11. hyster/o/salping/o/-oophor/ectomy

Word Building
1. culdocentesis
2. laparoscope
3. sonohysterography
4. hysterosalpigography
5. mammography
6. colposcope
7. transvaginal sonography
8. vaginal speculum
9. hormone replacement therapy
10. tubal ligation
11. cervical conization
12. cancer antigen-125 tumor marker
13. Papanicolau smear
14. biopsy
15. dilation and curettage
16. gynecology

Fill It In!
1. biopsy/Papanicolau smear/dilation and curettage
2. cancer antigen-125
3. vaginal speculum/cervical conization
4. tubal ligation
5. hormone replacement

Self Quiz 16.6
1. CIN
2. dilation and curettage
3. CIS
4. hormone replacement therapy
5. CA-125
6. premenstrual syndrome
7. ERT
8. toxic shock syndrome
9. PID
10. transvaginal sonography
11. GYN
12. biopsy
13. pap smear
14. anterior and posterior colporrhaphy
15. FBD
16. total abdominal hysterectomy/bilateral salpingo-oophorectomy

Chapter 17

Self Quiz 17.1

Definition
1. before

2. many
3. birth, labor
4. none
5. after
6. rupture
7. small

Word Root

1. amni, amnion
2. chori
3. embry
4. fet
5. gravid, cyes
6. lact
7. nat
8. omphal
9. par, part
10. puerper
11. ger, presby
12. ped
13. prim
14. toc

Self Quiz 17.2

Say It—Spell It!

1. lochia
2. meconium
3. embryogenic
4. lactogenic
5. gravida
6. para
7. puerpera
8. antepartum
9. gravidopuerperal
10. intrapartum
11. multigravida
12. multipara
13. nulligravida
14. nullipara
15. primigravida
16. primipara

Match It!

1. h
2. f
3. g
4. k
5. i
6. c
7. j
8. o
9. d
10. l
11. p
12. n
13. a
14. e
15. b
16. m
17. r
18. s
19. q
20. u
21. t

Break It Down!

1. ante/partum
   p   r
2. gravid/o/puerper/al
    r cv r   s
3. intra/partum
     p   r
4. multi/gravida
     p   r
5. multi/para
     p   r
6. nulli/gravida
     p   r
7. primi/para
      r   s
8. puerper/al

Fill It In!

1. pregnancy/cyesis/conception
2. gravida/para/premature/puerpera
3. neonate/childhood
4. puberty/adolescence
5. adulthood/senescence
6. prenatal development/embryo
7. fetus
8. amnion/amniotic fluid/placenta/ chorion/umbilical cord
9. parturition/labor
10. lochia/meconium

Self Quiz 17.3

Say It—Spell It!

1. amniorrhea
2. dystocia
3. hyperemesis gravidara
4. lactorrhea
5. polyhydramnios
6. psuedocyesis

Match It!

1. d
2. a
3. b
4. e
5. f
6. c

Break It Down!

1. dys/tocia
    p   s
2. hyper/emesis gravidar/a
    p   s   r s
3. lact/o/rrhea
    r cv s
4. poly/hydr/amni/o/s
   p   r   r cv s
5. pseud/o/cyes/is
    r cv   s

Word Building

1. lactorrhea
2. pseudocyesis
3. hyperemesis gravidara
4. polyhydramnios

5. amniorrhea
6. dystocia

Fill It In!

1. dystocia/hyperemesis gravidara
2. amniorrhea
3. pseudocyesis
4. lactorrhea

Self Quiz 17.4

Say It—Spell It!

1. amnionitis
2. amniorrhexis
3. chorioamnionitis
4. choriocarcinoma
5. embryotocia
6. erythroblastosis fetalis
7. hysterorrhexis
8. microcephaly
9. omphalitis
10. omphalocele
11. salpingocyesis
12. abortion
13. abruptio placentae
14. cervical effacement
15. congenital anomaly
16. esophageal atresia
17. placenta previa
18. preeclampsia
19. spina bifida

Match It!

1. c
2. e
3. g
4. d
5. f
6. b
7. a
8. m
9. j
10. h
11. r
12. i
13. o
14. q
15. n
16. k
17. s
18. u
19. p
20. l
21. t

Break It Down!

1. amnion/itis
    r   s
2. amni/o/rrhexis
   r cv r
3. chori/o/carcin/oma
   r cv r   s
4. embry/o/tocia
   r cv s

```
         r   cv    s
5.  hyster/o/rrhexis
         p     r     s
6.  micro/cephal/y
          r    cv  r   s
7.  salping/o/cyes/is
```

Word Building
1. omphalitis
2. hysterorrhexis
3. chorioamnionitis
4. choriocarcinoma
5. choriorrhexis
6. salpingocyesis
7. omphalocele
8. amnionitis

Fill It In!
1. abruptio placentae/miscarriage/abortion
2. breach
3. cervical effacement
4. congenital anomaly/cleft palate/ esophageal atresia/spina bifida
5. Down syndrome
6. rubella/hyaline membrane
7. ectopic pregnancy/placenta previa
8. preeclampsia/eclampsia

Self Quiz 17.5

Say It—Spell It!
1. amniocentesis
2. amniography
3. amnioscopy
4. amniotomy

5. cesarean section
6. episiotomy
7. fetometry
8. obstetrical sonography
9. pelvimetry
10. tocolytic
11. obstetrics
12. pediatrics
13. gerontology

Match It!
1. f
2. d
3. g
4. b
5. h
6. j
7. e
8. c
9. i
10. a

Break It Down!
```
         r  cv  s
1.  toc/o/lytic
         r  cv  s
2.  fet/o/metry
         r  cv  s
3.  amni/o/tomy
         r  cv  s
4.  pelv/i/metry
         r  cv  s
5.  amni/o/graphy
```

```
         r   cv    s
6.  amni/o/centesis
```

Word Building
1. amniocentesis
2. amniotomy
3. embryology
4. pediatrician
5. obstetrics
6. obstetrical sonography
7. episiotomy

Fill It In!
1. gerontologist
2. obstetrician
3. pediatrics
4. amniocentesis/obstetrical sonography
5. episiotomy/cesarean section

Self Quiz 17.6
1. date of birth
2. HMD
3. obstetrics
4. RDS
5. therapeutic abortion
6. LMP
7. cesarean section
8. EDD
9. pediatrics
10. GER
11. newborn
12. OB/GYN
13. spontaneous abortion
14. PIH

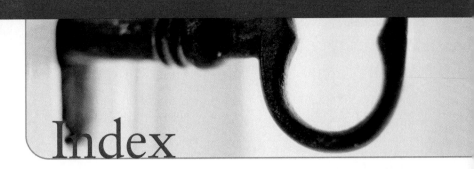

Index

[a]

Abbreviations
 blood and the lymphatic system, listed, 404
 cancer, listed, 80
 cardiovascular system, listed, 359
 digestive system, listed, 507
 ears, listed, 273
 endocrine system, listed, 310
 eyes, listed, 246
 female reproductive system, listed, 627–28
 human body, listed, 51
 integumentary system, listed, 115
 male reproductive system, listed, 584
 musculoskeletal system, listed, 165
 nervous system, listed, 212
 obstetrics and human development, listed, 666
 respiratory system, listed, 455
 urinary system, listed, 549
Abdominal regions, 29–30, 31f
Abdominopelvic cavity, 30, 32f
Abnormal, 4, 6, 7
ABO blood typing system, 373
Abruptio placentae, 651f
Abscess, 98
Absorption, 466
Acetaminophen, 473
Achondroplasia, 147f
Acidosis, 302
Acne, 104f
Acquired immune response, 377–78
Acromegaly, 294f
Acronyms, 2
Actinic dermatitis, 105
Addison, Thomas, 294
Addison's disease, 294
Adenohypophysis, 283
Adolescence, 642
Adrenal cortex, 285
Adrenal glands, 285
Adrenaline, 285
Adrenal medulla, 285
Adrenocorticotrophic hormone (ACTH), 283
Adulthood, 642
Afferent nerves, 185
Agranulocytes, 375
AIDS (acquired immune deficiency syndrome), 107f, 648. see also HIV (human immunodeficiency virus)
Aldosterone, 285
Allergy skin tests, 388f
Alopecia, 99f
Alveolar glands, 597
Alveolar macrophage, 422

Alveoli, 419–22
Alzheimer, Alois, 194
Alzheimer's disease (AD), 194f
American Cancer Society, 69, 74, 574, 613, 623
American Heart Association, 340f
American Medical Association (AMA), 574
Amniocentesis, 661f
Amnion, 638
Amniotic fluid, 641
Amylase, 473
Amyloid plaques, 194f
Anaplasia, 69
Anatomical planes, 28–29, 30f
Anatomical position, 28
Anatomical regions, 29–30, 31f
Anatomy, 26. see also Human body
Androgens, 285
Andry, Nicholas, 143
Aneurysm, 335f
Angina pectoris, 340
Angiogram, 346f
Angioscopy, 347f
Anorexia, 395
Anterior, 28, 29f
Anterior chamber of eye, 224
Antibiotics, 384, 438
Antibodies, 375
Antidiuretic hormone (ADH), 283
Antigens, 375
Anus, 472
Aorta, 321, 322
Appendages, 30
Appendicitis, 482f
Appendix, 4, 472
Aqueous humor, 224, 238
Arachnoid, 180, 181f
Areola, 597
Aristotle, 2, 62, 319, 349
Arteries, 319, 320, 324
Arterioles, 324
Arteriopathy, 10–11
Arteriosclerosis, 14
Arteriovenous, 9
Arthrocentesis, 159f
Arthrologist, 127
Arthrology, 127
Arthropathy, 8
Arthroscopic surgery, 160f
Articulations. see Joints
Asthma, 431
Atelectasis, 437f
Atherectomy, 348f
Atherosclerosis, 14, 336f, 341
Atoms, 26
Atria, 321
Atrioventricular (AV) bundle, 323
Atrioventricular (AV) node, 323

Atrioventricular (AV) valves, 321
Audation, 222, 254, 255, 261
Audiologist, 261
Audiology, 261
Audiometry, 269f
Auricles, 255
Auscultation, 348f, 349, 442f
Autonomic nerves, 185
Axons, 178, 179f, 183, 185

[b]

Bacteriology, 384
Balloon angioplasty, 341, 346f
Bartholin's glands, 597
Basal cell carcinoma, 104f
Basophils, 375
B cells, 375, 377
Benign prostatic hyperplasia (BPH), 566, 570f, 574
Benign tumors, 69
Biceps brachii, 133, 136
Bicuspid valve, 321
Bilateral, 4
Bile, 473
Biliary ducts, 473
Biopsy (Bx), 618f
Bladder, urinary, 520
Blepharoptosis, 230f
Blind spot, 226
Blood. see also Cardiovascular system
 ABO typing system, 373
 agranulocytes, 375
 antibodies, 375
 antigens, 375
 basophils, 375
 B cells, 375
 clots, 373, 374f
 coagulation, 373
 color of, 373
 as diagnostic tool, 383
 eosinophils, 375
 erythrocytes, 372
 fibrinogen, 372
 granulocytes, 375
 hematopoiesis, 373, 374f
 hemoglobin, 372–73
 immune response, 375
 leukocytes, 373, 375
 loss of, 383
 lymphocytes, 375
 macrophages, 375
 monocytes, 375
 neutrophils, 375
 phagocytosis, 375
 plasma, 372

Blood (*cont.*)
  platelets, 373
  red blood cells (RBCs), 372, 373f
  red bone marrow, 373
  Rh typing system, 373
  serum, 372
  stem cells, 373
  T cells, 375
  thrombocytes, 373
  typing, 373
  white blood cells (WBCs), 373
Blood and the lymphatic system. *see also*
    Blood; Lymphatic system
  abbreviations, listed, 404
  allergy skin tests, 388f
  antibiotics, 384
  bacteriology, 384
  blood transfusions, 399f
  diphtheria, 388, 389f
  diseases and disorders, listed, 387–93
  hematologist, 383
  hematology, 383
  hematopathologist, 383
  HIV (human immunodeficiency virus),
    384, 394–95, 657
  immunology, 383–84
  infectious diseases, 383
  interrelationship between, 370
  leukemia, 391f
  lymph, formation of, 370, 372
  malaria, 391f, 392
  mononucleosis, 392f
  prefixes, listed, 370
  roots, listed, 370, 378–79
  sickle cell anemia, 393f
  suffixes, listed, 371
  symptoms and signs, listed, 385
  toxicology, 384
  treatments, procedures, and devices,
    listed, 398–401
  vaccines, immunization with, 400f, 401
  viral infections, 384
  virology, 384
  vocabulary words, listed, 380
  word parts, listed, 370–71
Blood-brain barrier, 183, 190
Blood circulation, 318, 320, 321–22, 323
Blood pressure, 324
Blood transfusions, 399f
Blood vessels, 323–24
Body cavities, 30, 32f
Bone matrix, 128
Bowman's capsule (BC), 518–19
Brachial region, 29, 31f
Brain
  activities, 180
  amyloid plaques, 194f
  blood-brain barrier, 183, 190
  bood flow, importance of, 180
  cerebellum, 181, 182
  cerebral cortex, 181, 255
  cerebral hemispheres, 181
  cerebrum, 181
  corpus callosum, 181
  cranial nerves, 180, 183
  diencephalon, 181, 182–83
  gray and white matter, 180
  hypothalmus, 183, 282
  lobes, 181–82

main parts of, 182f
  medulla, 183
  nervous system, as part of, 178, 179f
  neurofibrillary tangles, 194f
  pons, 183
  stem, 181, 183
  thalmus, 183
  ventricles, 183, 202
  visual cortex, 229
  weight of, 180
Brain stem, 181, 183
Breast biopsy, 614
Breast cancer, 608f, 614
Breast nipples, 597
Bronchi, 418–19
Bronchial tree, 418–19, 420f
Bronchioles, 418–19
Bronchogenic carcinoma, 432f
Bronchoscopy, 443f
Building blocks, of body. *see under* Human
    Body
Bulbourethral glands, 559, 561
Bundle of His, 323
Bunions, 146
Bursae, 131

[c]

Caesar, Julius, 661
Calcitonin (CT), 284
Canal of Schlemm, 238
Cancer
  abbreviations, listed, 80
  anaplasia, 69
  basal cell carcinoma, 104f
  benign versus malignant, 69
  breast, 608f, 614
  bronchogenic carcinoma, 432f
  Cancer antigen-125 tumor marker (CA-
    125), 613
  carcinogens, 74
  carcinoma in situ (CIS) of the cervix,
    613
  as cause of death, annually in U.S., 69,
    74
  cervical, 608f, 613
  colorectal, 484f
  constructed terms, rules for assembling,
    69
  diseases and disorders, listed, 73–74
  DNA (deoxyribonucleic acid), 69,
    74–75
  dysplasia, 69
  endometrial, 610f, 613
  gastric, 486f
  gliomas, 74, 197f
  infiltrating ductal carcinoma (IDC), 614
  Kaposi's sarcoma, 107f, 395
  Latin word meaning, 69
  lipoma, 69
  liposarcoma, 69
  melanoma, 75, 107f
  metastasis, 69, 70f, 75, 383
  myoma, 69
  myosarcoma, 69
  neoplasms, 69, 75
  neurocarcinoma, 69

neuroma, 69
  oncogenes, 74
  oncologist, 69
  oncology, 69
  osteosarcoma, 153f
  ovarian, 611f
  ovarian cancer, 614
  Pap (Papanicolau) smear, 613, 623
  prostate, 572f, 574
  sarcomas, 69, 74
  squamous cell carcinoma, 109f
  suppressor genes, 74–75
  symptoms and signs, listed, 71
  treatments, procedures, and devices,
    listed, 78
  tumors, formation of, 69, 70f
  types of, naming, 69
  uterine, 613
Cancer antigen-125 tumor marker (CA-
    125), 613
Candidiasis, 395
Capillaries, 320, 322, 324
Carbuncles, 104f
Carcinogens, 74
Carcinoma in situ (CIS) of the cervix, 613
Cardia, 471
Cardiac arrest, 341
Cardiac catheterization, 349f
Cardiac muscle, 63, 64f
Cardiac output (CO), 322
Cardiac pacemaker, 350f
Cardiologist, 332
Cardiology, 332
Cardiopulmonary resuscitation (CPR), 447
Cardiovascular system
  abbreviations, listed, 359
  aneurysm, 335f
  angina pectoris, 340
  angiogram, 346f
  angioscopy, 347f
  arteries, 319, 320, 324
  arterioles, 324
  atherectomy, 348f
  atherosclerosis, 336f, 341
  auscultation, 348f, 349
  balloon angioplasty, 341, 346f
  blood circulation, 318, 320, 321–22, 323
  blood pressure, 324
  blood vessels, 323–24
  capillaries, 320, 322, 324
  cardiac arrest, 341
  cardiac catheterization, 349f
  cardiac output (CO), 322
  cardiac pacemaker, 350f
  cardi and vascul (word roots), 320
  cardiologist, 332
  cardiology, 332
  cardiopulmonary resuscitation (CPR),
    447
  coronary artery bypass graft (CABG),
    341, 351f
  coronary circulation, 322
  coronary stent, 351f
  defibrillation, 352f
  diastole, 324
  diseases and disorders, listed, 335–40
  Doppler sonography, 353f
  electrocardiography (ECG or EKG), 354f
  embolus, 341

endocarditis, 338f
endothelium, 324
heart. *see* Heart
heart attack, 341
heart disease, 340–41
heart transplants, 341
interstitial fluid, 324
myocardial infarction (MI), 339f, 340–41
prefixes, listed, 318
pulmonary circulation, 322
roots, listed, 318–19, 325–27
sphygmomanometry, 355f
suffixes, listed, 319
symptoms and signs, listed, 333
systemic circulation, 322
systole, 324
thrombus, 341
treatments, procedures, and devices, listed, 346–56
valvuloplasty, 356f
varicosis, 340f
vasoconstriction, 324
vasodilation, 324
veins, 320, 324
venules, 324
vocabulary words, listed, 327
word parts, listed, 318–19
Carpal tunnel syndrome (CTS), 147f
Cartilaginous joints, 131
Cataracts, 233, 241f
Catheter, 544
CAT (computed axial tomography) scans, 2, 44–45, 196f, 478
Caudal, 28
Cavities, 30, 32f
CD-4 receptors, 394
Cecum, 472
Cell body, of neuron, 178, 179f, 180
Cell membrane, 61
Cells. *see also* Blood; Cancer; Lymphatic system; Tissues
    B cells, 375, 377
    cell membrane, 61
    chromosomes, 62
    cytologist, 58
    cytology, 58
    cytoplasm, 61
    defined, 28, 58
    DNA (deoxyribonucleic acid), 61
    genes, 61
    hepatic, 473
    metabolism, 282
    microglia, 190
    neuroglial, 63, 178
    neurons, 63, 94, 178–79, 180
    nuclei, 61–62
    organelles, 61
    osteoblasts, 128
    osteoclasts, 128–29
    osteocytes, 128
    phagocytic white blood, 110, 375
    protein synthesis, 282
    Schwann, 178
    secretory, 62
    target, 282
    T cells, 375, 377
    word origin, 58
    word parts, listed, 58–59

Cellulitis, 104f
Centers for Disease Control (CDC), 190
Central nervous system (CNS)
    arachnoid, 180, 181f
    brain. *see* Brain
    cerebrospinal fluid (CSF), 183
    dura mater, 180, 181f
    lumbar puncture (LP), 183, 207f
    meninges, 180, 181f
    roots and nerves, spinal, 183
    spinal cord, 183, 184f
    subarachnoid space, 180, 181f
Cephalic, 28, 29f
Cephalic region, 29, 31f
Cerebellum, 181, 182
Cerebral aneurysm, 206f
Cerebral angiography, 205f
Cerebral cortex, 181, 255
Cerebral hemispheres, 181
Cerebrospinal fluid (CSF), 183, 202
Cerebrovascular accident (CVA), 190, 191f, 202
Cerebrum, 181
Cerumen, 255
Cervical canal, 595
Cervical cancer, 608f, 613
Cervical conization, 613
Cervical intraepithelial neoplasia (CIN), 613
Cervical region, 29, 31f
Cervix, 595
Cesarean section, 661
Chalazion, 233
Chest x-ray (CXR), 444f
Childhood, 642
Cholecystitis, 482
Cholelithiasis, 483f
Chorion, 638
Choroid, 224, 225
Chromosomes, 62
Cilia, 418
Ciliary muscles, 224
Circumcision, 562, 577f
Cirrhosis, 483f
Clavicle, 129
Cleft palate, 652f
Clitoris, 597
Closed fractures, 156
Clots, 373, 374f
Coagulation, 373
Coccyx, 129
Cochlea, 4, 256–57
Coitus, 559
Colitis, 484f
Collagen, 92, 128
Colles fracture, 156
Colon, 472
Colorectal cancer, 484f
Combining forms, 9–10
Combining vowels, 9
Common bile duct, 473
Compound fractures, 156
Conception, 638
Cones, 225
Congenital anomalies, 648
Conjunctiva, 224
Conjunctivitis, 234f
Connective tissues, 62–63, 128, 183
Constructed suffixes, 59

Constructed terms, 3, 69
Contact dermatitis, 105
Contraceptive diaphragm, 597
Cornea, 224
Coronal plane, 29, 30f
Coronary artery bypass graft (CABG), 341, 351f
Coronary circulation, 322
Coronary sinus, 321
Coronary stent, 351f
Corpus callosum, 181
Corynebacterium diphtheriae, 388, 389f
Costal cartilages, 131
CPR (cardiopulmonary resuscitation), 447
Cranial nerves, 180, 183
Craniectomy, 206f
Creatinine, 524
Crohn, B. B., 485
Crohn's disease, 484f, 485
Cryptorchidism, 569, 570f
Culdocentesis, 618f
Culdoscopy, 618f
Cushing's syndrome, 296f
Cuticle, 92–93
Cyesis, 638
Cystoscopy, 539f
Cystostomy, 539f
Cytologist, 58
Cytology, 58
Cytoplasm, 61

[d]

Debridement, 113f
Decubitus ulcer, 105f
Defecation, 466
Defibrillation, 352f
Dendrites, 178
Dermatitis, 105
Dermatologist, 98
Dermatology, 97–98
Dermis, 92
Diabetes insipidus (DI), 296
Diabetes mellitus (DM), 296, 297f, 302
Diabetic nephropathy, 297f
Diabetic retinopathy, 297f
Diagnosis
    CAT (computed axial tomography) scans, 44–45, 196f, 478
    CT scan, chest, 443f
    endoscopy, 44, 45f
    MRI (magnetic resonance imaging), 45–46, 198f, 200f, 208f, 478
    PET (positron emission tomography) scans, 45, 46f, 194f, 197f
    sonography, 46
    ultrasound imaging, 46
    urine testing, 524
    ventilation-perfusion scanning, 451f
Diaphragm, 2, 30, 32f, 414
Diarrhea, 479
Diastole, 324
Diencephalon, 181, 182–83
Digestion, 466
Digestive flora, 478

Digestive system. *see also* Gastrointestinal (GI) tract
  abbreviations, listed, 507
  absorption, 466
  amylase, 473
  anoplasty, 497f
  appendicitis, 482f
  barium enema (BE), 497f
  bile, 473
  biliary ducts, 473
  CAT (computed axial tomography) scans, 478
  cholecystectomy, 498
  cholecystitis, 482
  cholelithiasis, 483f
  cirrhosis, 483f
  colitis, 484f
  colonoscopy, 499f
  colorectal cancer, 484f
  common bile duct, 473
  Crohn's disease, 484f, 485
  defecation, 466
  diarrhea, 479
  digestion, 466
  digestive flora, 478
  diseases and disorders, listed, 481–91
  diverticulitis, 485f
  E. coli, 478, 479
  gallbladder, 471f, 473
  gastric cancer, 486f
  gastroenterologist, 478
  gastroscopy, 500f
  glossitis, 487f
  head and neck specialist, 478
  hepatic cells, 473
  hepatitis types (A, B, C, D, and E), 487
  hepatobiliary specialist, 478
  hepatoma, 488f
  hiatal hernia, 488f
  icterus, 480
  ileostomy, 501f
  ingestion, 466
  internal medicine, 478
  intussusception, 489f
  jaundice, 473, 480
  laparoscopy, 502f
  liver, 471f, 473
  mastication, 466, 470
  MRI (magnetic resonance imaging), 478
  oncologist, 478
  pancreas, 473
  pancreatic juice, 473
  parotid glands, 471f, 473
  polyposis, 490f
  polyps, 490f
  prefixes, listed, 466
  proctologist, 478
  roots, listed, 467, 474–75
  saliva, 473
  salivary glands, 473
  sublingual glands, 471f, 473
  submandibular glands, 471f, 473
  suffixes, listed, 467
  swallowing, 466
  swallow reflex, 470
  symptoms and signs, listed, 479–80
  treatments, procedures, and devices, listed, 496–503
  upper GI (UGI) series, 503f
  vocabulary words, listed, 475
  volvulus, 491f
  word parts, listed, 466–67
Digital rectal exam (DRE), 574, 578f
Diphtheria, 388, 389f
Directional terms, 28, 29f
Disease
  defined, 41
  diagnosis. *see* Diagnosis
  inflammation, 44
  pathologist, 41
  pathology, 41
  sequelae, 44
  trauma, 44
Distal, 28, 29f
Diverticulitis, 485f
DNA (deoxyribonucleic acid), 61, 69, 74–75, 92, 638
Doppler sonography, 353f
Dorsal, 28, 29f
Dorsal cavity, 30
Ductus deferens, 560
Ductus epididymidis, 560
Duodenum, 471–72
Dura mater, 180, 181f
Dysplasia, 69

[e]

Ears
  abbreviations, listed, 273
  audation, 222, 254, 255, 261
  audiologist, 261
  audiology, 261
  audiometry, 269f
  auricles, 255
  cerumen, 255
  cochlea, 256–57
  diseases and disorders, listed, 264–66
  ENT (ear, nose, and throat), 261
  equilibrium, 255, 257, 261
  Eustachian tube, 256, 266
  external auditory canal, 255
  incus, 256
  inner ear, 256
  labyrinth, 256–57
  labyrinthectomy, 269f
  malleus, 256
  mastoid process, 255
  middle ear, 256
  myringitis, 265f
  myringoplasty, 266
  organ of Corti, 257
  ossicles, 256
  otitis media (OM), 265f, 266
  otologist, 261
  otology, 261
  otorhinolaryngologist, 261
  otorhinolaryngology, 261
  otoscopy, 270f
  outer ear, 255
  oval window, 257
  palatine tonsils, 266
  prefixes, listed, 254
  roots, listed, 254, 258
  semicircular canals, 256, 257
  sound wave transmission, 256, 257, 258f
  stapes, 256
  suffixes, listed, 254
  symptoms and signs, listed, 262
  treatments, procedures, and devices, listed, 269–70
  tympanic cavity, 256
  tympanic membrane, 256, 257f, 266
  tympanoplasty, 266
  vestibule, 256, 257
  vocabulary words, listed, 259
  word parts, listed, 254
Ecchymosis, 106f
Eclampsia, 652
E. coli, 478, 479, 603
Ectopic pregnancies, 653f
Efferent nerves, 185
Ejaculation, 559, 561
Ejaculatory duct, 561
Elastin, 92
Electrocardiography (ECG or EKG), 354f
Electroencephalogram (EEG), 206f
Electromyography (EMG), 161f
Embolus, 341
Embryo, 638, 640f, 643
Emmetropia, 231f
Emphysema, 433f
Encephalitis, 196f
Endocarditis, 8, 338f
Endocardium, 321
Endocrine glands. *see also* Endocrine system; Hormones
  adenohypophysis, 283
  adrenal cortex, 285
  adrenal glands, 285
  adrenal medulla, 285
  anterior lobe, pituitary gland, 283
  distribution, throughout body, 283f
  gonads, 287
  hypophysis, 282–83
  islets of Langerhans, 286, 302
  neurohypophysis, 283
  ovaries, 287
  pancreas, 285–86, 287
  parathyroid glands, 284, 285f
  pineal gland, 284
  pituitary gland, 282–83, 284f
  posterior lobe, pituitary gland, 283
  suprarenals, 285
  testes, 287
  thymus, 286
  thyroid gland, 284, 285f
Endocrine system
  abbreviations, listed, 310
  acidosis, 302
  acromegaly, 294f
  Addison's disease, 294
  blood glucose measurement, 306f
  Cushing's syndrome, 296f
  diabetes insipidus (DI), 296
  diabetes mellitus (DM), 296, 297f, 302
  diabetic nephropathy, 297f
  diabetic retinopathy, 297f
  diseases and disorders, listed, 293–301
  endocrinologist, 290
  endocrinology, 290

endocrinopathy, 290
exophthalmos, 291f
glands. *see* Endocrine glands
goiter, 291f
Graves' disease, 291f
homeostasis, 280
hormones, 282. *see also* Hormones
hperthyroidism, 299f
hyperglycemia, 302
hypersecretion, 290
hyposecretion, 290
hypothyroidism, 299f
islets of Langerhans, 286, 302
maturity-onset diabetes, 302
metabolism, 282
myxedema, 301f
prefixes, listed, 280
protein synthesis, 282
roots, listed, 280, 287
suffixes, listed, 281
symptoms and signs, listed, 290–91
syndrome, 290
target cells, 282
thyroidectomy, 307f
thyroid scan, 306f
treatments, procedures, and devices,
    listed, 305–07
type I diabetes (insulin-dependent),
    302
type II diabetes (noninsulin-dependent),
    302
vocabulary words, listed, 288
word parts, listed, 280–81
Endocrinologist, 290
Endocrinology, 290
Endocrinopathy, 290
Endometrial cancer, 610f, 613
Endometriosis, 610f
Endometrium, 595–96
Endoscopy, 44, 45f
Endothelium, 324
ENT (ear, nose, and throat), 261
Eosinophils, 375
Epicardium, 320–21
Epidermis, 91–92, 110
Epididymis, 559, 560
Epigastric region, 29, 31f
Epiglottis, 418
Epilepsy, 196
Epinephrine, 285
Epiphyseal plate, 131
Epispadias, 529f
Epithelial tissues, 62, 91
Epithelium, 62
Eponychium, 93
Eponyms, 2
Equilibrium, 255, 257, 261
Erasistratus, 180
Erection, 562
Erythroblastosis fetalis, 654f
Erythrocytes, 372
Esophageal atresia, 654f
Esophagus, 470–71
Estrogen, 285, 287, 592, 594
Eustachian tube, 256, 266
Exophthalmos, 291f
Expiration, 414
External auditory canal, 255

External genitalia
    female reproductive system, 596f, 597
    male reproductive system, 562
External urethral orifice, 521
External urethral sphincter, 520–21
Eyelid, 224
Eyes
    abbreviations, listed, 246
    anterior chamber, 224
    aqueous humor, 224, 238
    blepharoptosis, 230f
    blind spot, 226
    canal of Schlemm, 238
    cataracts, 233, 241f
    chalazion, 233
    choroid, 224, 225
    ciliary muscles, 224
    cones, 225
    conjunctiva, 224
    conjunctivitis, 234f
    cornea, 224
    emmetropia, 231f
    eyelid, 224
    fibrous layer, 224
    fovea centralis, 225–26
    glaucoma, 235f, 238
    hordeolum, 235f
    intraocular pressure, 238
    iris, 224
    keratoplasty, 242f
    keratotomy, 244
    lacrimal glands, 224
    LASIK (laser-assisted in situ
        keratomileusis), 244
    lens, 224
    macula, 226
    meibomian glands, 224, 233
    myopia, 231f, 236
    nervous layer, 225
    ophthalmologist, 229
    ophthalmology, 229
    ophthalmoscopy, 243f
    optic disc, 226
    optic nerve, 226, 238
    optometrist, 229
    optometry, 229, 243f
    orbit, 224
    photoreceptors, 225
    photorefractive keratotomy (PRK), 244
    posterior cavity, 224
    prefixes, listed, 222
    pupil, 224
    radial keratotomy (RK), 244
    refractive errors and treatment options,
        231f
    retina, 225
    retinopathy, 237f
    rods, 225
    roots, listed, 222, 226
    sclera, 224
    strabismus, 237f
    suffixes, listed, 223
    symptoms and signs, listed, 230
    thalmus, 229
    trabecular meshwork, 238
    vascular layer, 224
    vision, 222
    visual cortex, 229

    vitreous humor, 224–25
    vocabulary words, listed, 227
    word parts, listed, 222–23

[f]

Fallopian tubes, 594, 595
Fallopius, Gabrielle, 256
Fascia, 133
Feces, 472
Female reproductive system
    abbreviations, listed, 627–28
    alveolar glands, 597
    areola, 597
    Bartholin's glands, 597
    biopsy (Bx), 618f
    breast biopsy, 614
    breast cancer, 608f, 614
    Cancer antigen-125 tumor marker
        (CA-125), 613
    carcinoma in situ (CIS) of the cervix,
        613
    cervical cancer, 608f, 613
    cervical conization, 613
    cervical intraepithelial neoplasia (CIN),
        613
    clitoris, 597
    contraceptive diaphragm, 597
    culdocentesis, 618f
    culdoscopy, 618f
    diseases and disorders, listed, 607–13
    E. coli, 603
    endometrial cancer, 610f, 613
    endometriosis, 610f
    estrogen, 592, 594
    external genitalia, 596f, 597
    fallopian tubes, 594, 595
    fertilization, 592
    fibrocystic breast disease (FBD), 610f
    fibroid tumors, 610f
    fistula, 611f
    fornix, 596, 597
    graafian follicle, 594
    GYN clinics, 603
    gynecologist, 603
    gynecology, 603
    hormone replacement therapy (HRT),
        613
    human papilloma viruses (HPVs), 613
    hydrosalpinx, 604–05
    hymen, 596
    hysterectomy, 613, 614, 619f
    hysterosalpingogram (HSG), 620f
    hysterosalpingo-oophorectomy, 619f
    infection, 603
    infiltrating ductal carcinoma (IDC), 614
    infundibulum, 595
    labia, majora and minora, 597
    laparoscopy, 621f
    lumpectomy, 614
    mammary glands, 597
    mammography, 614, 621f
    mastectomy, 622f
    menopause, 594, 613
    modified radical mastectomy, 614
    mons pubis, 597

Female reproductive system (*cont.*)
nipples, 597
oocytes, 592
osteoporosis, 613
ova (ovum), 592, 594
ovarian cancer, 611f, 614
ovarian cortex and medulla, 594
ovarian cycle, 594
ovarian follicles, 594
ovaries, 594, 595f
oviducts, 595
ovulation, 594
panhysterectomy, 619f
Pap (Papanicolau) smear, 613, 623
perimetritis, 612f
perineum, 597
peritoneal cavity, 594
prefixes, listed, 592
progesterone, 592, 594
prolapsed uterus, 612f
puberty, 596
radical mastectomy, 614
roots, listed, 592, 598
salpingo-oophorectomy, 614, 619f
STDs (sexually transmitted diseases),
603
suffixes, listed, 593
symptoms and signs, listed, 604–05
total hysterectomy, 614
transvaginal sonography (TVS), 614
treatments, procedures, and devices,
listed, 617–24
tubal ligation, 624f
uterine cancer, 613
uterine tubes, 595
uterus. *see* Uterus
vagina, 596
vaginal orifice, 596
vaginal speculum, 624f
vaginitis, 613f
vestibule, 597
vocabulary words, listed, 599
vulva, 597
word parts, listed, 592–93
Femoral region, 29, 31f
Fertilization, 592, 638, 640f
Fetal alcohol syndrome (FAS), 657
Fetus, 638, 643
Fibrinogen, 372
Fibrocystic breast disease (FBD), 610f
Fibroid tumors, 610f
Fibrous joints, 131
Fibrous layer, 224
Fistula, 611f
Flash cards, 15
Fleming, Alexander, 384
Follicle-stimulating hormone (FSH), 283
Fornix, 596, 597
Fovea centralis, 225–26
Fractures
closed (simple) fracture, 156
Colles, 156
open (compound) fracture, 156
secondary categories, 156, 157f
Frontal plane, 29, 30f
Fundus
of stomach, 471
of uterus, 595
Furuncle, 99f

[g]

Gallbladder, 471f, 473
Ganglia, 179f, 185
Gastrectomy, 491
Gastric cancer, 486f
Gastric juice, 471
Gastric ulcers, 471, 489f, 491–92
Gastritis, 8
Gastroenterologist, 478
Gastrointestinal (GI) tract. *see also*
Digestive system
anus, 472
appendix, 472
body of stomach, 471
cardia, 471
cecum, 472
colon, 472
duodenum, 471–72
esophagus, 470–71
feces, 472
fundus, 471
gastrectomy, 491
gastric juice, 471
gastric ulcers, 471, 489f, 491–92
hard palate, 470
Helicobacter pylori, 492
hydochloric acid (HCl), 471
ileum, 471–72
jejunum, 471–72
large intestine, 472
oral cavity, 470
palate, 470
pepsin, 471
pepsinogen, 471
peptic ulcers, 471, 489f, 491–92
peristalsis, 470
peritoneum, 471
pharynx, 470
pyloric valve, 471
pyloroplasty, 491
pylorus, 471
rectum, 472
small intestine, 471–72
soft palate, 470
stomach, 471
teeth, 470
tongue, 470
uvula, 470
vagotomy, 491
villi, 471
Gastrology, 9
General practitioner (GP), 647
Genes, 61
Geriatrics, 647
Gerontologist, 648
Gerontology, 647
Glands, secretory function of, 62. *see also*
Digestive system; Endocrine glands;
Eyes; Female reproductive system;
Integumentary system; Male
reproductive system
Glans penis, 562
Glaucoma, 235f, 238
Glioblastoma multiforme, 197f
Gliomas, 74, 197f
Glomerulonephritis, 533
Glomerulus, 519

Glossitis, 487f
Glottis, 418
Glucagon, 286, 473
Glucocorticoids, 285
Gluteal region, 29
Goiter, 291f
Gonads, 287
Gout, 147, 148f
Graafian follicle, 594
Granulocytes, 375
Graves' disease, 291f
Gray matter, 179f, 180, 183
Growth hormone (GH), 283
Gustation, 222
GYN clinics, 603
Gynecologist, 603
Gynecology, 603, 647

[h]

Hair, 92, 93f
Hair follicles, 92, 93f
Hair root, 92, 93f
Hair shaft, 92, 93f
Hard palate, 470
Head and neck specialist, 478
Hearing. *see* Audation
Heart. *see also* Cardiovascular system
aorta, 321, 322
atria, 321
atrioventricular (AV) bundle, 323
atrioventricular (AV) node, 323
atrioventricular (AV) valves, 321
bicuspid valve, 321
bundle of His, 323
coronary sinus, 321
endocardium, 321
epicardium, 320–21
external anatomy, 322f
heart conduction system, 323
internal anatomy, 323f
mitral valve, 321, 327
myocardium, 321
parietal pericardium, 320
pericardial cavity, 320
pericardial sac, 320
pulmonary trunk, 321
pulmonary veins, 321
semilunar (SL) valves, 321
sinoatrial (SA) node, 323
tricuspid valve, 321
vena cavae, 321
ventricles, 321
visceral pericardium, 320
Heart attack, 341
Heart conduction system, 323
Heart disease, 340–41
Heart transplants, 341
Heimlich maneuver, 447
Helicobacter pylori, 492
Helper T cells, 377, 394–95
Hematologist, 383
Hematology, 383
Hematopathologist, 383
Hematopoiesis, 373, 374f
Hematuria, 526f
Hemodialysis (HD), 533–34

Hemoglobin, 372–73
Hepatic cells, 473
Hepatitis types (A, B, C, D, and E), 487
Hepatobiliary specialist, 478
Hepatoma, 488f
Herniated disk, 148f
Herpes, 106f, 395
Hiatal hernia, 488f
Hilum, 518
Hippocrates, 2, 196, 284
Histologist, 58
Histology, 58
HIV (human immunodeficiency virus), 384,
    394–95, 657
Hodgkin, William, 2
Hodgkin's lymphoma, 2
Homeostasis, 26, 91, 94, 97, 128, 129,
    178, 280
Hooke, Robert, 58
Hordeolum, 235f
Hormone replacement therapy (HRT), 613
Hormones. *see also* Endocrine glands;
        Endocrine system
    adrenaline, 285
    adrenocorticotrophic hormone (ACTH),
        283
    aldosterone, 285
    androgens, 285
    antidiuretic hormone (ADH), 283
    calcitonin (CT), 284
    epinephrine, 285
    estrogen, 285, 287
    follicle-stimulating hormone (FSH), 283
    glucagon, 286
    glucocorticoids, 285
    growth hormone (GH), 283
    insulin, 286
    luteinizing hormone (LH), 283
    melanocyte-stimulating hormone
        (MSH), 283
    melatonin, 284
    norepinephrine, 285
    oxytocin (OT), 283
    parathyroid hormone (PTH), 284
    progesterone, 287
    prolactin (PRL), 283
    testosterone, 287
    thymosin, 286
    thyroid-stimulating hormone (TSH),
        283
    thyroxine (T_4), 284
    triiodothyronine (T_3), 284
Hperthyroidism, 299f
Human body
    abbreviations, listed, 51
    abdominal regions, 29–30, 31f
    anatomy, 26
    appendages, 30
    atoms and molecules, 26
    building blocks, 26–28, 61
    cavities, 30, 32f
    cells, 28
    directional terms, 28, 29f
    diseases and disorders, listed, 43–44. *see
        also* Diagnosis; Disease
    homeostasis, 26
    organisms, 28
    organs, 28
    organ systems, 28

physiology, 26
planes, anatomical, 28–29, 30f
prefixes, listed, 24
regions, anatomical, 29–30, 31f
roots, listed, 24–25, 33–35
suffixes, listed, 25
symptoms and signs, listed, 42
tissues, 28
treatments, procedures, and devices,
    listed, 48–49
trunk, 30
viscera, 30
vocabulary words, listed, 35–37
word parts, listed, 24–25
Human development. *see* Obstetrics and
    human development
Human papilloma viruses (HPVs), 613
Humerus, 129
Hydorchloric acid (HCl), 471
Hydrocele, 571f
Hydrocephalus, 202
Hydronephrosis, 529f
Hydrosalpinx, 604–05
Hymen, 596
Hyperglycemia, 302
Hypersecretion, 290
Hypertension, 4, 6
Hypochondriac region, 29, 31f
Hypogastric region, 29, 31f
Hypophysis, 282–83
Hyposecretion, 290
Hypospadias, 529f
Hypothalmus, 183, 282
Hypothyroidism, 299f
Hysterectomy, 613, 614, 619f
Hysterosalpingogram (HSG), 620f
Hysterosalpingo-oophorectomy, 619f

[i]

Icterus, 480
Ileum, 14, 471–72
Iliac region, 29, 31f
Ilium, 14
Immune response, 375, 376–78
Immunity, 378
Immunology, 383–84
Impetigo, 107f
Incentive spirometer, 445f
Incus, 256
Infancy, 642
Infection, 377, 390f, 524, 533f, 603
Infectious diseases, 383
Inferior, 28, 29f
Infiltrating ductal carcinoma (IDC), 614
Inflammation, 44, 110, 377, 390f
Infundibulum, 595
Ingestion, 466
Inguinal region, 29, 31f
Inhalation, 414
Innate immune response, 377
Inner ear, 256
In situ, 607
Inspiration, 414
Insulin, 286, 473
Integumentary system. *see also* Skin
    abbreviations, listed, 115

abscess, 98
acne, 104f
alopecia, 99f
basal cell carcinoma, 104f
carbuncles, 104f
cellulitis, 104f
components, 88
cuticle, 92–93
decubitus ulcer, 105f
dermatitis, 105
dermatologist, 98
dermatology, 97–98
diseases and disorders, listed,
    104–09
ecchymosis, 106f
eponychium, 93
functions, 91, 93–94
furuncle, 99f
hair, 92, 93f
herpes, 106f
impetigo, 107f
Kaposi's sarcoma, 107f, 395
keloid, 100f
keratin, 91–92, 93
lunula, 92
melanoma, 107f
nail body, 92
nails, 92–93
nevus, 100f
onychomycosis, 107f
paronychia, 108f
pediculosis, 108f
prefixes, listed, 89
psoriasis, 108f
purpura, 100f
roots, listed, 89, 94–95
scleroderma, 108f
sebaceous glands, 93
sebum, 93
sensory receptors, 93f, 94, 185
skin signs, common, 101f
squamous cell carcinoma, 109f
suffixes, listed, 89
sweat glands, 88f, 93–94
symptoms and signs, listed, 98–101
tinea, 109f
treatments, procedures, and devices,
    listed, 112–13
vocabulary words, listed, 95
word parts, listed, 89
Internal medicine, 478
Internal urethral sphincter, 520
Interstitial cells, 560
Interstitial fluid, 324, 375
Intervertebral discs, 131
Intracranial pressure, 202
Intraocular pressure, 238
Intravenous, 6, 11
Intussusception, 489f
Iris, 224
Islets of Langerhans, 286, 302

[j]

Jaundice, 473, 480
Jejunum, 471–72
Jenner, Edward, 401

Joints. *see also* Skeletal system
  bursae, 131
  cartilaginous, 131
  costal cartilages, 131
  epiphyseal plate, 131
  fibrous, 131
  intervertebral discs, 131
  knee, 131f
  ligaments, 131
  menisci, 131
  symphysis pubis, 131
  synovial, 131
  synovial fluid, 131
  word origin, 127

[k]

Kaposi's sarcoma, 107f, 395
Keloid, 100f
Keratin, 91–92, 93, 110
Keratoplasty, 242f
Keratotomy, 244
Kidneys. *see also* Urinary system
  Bowman's capsule (BC), 518–19
  filtration, 519
  glomerulus, 519
  hemodialysis (HD), 533–34
  hilum, 518
  kidney transplant, 533, 542f
  location and size, 518
  nephrologist, 525
  nephrology, 525
  nephrons, 518
  reabsorption, 520
  renal artery, 518
  renal corpuscle, 519
  renal cortex, 518
  renal medulla, 518
  renal pelvis, 518
  renal tubule, 519–20
  renal veins, 518
  secretion, 520
  ureters, 518
  urine formation, 519–20
Kidney transplant, 533, 542f

[l]

Labia, majora and minora, 597
Labor, 638, 641f, 644
Labyrinth, 256–57
Labyrinthectomy, 269f
Lacrimal glands, 224
Laparoscopy, 621f
Large intestine, 472
Larynx, 418
LASIK (laser-assisted in situ
  keratomileusis), 244
Lateral, 28, 29f
Legionnaire's disease, 434
Lens, 224
Leukemia, 391f
Leukocytes, 373, 375
Ligaments, 131
Lipoma, 69

Liposarcoma, 69
Lithotripsy, 540f
Liver, 471f, 473
Lobes, 181–82, 422
Lower respiratory tract, 418–19
Lumbar puncture (LP), 183, 207f
Lumbar region, 29–30, 31f
Lumpectomy, 614
Lungs, 422
Lunula, 92
Luteinizing hormone (LH), 283
Lymph, 370, 371, 375
Lymphatic capillaries, 375
Lymphatic nodules, 375
Lymphatic system. *see also* Blood and the
    lymphatic system
  acquired immune response, 377–78
  B cells, 377
  CD-4 receptors, 394
  functions, 376, 383
  helper T cells, 377, 394–95
  immune response, 376–78
  immunity, 378
  infection, 377, 390f
  inflammation, 377, 390f
  innate immune response, 377
  interstitial fluid, 375
  lymph, 370, 371, 375
  lymphatic capillaries, 375
  lymphatic nodules, 375
  lymphatic trunks, 375
  lymph nodes, 375, 376f, 377
  lymphocytes, 377
  macrophages, 377, 378f
  metastasis, 383
  monocytes, 377
  neutrophils, 377
  pathogens, 376–78
  phagocytic white blood cells, 377
  plasma cells, 377–78
  spleen, 375, 377
  T cells, 377
  thoracic duct, 375
  thymus gland, 375
  tonsils, 375
  toxins, 376–77
Lymphatic trunks, 375
Lymph nodes, 375, 376f, 377
Lymphocytes, 375, 377
Lymphoma, Hodgkin's, 2
Lysis, 539

[m]

Macrophages, 375, 377, 378f, 422
Macula, 226
Malaria, 391f, 392
Male reproductive system
  abbreviations, listed, 584
  benign prostatic hyperplasia (BPH), 566,
    570f, 574
  bulbourethral glands, 559, 561
  circumcision, 562, 577f
  coitus, 559
  cryptorchidism, 569, 570f
  digital rectal exam (DRE), 574, 578f
  diseases and disorders, listed, 569–73

  ductus deferens, 560
  ductus epididymidis, 560
  ejaculation, 559, 561
  ejaculatory duct, 561
  epididymis, 559, 560
  erection, 562
  external genitalia, 562
  glands, 561
  glans penis, 562
  hydrocele, 571f
  interstitial cells, 560
  orchidectomy, 578f
  organs, 559, 560f
  orgasm, 559
  penile implants, 579f
  penis, 561, 562
  phimosis, 572f
  pituitary gland, 560
  prefixes, listed, 558
  prepuce, 562
  Proscar, 574
  prostate cancer, 572f, 574
  prostatectomy, 579f
  prostate gland, 559, 561
  prostate-specific antigen (PSA), 574
  roots, listed, 558, 563
  scrotum, 559, 562
  semen, 561
  seminal duct, 560
  seminal vesicles, 559, 561
  seminiferous tubules, 560
  sexual climax, 559
  spermatic cord, 560
  spermatogenesis, 560
  spermatozoa, 558
  STDs (sexually transmitted diseases),
    566, 570f
  suffixes, listed, 558
  symptoms and signs, listed, 567
  syphilis, 573
  testes (testis), 559, 561f
  testicular torsion, 573f
  testosterone, 558, 560
  treatments, procedures, and devices,
    listed, 577–81
  tubules, 560–61
  TUIP (transurethral incision of the
    prostate gland), 574
  TUMT (transurethral microwave ther-
    motherapy), 574
  TURP (transurethral resection of the
    prostate gland), 574, 580f
  urethra, 559
  urinary meatus, 561
  urologist, 566
  varicocele, 573f
  vas deferens, 559, 560
  vasectomy, 581f
  venereal diseases, 566
  vocabulary words, listed, 563
  word parts, listed, 558
Malignant, 69
Malleus, 256
Mammary glands, 597
Mammography, 614, 621f
Mandible, 129
Marshall, Barry, 491–92
Mastectomy, 622f
Mastication, 466, 470

Mastoid process, 255
Maturity-onset diabetes, 302
Maxilla, 129
Mechanical ventilation, 446f
Medial, 28, 29f
Medical terminology. *see also* Word parts
    acronyms, 2
    constructed terms, 2–3, 69
    defined, 2
    eponyms, 2
    flash cards, use of, 15
    Greek and Latin, use of, 2
    history, 2
    study tips, 15–16
    vocabulary words, 3
Medical terms. *see also* Abbreviations;
    Vocabulary words; Word parts
    blood and the lymphatic system, listed,
        385, 387–93, 398–401
    cancer, listed, 71, 73–74, 78
    cardiovascular system, listed, 333,
        335–40, 346–56
    constructing, 12–14
    defining and interpreting, 10–12
    digestive system, listed, 479–80,
        481–91, 496–503
    ears, listed, 262, 264–66, 269–70
    endings, singular and plural, 14–15
    endocrine system, listed, 290–91,
        293–301, 305–07
    eyes, listed, 230, 233–37, 241–43
    female reproductive system, listed,
        604–05, 607–13, 617–24
    human body, listed, 42, 43–44, 48–49.
        see also Diagnosis; Disease
    integumetary system, listed, 98–101,
        104–09, 112–13
    male reproductive system, listed, 567,
        569–73, 577–81
    musculoskeletal system, listed, 144,
        146–56, 159–62
    nervous system, listed, 192, 194–201,
        205–09
    obstetrics and human development,
        listed, 649, 651–56, 660–63
    pronunciation, 14
    respiratory system, listed, 427–28,
        431–38, 442–51
    in situ, 607
    spelling, 14, 16
    urinary system, listed, 525–26, 528–33,
        538–45
Medulla, 183
Meibomian glands, 224, 233
Melanin, 92
Melanocyte-stimulating hormone (MSH),
    283
Melanoma, 75, 107f
Melatonin, 284
Menarche, 596
Meninges, 180, 181f
Meningioma, 198f
Meningitis, 199f
Meningocele, 199f
Menisci, 131
Menopause, 594, 596, 613
Menses, 596
Menstrual cycle, 596
Menstruation, 596

Metabolism, 282
Metastasis, 69, 70f, 75, 383
Microglia, 190
Micturition, 521
Middle ear, 256
Minos, King of Crete, 257
Mitral valve, 321, 327
Modified radical mastectomy, 614
Molecules, 26
Monocytes, 375, 377
Mononucleosis, 392f
Mons pubis, 597
Motor nerves, 185
Mouth-to-mouth resuscitation, 447
MRI (magnetic resonance imaging), 45–46,
    198f, 200f, 208f, 478
Mucous membrane, 418
Mucus, 418
Multiple sclerosis (MS), 200f
Muscle tissue, 63, 64f
Muscular system. *see also* Musculoskeletal
        system
    biceps brachii, 133, 136
    fascia, 133
    major muscles, human body, 132–33f
    movement, 132
    muscle actions, 133, 135
    skeletal muscle fibers, 133, 134f
    structure, of muscles, 133, 134f
    tendons, 132
    tissues, types of, 134f
    word origins, 132
Musculoskeletal system. *see also* Joints;
        Muscular system; Skeletal system
    abbreviations, listed, 165
    achondroplasia, 147f
    arthrocentesis, 159f
    arthroscopic surgery, 160f
    bones, joints, and muscles, naming,
        135–36
    bunions, 146
    carpal tunnel syndrome (CTS), 147f
    diseases and disorders, listed, 146–56
    electromyography (EMG), 161f
    gout, 147, 148f
    herniated disk, 148f
    orthopedics, 143
    orthopedist, 143
    osteoarthritis, 151f
    osteoporosis, 152f
    osteosarcoma, 153f
    prefixes, listed, 124
    rheumatoid arthritis (RA), 154f
    roots, listed, 124–25, 136–38
    rotator cuff tendonitis, 155f
    spinal disfigurements, 149f
    sprains, 155f
    suffixes, listed, 125
    symptoms and signs, listed, 144
    treatments, procedures, and devices,
        listed, 159–62
    vocabulary words, listed, 139–40
    word parts, listed, 124–25
Mycobacterium tuberculosis, 438–39
Myelin sheath, 178, 180
Myocardial infarction (MI), 339f, 340–41
Myocardium, 321
Myoma, 69
Myometrium, 595

Myopia, 231f, 236
Myosarcoma, 69
Myringitis, 265f
Myringoplasty, 266
Myxedema, 301f

[n]

Nail body, 92
Nails, 92–93
Nasal cavity, 418
Nasal septum, 418
Neonate, 641
Neoplasms, 69, 75
Nephroblastoma, 530f
Nephrolithiasis, 531f
Nephrologist, 525
Nephrology, 525
Nephrons, 518
Nerve impulses, 178
Nerves, 63, 94, 178, 179f, 180, 183,
    185
Nervous layer, 225
Nervous system, 205–08
    abbreviations, listed, 212
    Alzheimer's disease (AD), 194f
    axons, 178, 179f, 183, 185
    brain, 178, 179f. *see also* Brain
    cell body, of neuron, 178, 179f
    central nervous system (CNS), 178,
        179f. *see also* Central nervous system
        (CNS)
    cerebral aneurysm, 206f
    cerebral angiography, 205f
    cerebrospinal fluid (CSF), 183, 202
    cerebrovascular accident (CVA), 190,
        191f, 202
    craniectomy, 206f
    dendrites, 178
    diseases and disorders, listed,
        194–201
    electroencephalogram (EEG), 206f
    encephalitis, 196f
    epilepsy, 196
    gliomas, 197f
    gray matter, 179f, 180, 183
    homeostasis, 178
    hydrocephalus, 202
    intracranial pressure, 202
    lumbar puncture (LP), 183, 207f
    meningioma, 198f
    meningitis, 199f
    meningocele, 199f
    microglia, 190
    multiple sclerosis (MS), 200f
    myelin sheath, 178, 180
    nerve impulses, 178
    nerves, 178, 179f, 180, 183, 185
    neuroglial cells, 178
    neurologist, 190
    neurology, 190
    neurons, 178–79, 180
    neuroscience, 190
    neuroscientist, 190
    neurosurgeons, 190
    neurotransmitters, 179–80
    organization of, 178, 179f

Nervous system (*cont.*)
  peripheral nervous system (PNS), 178, 179f. *see also* Peripheral nervous system (PNS)
  prefixes, listed, 176
  psychiatrists, 190
  psychologists, 190
  roots, listed, 176, 186–87
  Schwann cells, 178
  spina bifida, 199f
  stroke, 190, 191f, 202
  suffixes, listed, 177
  symptoms and signs, listed, 192
  synapses, 179
  tissue, 178–79, 180f, 183
  treatments, procedures, and devices, listed, 205–09
  vocabulary words, listed, 187
  white matter, 179f, 180, 183
  word parts, listed, 176–77
Nervous tissue, 63, 64f, 178–79, 180f, 183
Neurocarcinoma, 69
Neurofibrillary tangles, 194f
Neuroglial cells, 63, 178
Neurohypophysis, 283
Neurologist, 190
Neurology, 190
Neuroma, 69
Neurons, 63, 94, 178–79, 180f
Neuroscience, 190
Neuroscientist, 190
Neurosurgeons, 190
Neurotransmitters, 179–80
Neutrophils, 375, 377
Nevus, 100f
Nipples, 597
Norepinephrine, 285
Nose, 418
Nose and throat specialist, 426
Nucleus, 61

[o]

OB (obstetrics), 647
OB/GYN (obstetrics/gynecology), 647
Obstetrician, 647
Obstetrics and human development
  abbreviations, listed, 666
  abruptio placentae, 651f
  AIDS (acquired immune deficiency syndrome), 648
  amniocentesis, 661f
  cesarean section, 661
  cleft palate, 652f
  congenital anomalies, 648
  diseases and disorders, listed, 651–56
  eclampsia, 652
  ectopic pregnancies, 653f
  episiotomy, 662f
  erythroblastosis fetalis, 654f
  esophageal atresia, 654f
  fetal alcohol syndrome (FAS), 657
  fetometry, 662f
  general practitioner (GP), 647
  geriatrics, 647
  gerontologist, 648
  gerontology, 647

  gynecology, 647
  HIV (human immunodeficiency virus), 657
  OB (obstetrics), 647
  OB/GYN (obstetrics/gynecology), 647
  obstetrical sonography, 663f
  obstetrician, 647
  omphalocele, 655f
  pediatrician, 647
  pediatrics, 647
  placental blood barrier, 656–57
  placenta previa, 655f
  postnatal development, 641–42. *see also* Postnatal development
  prefixes, listed, 636
  prenatal development, 638–41. *see also* Prenatal development and pregnancy
  roots, listed, 636–37, 643
  rubella, 648, 656
  salpingocyesis, 656f
  spina bifida, 656f
  suffixes, listed, 637
  symptoms and signs, listed, 649
  thalidomide, 657
  toxoplasmosis, 656–57
  treatments, procedures, and devices, listed, 660–63
  vocabulary words, listed, 639, 644
  word parts, listed, 636–37
Omphalocele, 655f
Oncogenes, 74
Oncologist, 69, 426, 478
Oncology, 69
Onychomycosis, 107f
Oocytes, 592
Open fractures, 156
Ophthalmologist, 229
Ophthalmology, 229
Ophthalmoscopy, 243f
Optic disc, 226
Optic nerve, 226, 238
Optometrist, 229
Optometry, 229, 243f
Orbit, 224
Orchidectomy, 578f
Organelles, 61
Organisms, 28
Organ of Corti, 257
Organs, 28
Organ systems, 28
Orgasm, 559
Orthopedics, 143
Orthopedist, 143
Ossicles, 256
Osteoarthritis, 151f
Osteoblasts, 128
Osteoclasts, 128–29
Osteocytes, 128
Osteologist, 127
Osteology, 127
Osteopathy, 9, 12–13
Osteoporosis, 152f, 613
Osteosarcoma, 153f
Otitis media (OM), 265f, 266
Otologist, 261
Otology, 261
Otorhinolaryngologist, 261
Otorhinolaryngology, 261
Otoscopy, 270f

Outer ear, 255
Ova (ovum), 592, 594
Oval window, 257
Ovarian cancer, 611f, 614
Ovarian cortex, 594
Ovarian cycle, 594
Ovarian follicles, 594
Ovarian medulla, 594
Ovaries, 287, 594, 595f
Oviducts, 595
Ovulation, 594
Oxytocin (OT), 283, 638

[p]

Pacemaker, 350f
Palate, 470
Palatine tonsils, 266
Pancreas, 285–86, 287, 473
Pancreatic juice, 473
Panhysterectomy, 619f
Papanicolau, George, 623
Pap (Papanicolau) smear, 613, 623
Paranasal sinuses, 418
Parathyroid glands, 284, 285f
Parathyroid hormone (PTH), 284
Parietal pericardium, 320
Parietal pleura, 422
Paronychia, 108f
Parotid glands, 471f, 473
Parturition, 638
Pathogens, 376–78
Pathologist, 41
Pathology, 41
Pediatrician, 647
Pediatrics, 647
Pediculosis, 108f
Penicillin, 384
Penicillium mold, 384
Penile implants, 579f
Penis, 561, 562
Pepsin, 471
Pepsinogen, 471
Peptic ulcers, 471, 489f, 491–92
Pericardial cavity, 320
Pericardial sac, 320
Perimetritis, 612f
Perimetrium, 595
Perineum, 597
Peripheral nervous system (PNS)
  afferent nerves, 185
  autonomic nerves, 185
  connective tissue, 183
  efferent nerves, 185
  ganglia, 179f, 185
  motor nerves, 185
  nerves, 183, 185
  sensory nerves, 185
  sensory receptors, 185
  somatic nerves, 185
Peristalsis, 471
Peritoneal cavity, 594
Peritoneum, 471
PET (positron emission tomography) scans, 45, 46f, 194f, 197f
Phagocytic white blood cells, 110, 375, 377
Phagocytosis, 375

Phalanges, 129
Pharynx, 418, 470
Phimosis, 572f
Photoreceptors, 225
Photorefractive keratotomy (PRK), 244
Physiology, 26. *see also* Human body
Pineal gland, 284
Pituitary gland, 282–83, 284f, 560
Placenta, 596, 638
Placental blood barrier, 656–57
Placenta previa, 655f
Plasma, 372
Plasma cells, 377–78
Platelets, 373
Plato, 593
Pleural cavity, 422
Pneumoconiosus, 435f
Pneumocystis carinii pneumonia (PCP), 395
Pneumonia, 395, 436f
Pneumothorax, 437f
Polycystic kidney, 532f
Polyposis, 490f
Polyps, 490f
Pons, 183
Posterior, 28, 29f
Posterior cavity, 224
Postnatal development
    adolescence, 642
    adulthood, 642
    childhood, 642
    infancy, 642
    neonate, 641
    puberty, 642
    senescence, 642
Prefixes
    blood and the lymphatic system, listed, 370
    cardiovascular system, listed, 318
    cells and tissues, listed, 58
    commonly used, listed, 6–7
    defined, 6
    digestive system, listed, 466
    ears, listed, 254
    endocrine system, listed, 280
    eyes, listed, 222
    female reproductive system, listed, 592
    human body, listed, 24
    integumentary system, 89
    male reproductive system, listed, 558
    musculoskeletal system, listed, 124
    obstetrics and human development, listed, 636
    respiratory system, listed, 414
    urinary system, listed, 516
Pregnancy. *see* Prenatal development and pregnancy
Prenatal development and pregnancy
    amnion, 638
    amniotic fluid, 641
    chorion, 638
    conception, 638
    cyesis, 638
    DNA (deoxyribonucleic acid), 638
    embryo, 638, 640f, 643
    fertilization, 638, 640f
    fetus, 638, 643
    labor, 638, 641f, 644
    obstetrics, 638
    oxytocin (OT), 638

parturition, 638
placenta, 638, 656–57
puerperium, 641
trimesters, 638
umbilical cord, 638
yolk sac, 638
zygote, 638
Prepuce, 562
Proctologist, 478
Progesterone, 287, 592, 594
Prolactin (PRL), 283
Prolapsed uterus, 612f
Proscar, 574
Prostate cancer, 572f, 574
Prostatectomy, 579f
Prostate gland, 521, 559, 561
Prostate-specific antigen (PSA), 574
Protein synthesis, 282
Proximal, 28, 29f
Psoriasis, 108f
Psychiatrists, 190
Psychologists, 190
Puberty, 596, 642
Puerperium, 641
Pulmonary angiography, 448f
Pulmonary circulation, 322
Pulmonary embolism, 448f
Pulmonary specialist, 426
Pulmonary trunk, 321
Pulmonary tuberculosis (TB). *see* Tuberculosis (TB)
Pulmonary veins, 321
Pulse oximetry, 447f
Pupil, 224
Purpura, 100f
Pyelonephritis, 532f
Pyloric valve, 471
Pyloroplasty, 491
Pylorus, 471
Pyuria, 526f

[r]

Radial keratotomy (RK), 244
Radical mastectomy, 614
Rectouterine pouch, 595
Rectum, 472
Red blood cells (RBCs), 372, 373f
Red bone marrow, 128, 373
Red Cross, 372
Renal artery, 518
Renal corpuscle, 519
Renal cortex, 518
Renal failure, acute and chronic, 533
Renal medulla, 518
Renal pelvis, 518
Renal transplant. *see* Kidney transplant
Renal tubule, 519–20
Renal veins, 518
Reproductive systems. *see* Female reproductive system; Male reproductive system
Respiration, 414
Respiratory membrane, 421
Respiratory system
    abbreviations, listed, 455
    alveolar macrophage, 422

alveoli, 419–22
asthma, 431
atelectasis, 437f
auscultation, 442f
bronchi, 418–19
bronchial tree, 418–19, 420f
bronchioles, 418–19
bronchogenic carcinoma, 432f
bronchoscopy, 443f
cardiopulmonary resuscitation (CPR), 447
chest x-ray (CXR), 444f
cilia, 418
conducting portion, 418–19
CT scan, chest, 443f
diaphragm, 414
diseases and disorders, listed, 431–38
emphysema, 433f
epiglottis, 418
expiration, 414
glottis, 418
Heimlich maneuver, 447
incentive spirometer, 445f
inhalation, 414
inspiration, 414
larynx, 418
Legionnaire's disease, 434
lobes, 422
lower respiratory tract, 418–19
lungs, 422
mechanical ventilation, 446f
mouth-to-mouth resuscitation, 447
mucous membrane, 418
mucus, 418
nasal cavity, 418
nasal septum, 418
nose, 418
nose and throat specialist, 426
oncologist, 426
organs, 417–18
paranasal sinuses, 418
parietal pleura, 422
pharynx, 418
pleural cavity, 422
pneumoconiosus, 435f
pneumonia, 436f
pneumothorax, 437f
prefixes, listed, 414
pulmonary angiography, 448f
pulmonary embolism, 448f
pulmonary specialist, 426
pulse oximetry, 447f
respiration, steps of, 414
respiratory membrane, 421
respiratory portion, 419–22
respiratory therapist, 426
resuscitation, 447
roots, listed, 415, 422–23
spirometry, 448f
sputum, 418
suffixes, listed, 415
surfactant, 421
symptoms and signs, listed, 427–28
TB skin test, 438, 450f
thoracotomy, 450f
trachea, 418
tracheostomy, 451f
treatments, procedures, and devices, listed, 442–51

Respiratory system (*cont.*)
    tuberculosis (TB), 437f, 438–39
    upper respiratory tract, 418
    ventilation, 414
    ventilation-perfusion scanning, 451f
    visceral pleura, 422
    vocabulary words, listed, 424
    vocal cords, 419f
    word parts, listed, 414–15
Respiratory therapist, 426
Resuscitation, 447
Retina, 225
Retinopathy, 237f
Retrograde pyelogram, 542f
Rh blood typing system, 373
Rheumatoid arthritis (RA), 154f
Rhitidoplasty, 113f
Ringworm, 109f
Rods, 225
Rotator cuff tendonitis, 155f
Rubella, 648, 656

[S]

Sacred Disease (Hippocrates), 196
Sagittal plane, 29, 30f
Saliva, 473
Salivary glands, 473
Salpingocyesis, 656f
Salpingo-oophorectomy, 614, 619f
Sarcomas, 69, 74
Scabs, 110
Scar tissue, 110
Schwann, Theodor, 178
Schwann cells, 178
Sclera, 224
Scleroderma, 108f
Scrotum, 559, 562
Sebaceous glands, 93
Sebum, 93
Secretory cells, 62
Semen, 561
Semicircular canals, 256, 257
Semilunar (SL) valves, 321
Seminal duct, 560
Seminal vesicles, 559, 561
Seminiferous tubules, 560
Senescence, 642
Sensory nerves, 94, 185
Sensory receptors, 93f, 94, 185, 222
Sequelae, 44
Serum, 372
Sexual climax, 559
Sexually transmitted diseases (STDs). *see*
    STDs (sexually transmitted diseases)
Sickle cell anemia, 393f
Simple fractures, 156
Sinoatrial (SA) node, 323
Skeletal muscle, 63, 64f, 133, 134f
Skeletal system. *see also* Musculoskeletal
    system
    arthrologist, 127
    arthrology, 127
    bone matrix, 128
    bones, internal components, 128
    bones of, 129–30f
    clavicle, 129

    coccyx, 129
    collagen, 128
    exercise, effect of, 128
    fractures, 156, 157f. *see also* Fractures
    functions, 127–28
    homeostasis, 129
    humerus, 129
    joints. *see* Joints
    mandible, 129
    mastoid process, 255
    maxilla, 129
    osteoblasts, 128
    osteoclasts, 128–29
    osteocytes, 128
    osteologist, 127
    osteology, 127
    phalanges, 129
    red bone marrow, 128, 373
    skeleton and bones, word origins of,
        127, 129
Skin. *see also* Integumentary system
    anatomy, 88f
    burns, 97, 110
    collagen, 92
    color, 92
    debridement, 113f
    dermis, 92
    elastin, 92
    epidermis, 91–92, 110
    grafts, 110
    inflammation, 110
    keratin, 91–92, 110
    layers, 91–92
    melanin, 92
    as protective barrier, 91, 110
    replacement, of epidermis, 91
    rhitidoplasty, 113f
    scabs, 110
    scar tissue, 110
    sensory perception/reception, 91
    subcutaneous layer, 92
    temperature regulation, 91, 93
    wound repair, 110
Skin signs, common, 101f
Small intestine, 471–72
Smooth muscle, 63, 64f
Soft palate, 470
Somatic nerves, 185
Sonography, 46
Sound wave transmission, 256, 257, 258f
Special senses, 222
Spermatic cord, 560
Spermatogenesis, 560
Spermatozoa, 558
Sphygmomanometry, 355f
Spina bifida, 199f, 656f
Spinal cord, 183, 184f
Spinal disfigurements, 149f
Spinal nerves, 183
Spinal roots, 183, 184f
Spirometry, 448f
Spleen, 375, 377
Sprains, 155f
Sputum, 418
Squamous cell carcinoma, 109f, 395
Stapes, 256
STDs (sexually transmitted diseases), 566,
    570f, 603
Stem cells, 110, 373

Stent, 351f
Stomach, 471
Strabismus, 237f
Stroke, 190, 191f, 202
Subarachnoid space, 180, 181f
Subcutaneous layer, 92
Sublingual glands, 471f, 473
Submandibular glands, 471f, 473
Suffixes
    blood and the lymphatic system, listed,
        371
    -capnia, 415
    cardiovascular system, listed, 319
    cells and tissues, listed, 59
    commonly used, listed, 8–9
    constructed, 59
    defined, 7–8
    digestive system, listed, 467
    ears, listed, 254
    endocrine system, listed, 281
    eyes, listed, 223
    female reproductive system, listed, 593
    -graphy versus -gram, 205–08
    human body, listed, 25
    integumentary system, 89
    male reproductive system, listed, 558
    musculoskeletal system, listed, 125
    obstetrics and human development,
        listed, 637
    respiratory system, listed, 415
    urinary system, listed, 517
Superior, 28, 29f
Suppressor genes, 74–75
Suprarenals, 285
Surfactant, 421
Swallowing, 466
Swallow reflex, 470
Sweat glands, 88f, 93–94
Symphysis pubis, 131
Symptoms and signs, 42
Synapses, 179
Syndrome, 290
Synovial fluid, 131
Synovial joints, 131
Syphilis, 573
Systemic circulation, 322
Systole, 324

[t]

Target cells, 282
TB skin test, 438, 450f
T cells, 375, 377
Teeth, 470
Tendons, 132
Testes, 287, 559, 561f
Testicular torsion, 573f
Testosterone, 287, 558, 560
Thalidomide, 657
Thalmus, 183, 229
Thoracic duct, 375
Thoracic region, 29, 31f
Thoracotomy, 450f
Thrombocytes, 373
Thrombus, 341
Thymosin, 286
Thymus, 286

Thymus gland, 375
Thyroidectomy, 307f
Thyroid gland, 284, 285f
Thyroid scan, 306f
Thyroid-stimulating hormone (TSH), 283
Thyroxine (T₄), 284
Tinea, 109f
Tissues. *see also* Cancer; Cells
  connective, 62–63, 128, 183
  defined, 28, 58, 62
  epithelial (epithelium), 62, 91
  histologist, 58
  histology, 58
  muscle, 63, 64f. *see also* Muscular
    system
  nervous, 63, 64f, 178–79, 180f, 183. *see
    also* Nervous system
  red bone marrow, 128
  secretion, 62
  word origin, 58
  word parts, listed, 58–59
Tongue, 470
Tonsils, 375
Total hysterectomy, 614
Toxicology, 384
Toxins, 376–77
Toxoplasma gondii, 656–57
Toxoplasmosis, 395, 656–57
Trabecular meshwork, 238
Trachea, 418
Tracheostomy, 451f
Transvaginal sonography (TVS), 614
Transverse plane, 29, 30f
Trauma, 44
Tricuspid valve, 321
Trigone, 520
Triiodothyronine (T₃), 284
Trimesters, 638
Trunk, 30
Tubal ligation, 624f
Tuberculosis (TB), 395, 437f, 438–39
TUIP (transurethral incision of the prostate
  gland), 574
Tumors, 69, 70f
TUMT (transurethral microwave
  thermotherapy), 574
TURP (transurethral resection of the
  prostate gland), 574, 580f
Tylenol, 473
Tympanic cavity, 256
Tympanic membrane, 256, 257f, 266
Tympanoplasty, 266
Type I diabetes (insulin-dependent), 302
Type II diabetes (noninsulin-dependent),
  302

[u]

Ultrasound imaging, 46
Umbilical cord, 638
Umbilical region, 30, 31f
Upper respiratory tract, 418
Ureters, 518, 520
Urethra, 520, 521, 559
Urethral sphincters, internal and external,
  520–21
Urinary bladder, 520

Urinary catheterization, 544f
Urinary meatus, 521, 561
Urinary system
  abbreviations, listed, 549
  cystoscopy, 539f
  cystostomy, 539f
  diseases and disorders, listed, 528–33
  epispadias, 529f
  excretion, 516
  external urethral orifice, 521
  external urethral sphincter, 520–21
  glomerulonephritis, 533
  hematuria, 526f
  hemodialysis (HD), 533–34
  hydronephrosis, 529f
  hypospadias, 529f
  infections, 524, 533f
  internal urethral sphincter, 520
  kidneys, 516. *see also* Kidneys
  kidney transplant, 533, 542f
  lithotripsy, 540f
  lysis, 539
  micturition, 521
  nephroblastoma, 530f
  nephrolithiasis, 531f
  polycystic kidney, 532f
  prefixes, listed, 516
  prostate gland, 521
  pyelonephritis, 532f
  pyuria, 526f
  renal failure, acute and chronic, 533
  retrograde pyelogram, 542f
  roots, listed, 516, 521–22
  suffixes, listed, 517
  symptoms and signs, listed, 525–26
  treatments, procedures, and devices,
    listed, 538–45
  trigone, 520
  ureters, 520
  urethra, 520, 521
  urinary bladder, 520
  urinary catheterization, 544f
  urinary meatus, 521
  urinary tract infection (UTI), 533f
  urine formation, 519–20
  urine testing, as diagnostic, 524
  urinometer, 543f
  urologist, 525
  urology, 524
  vocabulary words, listed, 522
  voiding, 521
  word parts, listed, 516–17
Urinary tract infection (UTI), 533f
Urine formation, 519–20
Urinometer, 543f
Urologist, 525, 566
Urology, 524
Uterine cancer, 613
Uterine cavity, 595
Uterine tubes, 595
Uterus
  body (or corpus), 595
  cervical canal, 595
  cervix, 595
  endometrium, 595–96
  external os, 595
  fundus, 595
  menarche, 596
  menopause, 596

  menses, 596
  menstrual cycle, 596
  menstruation, 596
  myometrium, 595
  perimetrium, 595
  placenta, 596
  prolapsed, 612f
  rectouterine pouch, 595
  size and location, 595
  uterine cavity, 595
  word origin, 593
Uvula, 4, 5f, 470

[v]

Vaccines, 400f, 401
Vagina, 596
Vaginal orifice, 596
Vaginal speculum, 624f
Vaginitis, 613f
Vagotomy, 491
Valvuloplasty, 356f
Varicocele, 573f
Varicosis, 340f
Vascular layer, 224
Vas deferens, 559, 560
Vasectomy, 581f
Vasoconstriction, 324
Vasodilation, 324
Veins, 320, 324
Vena cavae, 321
Venereal diseases, 566. *see also* STDs
  (sexually transmitted diseases)
Ventilation, 414, 446f
Ventilation-perfusion scanning, 451f
Ventral, 28, 29f
Ventral cavity, 30
Ventricles
  brain, 183, 202
  heart, 321
Venules, 324
Vestibule, 256, 257, 597
Villi, 471
Viral infections, 384
Virology, 384
Viscera, 30
Visceral pericardium, 320
Visceral pleura, 422
Vision, 222
Visual cortex, 229
Vitreous humor, 224–25
Vocabulary words
  blood and the lymphatic system, listed,
    380
  cardiovascular system, listed, 327
  cells and tissues, listed, 65–66
  defined, 3
  digestive system, listed, 475
  ears, 259
  endocrine system, listed, 287
  eyes, listed, 227
  female reproductive system, listed, 599
  human body, listed, 35–37
  integumentary system, listed, 95
  male reproductive system, listed, 563
  musculoskeletal system, listed, 139–40
  nervous system, listed, 187

Vocabulary words (*cont.*)
  obstetrics and human development, listed, 639, 644
  respiratory system, listed, 424
  urinary system, listed, 522
Vocal cords, 419f
Voiding, 521
Volvulus, 491f
Vulva, 597

[W]

White blood cells (WBCs), 373
White matter, 179f, 180, 183
Word parts. *see also* Medical terminology; Medical terms
  blood and the lymphatic system, listed, 370
  cardiovascular system, listed, 318–19
  cells and tissues, listed, 58–59
  combining vowels and forms, 9–10
  constructed terms, 3
  digestive system, listed, 466–67
  ears, listed, 254
  endocrine system, listed, 280–81
  eyes, listed, 222–23

female reproductive system, listed, 592–93
four types, listed, 3
Greek and Latin, 2–3, 4
human body, listed, 24–25
male reproductive system, listed, 558
musculoskeletal system, listed, 124–25
obstetrics and human development, listed, 636–37
prefixes, 6–7. *see also* Prefixes
purpose, 2
respiratory system, listed, 414–15
roots, 4–6. *see also* Word roots
suffixes, 7–9, 59. *see also* Suffixes
urinary system, listed, 516–17
Word roots
  blood and the lymphatic system, listed, 370, 378–79
  cardi and vascul, 320
  cardiovascular system, listed, 318–19, 325–27
  cells and tissues, listed, 59, 65
  commonly used, listed, 5
  defined, 4
  digestive system, listed, 467, 474–75
  ears, listed, 254, 258
  endocrine system, listed, 280, 287
  eyes, listed, 222, 226

female reproductive system, listed, 592, 598
Greek and Latin, 4
human body, listed, 24–25, 33–35
integumentary system, listed, 89, 94–95
male reproductive system, listed, 558, 563
musculoskeletal system, listed, 124–25, 136–38
nervous system, listed, 176, 186–87
obstetrics and human development, listed, 636–37, 643
orchi/o, 558
respiratory system, listed, 415, 422–23
urinary system, listed, 516, 521–22
Wound repair, 110

[Y]

Yolk sac, 638

[Z]

Zygote, 638

SINGLE PC LICENSE AGREEMENT AND LIMITED WARRANTY

READ THIS LICENSE CAREFULLY BEFORE OPENING THIS PACKAGE. BY OPENING THIS PACKAGE, YOU ARE AGREEING TO THE TERMS AND CONDITIONS OF THIS LICENSE. IF YOU DO NOT AGREE, DO NOT OPEN THE PACKAGE. PROMPTLY RETURN THE UNOPENED PACKAGE AND ALL ACCOMPANYING ITEMS TO THE PLACE YOU OBTAINED THEM. *THESE TERMS APPLY TO ALL LICENSED SOFTWARE ON THE DISK EXCEPT THAT THE TERMS FOR USE OF ANY SHAREWARE OR FREEWARE ON THE DISKETTES ARE AS SET FORTH IN THE ELECTRONIC LICENSE LOCATED ON THE DISK:*

1. GRANT OF LICENSE and OWNERSHIP: The enclosed computer programs and data ("Software") are licensed, not sold, to you by Pearson Education, Inc. ("We" or the "Company") and in consideration of your purchase or adoption of the accompanying Company textbooks and/or other materials, and your agreement to these terms. We reserve any rights not granted to you. You own only the disk(s) but we and/or our licensors own the Software itself. This license allows you to use and display your copy of the Software on a single computer (i.e., with a single CPU) at a single location for <u>academic</u> use only, so long as you comply with the terms of this Agreement. You may make one copy for back up, or transfer your copy to another CPU, provided that the Software is usable on only one computer

2. RESTRICTIONS: You may <u>not</u> transfer or distribute the Software or documentation to anyone else. Except for backup, you may <u>not</u> copy the documentation or the Software. You may <u>not</u> network the Software or otherwise use it on more than one computer or computer terminal at the same time. You may <u>not</u> reverse engineer, disassemble, decompile, modify, adapt, translate, or create derivative works based on the Software or the Documentation. You may be held legally responsible for any copying or copyright infringement which is caused by your failure to abide by the terms of these restrictions.

3. TERMINATION: This license is effective until terminated. This license will terminate automatically without notice from the Company if you fail to comply with any provisions or limitations of this license. Upon termination, you shall destroy the Documentation and all copies of the Software. All provisions of this Agreement as to limitation and disclaimer of warranties, limitation of liability, remedies or damages, and our ownership rights shall survive termination.

4. LIMITED WARRANTY AND DISCLAIMER OF WARRANTY: Company warrants that for a period of 60 days from the date you purchase this SOFTWARE (or purchase or adopt the accompanying textbook), the Software, when properly installed and used in accordance with the Documentation, will operate in substantial conformity with the description of the Software set forth in the Documentation, and that for a period of 30 days the disk(s) on which the Software is delivered shall be free from defects in materials and workmanship under normal use. The Company does not warrant that the Software will meet your requirements or that the operation of the Software will be uninterrupted or error-free. Your only remedy and the Company's only obligation under these limited warranties is, at the Company's option, return of the disk for a refund of any amounts paid for it by you or replacement of the disk. THIS LIMITED WARRANTY IS THE ONLY WARRANTY PROVIDED BY THE COMPANY AND ITS LICENSORS, AND THE COMPANY AND ITS LICENSORS DISCLAIM ALL OTHER WARRANTIES, EXPRESS OR IMPLIED, INCLUDING WITHOUT LIMITATION, THE IMPLIED WARRANTIES OF MERCHANTABILITY AND FITNESS FOR A PARTICULAR PURPOSE. THE COMPANY DOES NOT WARRANT, GUARANTEE OR MAKE ANY REPRESENTATION REGARDING THE ACCURACY, RELIABILITY, CURRENTNESS, USE, OR RESULTS OF USE, OF THE SOFTWARE.

5. LIMITATION OF REMEDIES AND DAMAGES: IN NO EVENT, SHALL THE COMPANY OR ITS EMPLOYEES, AGENTS, LICENSORS, OR CONTRACTORS BE LIABLE FOR ANY INCIDENTAL, INDIRECT, SPECIAL, OR CONSEQUENTIAL DAMAGES ARISING OUT OF OR IN CONNECTION WITH THIS LICENSE OR THE SOFTWARE, INCLUDING FOR LOSS OF USE, LOSS OF DATA, LOSS OF INCOME OR PROFIT, OR OTHER LOSSES, SUSTAINED AS A RESULT OF INJURY TO ANY PERSON, OR LOSS OF OR DAMAGE TO PROPERTY, OR CLAIMS OF THIRD PARTIES, EVEN IF THE COMPANY OR AN AUTHORIZED REPRESENTATIVE OF THE COMPANY HAS BEEN ADVISED OF THE POSSIBILITY OF SUCH DAMAGES. IN NO EVENT SHALL THE LIABILITY OF THE COMPANY FOR DAMAGES WITH RESPECT TO THE SOFTWARE EXCEED THE AMOUNTS ACTUALLY PAID BY YOU, IF ANY, FOR THE SOFTWARE OR THE ACCOMPANYING TEXTBOOK. BECAUSE SOME JURISDICTIONS DO NOT ALLOW THE LIMITATION OF LIABILITY IN CERTAIN CIRCUMSTANCES, THE ABOVE LIMITATIONS MAY NOT ALWAYS APPLY TO YOU.

6. GENERAL: THIS AGREEMENT SHALL BE CONSTRUED IN ACCORDANCE WITH THE LAWS OF THE UNITED STATES OF AMERICA AND THE STATE OF NEW YORK, APPLICABLE TO CONTRACTS MADE IN NEW YORK, AND SHALL BENEFIT THE COMPANY, ITS AFFILIATES AND ASSIGNEES. HIS AGREEMENT IS THE COMPLETE AND EXCLUSIVE STATEMENT OF THE AGREEMENT BETWEEN YOU AND THE COMPANY AND SUPERSEDES ALL PROPOSALS OR PRIOR AGREEMENTS, ORAL, OR WRITTEN, AND ANY OTHER COMMUNICATIONS BETWEEN YOU AND THE COMPANY OR ANY REPRESENTATIVE OF THE COMPANY RELATING TO THE SUBJECT MATTER OF THIS AGREEMENT. If you are a U.S. Government user, this Software is licensed with "restricted rights" as set forth in subparagraphs (a)-(d) of the Commercial Computer-Restricted Rights clause at FAR 52.227-19 or in subparagraphs (c)(1)(ii) of the Rights in Technical Data and Computer Software clause at DFARS 252.227-7013, and similar clauses, as applicable.

Should you have any questions concerning this agreement or if you wish to contact the Company for any reason, please contact in writing: Prentice-Hall, New Media Department, One Lake Street, Upper Saddle River, NJ 07458.